Modern Business Statistics 7e DATAfiles

Chapter 1

CompactSUV	Exercise 25
Nations	Table 1.1
Rogers	Table 1.5 & Figure 1.8

Chapter 2

Airports	Exercise 19
AirSurvey	Exercise 7
AptitudeTest	Table 2.8
Audit	Table 2.4
BaseBallHall	Exercise 8
BBB	Exercise 48
BestPayingDegrees	Exercise 25
BrandValue	Table 2.12
CEOTime	Exercise 20
Colleges	Table 2.18
Crosstab	Exercise 27
Crosstab2	Exercise 28
CutRate	Case Problem 4
ElectricVehicles	Exercise 57
Electronics	Table 2.14
Endowments	Exercise 21
EngineeringSalary	Exercise 24
FortuneBest100	Exercise 52
Franchise	Exercise 22
Frequency	Exercise 11
FuelData2018	Table 2.13
Grogan	Table 2.26
HotelRatings	Exercise 10
Hypertension	Exercise 41
Majors	Exercise 9
ManagerTime	Exercise 43
Marathon	Exercise 26
MarketIndexes	Exercise 23
MedianHousehold	Exercise 45
Movies2016	Table 2.20
MPG	Exercise 39
Names2018	Exercise 5
NBAPlayerPts	Exercise 18
NetworkShows	Exercise 6
PelicanStores	Table 2.19
Population2012	Exercise 46
QueenCity	Case Problem 3
Restaurant	Table 2.9
SAT2019	Exercise 44
Scatter	Exercise 36
Snow	Exercise 40
SoftDrink	Table 2.1
StartUps	Exercise 47
StocksBeta	Table 2.17
Televisions	Exercise 42
Websites	Exercise 4
Zoo	Exercise 58

Chapter 3

AdmiredCompanies	Exercise 53
Advertising	Exercise 32
AdvertisingSpend	Exercise 9
AfricanElephants	Table 3.13
AsiaMBA	Case Problem 3
BestCities	Exercise 43
BestPrivateColleges	Exercise 61
BorderCrossings	Exercise 54
CellPhoneExpenses	Exercise 31
CellService	Exercise 52
Coaches	Exercise 63
eICU	Exercise 7
Electronics	Table 3.6
Flights	Exercise 27
FoodIndustry	Exercise 69
Grogan	Figure 3.20
HeavenlyChocolates	Table 3.12
iPads	Exercise 45
JacketRatings	Exercise 10
MajorSalaries	Figure 3.14
Movies2016	Table 3.10
MutualFund	Table 3.2
NCAA	Exercise 44
NFLTeamValue	Exercise 71
OnlineGame	Exercise 12
PanamaRailroad	Exercise 75
PelicanStores	Table 3.9
PharmacySales	Exercise 51
Runners	Exercise 50
Russell	Exercise 60
SFGasPrices	Exercise 26
Sleep	Exercise 65
Smartphone	Exercise 66
SmokeDetectors	Exercise 59
SpringTraining	Exercise 72
StartingSalaries	Table 3.1
StockComparison	Exercise 57
TelevisionViewing	Exercise 11
Transportation	Exercise 66
Travel	Exercise 70
UnemploymentRates	Exercise 14
VarattaSales	Exercise 28
WaitTracking	Exercise 64

Chapter 4

CodeChurn	Exercise 10
Judge	Table 4.8
MarketBasket	Case Problem 2

Chapter 5

Coldstream12	Exercise 17

Chapter 7

AmericanLeague	Exercise 3
EAI	Section 7.1
Morningstar	Exercise 10
NationalLeague	Figure 7.1
ShadowStocks	Exercise 50

Chapter 8

35MPH	Exercise 65
Auto	Case Problem 3
AutoInsurance	Exercise 20
BlackPanther	Exercise 22
CasualDining	Exercise 38
CorporateBonds	Exercise 16
DrugCost	Exercise 52
FedSickHours	Exercise 45
FedTaxErrors	Exercise 44
FloridaFraud	Exercise 67
GulfProp	Table 8.9
HongKongMeals	Exercise 19
Houston	Exercise 5
JobSearch	Exercise 18
Lloyd's	Section 8.1
Miami	Exercise 17
NewBalance	Table 8.3
Obesity	Exercise 53
Professional	Table 8.8
RightDirection	Exercise 37
Scheer	Table 8.4
Setters	Exercise 6
SleepHabits	Exercise 51
TeeTimes	Section 8.4
TeleHealth	Exercise 21
TobaccoFires	Exercise 9
TravelTax	Exercise 6
UnderEmployed	Exercise 66

Chapter 9

AirRating	Section 9.4
Bayview	Case Problem 2
BritainMarriages	Exercise 54
ChannelSurfing	Exercise 64
ChildCare	Exercise 30
Coffee	Section 9.3
Eagle	Exercise 43
FedEmail	Exercise 46
Fowle	Exercise 21
GolfTest	Section 9.3
HomeState	Exercise 39
LawSuit	Exercise 44
Orders	Section 9.4
Quality	Case Problem 1
ResidentialWater	Exercise 29
SocialNetwork	Exercise 47
TSAWaitTimes	Exercise 66
UsedCars	Exercise 32
WeeklyHSGradPay	Exercise 55
WomenGolf	Section 9.5

Chapter 10

BusinessTravel	Exercise 24
CheckAcct	Section 10.2
CollegeCosts	Exercise 13
ComputerNews	Exercise 46
ExamScores	Section 10.1
Golf	Case Problem
GolfScores	Exercise 26
HomeStyle	Section 10.1
Hotel	Exercise 6
IntHotels	Exercise 15
LateFlights	Exercise 18
Matched	Table 10.2
Mutual	Exercise 40
SATMath	Exercise 16
SoftwareTest	Table 10.1
StockQuarter	Exercise 22
SUVLease	Exercise 39
TaxPrep	Section 10.4
TestScores	Exercise 25
Twins	Exercise 42

Chapter 11

Bags	Exercise 19
BatteryLife	Exercise 21
BusTimes	Section 11.1
CoachSalary	Exercise 5
Costco	Exercise 10
Detergent	Section 11.1
EconGMAT	Exercise 11
Halloween	Exercise 7
MeticulousDrills	Case Problem 2
SchoolBus	Section 11.2
StockPriceChange	Exercise 8
Training	Case Problem 1
TravelCosts	Exercise 25

Chapter 12

Ambulance	Exercise 30
AutoLoyalty	Figure 12.5
AutoQuality	Exercise 12
BBB	Exercise 25
BBG	Case Problem 3
BeerPreference	Table 12.2
FuentesChips	Case Problem 2
M&M	Exercise 4
Millennials	Exercise 11
NYReform	Case Problem 1
PairwiseComparisons	Table 12.8
Research	Figure 12.2
SocialMedia	Exercise 23
WorkforcePlan	Exercise 10

American Medical Association
Physicians dedicated to the health of America

Guides
to the Evaluation *of* Permanent Impairment

Fifth Edition

Linda Cocchiarella, MD, MSc, AMA Medical Editor
Gunnar B. J. Andersson, MD, PhD, Senior Medical Editor

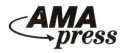

Guides to the Evaluation of Permanent Impairment,
Fifth Edition

First Edition—1971
Second Edition—1984
Third Edition—First Printing December 1988
            Second Printing February 1989
Third Edition (Revised)—December 1990
Fourth Edition—June 1993
Fifth Edition—First Printing November 2000
            Second Printing February 2002
            Third Printing January 2004
            Fourth Printing July 2004
            Fifth Printing January 2005
            Sixth Printing June 2005
Printed in the United States of America

Internet address: www.ama-assn.org

This book is for informational purposes only. It is not intended to
constitute legal or financial advice. If legal, financial, or other
professional advice is required, the services of a competent professional
should be sought.

Additional copies of this book may be ordered by calling 800 621-8335.
Mention product number OP025400.

ISBN 1-57947-085-8

BQ63:05-P-051:6/05

Preface

The American Medical Association (AMA) *Guides to the Evaluation of Permanent Impairment* (*Guides*) has become the most commonly used source for assessing and rating an individual's permanent impairment in the United States and, increasingly, abroad. Balancing the tradition of the *Guides* with the need for a scientific update, the fifth edition of the *Guides* has retained the focus of earlier editions, while incorporating updates in diagnostic criteria, clarifying key definitions and applications of the *Guides,* and enhancing readability, accessibility, and consistency. The updated scientific criteria are a blend of evidence-based medicine and specialty society consensus recommendations.

Although this preface cannot describe all of the updates to the fifth edition, we would like to emphasize certain features. Chapters have been reorganized, when possible, to follow a consistent format. Features include:

- **Chapter Outlines**—an outline of main chapter headings precedes each chapter for quick reference
- **Boldface Glossary Terms**—key impairment terms that are defined in the Glossary are boldface on first significant text occurrence
- **Principles of Assessment**—an overview of impairment assessment for each body system
- **Interpretation of Symptoms and Signs**—a description and interpretation of common signs and symptoms present for body system disorders
- **Description of Clinical Procedures**—a summary of common clinical procedures used to investigate system-specific impairment
- **Criteria for Rating Permanent Impairment**—clinical criteria used to determine impairment ratings
- **Case Studies**—expanded from earlier editions; succinct format; clinically relevant
- **Impairment Evaluation Summary**—summary of key conditions and their clinical assessment, with references to the main tables in the chapter

- **Bibliography and Key References**—some with annotations

The updates in content and diagnostic criteria reflect recommendations from members of leading specialty societies. Many specialty societies recommended members of their society who subsequently became chapter chairs, contributors, and reviewers. These members often served as liaisons and interpreters, applying guidelines from their specialty society to the clinical assessment of permanent impairment.

The AMA is grateful for the valued input and content recommendations from the American Medical Association Federation Members, including input from members of the following:

American Academy of Dermatology
American Academy of Gastroenterology
American Academy of Hand Surgery
American Academy of Neurology
American Academy of Occupational and Environmental Medicine
American Academy of Orthopaedic Surgeons
American Academy of Otolaryngology-Head and Neck Surgery
American Academy of Pain Medicine
American Academy of Physical Medicine and Rehabilitation
American Academy of Respiratory Diseases
American Association for Hand Surgery
American Association for Thoracic Surgery
American Association of Clinical Endocrinologists
American Cardiology Society
American College of Obstetricians and Gynecologists
American College of Occupational and Environmental Medicine
American College of Physicians/American Society of Internal Medicine
American College of Rheumatology

American Opthalmology Society
American Orthopaedic Association
American Psychiatric Association
American Society for Surgery of the Hand
American Society of Hand Therapists
American Thoracic Society
International Federation of Societies for Surgery
    of the Hand
North American Spine Society

Input from other non-AMA member associations was
also essential, including the International Association
of Industrial Boards and Commissioners, American
Academy of Disability Evaluating Physicians,
American Pain Society, American Thoracic
Association, and International Society for Low Vision
Research and Rehabilitation (ISLRR). Staff from the
Journal of the American Medical Association (*JAMA*)
provided guidance and perspective concerning con-
tent and editorial issues.

The editors wish to thank B. J. Anderson, JD, of the
AMA legal group and Donald R. Bennett, MD, PhD,
for their guidance, as well as the executive, steering,
and senior advisory committees who participated in
the early planning stages of the revision for their
input. A list of those individuals is available from the
AMA on request. The editors also wish to thank the
editorial, production, and marketing staff members at
the AMA, the Think Design Group, and the freelance
editors who developed and edited the manuscript,
designed this edition, shepherded the book through
production and manufacturing, and planned and exe-
cuted the marketing program: Mary Lou White,
Barry Bowlus, Jean Roberts, Reg Schmidt, Robert
Miller, Rosalyn Carlton, Mary Ann Albanese,
Ronnie Summers, Cindi Anderson, Linda Woodard,
Robin Husayko, Ryan Bergin, David Arispe, Coralee
Montes, Steve Straus, Nicole Netter, and Gerry van
Raavensway. The editors are grateful for the integral
administrative and secretarial support of Nancy
Pabon and Gloria Roebuck at Rush-Presbyterian-
St Luke's Medical Center.

The editors acknowledge and appreciate the prior hard
work, dedication, and foundation provided by the editors of the prior edition, Theodore C. Doege and Alan
Engelberg, and the many users of the *Guides* who sub-
mitted recommendations concerning the revision.
Their input was essential to creating this edition of the
Guides and ensuring subsequent revisions will meet
the needs of the population this book serves.

Linda Cocchiarella, MD, MSc,
    AMA Medical Editor

Gunnar B. J. Andersson, MD, PhD,
    Senior Medical Editor

Chairs, Contributors, and Reviewers

Chapter Chairs

Margit Bleecker, MD, PhD
Center for Occupational and
  Environmental Neurology
Baltimore, Maryland
The Central and Peripheral Nervous
  System

Francis I. Catlin, MD, ScD
Baylor College of Medicine
Houston, Texas
Ear, Nose, Throat, and Related
  Structures

Linda Cocchiarella, MD, MSc
American Medical Association
Chicago, Illinois
Impairment Evaluation and
Records and Reports

August Colenbrander, MD
California Pacific Medical Center and
  Smith-Kettlewell Eye Research
  Institute
San Francisco, California
The Visual System

Edward Covington, MD
Cleveland Clinic
Cleveland, Ohio
Pain

Paul E. Epstein, MD
University of Pennsylvania
Philadelphia, Pennsylvania
The Respiratory System

Eugene Frenkel, MD
University of Texas Southwestern
  Medical Center
Dallas, Texas
The Hematopoietic System

Robert H. Haralson III, MD
Maryville, Tennessee
The Spine

Frank E. Jones, MD
Nashville, TN
The Upper Extremities

Philipp M. Lippe, MD
Stanford University
San Jose, California
Pain

James V. Luck, Jr, MD
Orthopaedic Hospital
Los Angeles, California
The Lower Extremities

James R. McPherson, MD
Mayo Clinic
Rochester, Minnesota
The Digestive System

Arthur T. Meyerson, MD
New York University School of
  Medicine
New York, New York
Mental and Behavioral Disorders

Inder Perkash, MD
Stanford University
Palo Alto, California
The Urinary and Reproductive
  Systems

Nelson G. Richards, MD
Richmond, Virginia
The Central and Peripheral Nervous
  System

Harvey A. Rubenstein, MD, FACP,
  FACE
Georgetown University School of
  Medicine
McLean, Virginia
The Endocrine System

Joseph Sataloff, MD, MSc, DSc
Thomas Jefferson University
Philadelphia, Pennsylvania
Impairment Evaluation and Records
  and Reports

Genevieve de Groot Swanson, MD,
Michigan State University
Grand Rapids, Michigan
The Upper Extremities

James S. Taylor, MD
Cleveland Clinic
Cleveland, Ohio
The Skin

Dennis C. Turk, PhD
University of Washington
Seattle, Washington
Pain

Nancy Webb, MD
Kelsey-Seybold Clinic
Houston, Texas
The Visual System

Scott Wright, MD
Mayo Clinic
Rochester, Minnesota
The Cardiovascular System: Heart and
  Aorta
The Cardiovascular System: Systemic
  and Pulmonary Arteries

Contributors

Gunnar B. J. Andersson, MD, PhD
Rush-Presbyterian-St Luke's Medical
  Center
Chicago, Illinois

William S. Beckett, MD
University of Rochester School of
  Medicine and Dentistry
Rochester, New York

Scott Brown, MD
Physical Medicine and Rehabilitation
Sinai Rehabilitation Center
Baltimore, Maryland

Neil Busis, MD
Pittsburgh Neurological Group
Pittsburgh, Pennsylvania

Seine Chiang, MD
University of Alabama
Birmingham, Alabama

Linda Cocchiarella, MD, MSc
American Medical Association
Chicago, Illinois

Robert Cofield, MD
Mayo Clinic
Rochester, Minnesota

Phillip Coogan, MD
Nashville, Tennessee

G. Theodore Davis, MD
Albuquerque, New Mexico

Robert Dobie, MD
National Institute on Deafness and
  Communicative Disorders
Bethesda, Maryland

Anthony Dorto, MD, DC
Hollywood, Florida

Kenneth W. Eckmann, MD
The Neurology Center
Wheaton, Maryland

Patricia G. Engasser, MD
Stanford University
University of California, San Francisco
Atherton, California

Loren H. Engrav, MD
University of Washington School of
  Medicine
Seattle, Washington

Blair C. Filler, MD
Orthopaedic Hospital
Los Angeles, California

John J. Gerhardt, MD
Portland, Oregon

Darlene G. Kelley, MD, PhD
Mayo Clinic
Rochester, Minnesota

Randall D. Lea, MD
Center of Orthopaedic Care &
  Evaluation Medicine
Baton Rouge, Louisiana

Barry S. Levinson, MD
University of Texas Southwestern
  Medical Center and Dallas Veterans
  Administration Medical Center
Dallas, Texas

James Lockey, MD
University of Cincinnati College of
  Medicine
Cincinnati, Ohio

John D. Loeser, MD
University of Washington
Seattle, Washington

Donlin Long, MD
Johns Hopkins University Medical
  Center
Baltimore, Maryland

C. G. Toby Mathias, MD
University of Cincinnati
Cincinnati, Ohio

Tom Mayer, MD
Dallas, Texas

Michael McGoon, MD
Mayo Clinic
Rochester, Minnesota

Rick Nishimura, MD
Mayo Clinic
Rochester, Minnesota

Rajan Perkash, MD
Stanford University
Sunnyvale, California

John Phair, MD
Northwestern University
Chicago, Illinois

Mohammed I. Ranavaya, MD
Chapmanville, West Virginia

David C. Randolph, MD, MPH
Cincinnati, Ohio

Edward A. Rankin
Washington, DC

James P. Robinson, MD, PhD
University of Washington
Seattle, Washington

Joel R. Saper, MD
Ann Arbor, Michigan

Robert Thayer Sataloff, MD, DMA
Thomas Jefferson University
Graduate Hospital
Philadelphia, Pennsylvania

Gabriel Sella, MD
Martins Ferry, Ohio

William S. Shaw, MD
Integrated Health Management
Denver, Colorado

George M. Smith, MD
G. M. Smith Associates, Inc
Aliso Viejo, California

Mark Taylor, MD
San Antonio, Texas

Martha Terris, MD
Stanford University
Palo Alto, California

Mark Utell, MD
University of Rochester
Rochester, New York

Jonathan Van Geest, PhD
American Medical Association
Chicago, Illinois

Reviewers

Peter Amadio, MD
Rochester, Minnesota

Aries Arditi, PhD
New York, New York

Ian Bailey, OD
University of California, Berkeley
Berkeley, California

John R. Balmes, MD
University of California, San
  Francisco
San Francisco, California

Peter S. Barth, PhD
University of Connecticut
Storrs, Connecticut

William Beckett, MD
University of Rochester
Rochester, New York

James L. Becton, MD
Augusta, Georgia

Janette Bertness, JD
Providence, Rhode Island

Peter V. Bieri, MD, FAADEP
Lawrence, Kansas

Stan Bigos, MD
University of Washington
Seattle, Washington

Martin Black, MD
Philadelphia, Pennsylvania

Sidney Blair, MD, FACS
Loyola University Medical Center
Maywood, Illinois

William Blair, MD
Iowa City, Iowa

Christopher R. Brigham, MD
Portland, Maine

Charles Brooks, MD, PC
Bellevue, Washington

Robert Buchanan, MD
Oklahoma City, Oklahoma

William B. Bunn, MD, JD, MPH
Northwestern University
Chicago, Illinois

John F. Burton, Jr, PhD, LLB
Rutgers: The State University of New
  Jersey
New Brunswick, New Jersey

Thomas N. Byrne, MD
New Haven, Connecticut

Daniel Barry Carr, MD
Boston, Massachusetts

Susan O. Cassidy, MD, JD
Madison, Connecticut

Robert Cohen, MD
Chicago, Illinois

Alan L. Colledge, MD
Salt Lake City, Utah

Anne L. Corn, EdD
Vanderbilt University
Nashville, Tennessee

James Culver, MD
Cleveland, Ohio

Steven Darnell, MBA
Camas, Washington

Stanley Dersinski, MD
Redwood City, California

Mary Dombovy, MD
Rochester, New York

Joseph Drozda, MD
Chesterfield, Missouri

Eleanor Faye, MD
New York, New York

Michael Feuerstein, PhD
Uniformed Services University
Bethesda, Maryland

Donald Fletcher, MD
Birmingham, Alabama

Linda Forst, MD, MPH
University of Illinois
Chicago, Illinois

Robert J. Gatchel, PhD
University of Texas
Dallas, Texas

Elizabeth Genovese-Stone, MD, MBA
Bala Cynwyd, Pennsylvania

Philip Harber, MD
University of California, Los Angeles
Los Angeles, California

Holly B. Hahn, MD
Indiana University
Indianapolis, Indiana

Scott Halderman, MD
Santa Ana, California

Stephen Hanauer, MD
University of Chicago
Chicago, Illinois

Rowland Hazard, MD
University of Vermont
Williston, Vermont

George E. Healy, Jr, MD
Providence, Rhode Island

Lea Hyvärinen, MD
Helsinki, Finland

Mariell Jessup, MD
University of Pennsylvania
Philadelphia, Pennsylvania

Norman Johanson-Phil, MD
Philadelphia, Pennsylvania

Alan Johnston, PhD
University of Melbourne
Melbourne, Australia

Morton Kasden, MD
Louisville, Kentucky

Richard Katz, MD
St Louis, Missouri

Gideon Letz, MD, MPH
San Francisco, California

Philip Levy, MD
Phoenix, Arizona

Stephen Lord, JD
Boise, Idaho

Dean S. Louis, MD
Ann Arbor, Michigan

Boris D. Lushniak, MD, MPH
NIOSH
Cincinnati, Ohio

Peter J. Mandel, MD
San Francisco, California

Robert Massof, PhD
Johns Hopkins University
Baltimore, Maryland

Mark Melhorn, MD
Wichita, Kansas

Kathryn Mueller, MD
Littleton, Colorado

John Niparko, MD
Johns Hopkins University
Baltimore, Maryland

Mohamed M. Panjabi, PhD
Yale University
New Haven, Connecticut

Arun Perkash, MD
Stanford University
Sunnyvale, California

Dante J. Pieramici, MD
Johns Hopkins University
Baltimore, Maryland

Carrie Redlich, MD, MPH
Yale University
New Haven, Connecticut

Robert D. Rondinelli, MD, PhD
University of Kansas
Kansas City, Kansas

Cecile S. Rose, MD, MHP
Denver, Colorado

Henry J. Roth, MD
Denver, Colorado

Spencer Rowland, MD
San Antonio, Texas

Brian Schulman, MD
Bethesda, Maryland

Marcia Scott, MD
Cambridge, Massachusetts

William Shaw, MD
Denver, Colorado

Elizabeth Sherertz, MD
Wake Forest University
Winston-Salem, North Carolina

Priscilla Short, MD
American Medical Association
Chicago, Illinios

Emily A. Spieler, JD
West Virginia University
Morgantown, West Virginia

Gordon Steinagle, DO
Buffalo, New York

Henry (Hal) Lee Stockbridge,
    MD, MPH
Olympia, Washington

William M. Swartz, MD
Pittsburgh, Pennsylvania

James Talmage, MD
Cookeville, Tennessee

Marc T. Taylor, MD
San Antonio, Texas

Michael I. Vender, MD
Arlington Heights, Illinois

Greg Wagner, MD
Morgantown, West Virginia

Mary Warren, OT
Kansas City, Missouri

American Medical Association Staff

Professional Standards

Clair M. Callan, MD, MBA
Vice President
Division of Science, Quality and
    Public Health

Arthur Elster, MD
Director of Clinical and Public Health
    Practice and Outcomes

Linda Cocchiarella, MD, MSc
Senior Scientist
AMA Medical Editor
*Guides to the Evaluation of Permanent
    Impairment,* Fifth Edition

Thomas Houston, MD
Director of Science and Public Health
    Advocacy Programs

Priscilla Short, MD
Director of Genetic Medicine

Jonathan Van Geest, PhD
Ethical Standards

Ryan Bergin, Editorial Assistant

Cynthia Colvin, Senior Secretary

Mary Haynes, Administrative
    Secretary

Mary Wilborn, Assistant to the
    Director

AMA Press

Tony Frankos, Vice President,
    Business Products

Mary Lou White, Editorial Director

Barry Bowlus, Senior Acquisitions
    Editor

Jean Roberts, Director, Production and
    Manufacturing

Reg Schmidt, Marketing Manager

Rosalyn Carlton, Senior Production
    Coordinator

Ronnie Summers, Senior Print
    Coordinator

Mary Ann Albanese, Image
    Coordinator

Office of the General Counsel

B. J. Anderson, JD

Bruce Blehart, JD

Andrea Cooper-Finkel, JD

Karla Kinderman, JD

Table of Contents

Chapter 6

The Digestive System   117

Chapter 7

The Urinary and
Reproductive Systems   143

Chapter 8

The Skin   173

Chapter 9

The Hematopoietic System   191

Chapter 10

The Endocrine System   211

Chapter 11

Ear, Nose, Throat, and
Related Structures   245

List of Tables and Figures

Chapter 5

The Respiratory System   87

Chapter 6

The Digestive Tract   117

Chapter 14

Mental and Behavioral Disorders   357

Chapter 15

The Spine   373

Chapter 16

The Upper Extremities   433

Chapter 17

The Lower Extremities   523

Philosophy, Purpose, and Appropriate Use of the *Guides*

1.1 History

The *Guides* was first published in book form in 1971
in response to a public need for a standardized,
objective approach to evaluating medical impairments. Sections of the first edition of the *Guides*
were originally published in the *Journal of the
American Medical Association*, beginning in 1958
and continuing until August 1970.[1] Since then, the
Guides has undergone four revisions, culminating in
the current, fifth edition. The purpose of this fifth
edition of the *Guides* is to update the diagnostic criteria and evaluation process used in impairment
assessment, incorporating available scientific evidence and prevailing medical opinion. Chapter
authors were encouraged to use the latest scientific
evidence from their specialty and, where evidence
was lacking, develop a consensus view. This chapter
was revised from the earlier edition in response to
specific requests from user groups concerning the
definitions, appropriate use, and scope of application
of the *Guides*.

The fifth edition includes most of the common conditions, excluding unusual cases that require individual consideration. Since this edition encompasses the most current criteria and procedures for impairment assessment, it is strongly recommended that physicians use this latest edition, the fifth edition, when rating impairment.

1.2 Impairment, Disability, and Handicap

1.2a Impairment

The *Guides* continues to define **impairment** as **"a loss, loss of use, or derangement of any body part, organ system, or organ function."**[2] This definition of impairment is retained in this edition. A medical impairment can develop from an illness or injury. An impairment is considered permanent when it has reached **maximal medical improvement (MMI),** meaning it is well stabilized and unlikely to change substantially in the next year with or without medical treatment. The term *impairment* in the *Guides* refers to **permanent impairment,** which is the focus of the *Guides*.

An impairment can be manifested objectively, for example, by a fracture, and/or subjectively, through fatigue and pain.[3] Although the *Guides* emphasizes objective assessment, subjective symptoms are included within the diagnostic criteria. According to the *Guides,* determining whether an injury or illness results in a permanent impairment requires a medical assessment performed by a physician. An impairment may lead to functional limitations or the inability to perform activities of daily living.

Table 1-1, adapted from a report by the AMA Council on Scientific Affairs, lists various definitions of impairment and disability used by four main authorities: the AMA *Guides*, the World Health Organization, the Social Security Administration, and a state workers' compensation statute.[4] Although a nationally accepted definition for impairment does not exist, the general concept of impairment is similar in the definitions of most organizations. Several terms used in the AMA definition, and their application throughout the *Guides*, will be discussed in this chapter and Chapter 2.

Loss, loss of use, or derangement implies a change from a normal or "preexisting" state. *Normal* is a range or zone representing healthy functioning and varies with age, gender, and other factors such as environmental conditions. For example, normal heart rate varies between a child and adult and according to whether the person is at rest or exercising. Multiple factors need to be considered when assessing whether a specific or overall function is normal. A normal value can be defined from an individual or population perspective.

When evaluating an individual, a physician has two options: consider the individual's healthy preinjury or preillness state or the condition of the unaffected side as "normal" for the individual if this is known, or compare that individual to a normal value defined by population averages of healthy people. The *Guides* uses both approaches. Accepted population values for conditions such as extremity range-of-motion or lung function are listed in the *Guides*; it is recommended that the physician use those values as detailed in the *Guides* when applicable. In other circumstances, for instance, where population values are not available, the physician should use clinical judgment regarding normal structure and function and estimate what is normal for the individual based on the physician's knowledge or estimate of the individual's preinjury or preillness condition.

Table 1-1 Definitions and Interpretations of Impairment and Disability

Organization	Impairment	Disability	Physicians' Role	Comments
Guides to the Evaluation of Permanent Impairment (5th ed, 2000)	A loss, loss of use, or derangement of any body part, organ system, or organ function.	An alteration of an individual's capacity to meet personal, social, or occupational demands because of an impairment.	Determine impairment, provide medical information to assist in disability determination.	An impaired individual may or may not have a disability.
World Health Organization (WHO) (1999)	Problems in body function or structure as a significant deviation or loss. Impairments of structure can involve an anomaly, defect, loss, or other significant deviation in body structures.	Activity limitation (formerly disability) is a difficulty in the performance, accomplishment, or completion of an activity at the level of the person. Difficulty encompasses all of the ways in which the doing of the activity may be affected.	Not specifically defined; assumed to be one of the decision-makers in determining disability through impairment assessment.	Emphasis is on the importance of functional abilities and defining context-related activity limitations.
Social Security Administration (SSA) (1995)	An anatomical, physiological, or psychological abnormality that can be shown by medically acceptable clinical and laboratory diagnostic techniques.	The inability to engage in any substantial, gainful activity by reason of any medically determinable physical or mental impairment(s), which can be expected to result in death or which has lasted or can be expected to last for a continuous period of not less than 12 months.	Determine impairment; may assist with the disability determination as a consultative examiner.	Physicians and nonphysicians need to work together to define situational disabilities.
State Workers' Compensation Law (typical)[5]	"Permanent impairment" is any anatomic or functional loss after maximal medical improvement has been achieved and which abnormality or loss, medically, is considered stable or nonprogressive at the time of evaluation. Permanent impairment is a basic consideration in the evaluation of permanent disability and is a contributing factor to, but not necessarily an indication of, the entire extent of permanent disability. (*Idaho Code* section 72-422)	"Temporary disability" means a decrease in wage-earning capacity due to injury or occupational disease during a period of recovery. (*Idaho Code* section 72-102[10] "Permanent disability" results when the actual or presumed ability to engage in gainful activity is reduced or absent because of permanent impairment and no fundamental or marked change in the future can be reasonably expected. (*Idaho Code* section 72-423)	"Evaluation (rating) of permanent impairment" is a medical appraisal of the nature and extent of the injury or disease as it affects an injured employee's personal efficiency in the activities of daily living, such as self-care, communication, normal living postures, ambulation, elevation, traveling, and nonspecialized activities of bodily members. (*Idaho Code* section 72-424)	Purpose is to provide sure and certain relief to those who become injured by accident or suffer effects of disease from exposure to hazards arising out of and in the course of employment.

Data from healthy populations, when available and widely referenced, are incorporated into chapters of the *Guides*. In some organ or body systems, such as respiratory, certain measurements of lung function have been standardized for age and gender. In other body systems, such as the musculoskeletal, age and gender differences are not reflected in most of the values. While there may be age and gender differences anticipated for some musculoskeletal values, such as range of motion in the spine and extremities, this edition of the *Guides* mainly reflects average range of motion from healthy populations of mixed age and gender. The normal values presented in the musculoskeletal section are based on a review of studies measuring range of motion, as cited in the text. Evaluating physicians may use their clinical judgment, however, and comment on any significant age or gender effect for a particular individual. For instance, the "normal" preinjury range of motion for a gymnast with hypermobility may exceed the listed normal values.

If an individual had previous measurements of function that were below or above average population values, the physician may discuss that prior value and any subsequent loss for the individual, as well as compare it to the population normal. For example, a highly functioning athlete with documented, above-normal lung function, who has sustained an injury and now has decreased lung function that is nonetheless similar to population averages, has experienced a loss in his or her lung function and has sustained an impairment. Based only on a population comparison, the athlete would be given a 0% impairment rating. However, it would be more appropriate in this instance for the physician to assign an impairment rating based on the degree of change from the athlete's preinjury to postinjury state.

In evaluating impairment, the *Guides* considers both anatomic and functional loss. Some chapters place a greater emphasis on either anatomic or functional loss, depending upon common practice in that specialty. *Anatomic loss* refers to damage to the organ system or body structure, while *functional loss* refers to a change in function for the organ or body system. An example of an anatomic deviation is development of heart enlargement; functional loss includes a loss in ejection fraction or the ability of the heart to pump adequately. Anatomic loss receives greater emphasis in the musculoskeletal system, as in measurements such as range of motion. Functional considerations receive greater emphasis in the mental and behavioral section.

The impairment criteria outlined in the *Guides* provide a standardized method for physicians to use to determine medical impairment. The impairment criteria include diagnostic criteria, incorporating anatomic and functional measures. The impairment criteria were developed from scientific evidence as cited and from consensus of chapter authors or of medical specialty societies.

Impairment percentages or **ratings** developed by medical specialists are consensus-derived estimates that reflect the severity of the medical condition and the degree to which the impairment decreases an individual's ability to perform common **activities of daily living (ADL),** *excluding* work. Impairment ratings were designed to reflect functional limitations and not disability. The **whole person impairment percentages** listed in the *Guides* estimate the impact of the impairment on the individual's overall ability to perform activities of daily living, *excluding work*, as listed in Table 1-2.

Table 1-2 Activities of Daily Living Commonly Measured in Activities of Daily Living (ADL) and Instrumental Activities of Daily Living (IADL) Scales [6,7]

Activity	Example
Self-care, personal hygiene	Urinating, defecating, brushing teeth, combing hair, bathing, dressing oneself, eating
Communication	Writing, typing, seeing, hearing, speaking
Physical activity	Standing, sitting, reclining, walking, climbing stairs
Sensory function	Hearing, seeing, tactile feeling, tasting, smelling
Nonspecialized hand activities	Grasping, lifting, tactile discrimination
Travel	Riding, driving, flying
Sexual function	Orgasm, ejaculation, lubrication, erection
Sleep	Restful, nocturnal sleep pattern

The medical judgment used to determine the original impairment percentages could not account for the diversity or complexity of work but could account for daily activities common to most people. Work is not included in the clinical judgment for impairment percentages for several reasons: (1) work involves many simple and complex activities; (2) work is highly individualized, making generalizations inaccurate; (3) impairment percentages are unchanged for stable conditions, but work and occupations change; and (4) impairments interact with such other factors as the worker's age, education, and prior work experience to determine the extent of work disability. For example, an individual who receives a 30% whole person impairment due to pericardial heart disease is considered from a clinical standpoint to have a 30% reduction in general functioning as represented by a decrease in the ability to perform activities of daily living. For individuals who work in sedentary jobs, there may be no decline in their work ability although their overall functioning is decreased. Thus, a 30% impairment rating does not correspond to a 30% reduction in work capability. Similarly, a manual laborer with this 30% impairment rating due to pericardial disease may be completely unable to do his or her regular job and, thus, may have a 100% work disability.

As a result, impairment ratings are not intended for use as direct determinants of work disability. When a physician is asked to evaluate work-related disability, it is appropriate for a physician knowledgeable about the work activities of the patient to discuss the specific activities the worker can and cannot do, given the permanent impairment.

Most impairment percentages in this fifth edition have been retained from the fourth edition because there are limited scientific data to support specific changes. It is recognized that there are limited data to support some of the previous impairment percentages as well. However, these ratings are currently accepted and should not be changed arbitrarily. In this edition, some percentages have been changed for greater scientific accuracy or to achieve consistency throughout the book.

A 0% whole person (WP) impairment rating is assigned to an individual with an impairment if the impairment has no significant organ or body system functional consequences and does not limit the performance of the common activities of daily living

indicated in Table 1-2. A 90% to 100% WP impairment indicates a very severe organ or body system impairment requiring the individual to be fully dependent on others for self-care, approaching death.

The activities of daily living, as originally developed for the *Guides* in the first and second editions,[1,6] signify common activities currently represented in scales of Activities of Daily Living and Instrumental Activities of Daily Living.[7] The *Guides* refers to common ADLs, as listed in Table 1-2. The ADLs listed in this table correspond to the activities that physicians should consider when establishing a permanent impairment rating. A physician can often assess a person's ability to perform ADLs based on knowledge of the patient's medical condition and clinical judgment. When the physician is estimating a permanent impairment rating, Table 1-2 can help to determine how significantly the impairment impacts these activities. Using the impairment criteria within a class and knowing the activities the individual can perform, the physician can estimate where the individual stands within that class.

There are many scales that measure ability to perform ADLs with greater degrees of accuracy. Many of these scales are concerned with more severe levels of disability, relevant to institutionalized patients and the elderly.[7] During the 1970s, the ADL concept was extended to consider problems experienced by those living in the community, a field that has come to be termed Instrumental Activities of Daily Living (IADL).[7] There is a continued effort to validate these scales; some of the more commonly utilized, validated IADL and ADL scales are listed in Table 1-3.[7] Scales vary in their appropriateness for a given individual, based upon the level of impairment, body systems affected, and degree of accuracy required. Some scales are most appropriate for an active, working population; others are more suited to a chronically ill, disabled population. Since there is no agreed-upon scale for a working population and physicians who use the *Guides* may evaluate different populations of individuals (ie, healthy or chronically ill), a physician may choose the most appropriate of any of the validated scales for a more in-depth assessment of ADL, to obtain further information to supplement clinical judgment, or to gain assistance in determining where an individual stands within an impairment range.

Table 1-3 Scales for Measurement of Instrumental Activities of Daily Living (IADL) and Activities of Daily Living (ADL)

IADL

Scale	Design/Description	Target Population	Measures	Comment
The OECD Long-Term Disability Questionnaire [8]	Summary of the impact of ill health on essential activities of daily living.	General population	• Eyesight • Hearing • Speaking • Carry an object of 5 kg for 10 meters • Run 100 meters • Walk 400 meters without resting • Move between rooms • Get in and out of bed • Dress and undress • Cut toenails • Bend and pick up a shoe from floor • Cut food • Bite and chew hard food	An early attempt to develop an international set of disability items; European content
The Health Assessment Questionnaire [9]	Measures difficulty in performing activities of daily living	Used to assess adult arthritics in a wide range of research settings to evaluate care	• Dressing and grooming • Arising • Eating • Walking • Hygiene • Reach • Grip • Outdoor activity	Widely used instrument; pays close attention to rigorous measures
The Functional Independence Measure [10]	Assesses physical and cognitive disability, monitors patient progress, and assesses outcomes of rehabilitation	General population	• Self-care • Sphincter control • Mobility • Locomotion • Communication • Social cognition	Based on the Barthel index

ADL

Scale	Design/Description	Target Population	Measures	Comment
The Barthel Index (Formerly the Maryland Disability Index) [11]	Measures functional independence in personal care and mobility; completed by health professionals	Used in patients with chronic conditions, before and after treatment	Ten-item version evaluates: • Feeding • Moving from wheelchair to bed and return • Personal toilet • Getting on and off toilet • Bathing self • Mobility • Ascending and descending stairs • Dressing • Controlling bowels • Controlling bladder	Measures what a patient does; widely applied

Scale	Description	Target Population	Measures	Comment
The Index of Independence in Activities of Daily Living [12]	Describes primary biological and psychosocial function; limited information on ambulation	Originally developed for elderly and chronically ill patients with strokes and fractured hips	Assesses independence in six activities: • Bathing • Dressing • Toileting • Transferring from bed to chair • Continence • Feeding	Widely used with children and adults, with the mentally retarded and the physically disabled, in the community and institutions
The Functional Status Rating System [13]	Based on a method developed to provide national statistics on hospital utilization and treatment outcomes	Rehabilitation patients	• **Functional Status in Self-Care** (eating/feeding, personal hygiene, toileting, bathing, bowel/bladder/skin management, bed activities, dressing) • **Functional Status in Mobility** (transfers, wheelchair skills, ambulation, stairs, community mobility) • **Functional Status in Communication** (reading, talking, motor communication, written language expression) • **Functional Status in Psychosocial Adjustment** (emotional adjustment, social support, adjustment to limitations) • **Functional Status in Cognitive Function** (attention span, judgment, reasoning, memory)	
The OARS Multidimensional Functional Assessment Questionnaire [14]	A combined 7 ADL and 7 IADL scale that covers functional and services assessment	General population, especially elderly	• Individual functioning (basic demographics, social, economic resources) • Mental health • Physical health • ADL • Services assessment (transportation, social/recreational)	Flexible instrument, reliable, and valid ADL and IADL sections
The Medical Outcomes Study Physical Functioning Measure [15]	An extended ADL scale that is sensitive to variations at relatively high levels of physical function	General population	• Vigorous activities (running, lifting heavy objects, strenuous sports) • Moderate activities (moving a table, pushing a vacuum cleaner, bowling, playing golf) • Lifting or carrying groceries • Climbing *several* flights of stairs • Climbing *one* flight of stairs • Bending, kneeling, or stooping • Walking *more than one mile* • Walking *several blocks* • Walking *one block* • Bathing or dressing self	Recognizes differences in people's values regarding functional ability by including a question on satisfaction with physical performance

1.2b Disability

The term *disability* has historically referred to a broad category of individuals with diverse limitations in the ability to meet social or occupational demands. However, it is more accurate to refer to the specific activity or role the "disabled" individual is unable to perform. Several organizations are moving away from the term *disability* and instead are referring to specific *activity limitations* to encourage an emphasis on the specific activities the individual can perform and to identify how the environment can be altered to enable the individual to perform the activities associated with various social or occupational roles. (Table 1-1).[4]

According to a 1997 Institute of Medicine Report, "disability is a relational outcome, reflecting the individual's capacity to perform a specific task or activity, contingent on the environmental conditions in which they are to be performed."[16] Disability is context-specific, not inherent in the individual, but a function of the interaction of the individual and the environment.

The World Health Organization (WHO) is revising its 1980 *International Classification of Impairments, Disabilities and Handicaps* and has released a draft document, *The International Classification of Impairments, Activities and Participation (ICIDH-2)*.[17] The term *disability* has been replaced by a neutral term, *activity*, and limits in ability are described as *activity limitations*. The change in terminology arose for several reasons: to choose terminology without an associated stigma, to avoid labeling, and to emphasize the person's residual ability. Representatives worldwide are reviewing this international classification scale of impairments, function, and activities.

The *Guides* continues to define **disability as an alteration of an individual's capacity to meet personal, social, or occupational demands or statutory or regulatory requirements because of an impairment.**[2] An individual can have a disability in performing a specific work activity but not have a disability in any other social role.[2] Physicians have the education and training to evaluate a person's health status and determine the presence or absence of an impairment. If the physician has the expertise and is well acquainted with the individual's activities and needs, the physician may also express an opinion about the presence or absence of a specific disability. For example, an occupational medicine physician who understands the job requirements in a particular workplace can provide insights on how the impairment could contribute to a workplace disability.

The impairment evaluation, however, is only one aspect of disability determination. A disability determination also includes information about the individual's skills, education, job history, adaptability, age, and environment requirements and modifications.[3] Assessing these factors can provide a more realistic picture of the effects of the impairment on the ability to perform complex work and social activities. If adaptations can be made to the environment, the individual may not be disabled from performing that activity.

Figure 1-1 The Relationship Among the Concepts of Normal Health, Impairment, Functional Limitation, and Activity Disability (Performance Limitation)

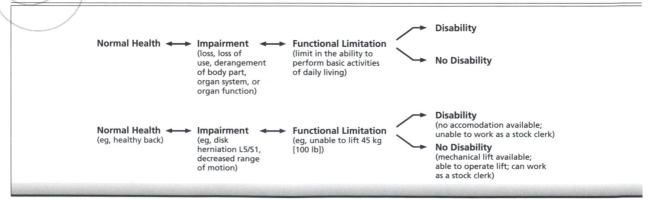

As discussed in this chapter and illustrated in Figure 1-1, medical impairments are not related to disability in a linear fashion. An individual with a medical impairment can have no disability for some occupations, yet be very disabled for others. For example, severe degenerative disk disease may impair the functioning of the spine of both a licensed practical nurse and a bank president in a similar fashion when performing their activities of daily living. However, in terms of occupation, the bank president is less likely to be disabled by this impairment than the licensed practical nurse. An individual who develops rheumatoid arthritis may be disabled from work as a tailor but may be able to work as a child care aide. A pilot who develops a visual impairment, correctable with glasses, may be able to perform all of his daily activities but is no longer able to fly a commercial plane. An individual with repeated hernias and repairs may no longer be able to lift more than 20 kg (40 lb) but could work in a factory where mechanical lifts are available.

The *Guides* is not intended to be used for direct estimates of work disability. Impairment percentages derived according to the *Guides* criteria do not measure work disability. Therefore, it is inappropriate to use the *Guides'* criteria or ratings to make direct estimates of work disability.

1.2c Handicap

Handicap is a term historically used in both a legal and a policy context to describe disability or people living with disabilities. Though the term continues to be used, generally it is being replaced with the preferred term *disability*.

1.3 The Organ System and Whole Body Approach to Impairment

The *Guides* impairment ratings reflect the severity and limitations of the organ/body system impairment and resulting **functional limitations.** Most organ/body systems chapters in the *Guides* provide impairment ratings that represent the extent of whole person impairment. In addition to listing whole person impairments, the musculoskeletal chapters provide regional impairment ratings (eg, upper extremity, lower extremity); regional ratings are then converted into whole person impairment ratings. Within some musculoskeletal regions, a consensus group developed weights to reflect the relative importance of certain regions. For example, different fingers or different areas of the spine are given different weights, representing their unique and relative importance to the region's overall functioning. These weights, which have gained acceptance in clinical practice, have been retained to enable regulatory authorities to convert from a regional body to whole person impairment when needed.

1.4 Philosophy and Use of the Combined Values Chart

The **Combined Values Chart** (p. 604) was designed to enable the physician to account for the effects of multiple impairments with a summary value. A standard formula was used to ensure that regardless of the number of impairments, the summary value would not exceed 100% of the whole person. According to the formula listed in the combined values chart, multiple impairments are combined so that the whole person impairment value is equal to or less than the sum of all the individual impairment values.

A scientific formula has not been established to indicate the best way to combine multiple impairments. Given the diversity of impairments and great variability inherent in combining multiple impairments, it is difficult to establish a formula that accounts for all situations. A combination of some impairments could decrease overall functioning more than suggested by just adding the impairment ratings for the separate impairments (eg, blindness and inability to use both hands). When other multiple impairments are combined, a less than additive approach may be more appropriate. States also use different techniques when combining impairments. Many **workers' compensation statutes** contain provisions that combine impairments to produce a summary rating that is more than additive. Other options are to combine (add, subtract, or multiply) multiple impairments based upon the extent to which they affect an individual's ability to perform activities of daily living. The current edition has retained the same combined values chart, since it has become the standard of practice in many jurisdictions. Other approaches, when published in scientific peer-reviewed literature, will be evaluated for future editions.

In general, impairment ratings within the same region are combined before combining the regional impairment rating with that from another region. For example, when there are multiple impairments involving abnormal motion, neurologic loss, and amputation of an extremity part, these impairments first should be combined for a regional extremity impairment. The regional extremity impairment then is combined with an impairment from another region, such as from the respiratory system. Spinal impairments in multiple regions are combined. Exceptions, as detailed in the musculoskeletal chapter, include impairments of the joints of the thumb, which are added, as are the ankle and subtalar joints in the lower extremity: both situations include complex motions.

1.5 Incorporating Science with Clinical Judgment

The *Guides* uses objective and scientifically based data when available and references these sources. When objective data have not been identified, estimates of the degree of impairment are used, based on clinical experience and consensus. Subjective concerns, including fatigue, difficulty in concentrating, and pain, when not accompanied by demonstrable clinical signs or other independent, measurable abnormalities, are generally not given separate impairment ratings. Chronic pain is discussed in Chapter 18. Physicians recognize the local and distant pain that commonly accompanies many disorders. Impairment ratings in the *Guides* already have accounted for commonly associated pain, including that which may be experienced in areas distant to the specific site of pathology. For example, when a cervical spine disorder produces radiating pain down the arm, the arm pain, which is commonly seen, has been accounted for in the cervical spine impairment rating.

The *Guides* does not deny the existence or importance of these subjective complaints to the individual or their functional impact. The *Guides* recommends that the physician ascertain and document subjective concerns. Because the presence and severity of subjective concerns varies among individuals with the same condition, the *Guides* has not yet identified an accepted method within the scientific literature to ascertain how these concerns consistently affect organ or body system functioning. The physician is encouraged to discuss these concerns and symptoms in the impairment evaluation.

Research is limited on the **reproducibility** and **validity** of the *Guides*.[18-20] Anecdotal reports indicate that adoption of the *Guides* results in a more standardized impairment assessment process. As relevant research becomes available, subsequent editions of the *Guides* will incorporate these evidence-based studies to improve the *Guides'* reliability and validity.

Given the range, evolution, and discovery of new medical conditions, the *Guides* cannot provide an impairment rating for all impairments. Also, since some medical syndromes are poorly understood and are manifested only by subjective symptoms, impairment ratings are not provided for those conditions. The *Guides* nonetheless provides a framework for evaluating new or complex conditions. Most adult conditions with measurable impairments can be evaluated under the *Guides*. In situations where impairment ratings are not provided, the *Guides* suggests that physicians use clinical judgment, comparing measurable impairment resulting from the unlisted condition to measurable impairment resulting from similar conditions with similar impairment of function in performing activities of daily living.

The physician's judgment, based upon experience, training, skill, thoroughness in clinical evaluation, and ability to apply the *Guides* criteria as intended, will enable an appropriate and reproducible assessment to be made of clinical impairment. Clinical judgment, combining both the "art" and "science" of medicine, constitutes the essence of medical practice.

1.6 Causation, Apportionment Analysis, and Aggravation

1.6a Causation

Physicians may be asked to provide an opinion about the likelihood that a particular factor (injury, illness, or preexisiting condition) caused the permanent impairment. Determining causation is important from a legal perspective, as it is a factor in determining liability.

The term **causation** has multiple meanings. *Dorland's Illustrated Medical Dictionary* lists 12 different types of "cause" including constitutional, exciting, immediate, local, precipitating, predisposing, primary, proximate, remote, secondary, specific, and ultimate.[21] For purposes of the *Guides,* causation means an identifiable factor (eg, accident or exposure to hazards of a disease) that results in a medically identifiable condition.

Medical or scientifically based causation requires a detailed analysis of whether the factor could have caused the condition, based upon scientific evidence and, specifically, experienced judgment as to whether the alleged factor in the existing environment did cause the permanent impairment.[22] Determining medical causation requires a synthesis of medical judgment with scientific analysis.

The legal standard for causation in civil litigation and in workers' compensation adjudication varies from jurisdiction to jurisdiction.[23] The physician needs to be aware of the different interpretations of causation and state the context in which the physician's opinion is being offered.

1.6b Apportionment Analysis

Apportionment analysis in workers' compensation represents a distribution or allocation of causation among multiple factors that caused or significantly contributed to the injury or disease and resulting impairment. The factor could be a preexisting injury, illness, or impairment. In some instances, the physician may be asked to apportion or distribute a permanent impairment rating between the impact of the current injury and the prior impairment rating. Before determining apportionment, the physician needs to verify that all the following information is true for an individual:

1. There is documentation of a prior factor.

2. The current permanent impairment is greater as a result of the prior factor (ie, prior impairment, prior injury, or illness).

3. There is evidence indicating the prior factor caused or contributed to the impairment, based on a reasonable probability (> 50% likelihood).

The apportionment analysis must consider the nature of the impairment and its possible relationship to each alleged factor, and it must provide an explanation of the medical basis for all conclusions and opinions. Most states have their own customized methods for calculating apportionment. Generally, the most recent permanent impairment rating is calculated, and then the prior impairment rating is calculated and deducted. The remaining impairment rating would be attributed or apportioned to the current injury or condition.

A common verbal formulation in the workers' compensation context might state, "in cases of permanent disability less than total, if the degree of disability resulting from an industrial injury or occupational disease is increased or prolonged because of a preexisting physical impairment, the employer shall be liable only for the additional disability from the injury or occupational disease."[5]

For example, in apportioning a spine impairment rating in an individual with a history of a spine condition, one should calculate the current spine impairment. Then calculate the impairment from any preexisting spine problem. The preexisting impairment rating is then subtracted from the present impairment rating to account for the effects of the former. This approach requires accurate and comparable data for both impairments.[23]

1.6c Aggravation

Aggravation, for the purposes of the *Guides,* refers to a factor(s) (eg, physical, chemical, biological, or medical condition) that alters the course or progression of the medical impairment. For example, an individual develops low back pain and sciatica associated with the finding of an L3-L4 herniated disk. Symptoms continue but are intermittent and do not interfere with performing activities of daily living. A few years later, the individual twists his body while lifting a heavy package and develops constant, severe, acute low back pain and sciatica. Imaging studies show no change in the herniated disk compared to earlier studies. The lifting is considered to have aggravated a preexisting condition.

Terms such as *causation, apportionment,* and *aggravation* may all have unique legal definitions in the context of the system in which they are used. The physician is advised to compare these definitions with terminology accepted by the appropriate state or system.

1.7 Use of the Guides

Because of the scope, depth, standardized approach, and foundation in science and medical consensus, the *Guides* is used worldwide to estimate adult permanent impairment. A survey completed in 1999 indicates that in the United States, 40 of 51 jurisdictions (50 states and the District of Columbia) use the *Guides* in workers' compensation cases because of statute or regulations, or by administrative/legal practice.[24]

The *Guides* is formally accepted through adoptive language in each jurisdiction's statutes (laws passed by a state legislature or the US Congress), court-made law (case law or precedent), or administrative agency regulation (rules promulgated by administrative agencies such as a state workers' compensation board). It is this statutory, judicial, or regulatory adoptive language that determines which edition of the *Guides* is mandated in a particular jurisdiction. Some states, such as Oregon and Florida, have developed their own impairment criteria, modeled on the concepts and material in the *Guides.* The *Guides* is also extensively used by the federal systems, eg, FECA (Federal Employees' Compensation Act). The most recent edition of the *Guides* is recommended as the latest blend of science and medical consensus.

Beyond the United States, the *Guides* is used in Canada, Australia, New Zealand, South Africa, and European countries for different applications, including workers' compensation, personal injury, and disability claim management. There is a growing international trend to adopt a standardized, medically accepted approach to impairment assessment such as in the *Guides.* As previously stated, the *Guides* is not to be used for direct financial awards nor as the sole measure of disability. The *Guides* provides a standard medical assessment for impairment determination and may be used as a component in disability assessment.

1.8 Impairment Evaluations in Workers' Compensation

In the United States, workers' compensation is a no-fault system for providing cash benefits, medical care, and rehabilitation services to individuals with work-related injuries and diseases. All 50 states and the District of Columbia have workers' compensation acts. Most acts share similar features, although no two are exactly alike. An employee normally must experience a "personal injury by accident arising out of and in the course of employment" to be eligible for benefits. All states provide benefits for workers with occupational diseases, but that coverage is restricted in many states. The claimant receives payments to compensate for lost wages due to temporary total, temporary partial, permanent total, and permanent partial disability. Survivors receive death benefits. For each category of benefits, the state prescribes a maximum and minimum weekly benefit. Many states stipulate partial compensation for a partial loss, based upon a proportion of the number of weeks' compensation allowed for total loss of the body part.[25] Determining eligibility of benefits and the extent of disability is specified by statute and case law.

Because schedules usually do not cover all conditions arising from injuries, many laws allow or require that, in unlisted cases of permanent disability, the jurisdiction must determine the percentage by which the "whole man" or "industrial use" of the employee's body was impaired. The board, commission, or court also must consider the nature of the injury and the employee's occupation, experience, training, and age and then award proportional compensation. Medical information is essential for the decision process in these cases.

Physicians who perform impairment and/or disability assessments for workers' compensation purposes need to identify the state workers' compensation law that applies to the situation, which is usually the state where the incident occurred. The physician needs to determine which edition of the *Guides* or other state guidelines are required for these assessments. This information can usually be obtained from the state workers' compensation board or the state medical society. If the *Guides* is recommended or *required*, copies may be ordered through the AMA (see copyright page) or other vendors.

Unfortunately, there is no validated formula that assigns accurate weights to determine how a medical condition can be combined with other factors, including education, skill, and the like, to calculate the effect of the medical impairment on future employment. Therefore, each commissioner or hearing official bases a decision on the assessment of the available medical and nonmedical information. The *Guides* may help resolve such a situation, but it cannot provide complete and definitive answers. Each administrative or legal system that bases disability ratings on permanent impairment defines its own process of converting impairment ratings into a disability rating that reflects the degree to which the impairment limits the capacity to meet personal, social, occupational, and other demands, or to meet statutory requirements. The *Guides* is a tool for evaluation of permanent impairment.[26, 27]

Impairment percentages derived from the *Guides* criteria should not be used as direct estimates of disability. Impairment percentages estimate the extent of the impairment on whole person functioning and account for basic activities of daily living, not including work. The complexity of work activities requires individual analyses. Impairment assessment is a necessary *first step* for determining disability.

1.9 Employability Determinations

Physicians with the appropriate skills, training, and knowledge may address some of the implications of the medical impairment toward work disability and future employment. The physician may be asked whether an impaired individual can return to work in a particular job. The employer can provide a detailed job analysis, with the actual and anticipated essential requirements of the job and a review of the work environment, including potential hazards and the need for personal protective equipment. The physician can then determine whether the individual's abilities match the job demands. The physician needs to determine that the individual, in performing essential job functions, will not either be endangered or endanger colleagues or the work environment. For example, it would be unsafe for an individual with a new, unstable seizure disorder to operate mechanical equipment. The physician and other responsible persons should keep in mind the potential for impairment aggravation, as well as the possibility of changing an individual's job responsibilities. After reviewing all the necessary information, the physician may then make an objective and reproducible assessment of the ability of the individual to safely perform the essential functions of the job.

More complicated are the cases in which the physician is requested to make a broad judgment regarding an individual's ability to return to any job in his or her field. A decision of this scope usually requires input from medical and nonmedical experts, such as vocational specialists, and the evaluation of both stable and changing factors, such as the person's education, skills, and motivation, the state of the job market, and local economic considerations.

Physicians who follow the procedures outlined in the *Guides,* who review the same information from medical and employment records, and who examine the same patient with a stable condition should obtain approximately the same findings.

1.10 Railroad and Maritime Workers

State workers' compensation laws are not the only means by which employees are compensated for injuries or illnesses. In 1908, Congress passed the Federal Employer's Liability Act (FELA), which put in place a comprehensive injury compensation system for railroad workers. FELA provides a modified tort system for injured railroad workers, and it supersedes state workers' compensation laws. The Jones Act, passed in 1920, covers compensation for maritime workers injured due to a ship owner's negligence. That law provides for the same rights and remedies that were extended through FELA.

A lawsuit filed under FELA must be based on the railroad's negligence in providing the employee with a safe workplace. An injured employee must prove that the railroad should have foreseen that a condition or activity might cause the injury or disease. The test determines whether the employer's negligence played any part in producing the injury. Recoverable amounts include those for necessary medical expenses, pain and suffering, loss of past earnings, and future losses due to diminished earning capacity. An important condition for recovery is that a physician must diagnose the effects of the injury.

Under FELA, all cases must go before a jury or judge, and there are no limits to the amount awarded. In contrast, the awards under state workers' compensation systems are fixed and limited. Under FELA, the jury decides on the degree of the injured person's disability. The physician is obligated to obtain a reliable history, confirm past employment by obtaining records, and collect all available medical information.

1.11 The Physician's Role Based on the Americans with Disabilities Act (ADA)

Physicians, particularly occupational physicians, are frequently asked questions pertaining to work disability and capacity, in light of increasing attention to compliance with the **Americans with Disabilities Act (ADA).** The ADA is a civil rights law that President Bush signed in 1990.[28] It was intended "to provide a clear and comprehensive national mandate to end discrimination against individuals with disabilities and bring those individuals into the economic and social mainstream of American life."[18] Under the ADA, individuals with disabilities are protected against discrimination in such diverse areas as employment, government service entitlement, and access to public accommodations (eg, health care services, lodging).

The ADA defines *disability* as a physical or mental impairment that substantially limits one or more of the major life activities of an individual; a record of impairment; or being regarded as having an impairment (see Table 1-1). A person needs to meet only one of the three criteria in the definition to gain the ADA's protection against discrimination. The physician's input often is essential for determining the first two criteria and valuable for determining the third.

To be deemed "disabled" for purposes of ADA protection, an individual generally must have a physical or mental impairment that substantially limits one or more major life activities. A "physical or mental impairment" could be any mental, psychological, or physiological disorder or condition, cosmetic disfigurement, or anatomical loss that affects one or more of the following body systems: neurologic, special sense organs, musculoskeletal, respiratory (including speech organs), reproductive, cardiovascular, hematologic and lymphatic, digestive, genitourinary, skin, and endocrine.[29]

Conditions that are temporary or not considered to be severe (eg, normal pregnancy) are not considered impairments under the ADA. Other nonimpairments include features and conditions such as hair or eye color, left-handedness, old age, sexual orientation, exhibitionism, pedophilia, voyeurism, sexual addiction, kleptomania, pyromania, compulsive gambling, gender identity disorders not resulting from physical impairment, smoking, and current illegal drug use or resulting psychoactive disorders.

On June 23, 1999, in answer to a case seeking refinement of the definition of "who is disabled" under the ADA, the Supreme Court stated that individuals who function normally with aids such as glasses or medication could not generally be considered disabled, despite their physical impairments.[30]

To have the protection of the ADA, a physical or mental impairment must substantially limit the ability to perform a "major life activity." Major life activities include "basic activities that the average person in the general population can perform with little or no difficulty," including caring for oneself, manual tasks, hearing, walking, learning, speaking, breathing, working, and reproduction. Major life activities do not have to occur frequently or be part of daily life.[31] Note that the major life activities listed here include work, unlike the *Guides'* impairment criteria.

The person must be presently, or perceived to be (not potentially or hypothetically), substantially limited in order to demonstrate a disability. It is difficult to determine if an impairment "substantially limits" a major life activity. An impairment's nature, extent, duration, impact, and effect on the individual are all considerations in assessing the "substantiality" of the limitations.[32]

For some major life activities, such as work, the physician may provide an opinion on the medical impairment's limitations. However, as indicated by the recent Supreme Court ruling, how much a limitation of a major life activity results in a determination of disability depends on the interaction between the remaining functional abilities and the possible types of accommodation being sought.[33]

The third criterion that may establish protection under the ADA is an erroneous perception that the individual is substantially limited in a major life activity or is being discriminated against on the basis of a real or perceived characteristic that does not substantially limit a major life activity.

It is the physician's responsibility to determine if the impairment results in functional limitations. The physician is responsible for informing the employer about an individual's abilities and limitations. It is the employer's responsibility to identify and determine if reasonable accommodations are possible to enable the individual's performance of essential job activities.

1.12 Summary

The purpose of this chapter is to discuss the philosophical assumptions and appropriate use of the *Guides*. The physician needs to comply with prescribed local, state, and federal practices for impairment evaluations. Generally, the physician evaluates all available information and provides as comprehensive a medical picture of the patient as possible, addressing the components listed in the Report of Medical Evaluation form discussed in Chapter 2. A complete impairment evaluation provides valuable information beyond an impairment percentage, and it includes a discussion about the person's abilities and limitations, including the ability to perform common activities as listed in Table 1-2. Combining the medical and nonmedical information, and including detailed information about essential work activities if requested, is a basis for improved understanding of the degree to which the impairment may affect the individual's work ability.

References

1. American Medical Association. Glossary. In: *Guides to the Evaluation of Permanent Impairment.* Chicago, Ill: American Medical Association; 1971.

2. American Medical Association. *Guides to the Evaluation of Permanent Impairment.* 4th ed. Chicago, Ill: American Medical Association; 1993.

3. Berkowitz M, Burton J. *Permanent Disability Benefits in Workers' Compensation.* Kalamazoo, Mich: Upjohn Institute for Employment Research; 1987.

4. Cocchiarella L, Deitchman M, Nielsen N. Establishing disability in various stages of HIV infection. Report of the Council on Scientific Affairs, American Medical Association. Paper presented at: Interim Meeting of the American Medical Association House of Delegates; December 1999; Chicago, Ill. Approved.

5. *Idaho Code* Section 406(1).

6. American Medical Association. *Guides to the Evaluation of Permanent Impairment.* 2nd ed. Chicago, Ill: American Medical Association; 1984.

7. McDowell I, Newell C. *Measuring Health: A Guide to Rating Scales and Questionnaires.* 2nd ed. New York, NY: Oxford University Press; 1996.

8. McWhinnie JR. Disability assessment in population surveys: results of the OECD common development effort. *Rev Epidemiol Sante Publique.* 1981;29:413-419.

9. Fries JF, Spitz PW, Young DY. The dimensions of health outcomes: the Health Assessment Questionnaire, disability and pain scales. *J Rheumatol.* 1982;9:789-793.

10. Hamilton BB, Granger CV, Sherwin FS, et al. A uniform national data system for medical rehabilitation. In: Fuhrer MJ, ed. *Rehabilitation Outcomes: Analysis and Measurement.* Baltimore, Md: Paul H. Brooks; 1987:137-147.

11. Mahoney FI, Wood OH, Barthel DW. Rehabilitation of chronically ill patients: the influence of complications on the final goal. *South Med J.* 1958;51:605-609.

12. Katz S, Akpom CA. A measure of primary sociobiological functions. *Int J Health Serv* 1976;6:493-507.

13. Forer SK. *Revised Functional Status Rating Instrument.* Glendale, Calif: Rehabilitation Institute, Glendale Adventist Medical Center; December 1981.

14. Fillenbaum GG. *Multidimensional Functional Assessment of Older Adults: The Duke Older Americans Resources and Services Procedures.* Hillsdale, NJ: Lawrence Erlbaum Associates; 1988.

15. Stewart AL, Kamberg CJ. Physical functioning measures. In: Stewart AL, Ware JE Jr, eds. *Measuring Functioning and Well-being: The Medical Outcomes Study Approach.* Durham, NC: Duke University Press; 1992:86-101.

16. Brandt EN Jr, Pope AM. *Enabling America: Assessing the Role of Rehabilitation Science and Engineering.* Washington, DC: National Academy Press; 1997.

17. World Health Organization. *ICIDH: International Classification of Impairments, Activities and Participation: A Manual of Dimensions of Disablement and Health. (Beta-2 Draft).* Available at: http://www.who.org/msa/mnh/ems/ icidh/introduction.htm. Accessed October 7, 1999.

18. Gloss DS, Wardle MG. Reliability and validity of American Medical Association's Guide to Ratings of Permanent Impairment. *JAMA.*1982;248:2292-2296.

19. Rondinelli RD, Dunn W, Hassanein KM, et al. A simulation of hand impairments: effects on upper extremity function and implications towards medical impairment rating and disability determination. *Arch Phys Med Rehabil.* 1997;78:1358-1363.

20. McCarthy ML, et al. Correlation between the measures of impairment, according to the modified system of the American Medical Association, and function. *J Bone Joint Surg Am.* 1998;80(7):1034-1042.

21. *Dorland's Illustrated Medical Dictionary*, 28th ed. Philadelpha, Pa: WB Saunders; 1994.

22. Rothman KJ, ed. *Modern Epidemiology.* 2nd ed. Philadelphia, Pa: Lippincott-Williams and Wilkins; 1998.

23. The Industrial Commission of Utah. *Utah's 1997 Impairment Guides.* Salt Lake City, Utah: The Industrial Commission of Utah; 1997

24. Barth PS, Niss M. *Permanent Partial Disability Benefits: Interstate Differences*: Workers Compensation Research Institute; 1999.

25. Bunn WB, Berté AP. The role of the physician in the worker's compensation process. In: Hadler NM, Bunn WB, eds. *Occupational Problems in Medical Practice.* New York, NY: Medical Publications, Inc; 1990:133-144.

26. Spieler EA, Barth PS, Burton JF Jr, Himmelstein J, Rudolph L. Recommendations to guide revision of the *Guides to the Evaluation of Permanent Impairment.* *JAMA.* 2000;283:519-523.

27. Cocchiarella L, Turk MA, Andersson G. Improving the evaluation of permanent impairment. *JAMA.* 2000; 283:532-533.

28. Americans with Disabilities Act, HR Rep No. 101-485, pt 3, at 23 (1990), reprinted in 1990 USCCN 445, 446.

29. 29 CFR 1630.2(h)(1)(1997); HR Rep No. 101-485, pt 3, at 28 (1990), reprinted in 1990 USCCN 445, 450.

30. *Sutton v United Airlines*, 97 US 1943 (1999).

31. Interpretive Guidance on Title One, ADA, 29 CFR App 1630.2.

32. 29 CFR 1630.2 (j) (2).

33. American Medical Association in Cooperation with the American Academy of Physical Medicine and Rehabilitation. *The Americans with Disabilities Act: A Practice of Accommodation.* Chicago, Ill: American Medical Association; 1998.

Chapter 2

Practical Application of the *Guides*

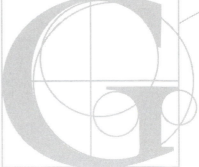

Introduction

This chapter describes how to use the *Guides* for consistent and reliable acquisition, analysis, communication, and utilization of medical information through a single set of standards. Two physicians, following the methods of the *Guides* to evaluate the same patient, should report similar results and reach similar conclusions. Moreover, if the clinical findings are fully described, any knowledgeable observer may check the findings with the *Guides* criteria. This chapter provides information about the practical application of the *Guides* and is to be used in conjunction with Chapter 1, which provides the conceptual framework upon which the instructions in this chapter are based.

2.1 Defining Impairment Evaluations

An **impairment evaluation** is a medical evaluation performed by a physician, using a standard method as outlined in the *Guides* to determine permanent impairment associated with a medical condition. An impairment evaluation may include a numerical impairment percentage or rating, as defined in the *Guides*. An impairment evaluation is not the same as an **independent medical evaluation (IME),** which is performed by an independent medical examiner who evaluates but does not provide care for the individual. Impairment evaluations may be less comprehensive than IMEs and may be performed by a treating physician or a nontreating physician, depending upon the state's requirements and the preferences of the individual, physician, and requesting party. Examples of an impairment evaluation and components of a comprehensive IME will be discussed later in this chapter.

2.2 Who Performs Impairment Evaluations?

Impairment evaluations are performed by a licensed physician. The physician may use information from other sources, such as hearing results obtained from audiometry by a certified technician. However, the physician is responsible for performing a medical evaluation that addresses medical impairment in the body or organ system and related systems. A state may restrict the type of practitioner allowed to perform an impairment evaluation, and some require additional state certification and other criteria, such as a minimum number of hours of practice, before the physician is approved as an impairment evaluator. The physician is encouraged to check with the local workers' compensation agency, industrial accident board, or industrial commission concerning their prerequisites.

2.3 Examiners' Roles and Responsibilities

The physician's role in performing an impairment evaluation is to provide an independent, unbiased assessment of the individual's medical condition, including its effect on function, and identify abilities and limitations to performing activities of daily living as listed in Table 1-2. Performing an impairment evaluation requires considerable medical expertise and judgment. Full and complete reporting provides the best opportunity for physicians to explain health status and consequences to patients, other medical professionals, and other interested parties such as claims examiners and attorneys. Thorough documentation of medical findings and their impact will also ensure that reporting is fair and consistent and that individuals have the information needed to pursue any benefits to which they are entitled.

The skills required for impairment evaluation are usually not taught during basic medical training, although some specialties such as occupational medicine, physical medicine and rehabilitation, and orthopedics have emphasized elements of the evaluation such as occupational, functional, or anatomical assessment.

In some cases, physicians may be asked to assess the medical impairment's impact on the individual's ability to work. In the latter case, physicians need to understand the essential functions of the occupation and specific job, as well as how the medical condition interacts with the occupational demands. In many cases, the physician may need to obtain additional expertise to define functional abilities and limitations, as well as vocational demands.

As an impairment evaluator, the physician has the responsibility to understand the regulations that pertain to medical practice in his or her specific area, as in workers' compensation or personal injury evaluations. It is also the responsibility of the physician to provide the necessary medical assessment to the party requesting the evaluation, with the examinee's consent. The physician needs to ensure that the examinee understands that the evaluation's purpose is medical assessment, not medical treatment. However, if new diagnoses are discovered, the physician has a medical obligation to inform the requesting party and individual about the condition and recommend further medical assessment.

2.4 When Are Impairment Ratings Performed?

An impairment should not be considered permanent until the clinical findings indicate that the medical condition is static and well stabilized, often termed the date of **maximal medical improvement (MMI)**. It is understood that an individual's condition is dynamic. Maximal medical improvement refers to a date from which further recovery or deterioration is not anticipated, although over time there may be some expected change. Once an impairment has reached MMI, a permanent impairment rating may be performed. The *Guides* attempts to take into account all relevant considerations in rating the severity and extent of permanent impairment and its effect on the individual's activities of daily living.

Impairments often involve more than one body system or organ system; the same condition may be discussed in more than one chapter. Generally, the organ system where the problems originate or where the dysfunction is greatest is the chapter to be used for evaluating the impairment. Thus, consult the vision chapter for visual problems due to optic nerve dysfunction. Refer to the extremity chapters for neurological and musculoskeletal extremity impairment from an injury. However, if the impairment is due to a stroke, the neurology chapter is most appropriate. Whenever the same impairment is discussed in different chapters, the *Guides* tries to use consistent impairment ratings across the different organ systems.

2.5 Rules for Evaluation

2.5a Confidentiality

Prior to performing an impairment evaluation, the physician obtains the individual's consent to share the medical information with other parties that will be reviewing the evaluation. If the evaluating physician is also that person's treating physician, the physician needs to indicate to the individual which information from his or her medical record will be shared.

2.5b Combining Impairment Ratings

To determine **whole person impairment,** the physician should begin with an estimate of the individual's most significant (primary) impairment and evaluate other impairments in relation to it. It may be necessary for the physician to refer to the criteria and estimates in several chapters if the impairing condition involves several organ systems. Related but separate conditions are rated separately and impairment ratings are combined unless criteria for the second impairment are included in the primary impairment. For example, an individual with an injury causing neurologic and muscular impairment to his upper extremity would be evaluated under the upper extremity criteria in Chapter 16. Any skin impairment due to significant scarring would be rated separately in the skin chapter and combined with the impairment from the upper extremity chapter. Loss of nerve function would be rated within either the musculoskeletal chapters or neurology chapter.

In the case of two significant yet unrelated conditions, each impairment rating is calculated separately, converted or expressed as a whole person impairment, then combined using the Combined Values Chart (p. 604). The general philosophy of the Combined Values Chart is discussed in Chapter 1.

2.5c Consistency

Consistency tests are designed to ensure reproducibility and greater accuracy. These measurements, such as one that checks the individual's lumbosacral spine range of motion (Section 15.9) are good but imperfect indicators of people's efforts. The physician must use the entire range of clinical skill and judgment when assessing whether or not the measurements or tests results are plausible and consistent with the impairment being evaluated. If, in spite of an observation or test result, the medical evidence appears insufficient to verify that an impairment of a certain magnitude exists, the physician may modify the impairment rating accordingly and then describe and explain the reason for the modification in writing.

2.5d Interpolating, Measuring, and Rounding Off

In deciding where to place an individual's impairment rating within a range, the physician needs to consider all the criteria applicable to the condition, which includes performing activities of daily living, and estimate the degree to which the medical impairment interferes with these activities. In some cases, the physician may need additional information to determine where to place an individual in the range.

As with any biological measurements, some variability and normal fluctuations are inherent in permanent impairment ratings. Two measurements made by the same examiner using the *Guides* that involve an individual or an individual's functions would be consistent if they fall within 10% of each other. Measurements should also be consistent between two trained observers or by one observer on two separate occasions, assuming the individual's condition is stable. Repeating measurements may decrease error and result in a measurement that is closer to average function. The final calculated whole person impairment rating, whether it is based on the evaluation of one organ system or several organ systems, should be rounded to the nearest whole number.

2.5e Pain

The impairment ratings in the body organ system chapters make allowance for any accompanying pain. Chronic pain, also called chronic pain syndrome, is discussed in the chapter on pain (Chapter 18).

2.5f Using Assistive Devices in Evaluations

If an individual's **prosthesis** or **assistive device** can be removed or its use eliminated relatively easily, the physician should usually test and evaluate the organ system without the device. For example, ask the patient to remove a hearing aid before testing auditory acuity. The examiner may choose also to test the system with the assistive device in place and then report both sets of results. The physician may also choose to report alterations in the individual's organ function with and without use of the device and challenges that are posed by using the device, if any.

If the assistive device is not easily removable, as with an implanted lens, evaluate the organ system's functioning with the device in place. Test the visual system with the patient's glasses or contact lenses in place if they are used.

2.5g Adjustments for Effects of Treatment or Lack of Treatment

In certain instances, the treatment of an illness may result in apparently total remission of the person's signs and symptoms. Examples include the treatment of hypothyroidism with levothyroxine and the treatment of type 1 diabetes mellitus with insulin. Yet it is debatable whether, with treatment, the patient has actually regained the previous status of normal good health. In these instances, the physician may choose to increase the impairment estimate by a small percentage (eg, 1% to 3%).

In some instances, as with organ transplant recipients who are treated with immunity-suppressing pharmaceuticals or persons treated with anticoagulants, the pharmaceuticals themselves may lead to impairments. In such an instance, the physician should use the appropriate parts of the *Guides* to evaluate impairment related to pharmaceutical effects. If information in the *Guides* is lacking, the physician may combine an estimated impairment percent based on the severity of the effect, with the primary organ system impairment, by means of the Combined Values Chart (p. 604).

A patient may decline surgical, pharmacologic, or therapeutic treatment of an impairment. If a patient declines therapy for a permanent impairment, that decision neither decreases nor increases the estimated percentage of the individual's impairment. However, the physician may wish to make a written comment in the medical evaluation report about the suitability of the therapeutic approach and describe the basis of the individual's refusal. The physician may also need to address whether the impairment is at maximal medical improvement without treatment and the degree of anticipated improvement that could be expected with treatment.

2.5h Changes in Impairment from Prior Ratings

Although a previous evaluator may have considered a medical impairment to be permanent, unanticipated changes may occur: the condition may have become worse as a result of aggravation or clinical progression, or it may have improved. The physician should assess the current state of the impairment according to the criteria in the *Guides*. If an individual received an impairment rating from an earlier edition and needs to be reevaluated because of a change in the medical condition, the individual is evaluated according to the latest information pertaining to the condition in the current edition of the *Guides*.

Valid assessment of a change in the impairment estimate would depend on the reliability of the previous estimate and the evidence upon which it was based. If a prior impairment evaluation was not performed, but sufficient historical information is available to currently estimate the prior impairment, the assessment would be performed based on the most recent *Guides* criteria. However, if the information is insufficient to accurately document the change, then the physician needs to explain that decision and should not estimate a change.

If apportionment is needed, the analysis must consider the nature of the impairment and its relationship to each alleged causative factor, providing an explanation of the medical basis for all conclusions and opinions. (Apportionment and causation are considered more fully in Chapter 1 and are briefly defined in the Glossary.) For example, in apportioning a spine impairment, first the current spine impairment rating is calculated, and then an impairment rating from any preexisting spine problem is calculated. The value for the preexisting impairment rating can be subtracted from the present impairment rating to account for the effects of the intervening injury or disease. Using this approach to apportionment requires accurate information and data to determine both impairment ratings. If different editions of the *Guides* are used, the physician needs to assess their similarity. If the basis of the ratings is similar, a subtraction is appropriate. If they differ markedly, the physician needs to evaluate the circumstances and determine if conversion to the earlier or latest edition of the *Guides* for both ratings is possible. The determination should follow any state guidelines and should consider whichever edition best describes the individual's impairment.

2.6 Preparing Reports

A clear, accurate, and complete report is essential to support a rating of permanent impairment. The following elements in **bold type** should be included in **all** impairment evaluation reports. Other elements listed in *italics* are commonly found within an IME or may be requested for inclusion in an impairment evaluation.

2.6a Clinical Evaluation

2.6a.1 Include a **narrative history** of the medical condition(s) with the onset and course of the condition, symptoms, findings on previous examination(s), treatments, and responses to treatment, including adverse effects. Include information that may be relevant to onset, such as an occupational exposure or injury. Historical information should refer to any relevant investigations. Include a detailed list of prior evaluations in the clinical data section.

2.6a.2 *Include a work history with a detailed, chronological description of work activities, specific type and duration of work performed, materials used in the workplace, any temporal associations with the medical condition and work, frequency, intensity, and duration of exposure and activity, and any protective measures.*

2.6a.3 Assess **current clinical status**, including current symptoms, review of symptoms, physical examination, and a list of contemplated treatment, rehabilitation, and any anticipated reevaluation.

2.6a.4 List **diagnostic study results** and outstanding pertinent **diagnostic studies**. These may include laboratory tests, electrocardiograms, exercise stress studies, radiographic and other imaging studies, rehabilitation evaluations, mental status examinations, and other tests or diagnostic procedures.

2.6a.5 Discuss the medical basis for determining whether the person is at **MMI.** If not, estimate and discuss the expected date of full or partial recovery.

2.6a.6 Discuss **diagnoses, impairments.**

2.6a.7 *Discuss causation and apportionment, if requested, according to recommendations outlined in Chapters 1 and 2.*

2.6a.8 Discuss impairment rating criteria, prognosis, residual function, and limitations. Include a discussion of the anticipated clinical course and whether further medical treatment is anticipated. Describe the residual function and the impact of the medical impairment(s) on the ability to perform activities of daily living *and, if requested, complex activities such as work.* List the types of affected activities (see Table 1-2). Identify any medical consequences for performing activities of daily living.

If requested, the physician may need to analyze different job tasks to determine if an individual has the residual function to perform that complex activity. The physician should also identify any medical consequence of performing a complex activity such as work.

2.6a.9 *Explain* any conclusion about the need for restrictions or accommodations for standard activities of daily living or *complex activities such as work.*

2.6b Calculate the Impairment Rating
Compare the medical findings with the impairment criteria listed within the *Guides* and calculate the appropriate impairment rating. Discuss how specific findings relate to and compare with the criteria described in the applicable *Guides* chapter. Refer to and explain the absence of any pertinent data and how the physician determined the impairment rating with limited data.

2.6c. Discuss How the Impairment Rating Was Calculated
2.6c.1 Include an explanation of each impairment value with reference to the applicable criteria of the *Guides*. Combine multiple impairments for a whole person impairment.

2.6c.2 Include a summary list of impairments and impairment ratings by percentage, including calculation of the whole person impairment.

On the following two pages is a standard form that the evaluator may use to ensure that all essential elements are included in the impairment evaluation report. The form may be reproduced without permission from the American Medical Association. Most chapters include a summary form that identifies the salient, specific features to consider for each category of organ system impairment.

Sample Report for Permanent Medical Impairment

Identifiers:

  Patient name: _____

  Address:_____

  Claim #:_____

  Date of birth: _____

  Date of injury or illness: _____

Examination date:_____

Dates of care by examining physician: _____

Examination location: _____

Examining physician: _____

Introduction: Purpose (impairment or IME evaluation, personal injury, workers' compensation) and procedures (who performed the exam, patient consent, location of examination)

_____

_____

_____

Narrative history: Chief complaints, history of injury or illness, occupational history, past medical history, family history, social history, review of systems

_____

_____

_____

Medical record review: Chronology of medical evaluation, diagnostic studies, and treatment for the injury or illness

_____

_____

_____

Physical examination:

_____

_____

_____

Diagnostic studies:

_____
_____
_____

Diagnoses and Impairments: (*If requested, discuss work relatedness, causation, apportionment, restrictions , accommodations, assistive devices*)

_____
_____
_____

Impairment Rating Criteria: MMI residual function, limitations of activities of daily living, prognosis

_____
_____
_____

Impairment Rating and Rationale Organ system and whole person impairment

Body part or system	Chapter No.	Table No.	% Impairment of the Whole Person
a.			
b.			
c.			
d.			

Calculated total whole person impairment:_____%. Discussion of rationale of impairment rating and any possible inconsistencies in the examination:

_____
_____

Recommendations: Further diagnostic or therapeutic follow-up care

_____
_____
_____

Work ability, work restrictions (If requested, review abilities and limitations in reference to essential job activities):

_____
_____
_____

Chapter 2

The Cardiovascular System: Heart and Aorta

Introduction

This chapter provides criteria for evaluating permanent impairments of the cardiovascular system and their effects on an individual's ability to perform the activities of daily living. The cardiovascular system consists of the heart, the aorta, the systemic arteries, and the pulmonary arteries. Impairment of the heart is the focus of this chapter; impairment of diseases of the aorta, the systemic arteries, and pulmonary arteries (including coronary and peripheral circulation) are included in Chapter 4.

The following sections have been revised from the fourth edition: (1) information about valvular heart disease reflecting newly published guidelines from the American Heart Association and American College of Cardiology; (2) information about coronary artery disease reflecting the important prognostic impact of left ventricular function on impairment in individuals with coronary artery disease, and the inclusion of silent ischemia and coronary artery spasm with regard to impairment; and (3) information about cardiomyopathy, including the impact of HIV-related conditions that affect cardiac function.

3.1 Principles of Assessment

Before using the information in this chapter, the *Guides* user should become familiar with Chapters 1 and 2 and the Glossary. Chapters 1 and 2 discuss the *Guides'* purpose, applications, and methods for performing and reporting impairment evaluations. The Glossary provides definitions of common terms used by many specialties in impairment evaluation.

3.1a Interpretation of Symptoms and Signs

Some impairment classes refer to limitations in the ability to perform daily activities because of symptoms. When this information is subjective and possibly misinterpreted, it should not serve as the sole criterion upon which decisions about impairment are made. Rather, the examiner should obtain objective data about the extent of the limitation and integrate the findings with the subjective data to estimate the degree of permanent impairment. See the functional classifications of cardiac disease in Table 3-1.

Exercise Testing

When feasible, the physician should attempt to quantify limitations due to symptoms by observing the individual during exercise.[2] A motor-driven treadmill with varying grades and speeds is the most widely used device for standardized exercise protocols. The protocols vary slightly, but they all attempt to relate the exercise to excess energy expended and to functional class. The excess energy expended is usually expressed in terms of the **"MET,"** which represents the multiples of resting metabolic energy used for any given activity. One MET is considered to be 3.5 mL (kg/min). The 70-kg man who burns 1.2 kcal/min while sitting at rest uses approximately 3 METS when walking 4 km/h.

Table 3-2 displays the relationship of excess energy expenditures in METS to functional class according to the protocols of several investigators. With all protocols, the exercise periods last for 2 or 3 minutes; the time periods are represented in the table by boxes with numbers giving the estimated METS involved.

Table 3-1 NYHA Functional Classification of Cardiac Disease*

Class	Description
I	Individual has cardiac disease but no resulting limitation of physical activity; ordinary physical activity does not cause undue fatigue, palpitation, dyspnea, or anginal pain.
II	Individual has cardiac disease resulting in slight limitation of physical activity; is comfortable at rest and in the performance of ordinary, light, daily activities; greater than ordinary physical activity, such as heavy physical exertion, results in fatigue, palpitation, dyspnea, or anginal pain.
III	Individual has cardiac disease resulting in marked limitation of physical activity; is comfortable at rest; ordinary physical activity results in fatigue, palpitation, dyspnea, or anginal pain.
IV	Individual has cardiac disease resulting in inability to carry on any physical activity without discomfort; symptoms of inadequate cardiac output, pulmonary congestion, systemic congestion, or anginal syndrome may be present, even at rest; if any physical activity is undertaken, discomfort is increased.

*Adapted from: Criteria Committee of the New York Heart Association. *Diseases of the Heart and Blood Vessels: Nomenclature and Criteria for Disease*. 6th ed. Boston, Mass: Little Brown & Co; 1964. This well-established classification is preferred over the newer classification introduced in the 7th edition.[1]

Table 3-2 Relationship of METS and Functional Class According to Five Treadmill Protocols*

METS	1.6	2	3	4	5	6	7	8	9	10	11	12	13	14	15	16
Treadmill tests																
Ellestad																
Miles per hour					1.7	3.0			4.0						5.0	
% grade					10	10			10						10	
Bruce																
Miles per hour					1.7		2.5		3.4				4.2			
% grade					10		12		14				16			
Balke																
Miles per hour				3.4	3.4	3.4	3.4	3.4	3.4	3.4	3.4	3.4	3.4	3.4	3.4	3.4
% grade				2	4	6	8	10	12	14	16	18	20	22	24	26
Balke																
Miles per hour			3.0	3.0	3.0	3.0	3.0	3.0	3.0	3.0	3.0	3.0				
% grade			0	2.5	5	7.5	10	12.5	15	17.5	20	22.5				
Naughton																
Miles per hour	1.0	2.0	2.0	2.0	2.0	2.0	2.0									
% grade	0	0	3.5	7	10.5	14	17.5									
METS	1.6	2	3	4	5	6	7	8	9	10	11	12	13	14	15	16

Clinical status		
Symptomatic patients	⟵————————⟶	
Diseased, recovered	⟵————————⟶	
Sedentary healthy	⟵————————⟶	
Physically active	⟵————————————————————⟶	
Functional class	IV ⟵—III—⟶ ⟵II⟶ ⟵——————— I and Normal ———————⟶	

*Adapted from: Fox SM III, Naughton JP, Haskell WL. Physical activity and the prevention of coronary heart disease. *Ann Clin Res.* 1971;3:404-432.[3]

Table 3-3 Energy Expenditure in METS During Bicycle Ergometry*

Body Weight		Work Rate on Bicycle Ergometer, kg m⁻¹ min⁻¹ (Watts)												
kg	(lb)	75 (50)	150 (75)	300 (100)	450 (125)	600 (150)	750 (175)	900 (200)	1050 (225)	1200 (250)	1350 (275)	1500 (300)	1650	1800
20	(44)	4.0	6.0	10.0	14.0	18.0	22.0							
30	(66)	3.4	4.7	7.3	10.0	12.7	15.3	17.9	20.7	23.3				
40	(88)	3.0	4.0	6.0	8.0	10.0	12.0	14.0	16.0	18.0	20.0	22.0		
50	(110)	2.8	3.6	5.2	6.8	8.4	10.0	11.5	13.2	14.8	16.3	18.0	19.6	21.1
60	(132)	2.7	3.3	4.7	6.0	7.3	8.7	10.0	11.3	12.7	14.0	15.3	16.7	18.0
70	(154)	2.6	3.1	4.3	5.4	6.6	7.7	8.8	10.0	11.1	12.2	13.4	14.0	15.7
80	(176)	2.5	3.0	4.0	5.0	6.0	7.0	8.0	9.0	10.0	11.0	12.0	13.0	14.0
90	(198)	2.4	2.9	3.8	4.7	5.6	6.4	7.3	8.2	9.1	10.0	10.9	11.8	12.6
100	(220)	2.4	2.8	3.6	4.4	5.2	6.0	6.8	7.6	8.4	9.2	10.0	10.8	11.6
110	(242)	2.4	2.7	3.4	4.2	4.9	5.6	6.3	7.1	7.8	8.5	9.3	10.0	10.7
120	(264)	2.3	2.7	3.3	4.0	4.7	5.3	6.0	6.7	7.3	8.0	8.7	9.3	10.0

*Source: American College of Sports Medicine. *Guidelines for Graded Exercise Testing and Exercise Prescription.* Philadelphia, Pa: Lea and Febiger; 1975:17.

A major problem with the use of any exercise-testing technique to attempt to quantify an individual's functional capacity is the marked variability in people's efforts and abilities. Therefore, while measuring the maximum oxygen consumption response, the health care professional should estimate and note the individual's cooperation and effort during the test; eg, some will continue longer than they should, while others will stop after minimal effort because they feel fatigued.

Functional Capacity
The functional capacity of an individual depends on age, gender, and level of training. The functional class determined by means of Tables 3-2 and 3-3 may not be applicable to people at the ends of the age spectrum, such as a 20-year-old athlete or an inactive 70-year-old woman. Therefore, it may be useful to calculate a "percentage functional aerobic capacity" that is achieved on an exercise test. Standard charts are available for the various exercise protocols that determine the percentage functional aerobic capacity based on total exercise duration, age, gender, and level of training.[4]

Left Ventricle Function
Knowledge of the status of the left ventricle is important to assess in the examination and evaluation of an individual with cardiac disease. Two phases of left ventricular (LV) function contribute to the person's symptoms and condition: systolic function, which is the ability of the heart to pump out blood during contraction; and diastolic function, the process by which the heart fills with blood during relaxation of the myocardium and a passive filling phase.[5]

Ejection Fraction
A clinically used measure of systolic function is the "ejection fraction" (EF), the percentage of blood the heart is able to eject during one beat. Echocardiography, radionuclide angiography, and left ventriculography are commonly used to measure the EF. A normal EF is greater than to 0.50; EFs of 0.40 to 0.50 indicate mild systolic dysfunction; 0.30 to 0.40, moderate systolic dysfunction; and < 0.30, severe systolic dysfunction.

Diastolic Dysfunction
Diastolic dysfunction may contribute to the signs and symptoms of heart failure (HF), but quantifying the degree of dysfunction is problematic. Diastolic dysfunction is usually diagnosed clinically by elevated filling pressures that result in HF in the absence of systolic dysfunction or valvular abnormalities. Echocardiography with cardiac Doppler is emerging as an accepted tool for the assessment of diastolic function.[3, 5-7]

3.1b Determination of Impairment
Impairment classes, as listed in Tables 3-5 through 3-11, are disease-specific and based on the NYHA classification system as listed in Table 3-1. The impairment classes reflect anatomic, physiologic, and functional abnormalities. For example, the information in Table 3-1 category I of the NYHA system is represented in the corresponding class 1 on Table 3-5. The classes listed in Tables 3-5 through 3-11 apply the NYHA functional classification to specific disease conditions. The percentages of impairment reflect the severity of the condition and the extent to which the condition limits the abilities to do activities of daily living.

In the illustrative examples of impairment in this chapter, any historic, physical examination, or laboratory information or data not described should be considered to be within normal limits.

In summary, an evaluation of the cardiovascular system that falls within normal range reflects an individual who performs all activities of daily living without cardiovascular symptoms, has some reserve capacity that allows comfortable exercise without the development of major cardiovascular symptoms, has an LV ejection fraction that falls within normal limits, and completes at least 80% of age- and gender-predicted functional aerobic capacity during exercise **stress testing.**

3.2 Valvular Heart Disease

Congenital, rheumatic, infectious, or traumatic factors or a combination of those factors may cause valvular heart disease. Valvular disease may result in (1) pressure hypertrophy of the left or right ventricle (RV), causing elevated filling pressures, myocardial ischemia, and eventual LV dysfunction with signs and symptoms of congestive heart failure (CHF); (2) volume hypertrophy of the LV or RV, causing ventricular dilatation and eventual irreversible myocardial dysfunction with signs and symptoms of CHF; (3) inflow obstruction to the ventricles causing congestion of organs, even in the absence of ventricular dysfunction; or (4) decreased cardiac output.[5]

Valvular heart disease can be detected and its severity assessed by means of a thorough history and physical examination and should be confirmed by either Doppler echocardiography or cardiac catheterization.[8] A valve gradient measures the pressure drop across a stenotic valve and is proportional to the severity of obstruction. Since the valve gradient is influenced by the cardiac output, the valve gradient calculates a valve area that takes into consideration both the pressure gradient and the cardiac output. There may be technical limitations to these derived variables. Their correlation with the severity of the stenosis is shown in Table 3-4.

The severity of a regurgitant valve lesion is more difficult to assess than that of a stenotic lesion. Physical examination and Doppler echocardiography may provide a qualitative assessment. Although Doppler echocardiography may help the physician determine a mild or severe regurgitant valve lesion, this technique's inherent limitations preclude an accurate assessment of intermediate grades of severity. Cardiac catheterization may be required for a semi-quantitative estimate of the valve lesion's severity; it can provide a view of the contrast medium's intensity as it crosses the regurgitating valve into the receiving heart chamber. To assess the severity of aortic valve regurgitation, obtain the estimate with aortic root angiography; to assess the severity of mitral valve regurgitation, obtain the estimate with left ventriculography.

Catheter-based interventional procedures, operative repair, or prosthetic valve replacement can reduce the severity of, but not fully repair, valvular heart disease. After any of these procedures, allow sufficient time to elapse from the date of surgery for maximum recovery and reconditioning of the heart, lungs, and other organs before estimating permanent impairment.

In addition, because medication may affect the severity of valvular heart disease, especially limitations due to symptoms, allow sufficient time for medication to be introduced and adjusted and to take effect before estimating permanent impairment.

Table 3-4 Severity of Valve Stenosis

Severity of Stenosis*	Mean Valve Gradient (mm Hg)	Valve Area ± (cm²)
Aortic valve		
Mild	<25	>1.5
Moderate	25-50	1.0-1.5
Severe	>50	<1.0
Mitral valve		
Mild	<5	>1.5
Moderate	5-10	1.0-1.5
Severe	>10	<1.0

* Severity of stenosis also may be indexed to body surface area.

Chapter 3

3.2a Criteria for Rating Permanent Impairment Due to Valvular Heart Disease

The impairment criteria for valvular heart disease are given in Table 3-5.

Table 3-5 Criteria for Rating Permanent Impairment Due to Valvular Heart Disease

Class 1 0%-9% Impairment of the Whole Person	Class 2 10%-29% Impairment of the Whole Person	Class 3 30%-49% Impairment of the Whole Person	Class 4 50%-100% Impairment of the Whole Person
Evidence by physical examination or laboratory studies of valvular heart disease *and* no symptoms in the performance of ordinary daily activities (functional class I; 5 METS; Table 3-2) or with moderately heavy exertion (7 to 10 METS) *and* does not require continuous treatment, except for intermittent prophylactic antibiotics for surgical or dental procedure to reduce risk of bacterial endocarditis *and* no evidence of CHF *and* no signs of ventricular dysfunction or dilation, and severity of stenosis or regurgitation estimated to be mild (METS >7; TMET [Bruce protocol] >6 min) *and* in the individual who has recovered from valvular heart surgery, all above criteria are met	Evidence by physical examination or laboratory studies of valvular heart disease, and no symptoms in performance of daily activities, but symptoms develop on moderately heavy physical exertion (functional class II) *or* requires moderate dietary adjustment or drugs to prevent symptoms or to remain free of signs of CHF or other consequences of valvular heart disease, such as syncope, chest pain, and emboli *or* signs or laboratory evidence of cardiac chamber dysfunction and/or dilation, severity of stenosis or regurgitation estimated to be moderate, and surgical correction not feasible or advisable; METS >5 but <7; TMET (Bruce protocol) >3 min *or* has recovered from valvular heart surgery and meets criteria for functional class II	Signs of valvular heart disease and slight to moderate symptomatic discomfort during performance of ordinary daily activities (functional class III) *and* dietary therapy or drugs do not completely control symptoms or prevent CHF *and* signs or laboratory evidence of cardiac chamber dysfunction or dilation, severity of stenosis or regurgitation estimated to be moderate or severe, and surgical correction not feasible; METS >2 but <5; TMET (Bruce protocol) >1 min but <3 min *or* has recovered from heart valve surgery but continues to meet criteria for functional class III	Signs by physical examination of valvular heart disease, and symptoms at rest or in performance of less than ordinary daily activities (functional class IV) *and* dietary therapy and drugs cannot control symptoms or prevent signs of CHF *and* signs or laboratory evidence of cardiac chamber dysfunction or dilation, severity of stenosis or regurgitation estimated to be moderate or severe, and surgical correction not feasible; METS <2; TMET (Bruce protocol) <1 min *or* recovered from valvular heart surgery but continues to meet criteria for functional class IV

Class 1
0%-9% Impairment of the Whole Person
Evidence by physical examination or laboratory studies of valvular heart disease
and
no symptoms in the performance of ordinary daily activities (functional class I; 5 METS; Table 3-2) or with moderately heavy exertion (7 to 10 METS)
and
does not require continuous treatment, except for intermittent prophylactic antibiotics for surgical or dental procedure to reduce risk of bacterial endocarditis
and
no evidence of CHF
and
no signs of ventricular dysfunction or dilation, and severity of stenosis or regurgitation estimated to be mild (METS >7; TMET [Bruce protocol] >6 min)
and
in the individual who has recovered from valvular heart surgery, all of above criteria are met

Example 3-1
0% to 9% Impairment Due to Valvular Heart Disease

Subject: 22-year-old woman.

History: Midsystolic click and late systolic murmur.

Current Symptoms: None. No signs of cardiac enlargement, HF, or cardiac rhythm disturbance.

Physical Exam: Slight pectus excavatum.

Clinical Studies: ECG: normal; echocardiogram: mitral valve prolapse, normal left atrium (LA) and LV size and function.

Diagnosis: Mitral valve prolapse syndrome.

Impairment Rating: 0% impairment of the whole person.

Comment: If definite T-wave abnormalities, or slight enlargement of the LA or LV, then estimate valve disorder impairment at 1% to 9%, depending on the severity of the abnormality. If aortic regurgitation murmur but no symptoms or signs of cardiac enlargement and CHF, then estimate is lower. LV size and function may be present; assess with 2-dimensional echocardiography (2DE) or radionuclide angiography to rule out significant LV dilation or dysfunction.

Example 3-2
0% to 9% Impairment Due to Valvular Heart Disease

Subject: 38-year-old-woman.

History: Systolic murmur on insurance physical exam. Played collegiate sports. Marathon runner.

Current Symptoms: Denies dyspnea, angina, palpitations, or fatigue.

Physical Exam: Blood pressure (BP): normal; pulse rate (PR): 52 BPM; mid-peaking systolic ejection murmur.

Clinical Studies: Echocardiogram: bicuspid aortic valve; mean gradient of 22 mm Hg; valve area 1.5 cm^2. ECG: tall R-waves and slight ST depression in precordial leads V_5 and V_6 in excess of 25 mm. Chest roentgenogram: normal.

Diagnosis: Asymptomatic mild aortic stenosis secondary to a bicuspid aortic valve with electrocardiographic evidence of LV hypertrophy.

Impairment Rating: 1% to 9% impairment of the whole person.

Comment: Antibiotic prophylaxis before dental or surgical procedure to minimize risk of bacterial endocarditis. Periodic cardiac follow-up for progression of aortic stenosis. Aortic valve surgery necessary later in life.

> **Class 2**
> **10%-29% Impairment of the Whole Person**
>
> Evidence by physical examination or laboratory studies of valvular heart disease, and no symptoms in performance of daily activities, but symptoms develop on moderately heavy physical exertion (functional class II)
>
> *or*
>
> requires moderate dietary adjustment or drugs to prevent symptoms or to remain free of signs of CHF or other consequences of valvular heart disease, such as syncope, chest pain, and emboli
>
> *or*
>
> signs or laboratory evidence of cardiac chamber dysfunction and/or dilation, severity of stenosis or regurgitation estimated to be moderate, and surgical correction not feasible or advisable; METS >5 but <7; TMET (Bruce protocol) >3 min
>
> *or*
>
> has recovered from valvular heart surgery and meets criteria for functional class II

Example 3-3
10% to 29% Impairment Due to Valvular Heart Disease

Subject: 66-year-old woman.

History: Progressive HF; culminated in several syncopal episodes 3 years ago. Severe calcific stenosis of the aortic valve; depressed systolic function. Aortic valve replacement with large St. Jude's bileaflet prosthesis.

Current Symptoms: Returned to normal life; walks 2 miles daily. Maintenance: oral anticoagulants. Prothrombin time level every 3 weeks. Antibiotics before dental or operative procedures; no other medication.

Physical Exam: BP and PR: normal. No signs of HF. Slightly sustained apical impulse. 1/6 early systolic murmur in first right intercostal space. S_1: normal; S_2: crisp, closing click of the prosthetic valve.

Clinical Studies: ECG: rhythm, QRS pattern normal; low T waves in I, L, V_5, and V_6. Chest roentgenogram: slight prominence heart apex; prosthesis properly positioned: no evidence of pulmonary congestion. Echocardiogram: normal size ventricles; thickening of LV wall; prosthesis properly positioned, mean gradient 10 mm Hg across the prosthesis; slight regurgitation. LV systolic function mildly depressed; 0.45 LVEF.

Diagnosis: Calcific aortic stenosis, probably related to congenital bicuspid aortic valve, and valve replacement.

Impairment Rating: 20% impairment of the whole person.

Comment: Impairment greater if (1) a diastolic decrescendo murmur; (2) the systolic gradient across the prosthesis > Doppler-derived normal values for the type of prosthesis; or (3) mild recurrent dyspnea. Cardiac catheterization not necessary for estimate.

Example 3-4
10% to 29% Impairment Due to Valvular Heart Disease

Subject: 63-year-old man.

History: Mild CHF and aortic regurgitation 5 years ago. Restricts salt intake; no cardiac medications. Golfs regularly.

Current Symptoms: None.

Physical Exam: BP: 160/50 mm Hg; PR: 70 BPM; bounding peripheral pulses, lungs clear, apex impulse slightly lateral to midclavicular line (MCL); S_1 and S_2 normal; 3/6 harsh aortic ejection murmur; 3/6 long decrescendo diastolic murmur.

Clinical Studies: ECG: borderline voltage for left ventricular hypertrophy (LVH). Chest roentgenogram: no cardiomegaly or pulmonary congestion. Echocardiogram: normal size aortic root; trileaflet aortic valve; fluttering anterior leaflet of the mitral valve; normal LV systolic function with moderate dilation. Doppler: moderately severe aortic regurgitation; no stenosis.

Diagnosis: Moderately severe aortic regurgitation of uncertain cause.

Impairment Rating: 20% to 29% impairment of the whole person.

Comment: Asymptomatic but impaired. Higher estimate if LV systolic dysfunction. Cardiac catheterization, angiography were not necessary for estimate. Elevated BP needs treatment. If elevation of BP persists after treatment, then estimate impairment due to hypertension per Table 4-2.

<table>
<tr><td>Class 3
30%-49% Impairment of the Whole Person</td></tr>
<tr><td>Signs of valvular heart disease and slight to moderate symptomatic discomfort during performance of ordinary daily activities (functional class III)</td></tr>
<tr><td>and</td></tr>
<tr><td>dietary therapy or drugs do not completely control symptoms or prevent CHF</td></tr>
<tr><td>and</td></tr>
<tr><td>signs or laboratory evidence of cardiac chamber dysfunction or dilation, severity of stenosis or regurgitation estimated to be moderate or severe, and surgical correction not feasible; METS >2 but <5; TMET (Bruce protocol) >1 min but < 3 min</td></tr>
<tr><td>or</td></tr>
<tr><td>has recovered from heart valve surgery but continues to meet criteria for functional class III</td></tr>
</table>

Example 3-5
30% to 49% Impairment Due to Valvular Disease

Subject: 71-year-old man.

History: Nonresponsive thrombocytopenia. Moderate exertional dyspnea for 2 years despite diuretics and digoxin.

Current Symptoms: Comfortable at rest; becomes short of breath (SOB) when climbing to second floor. Sleeps on two pillows; has not awakened SOB since diuretic increase 1 year earlier. Lies flat comfortably.

Physical Exam: BP: 110/80 mm Hg; PR: irregular—84 BPM. Venous pressure (VP): normal; no edema. Harsh breath sounds at each base; no rales. Apical impulse: large, hyperdynamic, displaced to the anterior axillary line. Slight parasternal heave. S_1, S_2: loud; 4/6 holosystolic murmur at lower sternal border, apex, and left axilla. Audible S_3.

Clinical Studies: ECG: atrial fibrillation; irregular ventricular response 80/min. Low T waves; QRS pattern normal. Chest roentgenogram: cardiomegaly; large LA. Upper lobes vasculature prominent. Echocardiogram: 2DE: flail mitral leaflet. Doppler: Severe mitral regurgitation; estimated peak systolic pulmonary arterial pressure (PAP) 50 mm Hg. Mild LV and moderate LA enlargement; hyperdynamic systolic function.

Diagnosis: Severe mitral regurgitation due to mitral valve prolapse with a flail leaflet. Atrial fibrillation with a controlled ventricular response at rest.

Impairment Rating: 40% to 49% impairment of the whole person.

Comment: Greater exercise tolerance and less cardiomegaly for lower impairment. If reduced systolic function, increase impairment. Cardiac catheterization not necessary for estimate. Consider surgical treatment.

Example 3-6
30% to 49% Impairment Due to Valvular Heart Disease

Subject: 60-year-old woman.

History: Seamstress; surgical replacement of aortic and mitral valves 1 year earlier. Little stamina despite oral anticoagulants, digoxin, diuretics, salt restrictions. Tired easily; rested each afternoon. Sometime ankle edema resolved after extra diuretic.

Current Symptoms: No nocturnal dyspnea; sleeps with one pillow. Light housework possible; not well enough to return to work. Weight 6.8 kg (15 lb) below preoperative weight.

Physical Exam: Comfortable lying flat. BP: 110/70 mm Hg; PR: irregular—80 BPM. Venous pressure: normal; no edema. Lungs: clear.

Clinical Studies: Apical impulse: enlarged, sustained through systole at anterior axillary line; no parasternal heave; normal prosthetic valve sounds; 1/6 early systolic murmur in first right intercostal space, along the left sternal border. ECG: atrial fibrillation; irregular ventricular response 80/min. Completes stage I Bruce protocol on treadmill; fatigue and SOB at stage II (5 METS). Chest roentgenogram: cardiomegaly; LV, LA enlargement. Upper lobes vasculature prominent. Echocardiogram: no prosthetic valve malfunction or displacement. Ventricles, LA slightly enlarged. LV systolic function normal.

Diagnosis: Aortic and mitral valve disease, probably rheumatic in origin; surgical replacement of valves.

Impairment Rating: 40% to 49% impairment of the whole person.

Comment: Bruce protocol: class I if exertion > 6 minutes; class II if 3 to 6 minutes; class III if 1 to 3 minutes; and class IV if < 1 minute.

> **Class 4**
> **50%-100% Impairment of the Whole Person**
>
> Signs by physical examination of valvular heart disease, and symptoms at rest or in performance of less than ordinary daily activities (functional class IV)
>
> *and*
>
> dietary therapy and drugs cannot control symptoms or prevent signs of CHF
>
> *and*
>
> signs or laboratory evidence of cardiac chamber dysfunction or dilation, severity of stenosis or regurgitation estimated to be moderate or severe, and surgical correction not feasible; METS <2; TMET (Bruce protocol) <1 min
>
> *or*
>
> recovered from valvular heart surgery but continues to meet criteria for functional class IV

Example 3-7
50% to 100% Impairment Due to Valvular Heart Disease

Subject: 50-year-old man.

History: Mitral valve replacement 2 years earlier; advanced symptoms and signs of CHF caused pulmonary and systemic circulation congestion. Activities remained limited by dyspnea on minimal exertion despite restriction of activities and salt intake, and digoxin and diuretics. Vigorous diuretic use eliminated peripheral edema but resulted in chemical evidence of prerenal azotemia.

Current Symptoms: Walks a city block at a normal pace, drives, and sleeps comfortably; breathless after climbing one flight of stairs.

Physical Exam: Comfortable; BP: 110/70 mm Hg; PR: irregular—80 BPM. Venous pressure: normal; no peripheral edema. Lung sounds: rales at the left base. Apical impulse: normal; parasternal heave. Prosthetic valve sounds: normal; 1/6 holosystolic murmur at the apex.

Clinical Studies: ECG: atrial fibrillation; irregular ventricular response 80 BPM; low T waves. Chest roentgenogram: cardiomegaly; enlarged LV, RV, LA. Prominent pulmonary vasculature in all lung fields; no Kerley B lines. Properly positioned prosthetic valve. Echocardiogram: enlarged ventricles and LA. Moderate global reduction LV systolic function; LVEF 0.30. Well-seated prosthetic valve; normal mean gradient 5 mm Hg across the valve; normal mild degree of periprosthetic regurgitation. Cardiac catheterization and angiography: LV pressure: 110/18 mm Hg; mean LA pressure: 20 mm Hg. PAP: 45/18 mm Hg. LV angiogram: mild mitral regurgitation; reduction of ventricular contraction.

Diagnosis: Mitral valve replacement with a prosthesis; LV dysfunction, with probable rheumatic origin.

Impairment Rating: 70% to 79% impairment of the whole person.

Comment: Cardiac catheterization, though done, not essential for estimate.

Example 3-8
50% to 100% Impairment Due to Valvular Heart Disease

Subject: 45-year-old woman.

History: CHF for 10 years. Breathlessness and fatigue with minimal exertion, despite diuretics, digoxin, and, for the past year, a peripheral vasodilator. Slept on three pillows. Long-term ankle edema; protuberant abdomen for last year. Unable to do most activities of daily living without assistance.

Physical Exam: Pale and weak; thin, jaundiced face showed temporal depression. Breaths: 22/min; BP: 110/70 mm Hg; PR: irregular—80 BPM. Preferred sitting position. Neck veins distended to the mid-neck; prominent V waves. Lung sounds: rales at both lung bases: parasternal heave. 3/6 harsh, long, systolic murmur in second right intercostal space that stopped in late systole, then a long, loud, decrescendo diastolic murmur. Blowing holosystolic murmur at the lower sternal border; mid-diastolic rumble at the apex. Diminished S_1; S_2 loud in the second left intercostal space. Liver was large, pulsatile, approximately 12 cm. Ascites, pitting edema of the thighs, sacral area, and legs.

Clinical Studies: ECG: atrial fibrillation; irregular ventricular response: 80 BPM; low-voltage QRS and T waves. Chest roentgenogram: massive cardiomegaly suggesting enlargement of all chambers. Vascular prominence and Kerley B lines on both sides of the upper lobes. Echocardiogram: enlargement of all chambers; LVEF 0.20. 2DE: heavy calcification of aortic and mitral valves. Doppler: severe aortic stenosis, mitral regurgitation, tricuspid regurgitation, moderate aortic regurgitation, and mitral stenosis. PAP: 70 mm Hg.

Diagnosis: Aortic and mitral stenosis and regurgitation, and tricuspid regurgitation.

Impairment Rating: 90% to 99% impairment of the whole person.

3.3 Coronary Heart Disease

Coronary heart disease (CHD) is most commonly due to arteriosclerosis of the coronary arteries, resulting in reduced coronary blood flow. Other causes of limited or reduced coronary blood flow include coronary artery spasm, emboli, congenital abnormalities, and trauma. Inflammatory processes and arthritis also can obstruct the coronary arteries, especially the coronary ostia.

Reduced coronary flow resulting in transient ischemia or in permanent injury to the myocardium causes angina pectoris, which may impair a person's ability to perform activities of daily living. Infarction or diffuse fibrosis and a decrease in EF causes permanent injury. The degree of the patient's impairment is determined by the consequences of both the reduced coronary blood flow and the reduced ventricular function. In addition, reduced coronary blood flow and myocardial damage may cause cardiac arrhythmias. (See Section 3.6).[9]

The physician must obtain a detailed history to estimate the degree of impairment due to CHD. The physical examination contributes to the estimate of the disorder's severity, and especially to the estimate of the degree of ventricular function impairment. In most individuals, laboratory studies will also be necessary. Studies obtained at rest, during exercise, and after exercise are especially useful in examining people suspected of having CHD. Knowledge of ventricular function should usually be obtained for all individuals. If there is a normal examination, normal heart size on chest x-ray, and normal resting ECG, the EF should be normal. Coronary angiography may be necessary in some.[2,6,10]

Exercise training programs, cessation of cigarette smoking, use of medications, and surgical procedures can reduce but not eliminate impairment due to CHD. Allow sufficient time for these measures to have an effect before estimating permanent impairment.

3.3a Criteria for Rating Permanent Impairment Due to Coronary Heart Disease

Impairment criteria for CHD are given in Table 3-6.

Table 3-6a Criteria for Rating Permanent Impairment Due to Coronary Heart Disease

Class 1 0%-9% Impairment of the Whole Person	Class 2 10%-29% Impairment of the Whole Person	Class 3 30%-49% Impairment of the Whole Person	Class 4 50%-100% Impairment of the Whole Person
Because of serious implications of reduced coronary blood flow, it is not reasonable to classify degree of impairment as 0% through 9% in anyone who has symptoms of CHD corroborated by physical examination or laboratory tests; this class of impairment should be reserved for individuals with equivocal histories of angina pectoris on whom coronary angiography is performed, or for those on whom coronary angiography is performed for other reasons and in whom less than 50% reduction in cross-sectional area of coronary artery is found with a normal EF; METS determination is not applicable	History of MI or angina pectoris documented by appropriate laboratory studies, but at time of evaluation, no symptoms while performing ordinary daily activities or even moderately heavy physical exertion (functional class I) *and* may require moderate dietary adjustment or medication to prevent angina or to remain free of signs and symptoms of CHF *and* able to walk on treadmill or bicycle ergometer and obtain HR of 90% of predicted maximum HR (see Table 3-6b) without developing significant ST-segment shift, VT, or hypotension; if uncooperative or unable to exercise because of disease affecting another organ system, this requirement may be omitted; METS >7 *or* has recovered from coronary artery surgery or angioplasty, remains asymptomatic during ordinary daily activities, and able to exercise as outlined above; if taking a beta-adrenergic blocking agent, should be able to walk on treadmill to level estimated to cause energy expenditure of at least 7 METS as substitute for HR target	History of MI documented by appropriate laboratory studies, or angina pectoris documented by changes on resting or exercise ECG or radioisotope study suggestive of ischemia *or* either fixed or dynamic focal obstruction of at least 50% of coronary artery, angiography, and function testing *and* requires moderate dietary adjustment or drugs to prevent frequent angina or to remain free of symptoms and signs of CHF, but may develop angina pectoris after moderately heavy physical exertion (functional class II); METS >5 but <7 *or* has recovered from coronary artery surgery or angioplasty, continues to require treatment, and has symptoms described above	History of MI documented by appropriate laboratory studies, or angina pectoris documented by changes on resting ECG or radioisotope study highly suggestive of myocardial ischemia *or* either fixed or dynamic focal obstruction of at least 50% of one or more coronary arteries, demonstrated by angiography and function testing *and* requires moderate dietary adjustments or drugs to prevent angina or to remain free of symptoms and signs of CHF, but continues to develop symptoms of angina pectoris or CHF during ordinary daily activities (functional class III or IV); METS <5 *or* has recovered from coronary artery bypass surgery or angioplasty and continues to require treatment and have symptoms as described above

Table 3-6b Maximal and 90% of Maximal Achievable Heart Rate, by Age and Sex*

		Heart Rate (beats/min) by Age (y)							
		30	35	40	45	50	55	60	65
Men	Maximal	193	191	189	187	184	182	180	178
	90% Maximal	173	172	170	168	166	164	162	160
Women	Maximal	190	185	181	177	172	168	163	159
	90% Maximal	171	167	163	159	155	151	147	143

*Source: Sheffield LH. Exercise stress testing. In: Braunwald E, ed. *Heart Disease: A Textbook of Cardiovascular Medicine.* 3rd ed. Philadelphia, Pa: WB Saunders Co; 1988:227.

> **Class 1**
> **0%-9% Impairment of the Whole Person**
>
> Because of serious implications of reduced coronary blood flow, it is not reasonable to classify degree of impairment as 0% through 9% in anyone who has symptoms of CHD corroborated by physical examination or laboratory tests; this class of impairment should be reserved for individuals with equivocal histories of angina pectoris on whom coronary angiography is performed, or for those on whom coronary angiography is performed for other reasons and in whom less than 50% reduction in cross-sectional area of coronary artery is found with a normal EF; METS determination is not applicable

Example 3-9
0% to 9% Impairment Due to Coronary Heart Disease

Subject: 55-year-old woman.

History: Cigarette smoker; family history of CHD. CT scan: calcium score in the 99th percentile. Subsequently referred to physician.

Current Symptoms: Denies angina, dyspnea, or fatigue. Worried about dying of a heart attack because of mother's death from MI at 62.

Physical Exam: Mild hyperlipidemia (total cholesterol: 215 mg/dL; LDL: 135 mg/dL; HDL: 45 mg/dL). Physician concerned about possible significant CHD; referred her to local cardiovascular specialist. 9 minutes on Bruce protocol: 1.5 mm up-sloping ST depression in V_5; normal echo images.

Clinical Studies: Cardiac catheterization: diffuse 40% disease in left circumflex and right coronary arteries; LAD 30% lesion. 0.68 LVEF.

Diagnosis: Asymptomatic coronary artery disease (CAD).

Impairment Rating: 1% to 5% impairment of the whole person.

Comment: Mild atherosclerotic CAD according to catheterization and CT scan. Normal exercise tolerance; no symptoms of angina or exertional dyspnea. False-positive stress electrocardiogram result: no cardiac ischemia. Aggressive secondary prevention program (eg, smoking cessation, exercise counseling, and treatment of hyperlipidemia) could modify risk factors.

Example 3-10
0% to 9% Impairment Due to Coronary Heart Disease

Subject: 55-year-old man.

History: Referred to a cardiologist because of abnormal exercise thallium stress test. Denied angina pectoris or dyspnea.

Current Symptoms: Plays golf and tennis regularly; states he has "endurance he had in college." Nonsmoker; no history of hypertension, diabetes mellitus, or family history of CAD. Concerned because friend and fellow jurist died unexpectedly of a heart attack 2 months earlier. Wanted to know "definitively" if he had any significant CAD because he was then on a short list of possible Supreme Court Justice nominees.

Physical Exam: Normal, including BP and PR.

Clinical Studies: Exercise thallium: normal exercise tolerance (9.0 min, Bruce protocol); peak heart rate (HR): 180 BPM. Total cholesterol: 365 mg/dL; HDL: 45 mg/dL; triglycerides: 225 mg/dL; LDL cholesterol: 275 mg/dL. Catheterization: 50% lesions in proximal and distal LAD. RCA, LCx: scattered 20% and 30% luminal irregularities. 0.65 EF. ECG: Ischemic evidence at HR 170 (1.5 mm ST depression); image changes demonstrated ischemia in the distal anterior wall. Elevated lipids.

Diagnosis: Asymptomatic CAD with silent myocardial ischemia.

Impairment Rating: 5% to 9% impairment of the whole person.

Comment: Changes on the exercise thallium stress test indicate a silent myocardial ischemia in a small area of the myocardium. No functional limitations; only mild CAD; could start treatment for hyperlipidemia. Medical therapy could reduce slightly increased risk of acute MI due to mild CAD and hyperlipidemia.

Class 2
10%-29% Impairment of the Whole Person
History of MI or angina pectoris documented by appropriate laboratory studies, but at time of evaluation, no symptoms while performing ordinary daily activities or even moderately heavy physical exertion (functional class I)
and
may require moderate dietary adjustment or medication to prevent angina or to remain free of signs and symptoms of CHF
and
able to walk on treadmill or bicycle ergometer and obtain HR of 90% of predicted maximum HR without developing significant ST-segment shift, VT, or hypotension; if uncooperative or unable to exercise because of disease affecting another organ system, this requirement may be omitted; METS >7
or
has recovered from coronary artery surgery or angioplasty, remains asymptomatic during ordinary daily activities, and able to exercise as outlined above; if taking a beta-adrenergic blocking agent, should be able to walk on treadmill to level estimated to cause energy expenditure of at least 7 METS as substitute for HR target

Any of the exercise protocols in Table 3-2 may be used. The maximal and 90% of maximal predicted HR by age and sex group are presented in Table 3-7.

Table 3-7 Maximal and 90% of Maximal Achievable Heart Rate, by Age and Sex*

		Heart Rate (beats/min) by Age (y)							
		30	35	40	45	50	55	60	65
Men	Maximal	193	191	189	187	184	182	180	178
	90% Maximal	173	172	170	168	166	164	162	160
Women	Maximal	190	185	181	177	172	168	163	159
	90% Maximal	171	167	163	159	155	151	147	143

*Source: Sheffield LH. Exercise stress testing. In: Braunwald E, ed. *Heart Disease: A Textbook of Cardiovascular Medicine*. 3rd ed. Philadelphia, Pa: WB Saunders Co; 1988:227.

Example 3-11
10% to 29% Impairment Due to Coronary Heart Disease

Subject: 50-year-old man.

History: Service station attendant; acute MI 8 months earlier. Hospitalized for 10 days; serial ECGs: classic changes of an inferior wall infarction. Post-MI echocardiography: inferior wall motion abnormalities; 0.55 EF.

Current Symptoms: After recovery, returned to work. Follows diet to maintain weight of 72 kg (160 lb)—11 kg (24 lb) less than 1 year before. Asymptomatic; no medication.

Clinical Studies: Chest roentgenograms: normal. ECG: Q and flat T waves in 2, 3, and F. During exercise, HR: 152 BPM; BP: adequate rise. ECG: no pattern changes to indicate ischemia or arrhythmias.

Diagnosis: Recent inferior-wall MI.

Impairment Rating: 10% to 19% impairment of the whole person.

Comment: Greater impairment for uncomplicated recovery from anterior wall infarction, especially if LV systolic dysfunction.

Example 3-12
10% to 29% Impairment Due to Coronary Heart Disease

Subject: 52-year-old woman.

History: Service specialist for an insurance firm; coronary artery bypass surgery for angina relief 6 months earlier. Vein grafts in LAD, RCA. Preoperative coronary angiography: no significant obstruction in circumflex coronary artery; normal EF.

Current Symptoms: Did well postsurgery; worked for 14 months. Asymptomatic; avoids heavy physical exertion. Daily 0.3 g of aspirin; no other medications.

Physical Exam: Well-healed scar; normal heart.

Clinical Studies: Bruce protocol exercise test 10 days earlier; HR: 144 BPM; no ST-segment shifts or arrhythmias after 10 minutes of exercise. ECG: low T waves in I, L, V_4, V_5, and V_6; no Q waves. Chest roentgenogram: normal.

Diagnosis: CHD with coronary artery bypass surgery.

Impairment Rating: 10% to 19% impairment of the whole person.

Example 3-13
10% to 29% Impairment Due to Coronary Heart Disease

Subject: 48-year-old man.

History: Chest pain for 2 years interrupted his work-day. Pain accompanied by diaphoresis and dyspnea. Slightly elevated cholesterol: 245 mg/dL. Family history: 66-year-old father with heart disease.

Current Symptoms: Chest pain; palpitations.

Physical Exam: BP: 140/90 mm Hg; PR: 76 BPM. Occasional ectopic beat; otherwise normal heart sounds.

Clinical Studies: Exercise stress test: completed 14 minutes on treadmill; maximum HR: 172; no evidence of ischemia. Because of the symptoms and the man's persistence at asking for a second opinion, he was referred to a cardiologist. Cardiac catheterization: 40% stenosis in right coronary artery; no disease in the left system; 0.60 EF. Reassured that he did not have significant CAD, he returned to work. Symptoms persisted for another 6 months; mild palpitations began. Holter monitor: ST segment elevation during palpitation. Second cardiologist suspected coronary artery spasm because of the correlation between the symptoms and mental stress. Ergonovine testing: coronary spasm in the right coronary artery.

Diagnosis: Vasospastic angina pectoris; had coronary artery vasospasm and experienced symptoms only with significant mental stress.

Impairment Rating: 10% to 29% impairment of the whole person.

Comment: Coronary artery spasm–related symptoms and hyperlipidemia treatment possible with medication and psychological therapy to decrease stress. Although CAD not significantly obstructive, angina pectoris limited work ability; at risk for ischemia-related complications. Impairment could be adjusted by controlling the vasospastic angina with medical treatment or stress reduction techniques. Greater impairment score if vasospastic angina nonresponsive, more frequent, and less reactive to stress.

Class 3 30%-49% Impairment of the Whole Person
History of MI documented by appropriate laboratory studies, or angina pectoris documented by changes on resting or exercise ECG or radioisotope study suggestive of ischemia
or
either fixed or dynamic focal obstruction of at least 50% of coronary artery, angiography, and function testing
and
requires moderate dietary adjustment or drugs to prevent frequent angina or to remain free of symptoms and signs of CHF, but may develop angina pectoris after moderately heavy physical exertion (functional class II); METS >5 but <7
or
has recovered from coronary artery surgery or angioplasty, continues to require treatment, and has symptoms described above

Example 3-14
30% to 49% Impairment Due to Coronary Heart Disease

Subject: 58-year-old man.

History: First MI 6 months ago; multivessel PTCA.

Current Symptoms: Exertional angina while working on industrial refrigeration equipment. Discontinued exercise 2 weeks ago because of exertional dyspnea and angina. Symptoms develop after walking 1 mile in the morning before work. Beta-blocker and nitrate medications discontinued because he could not remember to take them.

Physical Exam: Normal.

Clinical Studies: ECG: ST segment depression and T-wave inversion in lateral precordial leads. Exercise thallium stress test: small area of apical ischemia at peak exercise workload of 6.8 METS. Cardiac catheterization: all previously treated blockages widely patent; no evidence of restenosis. 80% blockage in distal LAD too small to be treated with a percutaneous procedure. EF: 0.40; anterior wall motion abnormalities.

Diagnosis: Exertional angina pectoris secondary to CAD.

Impairment Rating: 30% to 35% impairment of the whole person.

Comment: Recovered from MI; continued angina pectoris at moderately high workloads. Medications would reduce or alleviate anginal symptoms and ischemia. Not a candidate for percutaneous or surgical revascularization because of the location and size of his one untreated coronary artery blockage.

Example 3-15
30% to 49% Impairment Due to Coronary Heart Disease

Subject: 62-year-old woman.

History: Quadruple coronary artery bypass surgery 13 months ago; experienced retrosternal chest discomfort during usual activities at a brisk pace.

Current Symptoms: Discomfort in the morning and outdoors in the cold. Enjoys walking, but usually experiences discomfort if she hurries up a steep hill going to church. Without rushing, she is asymptomatic, doing light household and other activities. On a diet; takes beta-adrenergic blocking agent and oral nitrates.

Physical Exam: Comfortable; no signs of CHF. BP: 110/70 mm Hg; PR: regular—62 BPM. Apical impulse: normal; no gallops or murmurs.

Clinical Studies: ECG: Low T waves in all leads. Chest roentgenogram: normal. After 6 minutes of exercise, HR: 118 BPM (ECG). During the last minute: retrosternal discomfort; 1 and 2 minutes afterward: 1.5 mm ST-segment depression in V_4-V_6. Coronary angiogram: 90% or greater obstruction of all three native coronary arteries. Patent grafts to the right, circumflex, and left anterior descending coronary arteries; occluded graft to the diagonal branch of the LAD. EF: 0.50.

Diagnosis: CHD and continued angina after coronary artery bypass surgery.

Impairment Rating: 30% to 39% impairment of the whole person.

Comment: Patent grafts to the major vessel territories of the myocardium. Monitor for subsequent occlusion.

Example 3-16
30% to 49% Impairment Due to Coronary Heart Disease

Subject: 55-year-old man.

History: Physician; anterior wall MI 6 months earlier with angina pectoris, diaphoresis, and dyspnea. ECG: new ST segment elevation in V_1 through V_6; elevated cardiac enzymes. Treated with thrombolytic and the usual adjunct medical therapies. Completed phase II cardiac rehabilitation, but never regained strength and stamina. Dyspnea on exertion after 20 to 30 minutes' brisk walk; unusually fatigued after each exercise session. Continued to practice medicine, but limited himself by not accepting any new patients. 6 weeks after hospital discharge, resting ECG: 105 BPM; < 1 mm ST elevation in V_3-V_6. Stress echocardiogram: reduced exercise tolerance; completed only 5.5 minutes on Bruce protocol. ECG with exercise: 4 mm of ST segment elevation.

Current Symptoms: Complained of exertional dyspnea after 20 minutes' exercise and significant fatigue in office practice by early afternoon despite medication.

Physical Exam: BP: 98/60; PR: 68. No venous pressure elevation; large, sustained impulse above and lateral to the left nipple centered in the third intercostal space at the anterior axillary line. S_4 gallop.

Clinical Studies: Echocardiogram: anteroapical LV aneurysm at rest; EF: 0.35; fell to 0.25 with exercise. Cardiac catheterization: occluded proximal LAD; no significant disease in LCx, RCA. Initially placed on an ACE inhibitor, nitrates, and low doses of furosemide and Coumadin. Low-salt diet. Beta-blocker 4 weeks later. ECG: 1-mm ST segment elevation in V_2-V_6. Chest roentgenogram: Cardiac enlargement; clear lung fields.

Diagnosis: Anterior LV aneurysm secondary to MI and CAD.

Impairment Rating: 45% to 49% impairment of the whole person.

Comment: LV aneurysm with secondary symptoms. Stable symptoms occurred with moderate activity. Maximal medical therapy. If symptoms worsen, future treatment includes aneurysm resection.

> **Class 4**
> **50%–100% Impairment of the Whole Person**
>
> History of MI documented by appropriate laboratory studies, or angina pectoris documented by changes on resting ECG or radioisotope study highly suggestive of myocardial ischemia
>
> *or*
>
> either fixed or dynamic focal obstruction of at least 50% of one or more coronary arteries, demonstrated by angiography and function testing
>
> *and*
>
> requires moderate dietary adjustments or drugs to prevent angina or to remain free of symptoms and signs of CHF, but continues to develop symptoms of angina pectoris or CHF during ordinary daily activities (functional class III or IV); METS <5
>
> *or*
>
> has recovered from coronary artery bypass surgery or angioplasty and continues to require treatment and have symptoms as described above

Example 3-17
50% to 100% Impairment Due to Coronary Heart Disease

Subject: 42-year-old man.

History: Inferior wall MI 2 years ago. Anteroseptal MI 15 months ago.

Current Symptoms: For past 6 months, almost daily, 1- to 10-minute episode of retrosternal discomfort on minimal exertion and at rest, despite adequate doses of beta-adrenergic blocking agents, oral and sublingual nitrates, and a calcium-channel blocking agent.

Physical Exam: Comfortable at rest. BP: 120/80 mm Hg; PR: 54 BPM. No signs of CHF. Apical impulse: enlarged, sustained, and displaced laterally to the anterior axillary line at the fifth intercostal space. S_1 soft; prominent S_4. 2/6 holosystolic murmur at apex.

Clinical Studies: ECG: Q waves in 2, 3, and F; QS pattern in V_1-V_3; QR in V_4; T waves low in all leads. Chest roentgenogram: marked cardiomegaly; upper lung fields vasculature prominent. During and after 2 minutes of exercise, pain and ST depression in I, L, V_5, and V_6. EF: fell from 0.30 to 0.25 (multigated blood pool scan).

Diagnosis: Angina pectoris and LV failure due to CHD.

Impairment Rating: 75% to 90% impairment of the whole person.

Comment: Needs assistance for most activities of daily living.

Example 3-18
50% to 100% Impairment Due to Coronary Heart Disease

Subject: 46-year-old woman.

History: Quadruple coronary artery bypass surgery 11 months earlier; daily pain, weakness, and breathlessness after minimal exertion.

Current Symptoms: Uses three pillows; awakes SOB; commonly sleeps sitting in a chair. Symptoms continue despite digitalis, diuretics, nitrates, calcium-channel blocking agents, and hydralazine.

Physical Exam: Evidence of weight loss. Preferred sitting position. BP: 110/70 mm Hg; HR: 92 BPM. Distended neck veins with abdominal hand pressure, even when upper part of the examining table at 45°. Apical impulse: enlarged, sustained, and displaced to the anterior axillary line; parasternal heave. Rales at both lung bases; dullness at right lung base. S_1 soft; prominent S_3. 2/6 holosystolic murmur at the apex.

Clinical Studies: ECG: QS in V_1-V_4; prominent Q waves in V_5 and V_6; low R waves throughout. Inverted T waves in I, L, and V_1-V_5; low elsewhere. Chest roentgenogram: marked cardiomegaly; increased vascular markings in upper lung fields; small, right-sided pleural effusion. Coronary angiography: total occlusion of LAD; 90% blockage right and circumflex coronary arteries. Patent grafts to RCA and one circumflex artery branch; no visualization of grafts to other circumflex artery branch and anterior descending artery. Ventriculogram: 0.20 EF; akinesis of entire anterior wall; poor contraction elsewhere.

Diagnosis: Angina pectoris and LV failure after coronary artery bypass surgery.

Impairment Rating: 90% to 100% impairment of the whole person.

Comment: Unable to perform most activities of daily living.

3.4 Congenital Heart Disease

Recently, surgical procedures designed to correct or improve the circulation of infants and children with congenital cardiac disorders have allowed many of the children to live to adulthood. Many of these surgically treated patients continue to have less than normal functioning of the heart and circulation and are therefore impaired.[11]

Congenital heart disease may be recognized by medical history and physical examination, but often the exact diagnosis and the individual's functional impairment require special studies, including ECG, chest roentgenogram, radioisotope studies, echocardiography, hemodynamic measurements, and angiography.[12] The functional classification of cardiac disease found in Table 3-1 is used in the classification for congenital heart disease listed below in Table 3-8.

3.4a Criteria for Rating Permanent Impairment Due to Congenital Heart Disease

Impairment criteria for congenital heart disease are given in Table 3-8.

Table 3-8 Criteria for Rating Permanent Impairment Due to Congenital Heart Disease

Class 1 0%-9% Impairment of the Whole Person	Class 2 10%-29% Impairment of the Whole Person	Class 3 30%-49% Impairment of the Whole Person	Class 4 50%-100% Impairment of the Whole Person
Evidence by physical examination or laboratory studies of congenital heart disease; has no symptoms in performance of ordinary daily activities or even on moderately heavy physical exertion *and* continuous treatment not required, although prophylactic antibiotics may be recommended after surgical procedures to reduce risk of bacterial endocarditis; remains free of signs of CHF and pain *and* no signs of cardiac chamber dysfunction or dilation; evidence of residual valvular stenosis or regurgitation estimated to be mild; no evidence of right-to-left shunt; a small left-to-right shunt may be present, but Qp/Qs < 1.5:1.0 *or* in individual who has recovered from corrective heart surgery, all above criteria are met	Evidence by physical examination or laboratory studies of congenital heart disease; has no symptoms in performance of ordinary daily activities, but has symptoms with moderately heavy physical exertion (functional class II) *or* requires moderate dietary adjustments or drugs to prevent symptoms or to remain free of signs of CHF or other consequences of congenital heart disease, such as syncope, chest pain, emboli, or cyanosis *or* signs or laboratory findings of cardiac chamber dysfunction or dilation, or severity of valvular stenosis or regurgitation estimated to be moderate; no evidence of right-to-left shunt; moderate-sized left-to-right shunt may be present with Qp/Qs < 2.0:1.0; or evidence of moderate elevation of pulmonary vascular resistance, which should be less than one-half systemic vascular resistance *or* has recovered from surgery for treatment of congenital heart disease and meets above criteria for impairment	Evidence by physical examination or laboratory studies of congenital heart disease; experiences symptoms during performance of ordinary daily activities (functional class III), despite dietary therapy and medication *and* signs or laboratory evidence of cardiac chamber dysfunction or dilation; or the severity of valvular stenosis or regurgitation estimated to be moderate or severe; or evidence of a right-to-left shunt or evidence of left-to-right shunt with pulmonary flow being greater than 2 times the systemic flow; or pulmonary vascular resistance elevated to greater than one-half systemic vascular resistance *or* has recovered from surgery for treatment of congenital heart disease but continues to have functional class 3 symptoms; or continues to have signs of CHF or cyanosis, and evidence of cardiomegaly and significant residual valvular stenosis or regurgitation; left-to-right shunt, right-to-left shunt, or elevated pulmonary vascular resistance	Signs of congenital heart disease and experiences symptoms of CHF at less than ordinary daily activities (functional class IV), despite dietary therapy and medication *and* evidence from physical examination or laboratory studies of cardiac dilation, or chamber dysfunction or dilation, or pulmonary vascular resistance remains elevated at greater than one-half systemic vascular resistance; or severity of valvular stenosis or regurgitation estimated to be moderate to severe; or left-to-right shunt with pulmonary flow being greater than 2 times systemic flow; or left-to-right shunt with pulmonary vascular resistance being elevated to greater than one-half systemic vascular resistance; or right-to-left shunt *or* has recovered from heart surgery for treatment of congenital heart disease and continues to have symptoms or signs of CHF causing impairment as outlined above

---

Class 1
0%-9% Impairment of the Whole Person

Evidence by physical examination or laboratory studies of congenital heart disease; has no symptoms in performance of ordinary daily activities or even on moderately heavy physical exertion

and

continuous treatment not required, although prophylactic antibiotics may be recommended after surgical procedures to reduce risk of bacterial endocarditis; remains free of signs of CHF and pain

and

no signs of cardiac chamber dysfunction or dilation; evidence of residual valvular stenosis or regurgitation estimated to be mild; no evidence of right-to-left shunt; a small left-to-right shunt may be present, but Qp/Qs < 1.5:1.0

or

in individual who has recovered from corrective heart surgery, all above criteria are met

---

Example 3-19
0% to 9% Impairment Due to Congenital Heart Disease

Subject: 25-year-old woman.

History: Repair of atrial septal defect 10 years earlier. No complications.

Current Symptoms: Asymptomatic and returned to an active life.

Physical Exam: Well-healed sternum wound without tenderness. No abnormal precordial pulsations or signs of CHF. S_1 normal; S_2 widely split; degree of splitting varies with respiration. No audible murmur.

Clinical Studies: ECG: incomplete right bundle-branch block pattern. Chest roentgenogram: normal. Echocardiogram: mild RV enlargement; reduced ventricular septum motion. 2DE: no atrial level shunt. Doppler: no atrial level shunt; systolic PAP normal. Cardiac catheterization, angiography: normal.

Diagnosis: Atrial septal defect with surgical closure.

Impairment Rating: 5% impairment of the whole person.

Comment: If very small postoperative left-to-right shunt, or mildly elevated residual PAP, then probable impairment of 6% to 9%. Cardiac catheterization, angiography unnecessary for evaluation.

Example 3-20
0% to 9% Impairment Due to Congenital Heart Disease

Subject: 22-year-old woman.

History: Loud left sternal border systolic murmur since childhood. Cardiac catheterization at 2 and 18 years old—20 mm Hg gradient between right ventricle and PA. Normal PAP and cardiac output; no evidence of shunts or CV symptoms.

Physical Exam: Comfortable; no signs of HF or cyanosis. No precordium heaves, thrills, or taps. S_1 normal; S_2 widely split; varies with respiration. 3/6 systolic murmur ends well short of S_2, loudest in second left intercostal space; early systolic click varies with respiration. No diastolic murmurs or gallops.

Clinical Studies: Chest roentgenogram: normal. ECG: normal.

Diagnosis: Mild pulmonary valve stenosis.

Impairment Rating: 9% impairment of the whole person.

Comment: Higher estimate if gradient > 40 mm Hg (Doppler echocardiography) or if ECG showed RV hypertrophy and a suitable surgical candidate. If asymptomatic with a small ventricular septal defect, estimate at upper end of class 1; but if bacterial endocarditis present, then estimate higher. If small atrial septal defect and normal pressures in all cardiac chambers and great vessels, or anomalous venous return from small lung segment, also estimate at upper end of class 1.

> **Class 2**
> **10%-29% Impairment of the Whole Person**
>
> Evidence by physical examination or laboratory studies of congenital heart disease; has no symptoms in performance of ordinary daily activities, but has symptoms with moderately heavy physical exertion (functional class II)
>
> *or*
>
> requires moderate dietary adjustments or drugs to prevent symptoms or to remain free of signs of CHF or other consequences of congenital heart disease, such as syncope, chest pain, emboli, or cyanosis
>
> *or*
>
> signs or laboratory findings of cardiac chamber dysfunction or dilation, or severity of valvular stenosis or regurgitation estimated to be moderate; no evidence of right-to-left shunt; moderate-sized left-to-right shunt may be present with Qp/Qs < 2.0:1.0; or evidence of moderate elevation of pulmonary vascular resistance, which should be less than one-half systemic vascular resistance
>
> *or*
>
> has recovered from surgery for treatment of congenital heart disease and meets above criteria for impairment.

Example 3-21
10% to 29% Impairment Due to Congenital Heart Disease

Subject: 42-year-old man.

History: Open-heart surgery for tetralogy of Fallot 15 years earlier. Procedure relieved pulmonary stenosis: pericardial patch placed in the right ventricular outflow tract (RVOT); ventricular septal defect closed.

Current Symptoms: Did well postoperatively without medication.

Physical Exam: Appeared healthy; BP: 110/70 mm Hg; PR: regular—70 BPM. No signs of CHF; precordium: normal. S_1: normal; S_2: louder than normal, followed by a mid-diastolic, scratchy murmur and a short, 2/6 ejection systolic murmur in the second and third left intercostal spaces.

Clinical Studies: ECG: right bundle-branch block. Chest roentgenogram: apical prominence left side of cardiac silhouette. Echocardiography: thickening of RV wall; dilation of RV cavity with diminished ventricular septal motion. Patent RVOT: 8-mm Hg gradient. Systolic RVP: 30 mm Hg. Doppler: no shunt.

Diagnosis: Tetralogy of Fallot with surgical relief of pulmonary valve stenosis and closure of the ventricular septal defect.

Impairment Rating: 15% to 20% impairment of the whole person.

Comment: If shunt evidence, then impairment estimate higher. Also, if conduit or prosthesis in pulmonary outflow tract, or if significant symptoms, impairment estimate higher. Cardiac catheterization unnecessary for estimate.

Example 3-22
10% to 29% Impairment Due to Congenital Heart Disease

Subject: 35-year-old woman.

History: Systolic murmur; abnormal cardiac sounds for many years. Led a relatively normal life; avoided participation in sports on the advice of physicians.

Current Symptoms: Weakness and fatigue with heavy exercise within last year, but still performs most daily activities without limitations. Palpitations never sustained; not associated with inadequate cerebral perfusion. No history of cyanosis, breathlessness, or peripheral edema.

Physical Exam: Comfortable; no cyanosis. Elevated venous pressure 15 cm without large V waves; enlarged liver width of 12 cm. Clear lungs. No precordium thrills, taps, or heaves. S_1: loud, followed by a very loud, sharp sound in early systole heard best along the left sternal border. S_2: loud, early diastolic sound heard best at midprecordium. Holosystolic murmur along the left sternal border increased in intensity with inspiration.

Clinical Studies: ECG: right bundle-branch block pattern; very low R wave in V_1. Broad, notched P wave in leads III and F; inverted T waves in V_1 and V_2. Occasional premature atrial beats. Chest roentgenogram: marked enlargement of cardiac silhouette, particularly to right of the sternum; normal pulmonary vasculature. Echocardiogram: features consistent with Ebstein's anomaly of the tricuspid valve. Tricuspid valve: markedly displaced into a small RV; severe regurgitation. Doppler: no right-to-left shunt. Cardiac catheterization, angiography: mean right atrial pressure 7 mm Hg; V waves 15 mm Hg. RVP and PAP: normal. No evidence of a shunt.

Diagnosis: Ebstein's anomaly of the tricuspid valve.

Impairment Rating: 25% impairment of the whole person.

Comment: If right-to-left shunt, then estimate considerably higher. If symptomatic cardiac arrhythmia, then estimate impairment according to arrhythmia criteria and combine with congenital heart disease impairment (see Combined Values Chart, p. 604). Cardiac catheterization unnecessary for estimate. Exercise testing might be useful for determining functional class.

Class 3
30%-49% Impairment of the Whole Person

Evidence by physical examination or laboratory studies of congenital heart disease; experiences symptoms during performance of ordinary daily activities (functional class III), despite dietary therapy and medication

and

signs or laboratory evidence of cardiac chamber dysfunction or dilation; or the severity of valvular stenosis or regurgitation estimated to be moderate or severe; or evidence of a right-to-left shunt or evidence of left-to-right shunt with pulmonary flow being greater than 2 times the systemic flow; or pulmonary vascular resistance elevated to greater than one-half systemic vascular resistance

or

has recovered from surgery for treatment of congenital heart disease but continues to have functional class 3 symptoms; or continues to have signs of CHF or cyanosis, and evidence of cardiomegaly and significant residual valvular stenosis or regurgitation; left-to-right shunt, right-to-left shunt, or elevated pulmonary vascular resistance

---

Example 3-23
30% to 49% Impairment Due to Congenital Heart Disease

Subject: 52-year-old woman.

History: Ebstein's anomaly of the tricuspid valve years ago. (Diagnosis made with echocardiography, cardiac catheterization, and angiography.) For several years, breathlessness increased during daily activities such as climbing stairs, mopping, or cleaning. Also complained of ankle edema and increased abdominal girth.

Current Symptoms: Diuretics diminished edema and ascites; salt restriction; takes digitalis.

Physical Exam: Appeared well; lips, fingernails appeared dusky. Markedly distended neck veins; slightly pulsatile, 14-cm-wide liver. Clear lungs. Precordium: active parasternal area; no heave. S_1: loud, followed by loud, early systolic sound along left sternal border; S_2: widely split, followed by early diastolic sound. Holosystolic murmur increased with inspiration, heard best left of the sternum. Diastolic murmur heard best during inspiration and along the left sternal border.

Clinical Studies: ECG: right bundle-branch block; low R waves in V_1; prominent P waves. Chest roentgenogram: greatly enlarged cardiac silhouette, especially right of the sternum. Pulmonary vasculature: normal. Echocardiogram: Ebstein's anomaly of the tricuspid valve—typical changes. Doppler: small right-to-left shunt across atrial septum.

Diagnosis: Ebstein's anomaly of the tricuspid valve.

Impairment Rating: 40% to 49% impairment of the whole person.

Example 3-24
30% to 49% Impairment Due to Congenital Heart Disease

Subject: 20-year-old man.

History: Blalock-Hanlon procedure in infancy. Mustard procedure for transposition of the great vessels 10 years ago. Did moderately well except for reduced stamina: tired easily and was unable to participate in such activities as tennis and hiking.

Physical Exam: Appeared healthy with no cyanosis; underweight. Neck veins distended; prominent A wave. No liver enlargement or peripheral edema. Clear lungs. Parasternal and apical heaves at precordium. Holosystolic murmur at left sternal border; S_4 present.

Clinical Studies: ECG: tall R-wave voltage in all precordial leads. Chest roentgenogram: moderate cardiomegaly. Echocardiogram: properly functioning intra-atrial baffle. Enlarged ventricular cavities; good ventricular function. Cardiac catheterization, angiography: elevated right mean atrial pressure 12 mm Hg; A waves 20 mm Hg. Systolic RVP and PAP: 30 to 35 mm Hg.

Diagnosis: Transposition of the great vessels and Mustard procedure.

Impairment Rating: 40% to 49% impairment of the whole person.

Comment: If significant arrhythmias complicated postoperative period, estimate according to the arrhythmia criteria and combine with congenital heart disease criteria (see Combined Values Chart, p. 604) to determine whole person impairment from cardiac disease.

Class 4
50%-100% Impairment of the Whole Person
Signs of congenital heart disease and experiences symptoms of CHF at less than ordinary daily activities (functional class IV), despite dietary therapy and medication
and
evidence from physical examination or laboratory studies of cardiac dilation, or chamber dysfunction or dilation, or pulmonary vascular resistance remains elevated at greater than one-half systemic vascular resistance; or severity of valvular stenosis or regurgitation estimated to be moderate to severe; or left-to-right shunt with pulmonary flow being greater than 2 times systemic flow; or left-to-right shunt with pulmonary vascular resistance being elevated to greater than one-half systemic vascular resistance; or right-to-left shunt
or
has recovered from heart surgery for treatment of congenital heart disease and continues to have symptoms or signs of CHF causing impairment as outlined above

Example 3-25
50% to 100% Impairment Due to Congenital Heart Disease

Subject: 35-year-old man.

History: Tetralogy of Fallot since childhood; Blalock-Taussig systemic to PA anastomosis ligated during a second operation years later. Muscle in the RVOT area removed to relieve pulmonary stenosis; ventricular septal defect closed. Did not do well after second operation—continued to tire easily. Significant peripheral edema and ascites responded to diuretics.

Current Symptoms: Comfortable during exertion for short periods; weak and breathless on more moderate exertion.

Physical Exam: Prominent V wave in neck veins. Liver 14 cm across. Palpable parasternal cardiac activity; no sustained heave. 3/6 holosystolic murmur along left sternal border; mid-diastolic murmur in the second left intercostal space. S_1: normal; S_2: single and loud.

Clinical Studies: ECG: right bundle-branch block. Chest roentgenogram: cardiomegaly and right pleural effusion. Echocardiogram: dilated, poorly functioning RV with severe tricuspid regurgitation. No residual RVOT obstruction. 2DE, Doppler: no residual ventricular septal defect.

Diagnosis: Tetralogy of Fallot with surgical relief of the pulmonary stenosis and closure of the ventricular septal defect, followed by development of tricuspid regurgitation and heart failure.

Impairment Rating: 80% to 90% impairment of the whole person.

Example 3-26
50% to 100% Impairment Due to Congenital Heart Disease

Subject: 23-year-old woman.

History: Eisenmenger's complex 10 years ago; regular follow-up visits. Cardiac catheterization, angiography: ventricular septal defect; pulmonary vascular resistance equal to systemic vascular resistance.

Current Symptoms: Recent activity markedly limited because of fatigue on minimal exertion. Recent peripheral edema responded to diuretics.

Physical Exam: Mild cyanosis intensified with exertion. Neck veins: prominent A waves; no jugular venous distention when placed at 45° angle. No enlargement or peripheral edema. Clear lungs. Forceful, sustained, parasternal heave. S_1: normal; S_2: narrowly split, marked increase in second component. Short, early systolic ejection murmur along left sternal border.

Clinical Studies: ECG: RV hypertrophy, peaked P waves in leads II, III, and F. Chest roentgenogram: RV hypertrophy; marked prominence of proximal portion of PA; greatly diminished pulmonary vascular markings in peripheral lung fields.

Diagnosis: Eisenmenger's complex with ventricular septal defect and elevated pulmonary vascular resistance.

Impairment Rating: 95% to 100% impairment of the whole person.

3.5 Cardiomyopathies

Cardiomyopathies, caused by a primary disease that affects the heart muscle, lead to impairment from abnormal ventricular function. Abnormal ventricular function may be the result of (1) systolic dysfunction, (2) diastolic dysfunction, or (3) a combination of both. An individual with these abnormalities may be asymptomatic or symptomatic due to pulmonary or systemic organ congestion and decreased cardiac output. In people with hypertrophic cardiomyopathy, a dynamic outflow tract obstruction and secondary mitral regurgitation may cause symptoms of exertional dyspnea, angina, and syncope. Because some cardiomyopathies are reversible, every effort should be made to identify the reversible forms and to treat them appropriately and prevent further deterioration. When the conditions are stable, the individual may be evaluated in terms of permanent impairment.[13-18]

Cardiomyopathies arise from many mechanisms, but the conditions may be divided into three major types: (1) dilated or congestive, (2) hypertrophic, and (3) restrictive. Careful history-taking and physical examination can reveal cardiomyopathies, but it is appropriate to confirm the diagnosis with echocardiography and selected laboratory studies.

3.5a Criteria for Rating Permanent Impairment Due to Cardiomyopathies

Impairment criteria for cardiomyopathies are given in Table 3-9.

Table 3-9 Criteria for Rating Permanent Impairment Due to Cardiomyopathies

Class 1 0%-9% Impairment of the Whole Person	Class 2 10%-29% Impairment of the Whole Person	Class 3 30%-49% Impairment of the Whole Person	Class 4 50%-100% Impairment of the Whole Person
Asymptomatic *and* no evidence of congestive heart failure (CHF) from physical examination or laboratory studies	Asymptomatic *and* moderate dietary adjustment or drug therapy necessary for individual to be free of symptoms and signs of CHF *or* has recovered from surgery for treatment of hypertrophic cardiomyopathy or has recovered from successful heart transplantation and meets above criteria	Symptoms of CHF on greater than ordinary daily activities (functional class II) *and* moderate dietary restriction or use of drugs necessary to minimize symptoms or to prevent appearance of signs of CHF or evidence of it by laboratory study *or* has recovered from surgery for treatment of hypertrophic cardiomyopathy or has recovered from successful heart transplantation and meets above criteria	Symptomatic during ordinary daily activities despite appropriate use of dietary adjustment and drugs (functional class III or IV) *or* persistent signs of CHF despite use of dietary adjustment and drugs *or* has recovered from surgery for treatment of hypertrophic cardiomyopathy or has recovered from successful heart transplantation and meets above criteria

Class 1
0%-9% Impairment of the Whole Person
Asymptomatic
and
no evidence of congestive heart failure (CHF) from physical examination or laboratory studies

Example 3-27
0% to 9% Impairment Due to Cardiomyopathy

Subject: 31-year-old man.

History: Admitted to hospital following syncope attack at detoxification center. Admitted to "a problem with alcohol"; refused chemical dependency treatment.

Current Symptoms: Denies exertional dyspnea, fatigue, angina, nocturnal dyspnea, and any history of syncope.

Physical Exam: Vital signs: normal; CV exam: normal.

Clinical Studies: Echocardiogram: 0.40 LVEF; mild global hypokinesis of all LV wall segments. Normal atrial dimensions and function, right heart size, function, and estimated PAP. Overnight telemetry monitoring: no arrhythmias to explain syncope.

Diagnosis: Syncope secondary to alcohol intoxication and asymptomatic LV dysfunction, presumably due to alcoholic cardiomyopathy.

Impairment Rating: 5% to 9% impairment of the whole person.

Comment: Evaluated for reversible causes. Impairment higher if symptomatic or condition limits daily activities.

Example 3-28
0% to 9% Impairment Due to Cardiomyopathy

Subject: 26-year-old woman.

History: Signs of pulmonary congestion 3 days postpartum; normal birth. Normotensive; no evidence of valvular heart disease. ECG: within normal limits except for sinus tachycardia. Echocardiogram: showed diffuse global hypokinesis; 0.30 EF. Successfully treated with digitalis and diuretics. Digitalis and diuretics discontinued 6 months before evaluation. Advised to avoid subsequent pregnancies; otherwise able to do all activities of daily living.

Current Symptoms: Asymptomatic for several months; resumed full activities.

Physical Exam: No CHF signs. BP: 110/70 mm Hg; PR: regular—70 BPM. Precordium quiet; no ventricular heaves. Heart sounds: normal.

Clinical Studies: ECG: normal. Chest roentgenogram: slight cardiomegaly; no chamber enlargement. Echocardiogram: slightly enlarged; mild global hypokinesis; 0.55 EF. Upon exercise, achieved 95% of functional aerobic capacity with ECG changes; EF fell to 0.50.

Diagnosis: Postpartum cardiomyopathy.

Impairment Rating: 9% impairment of the whole person.

Comment: If symptomatic, then estimate greater impairment. If normal heart size and EF normal at rest and increased on exercise, then estimate < 9%.

Class 2
10%-29% Impairment of the Whole Person

Asymptomatic

and

moderate dietary adjustment or drug therapy necessary for individual to be free of symptoms and signs of CHF

or

has recovered from surgery for treatment of hypertrophic cardiomyopathy or has recovered from successful heart transplantation and meets above criteria

---

Example 3-29
10% to 29% Impairment Due to Cardiomyopathy

Subject: 28-year-old man.

History: Hypertrophic cardiomyopathy with outflow obstruction. Septal myectomy 2 years ago for severe exertional dyspnea and lightheadedness. Individual's father had hypertrophic cardiomyopathy.

Current Symptoms: Active lifestyle; no further symptoms.

Physical Exam: Appeared healthy; no evidence of CHF. BP: 130/70 mm Hg; PR: regular—70 BPM. Brisk carotid pulses; sustained apical impulse. Soft 1/6 midsystolic murmur heard best along left sternal border; S_4 gallop.

Clinical Studies: ECG: prominent Q waves; high voltage. Chest roentgenogram: heart size normal. Echocardiogram: marked thickening of ventricular septum; some thickening of posterior ventricular wall. Mitral valve motion normal; 0.80 EF. Mild systolic anterior motion of mitral valve. Doppler: minimal 10-mm Hg gradient across the LVOT. 48-hour Holter monitor: no evidence of VT.

Diagnosis: Hypertrophic cardiomyopathy post–septal myectomy.

Impairment Rating: 20% impairment of the whole person.

Comment: Asymptomatic after successful myectomy; advised avoidance of strenuous physical exertion and importance of follow-up evaluation. If significant VT Holter, antiarrhythmic therapy possibly indicated. Impairment then estimated according to combined percentages from arrhythmia and cardiomyopathy criteria of impairment (see Combined Values Chart, p. 604).

Example 3-30
10% to 29% Impairment Due to Cardiomyopathy

Subject: 59-year-old man.

History: Greenskeeper on a golf course; longstanding, excessive alcohol use; nutritional deficiencies. Hospitalized previously with severe pulmonary congestion probably due to LV failure due to combination of excessive alcohol intake and poor nutrition.

Current Symptoms: Condition responded promptly to nutritional treatment, digitalis, diuretics, and ACE inhibitors. Avoided alcohol; returned to most activities. Regularly visited physician; continued ACE inhibitors and moderate salt restriction.

Physical Exam: Appeared comfortable; no signs of CHF. BP: 120/80 mm Hg; PR: regular—70 BPM. Precordium apical impulse larger than normal, slightly sustained, and displaced to anterior axillary line. No parasternal heave. S_1, S_2: normal. No S_3.

Clinical Studies: ECG: Small R waves, low T waves in lateral chest leads. Chest roentgenogram: moderate cardiomegaly; no specific chamber enlargement. Echocardiogram: 0.40 EF at rest and after exercise. Achieved 75% of functional aerobic capacity on exercise testing. No ECG changes during exercise.

Diagnosis: Cardiomyopathy, probably alcoholic and nutritional.

Impairment Rating: 25% impairment of the whole person.

Chapter 3

Class 3
30%-49% Impairment of the Whole Person
Symptoms of CHF on greater than ordinary daily activities (functional class II)
and
moderate dietary restriction or use of drugs necessary to minimize symptoms or to prevent appearance of signs of CHF or evidence of it by laboratory study
or
has recovered from surgery for treatment of hypertrophic cardiomyopathy or has recovered from successful heart transplantation and meets above criteria

Example 3-31
30% to 49% Impairment Due to Cardiomyopathy

Subject: 38-year-old man.

History: 3-month exertional dyspnea. HIV-positive for 5 years. Treatment with ace inhibitor; still experienced dyspnea (functional class II).

Current Symptoms: Stopped jogging after two blocks because of dyspnea. Denied cough, fever, chills, edema, orthopnea, and paroxysmal nocturnal dyspnea.

Physical Exam: BP: 130/80 mm Hg; PR: normal—88 BPM. Normal jugular venous pressure; clear lungs. Cardiac examination: soft S_1; normal S_2; no gallops or murmurs. Remainder of examination normal.

Clinical Studies: Chest roentgenogram: mild pulmonary congestion; suggested cardiomegaly. Stress testing: exercise tolerance of 3.8 minutes with development of 1 mm ST depression. Echocardiogram: reduced systolic function; 0.30 EF; mild LV enlargement. Mild (grade ¼) mitral regurgitation. Cardiac catheterization: noncritical CAD. Cardiac biopsy: no infiltrative cardiomyopathy.

Diagnosis: HIV cardiomyopathy.

Impairment Rating: 40% to 49% impairment due to cardiomyopathy; combine with HIV impairment (see Combined Values Chart, p. 604) to determine whole person impairment.

Comment: Significantly reduced exercise capacity; poor LV function. Concurrent cardiac disorders excluded for medical therapy. No cardiac surgery since no significant CAD or severe valvular disease.

Example 3-32
30% to 49% Impairment Due to Cardiomyopathy

Subject: 54-year-old woman.

History: Treated for symptoms of CHF and inadequate cardiac output for past 3 years. Cardiac catheterization and cineangiography 2 years ago; no evidence of coronary artery or valvular disease. Depressed ventricular function; elevated end-diastolic pressure 28 mm Hg; 0.30 EF. Subsequently treated with ACE inhibitors.

Current Symptoms: Condition stable for past year; able to do light housework and sedentary work. Breathlessness upon climbing a flight of stairs; prefers two pillows.

Physical Exam: BP: 110/70 mm Hg; PR: regular—70 BPM. Venous pressure normal; clear lungs. Apical impulse markedly enlarged, sustained, displaced laterally to anterior axillary line. Early diastolic impulse palpable after systolic impulse. Diminished S_1; normal S_2; prominent S_3.

Clinical Studies: ECG: low T waves in all leads. QS pattern in V_1, V_2. Chest roentgenogram: marked cardiomegaly; some distention of pulmonary vessels in upper lobes. Echocardiogram: LV: moderately dilated; LVEF 0.30; enlarged LA.

Diagnosis: Idiopathic cardiomyopathy.

Impairment Rating: 49% impairment of the whole person.

Comment: Reduced exercise capacity; poor LV function.

Class 4
50%-100% Impairment of the Whole Person
Symptomatic during ordinary daily activities despite appropriate use of dietary adjustment and drugs (functional class III or IV)
or
persistent signs of CHF despite use of dietary adjustment and drugs
or
has recovered from surgery for treatment of hypertrophic cardiomyopathy or has recovered from successful heart transplantation and meets above criteria

Example 3-33
50% to 100% Impairment Due to Cardiomyopathy

Subject: 62-year-old woman.

History: Increasing dyspnea and chest pressure with exertion for 2 years. Long-standing, poorly treated hypertension; no other medical problems. Heart murmur, hypertrophic cardiomyopathy; treated with large dosages of beta-blocker and calcium channel-blocker.

Current Symptoms: Still severely limited by symptoms; unable to walk up a half flight of stairs or do daily activities. Although dual-chamber pacemaker placed 6 months earlier, minimal change in symptoms.

Physical Exam: BP: 150/90 mm Hg; HR: 50 BPM. Venous pressure: normal; carotid brisk with bifid quality. LV impulse: sustained with a triple impulse.

Clinical Studies: Echocardiogram: severe septal hypertrophy; 0.70 EF; 70 mm Hg outflow tract obstruction. Severe mitral regurgitation secondary to systolic anterior motion of mitral valve. Chest roentgenogram: cardiomegaly with clear fields. ECG: sinus bradycardia with paced rhythm.

Diagnosis: Severe hypertrophic cardiomyopathy with outflow obstruction.

Impairment Rating: 70% to 79% impairment of the whole person.

Comment: Typical symptoms of hypertrophic cardiomyopathy related to outflow tract obstruction and diastolic dysfunction. No typical findings of "backward" HF present in individuals with dilated cardiomyopathies. If successful septal myectomy, then improved symptoms and classification.

Example 3-34
50% to 100% Impairment Due to Cardiomyopathy

Subject: 47-year-old man.

History: 3 months ago developed exertional dyspnea, orthopnea, and edema.

Current Symptoms: Evaluation for cardiac transplantation: dyspnea on exertion with one flight of stairs or ambulating > 25 feet. Meds: ACE inhibitor, diuretics, and beta-blocker. Unable to do many activities of daily living.

Physical Exam: Elevated venous pressures and rales in both lung fields. Cardiac examination: laterally displaced, sustained apical impulse; 2/6 apical holosystolic murmur. No peripheral edema.

Clinical Studies: ECG: normal sinus rhythm—90 BPM; low amplitude QRS complex throughout all leads. QS complexes present in II, III, and aVF. Chest roentgenogram: moderate cardiomegaly; mild pulmonary venous hypertension. Reduced LV function (0.32 EF) secondary to cardiac amyloidosis.

Diagnosis: Cardiac amyloidosis with CHF.

Impairment Rating: 80% to 89% impairment due to cardiomyopathy; combine with impairment due to organ system effects of amyloidosis (see Combined Values Chart, p. 604) to determine whole person impairment.

Comment: Level of impairment higher if more severe symptoms (dyspnea with minimal exertion, peripheral edema), history of syncope, or evidence of nonsustained ventricular tachyarrhythmias. Physical findings of HF despite medical therapy. If significant arrhythmias develop, evaluate according to arrhythmia criteria (see Combined Values Chart, p. 604).

3.6 Pericardial Heart Disease

Inflammation from diseases of the pericardium is associated with (1) systemic illnesses such as lupus erythematosus; (2) a reaction to mechanical forces, such as trauma or irradiation; (3) no obvious cause (idiopathic pericarditis); (4) infections, eg, viral, bacterial, fungal; or (5) open heart surgery (postcardiotomy syndrome). The pericardium may also be affected by tumors.

Recurrent pericarditis can lead to disabling episodes of fevers and pleuritic chest pain. Since chest pain is nonspecific, pericarditis evidence must be documented by echocardiography to show a pericardial effusion or by laboratory evidence of active inflammation, such as an increase in the erythrocyte sedimentation rate (ESR).

Constrictive pericarditis is the most common pericardial disorder leading to permanent impairment; surgical removal of the thickened pericardium may significantly reduce symptoms and improve the overall condition of the individual. Before assessing permanent impairment, it is mandatory to allow sufficient time for the person to recover from a surgical procedure and to reach maximal medical improvement.

Pain and compromised cardiac function because of tamponade may cause some impairment, but they are rare as causes of permanent impairment. Recurrent episodes of pericarditis with tamponade or pericardial disease related to tumors may lead to permanent impairment. Allow adequate time for resolution of an acute illness, generally a period of months, before assessing permanent impairment.

Diagnosis of pericardial disease is made by history-taking; identifying a pericardial fraction rub or early diastolic pericardial knock; demonstrating pericardial effusion, thickening, or calcification on an echocardiogram; showing a thickened pericardium with computerized tomography (CT) or magnetic resonance imaging (MRI); or findings at cardiac catheterization.

3.6a Criteria for Rating Permanent Impairment Due to Pericardial Heart Disease

Criteria for evaluating permanent impairment related to pericardial heart disease are given in Table 3-10.

Table 3-10 Criteria for Rating Permanent Impairment Due to Pericardial Heart Disease

Class 1 0%-9% Impairment of the Whole Person	Class 2 10%-29% Impairment of the Whole Person	Class 3 30%-49% Impairment of the Whole Person	Class 4 50%-100% Impairment of the Whole Person
No symptoms in performance of ordinary daily activities or moderately heavy physical exertion, but evidence from either physical examination or laboratory studies of pericardial heart disease *and* continuous treatment not required, and no signs of cardiac enlargement or of congestion of lungs or other organs *or* in an individual who has had surgical removal of the pericardium or a surgical window for drainage, no adverse consequences from the treatment and meets above criteria	No symptoms in performance of ordinary daily activities, but evidence from either physical examination or laboratory studies of pericardial heart disease *and* dietary adjustment or drugs required to keep individual free of symptoms and signs of CHF *or* has recovered from pericardiectomy and meets above criteria	Slight to moderate discomfort in performance of ordinary daily activities (functional class II) despite dietary or drug therapy, and has physician examination or laboratory studies of pericardial disease *and* physical signs present of increased venous pressure, or laboratory evidence of constrictive physiology on echocardiographic or hemodynamic evaluation *or* has recovered from surgery to remove pericardium but continues to have symptoms, signs, and laboratory evidence described above	Symptoms on performance of ordinary daily activities (functional class III or IV) despite appropriate dietary restrictions or drugs, and evidence from physical examination or laboratory studies of pericardial heart disease *and* has recovered from surgical pericardiectomy and continues to have symptoms, signs, and laboratory evidence described above

> **Class 1**
> **0%-9% Impairment of the Whole Person**
>
> No symptoms in performance of ordinary daily activities or moderately heavy physical exertion, but evidence from either physical examination or laboratory studies of pericardial heart disease
>
> *and*
>
> continuous treatment not required, and no signs of cardiac enlargement or of congestion of lungs or other organs
>
> *or*
>
> in an individual who has had surgical removal of the pericardium or a surgical window for drainage, no adverse consequences from the treatment and meets above criteria

Example 3-35
0% to 9% Impairment Due to Pericardial Heart Disease

Subject: 28-year-old man.

History: Acute pericarditis 15 months ago. Symptoms: acute, self-limited, febrile illness, with anterior chest pain and a pericardial friction rub.

Current Symptoms: Asymptomatic; returned to work and leading a normal life.

Physical Exam: Normal.

Clinical Studies: Echocardiogram: small pericardial effusion. Illness resolved with aspirin treatment.

Diagnosis: Acute benign idiopathic pericarditis.

Impairment Rating: 0% impairment of the whole person.

Comment: Could develop constrictive pericarditis, but most individuals have no permanent impairment.

Example 3-36
0% to 9% Impairment Due to Pericardial Heart Disease

Subject: 64-year-old woman.

History: Had successful pericardiocentesis for idiopathic pericardial effusion. Moderate symptoms resolved after treatment.

Current Symptoms: Asymptomatic from rigorous traveling to South America.

Physical Examination: Normal.

Clinical Studies: Chest roentgenogram: normal. Echocardiogram: normal.

Diagnosis: Resolved pericardial effusion following percutaneous pericardiocentesis with no recurrence.

Impairment Rating: 0% impairment of the whole person.

Comment: Self-limited illness; no effects on activities of daily living.

> **Class 2**
> **10%-29% Impairment of the Whole Person**
>
> No symptoms in performance of ordinary daily activities, but evidence from either physical examination or laboratory studies of pericardial heart disease
>
> *and*
>
> dietary adjustment or drugs required to keep the individual free of symptoms and signs of CHF
>
> *or*
>
> has recovered from pericardiectomy and meets above criteria

Example 3-37
10% to 29% Impairment Due to Pericardial Heart Disease

Subject: 32-year-old woman.

History: Viral pericarditis with fever and pleuritic pain 1 year ago. Echocardiogram: moderate-sized, circumferential, pericardial effusion, an elevated ESR and white blood cell count; no evidence of bacterial or fungal infection. Pericardial tap: no bacteria. Autoimmune workup: negative.

Current Symptoms: For past year, several recurrences of chest pain with effusions; unable to carry out daily activities. Treated with NSAIDs for 4-6 weeks each time. Condition stable for about 10 months.

Physical Exam: Comfortable; no signs or symptoms of CHF. Heart sounds normal; no murmurs or extra heart sounds. No audible pericardial rub.

Clinical Studies: ECG: flat T-wave abnormalities. Chest roentgenogram: normal size heart; clear lung fields. Echocardiogram: small residual pericardial effusion.

Diagnosis: Recurrent idiopathic pericarditis.

Impairment Rating: 15% impairment of the whole person.

Comment: If episodes more frequent, then consider long-term medication (eg, salicylates, NSAIDs, steroids, or colchicine).

Chapter 3

Example 3-38
10% to 29% Impairment Due to Pericardial Heart Disease

Subject: 60-year-old man.

History: Pericardiectomy for constrictive pericarditis 1 year ago.

Current Symptoms: No symptoms even with significant exertion. Denied peripheral edema, orthopnea, exertional dyspnea, or early satiety.

Physical Exam: BP: normal; no pulsus paradoxicus; normal CV examination and laboratory work.

Clinical Studies: Chest roentgenogram: small area of pericardial calcification appeared where pericardium incompletely stripped during surgery. Echocardiogram: mild LV enlargement; 0.50 EF; inspiratory changes in mitral inflow amplitude; early diastolic filling wave consistent with constrictive physiology.

Diagnosis: LV enlargement and constrictive pericarditis following surgical pericardectomy.

Impairment Rating: 20% to 29% impairment of the whole person.

Comment: Mild LV enlargement; persistent constrictive physiology following surgical pericardectomy. Level of impairment higher if any symptoms.

Class 3
30%-49% Impairment of the Whole Person

Slight to moderate discomfort in performance of ordinary daily activities (functional class II) despite dietary or drug therapy, and has physician examination or laboratory studies of pericardial disease

and

physical signs present of increased venous pressure, or laboratory evidence of constrictive physiology on echocardiographic or hemodynamic evaluation

or

has recovered from surgery to remove pericardium but continues to have symptoms, signs, and laboratory evidence described above

---

Example 3-39
30% to 49% Impairment Due to Pericardial Heart Disease

Subject: 45-year-old man.

History: Pericardiectomy for constrictive pericarditis 10 years earlier. Daily furosemide to prevent lower extremity edema.

Current Symptoms: Weakness and breathlessness with heavy physical exertion; works regularly.

Physical Exam: Venous pressure mildly elevated: 12 cm H_2O; no edema. BP and PR: normal. No ventricular heaves or thrills. S_1: normal; S_2: diminished. No extra sounds or rubs.

Clinical Studies: ECG: low-voltage QRS; T waves in all leads. Chest roentgenogram: considerable cardiomegaly; some calcification at posterior aspect of heart. Clear lung fields. Echocardiogram: pericardium thickening; moderate diminution of RV, LV contraction; 0.40 LVEF. Doppler: evidence of residual pericardial restraint. Mitral inflow; early diastolic filling wave amplitude demonstrated 50% variation with inspiration.

Diagnosis: Constrictive pericarditis with pericardiectomy.

Impairment Rating: 30% to 39% impairment of the whole person.

Comment: After pericardiectomy, possible residual elevation of venous pressure. If more activities limited, then level of impairment > 30% to 39%.

Example 3-40
30% to 49% Impairment Due to Pericardial Heart Disease

Subject: 48-year-old woman.

History: Tuberculosis after assignment in Central Africa. Developed intermittent pericardial effusions. Two to three dyspnea episodes and lower extremity edema annually. Pericardiocentesis for fluid removal. No chest pain. Refused surgical pericardiectomy; father died during similar procedure.

Current Symptoms: Asymptomatic since prior episode 3 months earlier.

Physical Exam: Currently normal.

Clinical Studies: Echocardiogram: thickened pericardium, constrictive physiology during asymptomatic periods; effusive constrictive physiology during symptomatic periods. Medications did not suppress symptoms.

Diagnosis: Recurrent pericarditis with symptomatic effusions.

Impairment Rating: 30% to 49% impairment of the whole person.

Comment: Recurrent pericardial effusions despite aggressive treatment. Impairment higher if symptoms more frequent or if LV dysfunction evident.

Class 4
50%–100% Impairment of the Whole Person

Symptoms on performance of ordinary daily activities (functional class III or IV) despite appropriate dietary restrictions or drugs, and evidence from physical examination or laboratory studies of pericardial heart disease

and

has recovered from surgical pericardiectomy and continues to have symptoms, signs, and laboratory evidence described above

---

Example 3-41
50% to 100% Impairment Due to Pericardial Heart Disease

Subject: 62-year-old man.

History: Profound ascites, peripheral edema, weight loss, signs of pulmonary congestion attributed to a pericardial effusion. Effusion drained, temporarily relieved severe ascites and peripheral edema. Fatigue and breathlessness continue with ordinary activity; unable to climb one flight of stairs without resting.

Current Symptoms: Edema, ascites returned. Able to walk on a level surface and do light activities of daily living.

Physical Exam: Comfortable. Neck veins elevated 20 cm H_2O; 2+ peripheral edema and ascites. Evidence of marked weight loss remained. No ventricular heaves, thrills, or taps in the precordium. Diminished heart sounds; no murmurs or extra sounds.

Clinical Studies: ECG: low voltage of the QRS and T waves. Chest roentgenogram: marked cardiomegaly; some upper lobe pulmonary vasculature distention. Echocardiogram: systolic ventricular function: normal; 0.55 LVEF. Doppler: constrictive pericarditis.

Diagnosis: Constrictive pericarditis following pericardial drainage.

Impairment Rating: 80% to 89% impairment of the whole person.

Comment: Drainage of pericardial effusion may cause limitations from residual constrictive pericarditis. If symptoms with minimal daily activities, or if signs of overt congestion at evaluation, then impairment possibly as high as 95% to 100% (total impairment). Complete pericardiectomy may result in symptom and class improvement.

Example 3-42
50% to 100% Impairment Due to Pericardial Heart Disease

Subject: 47-year-old woman.

History: Pericardiectomy for constrictive pericarditis 2 years ago. Continued dyspnea with minimal activities; dependent on others for self-care. Daily furosemide (160 mg twice a day), digitalis, and nitrates. Compression stockings caused symptomatic improvement.

Current Symptoms: Waking at night with breathlessness.

Physical Exam: BP: 115/80 mm Hg; fell to 85/45 mm Hg with inspiration. Neck veins elevated; did not fall with inspiration. Clear lung fields; distant heart sounds; audible S_3. Abdomen: moderate ascites and hepatomegaly. 2+ pitting edema in lower extremities and lower back region.

Clinical Studies: Echocardiogram: enlarged heart with reduced function; 0.30 EF. Constrictive physiology. No pericardial effusion. Laboratory studies: mild anemia; liver enzymes elevation consistent with congestive hepatomegaly.

Diagnosis: Constrictive pericarditis following surgical pericardiectomy and biventricular dysfunction with HF.

Impairment Rating: 90% to 100% impairment of the whole person.

Comment: Class IV symptoms; terminal prognosis.

3.7 Arrhythmias

An arrhythmia is one or more heartbeats generated at a site other than the sinus node. An impulse generated in the sinus node but not transmitted normally through the conducting system is a conduction defect arrhythmia. Arrhythmias may occur in individuals with structurally and functionally normal hearts or in those with any type of organic heart disease.

Because arrhythmias tend to fluctuate remarkably in frequency, the physician must adequately document and estimate the frequency with which an arrhythmia occurs. The associated symptoms can include syncope, weakness and fatigue, palpitations, dizziness, lightheadedness, chest heaviness, and shortness of breath, alone or in any combination.

The degree of impairment from cardiac arrhythmias often has to be combined with the degree of impairment due to underlying heart disease and then calculated according to the Combined Values Chart (p. 604). Before estimating the degree of permanent impairment, allow adequate time for the individual's condition to reach maximal medical improvement after instituting therapy.[19]

3.7a Criteria for Rating Permanent Impairment Due to Arrhythmias

Criteria for evaluating impairments related to arrhythmias are given in Table 3-11.

Table 3-11 Criteria for Rating Permanent Impairment Due to Arrhythmias

Class 1 0%-9% Impairment of the Whole Person	Class 2 10%-29% Impairment of the Whole Person	Class 3 30%-49% Impairment of the Whole Person	Class 4 50%-100% Impairment of the Whole Person
Asymptomatic during ordinary activities and a cardiac arrhythmia is documented by ECG, or has had an isolated syncopal episode *and* no documentation of three or more consecutive ectopic beats or periods of asystole > 1.5 seconds, and both atrial and ventricular rates are maintained between 50 and 100 beats per minute *and* no evidence of organic heart disease *or* has recovered from surgery or a catheter procedure to correct arrhythmia and above criteria are met	Asymptomatic during ordinary activities and a cardiac arrhythmia is documented by ECG, or has had an isolated syncopal episode *and* moderate dietary adjustment, use of drugs, or an artificial pacemaker required to prevent symptoms related to the arrhythmia *or* arrhythmia persists and there is organic heart disease *or* has recovered from surgery or a catheter procedure to correct arrhythmia or implantable cardioverter-defibrillator placement to treat arrhythmia and meets above criteria for impairment	Symptoms despite use of dietary therapy or drugs or of an artificial pacemaker, and a cardiac arrhythmia is documented with ECG *and* is able to lead an active life and symptoms due to arrhythmia are limited to infrequent palpitations and/or episodes of lightheadedness, presyncope, or temporary inadequate cardiac output *or* has recovered from surgery, a catheter procedure, or implantable cardioverter-defibrillator placement to treat arrhythmia and meets above criteria for impairment	Symptoms due to documented cardiac arrhythmia that are constant and interfere with ordinary daily activities (functional class III or IV) *or* frequent symptoms of inadequate cardiac output documented by ECG to be due to frequent episodes of cardiac arrhythmia *or* continues to have episodes of syncope that are either due to, or have a high probability of being related to, arrhythmia; to fit into this category of impairment, symptoms must be present despite use of dietary therapy, drugs, or artificial pacemakers *or* has recovered from surgery, a catheter procedure, or implantable cardioverter-defibrillator placement to treat arrhythmia and continues to have symptoms causing impairment outlined above

Class 1 0%-9% Impairment of the Whole Person
Asymptomatic during ordinary activities and a cardiac arrhythmia is documented by ECG, or has had an isolated syncopal episode *and* no documentation of three or more consecutive ectopic beats or periods of asystole > 1.5 seconds, and both atrial and ventricular rates are maintained between 50 and 100 beats per minute *and* no evidence of organic heart disease *or* has recovered from surgery or a catheter procedure to correct arrhythmia and above criteria are met

Class 2 10%-29% Impairment of the Whole Person
Asymptomatic during ordinary activities and a cardiac arrhythmia is documented by ECG, or has had an isolated syncopal episode *and* moderate dietary adjustment, use of drugs, or an artificial pacemaker required to prevent symptoms related to the arrhythmia *or* arrhythmia persists and there is organic heart disease *or* has recovered from surgery or a catheter procedure to correct arrhythmia or implantable cardioverter-defibrillator placement to treat arrhythmia and meets above criteria for impairment

Example 3-43
0% to 9% Impairment Due to Arrhythmias

Subject: 56-year-old man.

History: Frequent premature beats during annual physical examination.

Current Symptoms: None. Able to perform all activities of daily living.

Physical Exam: Remainder of exam normal.

Clinical Studies: ECG: frequent premature complexes.

Diagnosis: Atrial premature complexes.

Impairment Rating: 0% impairment of the whole person.

Example 3-44
0% to 9% Impairment Due to Arrhythmias

Subject: 21-year-old woman.

History: Syncopal spell while studying for final exam. Gastrointestinal illness for 3 days before episode. ER evaluation. HR: 110 BPM; BP with orthostatic drop: 110/65 mm Hg supine to 85/40 mm Hg standing, with presyncope. Didn't follow up for 3 months; no subsequent episodes.

Physical Exam: Normal now.

Clinical Studies: None.

Diagnosis: Orthostatic hypotension with vasovagal syncope.

Impairment Rating: 0% impairment of the whole person.

Comment: Isolated episode of dehydration-related syncope. No further evaluation necessary.

Example 3-45
10% to 29% Impairment Due to Arrhythmias

Subject: 62-year-old man.

History: 1-year history of atrial fibrillation with irregular ventricular response 75 BPM.

Current Symptoms: Asymptomatic.

Physical Exam: PR: 75 BPM.

Clinical Studies: ECG, chest roentgenogram, and echocardiogram: normal.

Diagnosis: Atrial fibrillation with controlled ventricular response.

Impairment Rating: 15% impairment of the whole person.

Comment: If medications needed to maintain ventricular response, then impairment estimate slightly higher.

Example 3-46
10% to 29% Impairment Due to Arrhythmias

Subject: 52-year-old man.

History: Recurring syncope 8 months ago; treated with insertion of a permanent pacemaker for complete heart block.

Current Symptoms: Asymptomatic.

Physical Exam: Appeared well. BP: 120/80 mm Hg; PR: 72 BPM. Normal heart sounds; no murmurs.

Clinical Studies: ECG: complete capture of the heart by artificial pacemaker at 72 BPM. Pacemaker sensed and properly inhibited rare premature ventricular beat.

Diagnosis: Adams-Stokes attacks in individual with complete heart block; managed with properly functioning artificial pacemaker.

Impairment Rating: 20% impairment of the whole person.

Class 3
30%-49% Impairment of the Whole Person

Symptoms despite use of dietary therapy or drugs or of an artificial pacemaker, and a cardiac arrhythmia is documented with ECG

and

is able to lead an active life and symptoms due to arrhythmia are limited to infrequent palpitations and/or episodes of lightheadedness, presyncope, or temporary inadequate cardiac output

or

has recovered from surgery, a catheter procedure, or implantable cardioverter-defibrillator placement to treat arrhythmia and meets above criteria for impairment

---

Example 3-47
30% to 49% Impairment Due to Arrhythmias

Subject: 44-year-old man.

History: Multiple, recurrent, 5- to 15-minute episodes of rapid heart rate accompanied by lightheadedness. Vagal-type maneuvers occasionally terminated episodes; spontaneous termination. No frank syncope. Occasional episode with verapamil LA 240 mg a day. Symptom free with verapamil LA 360 mg a day. Regimen continued for 13 months when impairment evaluated.

Current Symptoms: Episodes of rapid heart rate. Episodes cause weakness and prohibit any physical activity.

Physical Exam: PR: regular—86 BPM.

Clinical Studies: ECG: Holter monitoring: atrial tachycardia: 155 BPM during episode. Typical patterns of reentry atrioventricular (AV) nodal tachycardia.

Diagnosis: AV nodal reentry tachycardia with atrial tachycardia, adequately controlled by calcium-channel blocker.

Impairment Rating: 30% impairment of the whole person.

Comment: If palpitations continued with medications, or if rare episode associated with inadequate cerebral perfusion, then estimated impairment possibly as high as 49%.

Example 3-48
30% to 49% Impairment Due to Arrhythmias

Subject: 58-year-old man.

History: Asymptomatic LV dysfunction; out-of-hospital cardiac arrest 3 months ago. Returned for evaluation of implanted pacemaker-cardioverter-defibrillator. No syncope; five instances of profound palpitations followed by internal firing of the cardioverter-defibrillator system 45 seconds after symptom onset.

Current Symptoms: Internal shocks were "mildly disconcerting" at best. No HF or angina symptoms.

Physical Exam: PR: 80 BPM, normal pacing.

Clinical Studies: Pacemaker-cardioverter-defibrillator working well.

Diagnosis: Sustained VT.

Impairment Rating: 40% to 49% impairment of the whole person.

Comment: Infrequent discharges of internal defibrillator system in response to sustained VT. Leads somewhat active life; higher impairment if (*a*) shocks occurring weekly or more frequently, (*b*) LV dysfunction symptoms, or (*c*) episodes include syncope.

Class 4
50%-100% Impairment of the Whole Person
Symptoms due to documented cardiac arrhythmia that are constant and interfere with ordinary daily activities (functional class III or IV)
or
frequent symptoms of inadequate cardiac output documented by ECG to be due to frequent episodes of cardiac arrhythmia
or
continues to have episodes of syncope that are either due to, or have a high probability of being related to, arrhythmia; to fit into this category of impairment, symptoms must be present despite use of dietary therapy, drugs, or artificial pacemakers
or
has recovered from surgery, a catheter procedure, or implantable cardioverter-defibrillator placement to treat arrhythmia and continues to have symptoms causing impairment outlined above

Example 3-49
50% to 100% Impairment Due to Arrhythmias

Subject: 38-year-old woman.

History: Rapid heart action episodes for over 10 years with retrosternal pressure, fainting sensation, and general weakness. Several spells of unconsciousness, during which husband used CPR. Tachyarrhythmia ended spontaneously within 30 minutes; no external electrical conversion necessary. Many antiarrhythmic medications for past 5 months (ie, quinidine sulfate, 300 mg every 6 h; procainamide, 750 mg every 4 h; and propranolol, 160 mg twice daily) controlled arrhythmia fairly well. Previous verapamil use failed to prevent arrhythmia.

Current Symptoms: Episodes continue monthly, none associated with loss of consciousness. Occasional swelling of small joints in the hands respond to low corticosteroid doses.

Physical Exam: Cardiovascular: no evidence of valvular or myocardial disease.

Clinical Studies: Serologic abnormalities characteristic of systemic lupus erythematosis (SLE). ECG: normal pattern and rhythm; ECG during palpitations: rapid regular rhythm 200-250 BPM. Electrophysiologic studies: no abnormal conduction problems. VT easily induced; pattern similar to one during spontaneous episode.

Diagnosis: Recurrent VT.

Impairment Rating: 70% to 90% impairment of the whole person.

Comment: Impairment depends on frequency and symptomatic nature of episodes.

Example 3-50
50% to 100% Impairment Due to Arrhythmias

Subject: 42-year-old man.

History: Medications, pacemaker for syncope for past 8 years. Syncope continued daily without warning despite all efforts. Work limited; unable to conduct business meetings because of embarrassment about syncope unpredictability. Could not legally drive an automobile or use any power equipment that might endanger his safety if spell occurred.

Physical Exam: Normal.

Clinical Studies: Echocardiogram, exercise stress test: heart within normal limits.

Diagnosis: Recurrent syncope despite maximal therapy.

Impairment Rating: 75% to 90% impairment of the whole person.

Comment: Daily syncope with maximal therapy.

3.8 Cardiovascular Impairment Evaluation Summary

See Table 3-12 for an evaluation summary for the assessment of cardiovascular impairment.

Table 3-12 Cardiac Impairment Evaluation Summary

Disorder	History, Including Selected Relevant Symptoms	Examination Record	Assessment of Cardiac Function
General	Cardiovascular symptoms (eg, fatigue, palpitations, dyspnea, chest pain) and general symptoms; impact of symptoms on function and ability to do daily activities Prognosis if change anticipated Review medical history	Comprehensive physical examination; detailed cardiovascular system assessment	Data derived from relevant studies (eg, ECG, echocardiography, stress tests, cardiac catheterization)
Valvular Heart Disease	Discuss symptoms and any resulting limitation of physical activity (eg, angina) Address cardiac output, pulmonary and systemic congestion	Note rate, rhythm, heart sounds, and other organ function	Doppler echocardiography or cardiac catheterization
Coronary Heart Disease (CHD)	Angina pectoris; reduced ventricular function; limitation of physical activity due to fatigue; palpitations; dyspnea; anginal pain	Detailed history Note rate, rhythm, heart sounds, and other organ function	Coronary angiography; chest x-ray; ECG; EF; studies may be obtained at rest and during and after exercise
Congenital Heart Disease	Dyspnea; fatigue; palpitations; symptoms of end-organ dysfunction	Note rate, rhythm, heart sounds, and other organ function	ECG; chest roentgenogram; radioisotope studies; echocardiography; hemodynamic measurements; angiography
Cardiomyopathies	Exertional dyspnea; angina; syncope; pulmonary or systemic organ congestion	Note rate, rhythm, heart sounds, and other organ function	Echocardiography; ECG; chest roentgenogram; abnormal ventricular function; dynamic outflow tract obstruction
Pericardial Heart Disease	Chest pain Note active inflammation, increase in ESR	Note rate, rhythm, heart sounds (pericardial rub, early diastolic pericardial knock), and other organ function	ECHO-pericardial effusion, thickening, or calcification; thickened pericardium on CT scan or MRI; cardiac catheterization
Arrhythmias	Syncope; weakness and fatigue; palpitations; dizziness; chest heaviness; shortness of breath	Note rate, rhythm, heart sounds; document arrhythmia and estimate its frequency	ECG: frequent premature complexes, tachycardia Echocardiogram: atrial enlargement

Chapter 3

End-Organ Damage	Diagnosis(es)	Degree of Impairment
Include assessment of sequelae, including end-organ damage and impairment	Record all pertinent diagnosis(es); note if they are at maximal medical improvement; if not, discuss under what conditions and when stability is expected	Criteria outlined in this chapter
Assess relevant organs (eg, lungs, kidneys) for congestion or dysfunction	Aortic or mitral valve stenosis; mitral valve prolapse; aortic or mitral valve regurgitation; aortic and/or mitral valve disease; ventricular dysfunction	See Table 3-5
Assess relevant organs (eg, brain, lungs, kidneys, eyes, peripheral vascular system)	MI; angina pectoris; coronary artery vasospasm; ventricular failure	See Table 3-6
Assess relevant organs (eg, brain, lungs, kidneys, peripheral vascular system)	Valve stenosis, septal defects; valve anomalies; tetralogy of Fallot; Ebstein's anomaly; vessel transposition; Eisenmenger's complex	See Table 3-8
Assess relevant organs (eg, brain, lungs, kidneys, peripheral vascular system)	Dilated or congested; hypertrophic; restrictive	See Table 3-9
Assess relevant organs (eg, brain, lungs, kidneys, peripheral vascular system)	Constrictive or idiopathic pericarditis; tamponade; tumor; pericardial effusion; pericardial damage	See Table 3-10
Assess relevant organs (eg, brain, lungs, kidneys, peripheral vascular system)	Syncope; VT; atrial fibrillation; complete heart block; premature complexes	See Table 3-11

References

1. Criteria Committee of the New York Heart Association. *Diseases of the Heart and Blood Vessels: Nomenclature and Criteria for Disease.* 6th ed. Boston, Mass: Little Brown & Co; 1964.

2. Cheitlin MD, Alpert JS, Armstrong WF, et al. ACC/AHA guidelines for the clinical application of echocardiography. A report of the American College of Cardiology/American Heart Association Task Force on Practice Guidelines (Committee on Clinical Application of Echocardiography). Developed in collaboration with the American Society of Echocardiography. *Circulation.* 1997;95:1686-1744.

    Summarizes the utility of echocardiography in patients with heart disease.

3. Fox SM III, Naughton JP, Haskell WL. Physical activity and the prevention of coronary heart disease. *Ann Clin Res.* 1971;3:404-432.

4. Gibbons RJ, Balady GJ, Bricker JT, et al. ACC/AHA guidelines for exercise testing. A report of the American College of Cardiology/American Heart Association Task Force on Practice Guidelines (Committee on Exercise Testing). *J Am Coll Cardiol.* 1997;30:260+.

    Summarizes the most recent data on the prognostic and diagnostic utility of exercise testing for patients with heart disease.

5. Nishimura RA, Tajik AJ. Evaluation of diastolic filling of left ventricle in health and disease: Doppler echocardiography is the clinician's Rosetta Stone. *J Am Coll Cardiol.* 1997;30:8-18.

    A simplified approach to understanding the process of diastolic filling of the left ventricle and interpreting the Doppler flow velocity curves as they relate to this procedure. Specific therapy for diastolic dysfunction based on Doppler flow velocity curves is discussed.

6. Scanlon PJ, Faxon DP, Audet AM, et al. ACC/AHA guidelines for coronary angiography: executive summary and recommendations. A report of the American College of Cardiology/American Heart Association Task Force on Practice Guidelines (Committee on Coronary Angiography) developed in collaboration with the Society for Cardiac Angiography and Interventions. *Circulation.* 1999;99:2345-2357.

    Summarizes the latest data on the diagnostic utility of invasive catheterization in patients with heart disease.

7. ACC/AHA guidelines for the management of patients with valvular heart disease. A report of the American College of Cardiology/American Heart Association Task Force on Practice Guidelines (Committee on Management of Patients with Valvular Heart Disease). *J Am Coll Cardiol.* 1998;32:1486-1588.

    Summarizes the latest treatment and prognostic information for patients with valvular heart disease.

8. Jaffe WM, Roche AG, Coverdale HA, McAlister HF, Ormiston JA, Greene ER. Clinical evaluation versus Doppler echocardiography in quantitative assessment of valvular heart disease. *Circulation.* 1988;78:267-275.

    Tests the hypotheses that Doppler echocardiography has a higher accuracy than clinical evaluation in the detection of significant aortic and mitral valvular heart disease and that Doppler echocardiography is highly accurate as compared with cardiac catheterization for the assessment of valvular disease severity.

9. Lee KL, Woodlief LH, Topol EJ, et al. Predictors of 30-day mortality in the era of reperfusion for acute MI: results from an international trial of 41,021 patients. *Circulation.* 1995;91:1659-1668.

    Analyzes predictors of short-term mortality in acute MI and establishes the relative importance of a variety of prognostic variables.

10. Ryan TJ, Anderson JL, Antman EM, et al. ACC/AHA guidelines for the management of patients with acute MI. A report of the American College of Cardiology/American Heart Association Task Force on Practice Guidelines (Committee on Management of Acute MI). *J Am Coll Cardiol.* 1996;28:1328-1428.

    Summarizes the latest treatment recommendations and prognostic information for patients with acute MI.

11. Congenital heart disease after childhood: an expanding patient population [22nd Bethesda Conference, Maryland, October 18-19, 1990]. *J Am Coll Cardiol.* 1991;18:312-342.

    Summarizes a consensus opinion on adult congenital heart disease.

12 Nishimura RA, Miller FA Jr, Callahan MJ, Benassi RC, Seward JB, Tajik AJ. Doppler echocardiography: theory, instrumentation, technique, and application. *Mayo Clin Proc.* 1985;60:321-343.

    Doppler echocardiography is a valuable adjunct to a complete cardiovascular examination. Evaluation of other aspects of Doppler echocardiography, such as color-flow mapping and assessment of diastolic events, are also included.

13. Rihal CS, Nishimura RA, Hatle LK, et al. Systolic and diastolic dysfunction in patients with clinical diagnosis of dilated cardiomyopathy: relation to symptoms and prognosis. *Circulation.* 1994;90:2772-2779.

    In patients with the clinical diagnosis of dilated cardiomyopathy, markers of diastolic dysfunction correlated strongly with congestive symptoms, whereas variables of systolic function were the strongest predictors of survival. Consideration of both ejection fraction and deceleration time allowed identification of subgroups with divergent long-term prognoses.

14. Feldman AM. Can we alter survival in patients with congestive heart failure? *JAMA*. 1992;267:1956-1961.

Assesses the efficacy of pharmacologic therapy in improving survival in patients with congestive heart failure (CHF) in the context of recent investigational studies having mortality as an endpoint.

15. Levy D, Larson MG, Vasan RS, Kannel WB, Ho KK. The progression from hypertension to congestive heart failure. *JAMA*. 1996;275:1557-1562.

Reviews the relative and population-attributable risks of hypertension for the development of CHF, assesses the time course of progression from hypertension to CHF, and identifies the risk factors that contribute to the development of overt heart failure in hypertensive subjects.

16. Garg R, Yusuf S. Overview of randomized trials of angiotensin-converting enzyme inhibitors on mortality and morbidity in patients with heart failure [published erratum appears in *JAMA*. 1995;274:462. *JAMA*. 1995;273:1450-1456.

Evaluates the effect of angiotensin-converting enzyme (ACE) inhibitors on mortality and morbidity in patients with symptomatic CHF. Total mortality and hospitalization for CHF are significantly reduced by ACE inhibitors with consistent effects in a broad range of patients.

17. Hatle LK, Appleton CP, Popp RL. Differentiation of constrictive pericarditis and restrictive cardiomyopathy by Doppler echocardiography. *Circulation*. 1989;79:357-370.

A landmark publication that suggests that patients with constrictive pericarditis and restrictive cardiomyopathy can be differentiated by comparing respiratory changes in transvalvular flow velocities. In also adds that although baseline hemodynamics in the two groups were similar, characteristic changes were seen with respiration that suggest that differentiation of these disease states may also be possible from hemodynamic data.

18. Edwards BS. Recent advances in cardiac transplantation. *Curr Opin Cardiol*. 1990;5:295-299.

This review summarizes the issue of cardiac transplantation.

19. Gregoratos G, Cheitlin MD, Conill A, et al. ACC/AHA guidelines for implantation of cardiac pacemakers and antiarrhythmia devices: executive summary—a report of the American College of Cardiology/American Heart Association Task Force on Practice Guidelines (Committee on Pacemaker Implantation). *Circulation*. 1998;97:1325-1335.

Reviews the current indications for pacemaker therapy in patients with heart disease.

Chapter 3

The Cardiovascular System: Systemic and Pulmonary Arteries

Chapter 4

Introduction

This chapter provides criteria for evaluating permanent impairments of the systemic and pulmonary arteries as they affect an individual's ability to function and perform activities of daily living. The information regarding medical evaluation, analysis of findings, and impairment criteria in Chapter 3, The Cardiovascular System: Heart and Aorta, remain applicable for this chapter. See Table 3-1 for the functional classification of cardiac disease.

This chapter also integrates new findings in the rapidly changing specialty of cardiovascular disease. The following areas are new or revised from the fourth edition: (*a*) the addition of recent guidelines of the sixth report of the Joint National Committee on Prevention, Detection, Evaluation and Treatment of High Blood Pressure (JNC-6)[1]; (*b*) an expanded section on pulmonary hypertension that outlines guides for impairment assessment; and (*c*) the latest data for prognosis of individuals with pulmonary hypertension.

4.1 Hypertensive Cardiovascular Disease

The JNC-6 classifies hypertension, or elevated blood pressure, as an elevation of the systolic blood pressure to ≥ 140 mm Hg or diastolic blood pressure to >89 mm Hg on two or more separate readings.[1] (See Table 4-1 for the JNC-6 three-stage hypertension classification.) Hypertension, the leading cause of ambulatory office visits in the United States, can produce heart disease, stroke, and renal failure. The economic impact of heart disease and stroke exceeds $29 billion annually in the United States. The prevalence of hypertension and its complications make it a major public health concern, particularly in the Southeast and among African Americans.[2,3]

Hypertensive heart disease includes hypertension, hypertension-associated systolic and diastolic heart failure (HF), hypertension-associated angina, and hypertension-induced left ventricular (LV) hypertrophy. Hypertensive heart disease can be very debilitating and demands aggressive treatment. Preventive treatment strategies may reduce the risk of developing secondary cardiac changes, the symptoms associated with hypertension, and other organ dysfunction.[4-7]

4.1a Criteria for Rating Permanent Impairment Due to Hypertensive Cardiovascular Disease

Table 4-2 addresses the impairment classification for hypertensive cardiovascular disease. Cardiovascular complications of hypertension should be established before assigning a diagnosis of hypertensive cardiovascular disease. Because patients with hypertensive cardiovascular disease do not become symptomatic until the very late stages, the impairment classification requires information on the end-organ damage that may occur even in the absence of symptoms.

Table 4-1 Classification of Hypertension in Adults

Blood Pressure	Blood Pressure Categories			Hypertension Categories		
	Optimal	Normal	High-Normal	Stage 1	Stage 2	Stage 3
Systolic	<120 and	<130 and	130-139 or	140-159 or	160-179 or	≥180 or
Diastolic	<80	<85	85-89	90-99	100-109	≥110

[1] Adapted from the sixth report of the Joint National Committee on Prevention, Detection, Evaluation, and Treatment of High Blood Pressure. *Arch Intern Med.* 1997;157:2413-2446.

Table 4-2 Criteria for Rating Permanent Impairment Due to Hypertensive Cardiovascular Disease

Class 1 0%-9% Impairment of the Whole Person	Class 2 10%-29% Impairment of the Whole Person	Class 3 30%-49% Impairment of the Whole Person	Class 4 50%-100% Impairment of the Whole Person
Asymptomatic; stage 1 or 2 hypertension without medications **or** normal blood pressure on antihypertensive medication **and** no evidence of end-organ damage	Asymptomatic; stage 1 or 2 hypertension despite multiple medications **or** antihypertensive medication with any of the following: (1) proteinuria, urinary sediment abnormalities, no renal function impairment as measured by the blood urea nitrogen (BUN) and serum creatinine; (2) definite hypertensive changes on funduscopic examination in arterioles, eg, "copper" or "silver wiring," or arteriovenous crossing changes with or without hemorrhages and exudates; either abnormality suggests end-organ damage	Asymptomatic; stage 3 hypertension despite multiple medications **or** antihypertensive medication with any of the following: (1) proteinuria, urinary sediment abnormalities, renal function impairment as measured by the BUN and serum creatinine, and a decreased creatinine clearance of 20% to 50% normal; (2) LV hypertrophy by ECG or echocardiography but no symptoms of HF; either abnormality suggests more extensive end-organ damage	Antihypertensive medication with stages 1–3 and any of the following abnormalities: (1) proteinuria, urinary sediment abnormalities, renal function impairment as measured by the BUN and serum creatinine, and a creatinine clearance < 20% normal; (2) hypertensive cerebrovascular damage or episodic hypertensive encephalopathy; (3) LV hypertrophy, systolic dysfunction, and/or signs and symptoms of HF due to hypertension

---
Class 1
0%-9% Impairment of the Whole Person

Asymptomatic; stage 1 or 2 hypertension without medications

or

normal blood pressure on antihypertensive medication

and

no evidence of end-organ damage

Example 4-1
0% to 9% Impairment Due to Hypertensive Cardiovascular Disease

Subject: 55-year-old woman.

History: Essential hypertension 5 years ago. Medication: angiotensin II antagonist and diuretic. Normal BP readings prior to visit.

Current Symptoms: Asymptomatic; denies medication side effects.

Physical Exam: Normal; BP: 105/78 mm Hg.

Clinical Studies: ECG: normal.

Diagnosis: Essential hypertension with adequate control.

Impairment Rating: 0% to 3% impairment of the whole person.

Comment: Continue medication. Impairment based on hypertension pathological changes, medication needs, and impact on activities of daily living. If medication needs change, then reassess rating.

Example 4-2
0% to 9% Impairment Due to Hypertensive Cardiovascular Disease

Subject: 26-year-old man.

History: Hypertensive since 18; causative factors unknown. Asymptomatic; elevated blood pressure (BP) despite salt restriction, weight control, and regular exercise. Antihypertensive prescribed.

Current Symptoms: Discontinued medication last year; seeking consultation.

Physical Exam: Sitting BP: 160/95 mm Hg in each arm, 160/95 mm Hg in right leg. Good-quality arterial pulses. Same BP 1 week later. All other findings normal.

Clinical Studies: ECG: normal. Chest roentgenogram: normal. Serum electrolyte levels (BUN, serum creatinine) and urinalysis: normal.

Diagnosis: Essential hypertension.

Impairment Rating: 1% to 3% impairment of the whole person.

Comment: Mild hypertension; check BP after medication.

Class 2
10%-29% Impairment of the Whole Person

Asymptomatic; stage 1 or 2 hypertension despite multiple medications

or

antihypertensive medication with any of the following: (1) proteinuria, urinary sediment abnormalities, no renal function impairment as measured by the blood urea nitrogen (BUN) and serum creatinine; (2) definite hypertensive changes on funduscopic examination in arterioles, eg, "copper" or "silver wiring," or arteriovenous crossing changes with or without hemorrhages and exudates; either abnormality suggests end-organ damage

---

Example 4-3
10% to 29% Impairment Due to Hypertensive Cardiovascular Disease

Subject: 44-year-old man.

History: Obstructive sleep apnea, hypertension; beta-blockers, diuretics, and ACE inhibitor.

Current Symptoms: Mild exertional dyspnea while jogging.

Physical Exam: BP: 145/90 mm Hg. Otherwise within normal limits. Mild silver arteriole wiring.

Clinical Studies: Electrolytes: normal.

Diagnosis: Essential hypertension resistant to treatment with persistent stage I hypertension.

Impairment Rating: 10% to 15% impairment of the whole person due to hypertensive disease; combine with a rating due to sleep apnea to determine whole person impairment.

Comment: Higher impairment if higher BP or more limiting symptoms. Note interaction between hypertension and obstructive sleep apnea and the persistence of hypertension despite multiple medications. Also check echo as exertional dyspnea may reflect LVH, which would increase impairment.

Chapter 4

Example 4-4
10% to 29% Impairment Due to Hypertensive Cardiovascular Disease

Subject: 40-year-old woman.

History: Elevated BP during pregnancy at 32; normal BP 3 weeks, 12 months postpartum. Recent bleeding between menstrual periods. Several BP readings between 150/100 and 160/105 mm Hg. Elevated leg BP. Low-salt diet and exercise program did not effectively lower BP. Medication needed.

Current Symptoms: Occasional headaches.

Physical Exam: Otherwise normal.

Clinical Studies: ECG: normal. Chest roentgenogram: normal. Serum electrolyte, BUN, and creatinine levels: normal. Urinalysis: 2+, twice-confirmed proteinuria; sediment: one to three red blood cells per high-power field; 24-hr urine collection: 1400 mg protein.

Diagnosis: Essential hypertension with proteinuria.

Impairment Rating: 15% impairment of the whole person.

Comment: Monitor for further renal impairment or other end-organ damage.

Class 3
30%-49% Impairment of the Whole Person

Asymptomatic; stage 3 hypertension despite multiple medications

or

antihypertensive medication with any of the following: (1) proteinuria, urinary sediment abnormalities, renal function impairment as measured by the BUN, and serum creatinine, and a decreased creatinine clearance of 20 to 50% normal; (2) LV hypertrophy by ECG or echocardiography but no symptoms of HF; either abnormality suggests more extensive end-organ damage

---

Example 4-5
30% to 49% Impairment Due to Hypertensive Cardiovascular Disease

Subject: 48-year-old man.

History: Severe hypertension; intermittent therapeutic drugs. Current triple therapy: beta-blocker, vasodilator, and diuretic.

Current Symptoms: None. Remains mildly active.

Physical Exam: BP: 170/95 mm Hg in both arms; PR: 64 BPM. No signs of congestive heart failure (CHF). Fundus: increased light reflexes from arterioles and arteriovenous crossing depressions; no hemorrhages or exudates. Disk flat. Enlarged, sustained LV impulse in normal position. Normal S_1; S_2 increased in intensity; S_4 present.

Clinical Studies: ECG: LV hypertrophy; tall R and inverted T waves in lateral chest leads. Chest roentgenogram: mild cardiomegaly; pulmonary vasculature normal. Serum electrolyte levels and urinalysis: normal.

Diagnosis: Essential hypertension and hypertensive heart disease with documented LV hypertrophy.

Impairment Rating: 30% to 39% impairment of the whole person.

Example 4-6
30% to 49% Impairment Due to Hypertensive Cardiovascular Disease

Subject: 55-year-old man

History: Hypertension; beta-blocker and ACE-inhibitor. Well-controlled BP remained in normal range.

Current Symptoms: None. Remains mildly active.

Physical Exam: Normal except for S_4; sustained apical impulse.

Clinical Studies: ECG: LV hypertrophy. Echocardiogram: consistent; concentric, increased wall thickness. Normal systolic function; II/IV diastolic dysfunction.

Diagnosis: Hypertensive heart disease with LV hypertrophy and early diastolic dysfunction.

Impairment Rating: 30% to 39% impairment of the whole person.

Comment: Evidence of end-organ damage but asymptomatic; medication adequately controls hypertension and treats end-organ dysfunction. Higher impairment if *(a)* more symptoms, *(b)* additional medications required to control hypertension, or *(c)* greater evidence of additional end-organ damage.

Class 4
50%-100% Impairment of the Whole Person

Antihypertensive medication with stages 1–3 and any of the following abnormalities: (1) proteinuria, urinary sediment abnormalities, renal function impairment as measured by the BUN and serum creatinine, and a creatinine clearance < 20% normal; (2) hypertensive cerebrovascular damage or episodic hypertensive encephalopathy; (3) LV hypertrophy, systolic dysfunction, and/or signs and symptoms of HF due to hypertension

---

Example 4-7
50% to 100% Impairment Due to Hypertensive Cardiovascular Disease

Subject: 48-year-old man.

History: In hospital 8 months ago for 2 weeks of headaches, blurred vision, and breathlessness. BP: 260/160 mm Hg in arms and legs. Drowsy; no localizing neurologic signs. Fundi: arterial spasm, hemorrhages, and bilateral papilledema.

Current Symptoms: Asymptomatic.

Physical Exam: Papilledema cleared with treatment, remained asymptomatic. Normal heart, lungs, abdomen.

Clinical Studies: Chest roentgenogram: normal. ECG: Low T waves in lateral chest leads. BUN: 14.3 mmol/L (40 mg/dL); serum creatinine: 203 mmol/L (2.3 mg/dL). Urinalysis: abnormal: 3+ proteinuria, numerous red blood cells, occasional white blood cells. Diastolic BP remained >120 mm Hg despite three antihypertensives.

Diagnosis: Essential hypertension with a history of hypertensive encephalopathy.

Impairment Rating: 55% impairment of the whole person.

Comment: Lower impairment if diastolic pressure, renal function return to normal but not if any of other findings persist.

Example 4-8
50% to 100% Impairment Due to Hypertensive Cardiovascular Disease

Subject: 62-year-old woman.

History: 10 years' BP treatment. Elevated BP despite medication, salt restriction, and weight control. CHF 2 years ago; improved with digitalis and diuretics.

Current Symptoms: 6 months' marked tiredness and breathlessness with ordinary activity; ankle edema. Difficulty in performing most activities of daily living.

Physical Exam: BP: 180/100 mm Hg in arms and legs. Ankle and lower leg edema. Fundus: increased arteriole light reflexes, arteriovenous crossing compressions, no hemorrhages or exudates; flat disks. Apical impulse: enlarged, sustained, displaced to anterior axillary line. Normal S_1; increased S_2; S_3 and S_4 present. Rales at both lung bases.

Clinical Studies: ECG: deep S wave in V_2; normal R waves in V_5 and V_6. Low T waves in I, L, and V_4 through V_6. Chest roentgenogram: cardiomegaly; pulmonary vasculature prominent in upper lung fields. Serum electrolyte, BUN, creatinine levels, and urinalysis: normal. Echocardiogram: increased wall thickness; dilated LV cavity with global hypokinesis; 0.30 EF.

Diagnosis: Essential hypertension with CHF.

Impairment Rating: 80% impairment of the whole person.

Comment: Lower impairment after hypertension treatment if improvement in HF symptoms and EF. *Note:* Impairment class corresponds to cardiomyopathy impairment in Chapter 3. Here, the class 4 impairment for hypertensive cardiovascular disease (CVD) is not combined with cardiomyopathy since hypertensive CVD class 4 includes cardiomyopathy.

4.2 Diseases of the Aorta

Diseases of the aorta, less prevalent than heart disease, can be more acutely life threatening. Diseases of the aorta include atherosclerotic dilatation, dilatation and/or stenosis from a concurrent connective tissue disease or vasculitis, and atheroembolic complications from diffuse aortic atherosclerosis.

Aortic atherosclerotic dilatation can progress to a significant degree and cause dyspnea, wheezing, cough, recurrent pneumonia, and hemoptysis. Aortic dilatation can be associated with significant aortic regurgitation and can also enlarge to the point of rupture and death.

The physician must obtain a careful and detailed history to estimate aortic involvement. Physical examination and chest roentgenogram may suggest aortic enlargement, but often a more advanced imaging assessment is necessary. MRI, CT scan, and transesophageal imaging identify aortic aneurysms, aortic vasculitic involvement, and atheromatous emboli sources. Laboratory studies help establish the presence of atheroemboli.[8-13]

4.2a Criteria for Rating Permanent Impairment Due to Diseases of the Aorta

See Table 4-3 for the classification of whole person impairment due to diseases of the aorta.

Table 4-3 Criteria for Rating Permanent Impairment Due to the Diseases of the Aorta

Class 1 0%-9% Impairment of the Whole Person	Class 2 10%-29% Impairment of the Whole Person	Class 3 30%-49% Impairment of the Whole Person	Class 4 50%-100% Impairment of the Whole Person
Asymptomatic during ordinary activities; has evidence of mild aortic abnormality that is unlikely to progress	Asymptomatic during ordinary activities; has a known progressive aortic abnormality *or* recovered from aortic surgery, asymptomatic, and is not expected to be at risk for future aortic disease as a consequence of surgery	Mild to moderate symptoms from aortic abnormality despite medication *or* recovered from aortic surgery, continues mild to moderate symptoms, or at risk for recurrence of aortic abnormality	Moderate to severe symptoms due to aortic abnormality that persist despite medication and that interfere with activities of daily living (functional class 3 or 4) *or* recovered from aortic surgery but moderate to severe symptoms persist despite medication

Class 1 0%-9% Impairment of the Whole Person
Asymptomatic during ordinary activities; has evidence of mild aortic abnormality that is unlikely to progress

Example 4-9
0% to 9% Impairment Due to Disease of the Aorta

Subject: 60-year-old woman.

History: Mild hypertension; well-controlled with medications.

Current Symptoms: Denies cardiac symptoms.

Physical Exam: Unremarkable.

Clinical Studies: CT scan: mild ectasia of ascending aorta to 45 mm. No aortic regurgitation. No significant atherosclerosis. Laboratory: normal.

Diagnosis: Ectasia of the ascending aorta.

Impairment Rating: 0% impairment of the whole person.

Comment: Aortic ectasia unlikely to progress to aortic aneurysm; no effect on function. Evaluate for impairment from hypertension.

Example 4-10
0% to 9% Impairment Due to Disease of the Aorta

Subject: 55-year-old man.

History: Excellent health except for past tobacco use.

Current Symptoms: Asymptomatic.

Physical Exam: Normal.

Clinical Studies: Abdominal ultrasound: 3.9-cm abdominal aortic aneurysm.

Diagnosis: Asymptomatic abdominal aortic aneurysm.

Impairment Rating: 0% to 5% impairment of the whole person.

Comment: Small abdominal aortic aneurysm may or may not progress. Periodic ultrasound or CT scan. Higher impairment if symptomatic.

Class 2 10%-29% Impairment of the Whole Person
Asymptomatic during ordinary activities; has a known progressive aortic abnormality
or
recovered from aortic surgery, asymptomatic, and is not expected to be at risk for future aortic disease as a consequence of surgery

Example 4-11
10% to 29% Impairment Due to Disease of the Aorta

Subject: 60-year-old man.

History: Uncomplicated surgical repair of abdominal aortic aneurysm 5 years ago.

Current Symptoms: None.

Physical Exam: Normal.

Clinical Studies: Abdominal ultrasound: well-seated graft; aneurysm repair site normal.

Diagnosis: Abdominal aortic aneurysm with surgical repair; no evidence of recurrence.

Impairment Rating: 10% to 15% of the whole person.

Comment: Higher impairment if graft failure evidence, adjacent vasculature enlargement, or peripheral embolization from the graft.

Example 4-12
10% to 29% Impairment Due to Disease of the Aorta

Subject: 50-year-old man.

History: Mixed connective tissue disorder.

Current Symptoms: None at rest. Participating in community senior sports league causes symptoms.

Physical Exam: BP: 130/50 mm Hg; PR: 88 BPM; 1/6 diastolic murmur.

Clinical Studies: Transesophageal echocardiogram: proximal ascending aortic enlargement at 50 mm; mild aortic regurgitation.

Diagnosis: Proximal ascending aortic aneurysm, asymptomatic.

Impairment Rating: 10% to 20% impairment of the whole person.

Comment: Aortic aneurysm at increased risk of progression. Asymptomatic but annual follow-ups for aneurysm progression.

Class 3 30%-49% Impairment of the Whole Person
Mild to moderate symptoms from aortic abnormality despite medication
or
recovered from aortic surgery, continues mild to moderate symptoms, or at risk for recurrence of aortic abnormality

Example 4-13
30% to 49% Impairment Due to Disease of the Aorta

Subject: 48-year-old woman.

History: Twice experienced peripheral atheroembolic complications from diffuse aortic atherosclerosis. "Blue toe" resolved with treatment; mild renal insufficiency after subcutaneous heparin injections for deep vein thrombosis (DVT) prophylaxis following uncomplicated knee arthroscopic procedure.

Current Symptoms: Fatigue and pain on walking long distances.

Physical Exam: Embolic lesions on foot.

Clinical Studies: Transesophageal echocardiogram: "shaggy atheromatous" changes in distal descending thoracic aorta; one mobile atheromatous plaque 0.5 mm by 1.5 mm. Enlarged ascending aorta 54 mm in sinotubular junction. Stopped smoking; statin cholesterol-lowering agent for hyperlipidemia. Combination beta-blocker and alpha-blocker for aneurysm.

Diagnosis: Proximal ascending aortic aneurysm with diffuse atheromatous involvement of the descending aorta with two episodes of peripheral thromboembolism.

Impairment Rating: 30% to 40% impairment of the whole person.

Comment: Aortic aneurysm at increased risk of progression. Increased risk for further atheromatous emboli.

Chapter 4

Example 4-14
30% to 49% Impairment Due to Disease of the Aorta

Subject: 54-year-old man.

History: Ascending aortic aneurysm. Mildly enlarged proximal ascending aorta 48 mm; traumatic dissection repair primarily involved descending thoracic aorta. Mild preoperative aortic regurgitation; no aortic valve replacement.

Current Symptoms: Exertional dyspnea with exercise and after walking 1.5 blocks. Denies angina, orthopnea, and paroxysmal nocturnal dyspnea.

Physical Exam: BP: 140/45 mm Hg; PR: 92 BPM. Normal neck veins; 3/6 diastolic decrescendo murmur at upper sternal border—right > left. LV apical impulse laterally displaced, mildly sustained to palpation. Remainder of examination normal.

Clinical Studies: Chest roentgenogram: mild aortic ectasia and LV enlargement. Echocardiogram: class 3 aortic regurgitation; increased diastolic dimensions 58 cm. 0.62 LVEF. Transesophageal echocardiogram: enlarged ascending aorta 54 mm; secondary aortic regurgitation. Exercise stress test: 5.2 minutes on Bruce protocol; HR 144. Stopped because of dyspnea.

Diagnosis: Progressive symptomatic aortic regurgitation secondary to an ascending aortic aneurysm.

Impairment Rating: 30% to 49% impairment of the whole person.

Comment: Enlarging aortic aneurysm, aortic regurgitation secondary to aneurysm. Symptoms, significant limitation from aneurysm. Higher impairment if more symptoms or greater severity of valvular dysfunction. Overlap often seen among aortic, valvular, and cardiomyopathic heart diseases.

Class 4
50%-100% Impairment of the Whole Person
Moderate to severe symptoms due to aortic abnormality that persist despite medication and that interfere with activities of daily living (functional class 3 or 4)
or
patient recovered from aortic surgery but moderate to severe symptoms persist despite medication

Example 4-15
50% to 100% Impairment Due to Disease of the Aorta

Subject: 62-year-old man.

History: Surgical treatment of dissecting proximal aortic aneurysm 2 years ago; valved conduit. Postoperative complaint: exertional dyspnea; moderately severe aortic regurgitation. Symptoms persist despite beta-blocker, an ACE-inhibitor, and loop diuretic.

Current Symptoms: Dyspnea after 1 block of exertion; discontinued exercise. Requires nap every afternoon. No hypertension.

Physical Exam: BP: 150/85 mm Hg; PR: 96 BPM; 4/6 diastolic murmur at upper right sternal border.

Clinical Studies: Continued dissection of aorta distal to graft insertion.

Diagnosis: Moderately severe aortic regurgitation with exertional dyspnea following repair of proximal aortic dissection.

Impairment Rating: 60% to 70% impairment of the whole person.

Comment: Leakage of valved conduit and residual distal dissection. Symptoms are of moderately severe intensity (class 3).

Example 4-16
50% to 100% Impairment Due to Disease of the Aorta

Subject: 52-year-old man.

History: Diffuse aortic atherosclerosis; multiple atheroembolisms for 2 years. Lipid-lowering and potent antiplatelet medications. Nonsmoker for 8 years.

Current Symptoms: Moderate to severe exertional dyspnea (< 1 block); moderate edema. Some inconsistent claudication. Unable to perform most activities of daily living.

Physical Exam: Lower extremity livedo reticularis; pitting edema.

Clinical Studies: Three emergent surgical embolectomies. Moderate renal impairment.

Diagnosis: Severe, diffuse atheroemboli from aortic atherosclerosis with concurrent peripheral edema and moderate renal failure.

Impairment Rating: 60% to 80% impairment of the whole person.

Comment: Progressive condition; very symptomatic. No surgical therapies exist given diffuse nature of aortic atherosclerosis. Potential impairment from three body systems—aorta, kidney, and peripheral vascular—should be integrated in determining the total degree of impairment.

4.3 Vascular Diseases Affecting the Extremities

Peripheral vascular disease (PVD) that leads to permanent impairment usually includes (1) arterial disorders that reduce blood flow and lead to one or more of the following: intermittent claudication, pain at rest, minor trophic changes, ulceration, gangrene, extremity loss, or **Raynaud's phenomenon;** (2) venous disorders that lead to one or more of the following: pain, edema, induration, stasis dermatitis, or ulceration; or (3) lymphatic disorders that lead to chronic lymphedema and may be complicated by recurrent acute infection.

Arterial disorders are most commonly caused by arteriosclerosis, trauma, and inflammatory processes such as thromboangiitis obliterans. The venous system is most frequently affected by varicose veins, thrombosis, and chronic deep venous insufficiency. The lymphatic system may become impaired by inflammatory or neoplastic processes.

Noninvasive laboratory studies are valuable in confirming occlusive arterial disease or venous abnormalities of the extremities. To estimate functional impairment due to occlusive peripheral arterial disease, determine ankle or arm systolic pressure indices before, and 1 minute after, standard exercise (eg, walking on a treadmill at 2 miles per hour at a 10% grade for 5 minutes, or something less strenuous if the individual's symptoms warrant it).[14, 15]

Before evaluating impairment, establish a specific diagnosis of vascular disease. The impairment estimate depends on the extent, severity, and impact of the lesions rather than on the specific diagnosis.

Table 4-4 provides a classification of impairments due to peripheral vascular disease. Physical signs of vascular damage must be present and are the primary determinants in placing the the examinee into one of these classes. Raynaud's phenomenon consists of localized blanching of one or more fingers, followed by a period of cyanosis, followed by erythema. Pain on exposure to cold or generalized paleness of the fingers on exposure to cold do not in themselves indicate Raynuad's. When amputation due to peripheral vascular disease is involved, the impairment due to amputation should be evaluated separately and combined with the appropriate value in Table 4-4 using the Combined Values Chart (p. 604).

It is important to differentiate Raynaud's symptoms on the basis of obstructive physiology from those occurring because of vasoreactivity. Individuals with obstructive physiology will often experience symptoms more frequently and to a greater degree of severity. Establish the presence of obstructive physiology by objective testing. Arterial pressure ratios between the affected digits and the brachial pressure (finger/brachial index) are easily performed. A ratio of < 0.8 suggests obstructive physiology, even if Raynaud's symptoms are not present. Obstuctive physiology can also be established by the use of cutaneous laser Doppler flowmetry. This technique is established and can reliably assess microcirculation performance and real time changes in skin blood flow.[16]

4.3a Criteria for Rating Permanent Impairment Due to Vascular Diseases Affecting the Extremities

The criteria for evaluating impairment due to vascular diseases of the upper extremity are found in Table 4-4; for lower extremity, Table 4-5.

To translate an upper extremity impairment into a whole person impairment, multiply the upper extremity impairment by 0.6 or use Table 16-3 in the upper extremities chapter. To translate the lower extremity impairment to a whole person impairment, multiply the lower impairment by 0.4, or use Table 17-3 in the lower extremities chapter.

Table 4-4 Criteria for Rating Permanent Impairment of the Upper Extremity Due to Peripheral Vascular Disease

Class 1 0%-9% Impairment of the Upper Extremity	Class 2 10%-39% Impairment of the Upper Extremity	Class 3 40%-69% Impairment of the Upper Extremity	Class 4 70%-89% Impairment of the Upper Extremity	Class 5 90%-100% Impairment of the Upper Extremity
Neither intermittent claudication nor pain at rest *or* only transient edema *and* on physical examination, not more than the following findings are present: loss of pulses; minimal loss of subcutaneous tissue of fingertips; calcification of arteries as detected by radiographic examination; asymptomatic dilation of arteries or of veins, not requiring surgery and not resulting in curtailment of activity *or* Raynaud's symptoms with or without obstructive physiology (as documented by finger brachial indices of < 0.8 or low digital temperatures with decreased laser Doppler signals that do not normalize with warming of affected digits) that completely responds to lifestyle changes and/or medical therapy	Intermittent claudication on severe upper extremity usage *or* persistent edema of a moderate degree, controlled by elastic supports *or* vascular damage evidenced by a sign such as a healed, painless stump of an amputated digit showing evidence of persistent vascular disease, or a healed ulcer *or* Raynaud's phenomena with obstructive physiology (as documented by finger/brachial indices of < 0.8 or low digital temperatures with decreased laser Doppler signals that do not normalize with warming of affected digits) that incompletely responds to lifestyle changes and/or medical therapy	Intermittent claudication on mild upper extremity usage *or* marked edema that is only partially controlled by elastic supports *and* vascular damage evidenced by a healed amputation of two or more digits of one extremity, with evidence of persisting vascular disease or superficial ulceration	Intermittent claudication on mild upper extremity usage *or* marked edema that cannot be controlled by elastic supports *or* vascular damage as evidenced by signs such as an amputation at or above a wrist, or amputation of two or more digits of both extremities with evidence of persistent vascular disease; or persistent widespread or deep ulceration involving one extremity	Severe and constant pain at rest *or* vascular damage evidenced by signs such as amputation at or above the wrists of both extremities, or amputation of all digits of both extremities with evidence of persistent, widespread, or deep ulceration involving both upper extremities

Class 1 0%-9% Impairment of the Upper Extremity
Neither intermittent claudication nor pain at rest *or* only transient edema *and* on physical examination, not more than the following findings are present: loss of pulses; minimal loss of subcutaneous tissue of fingertips; calcification of arteries as detected by radiographic examination; asymptomatic dilation of arteries or of veins, not requiring surgery and not resulting in curtailment of activity *or* Raynaud's symptoms with or without obstructive physiology (as documented by finger brachial indices of < 0.8 or low digital temperatures with decreased laser Doppler signals that do not normalize with warming of affected digits) that completely responds to lifestyle changes and/or medical therapy

Example 4-17
0% to 9% Impairment of the Upper Extremity

Subject: 25-year-old man.

History: Raynaud's phenomenon of fingers for 1 year.

Current Symptom's: Fingers blanch and painful when exposed to cold or stress. Some impairment in performing activities of daily living.

Physical Exam: Normal. Blanching of digits due to exposure to temperatures $< 0°C$ ($32°F$) or extreme emotional stress; 1 mg of prazosin twice daily relieved problem, except on rare occasions.

Clinical Studies: Finger/brachial index = 0.6.

Diagnosis: Raynaud's phenomenon, with obstructive physiology.

Impairment Rating: 5% to 9% impairment of the upper extremity.

Comment: Some interference with activities of daily living.

<table>
<tr><td>

Class 2
10%-39% Impairment of the Upper Extremity

Intermittent claudication on severe upper extremity usage

or

persistent edema of a moderate degree, controlled by elastic supports

or

vascular damage evidenced by a sign such as a healed, painless stump of an amputated digit showing evidence of persistent vascular disease, or a healed ulcer

or

Raynaud's phenomena with obstructive physiology (as documented by finger/brachial indices of < 0.8 or low digital temperatures with decreased laser Doppler signals that do not normalize with warming of affected digits) that incompletely responds to lifestyle changes and/or medical therapy

</td><td>

Class 3
40%-69% Impairment of the Upper Extremity

Intermittent claudication on mild upper extremity usage

or

marked edema that is only partially controlled by elastic supports

and

vascular damage evidenced by a healed amputation of two or more digits of one extremity, with evidence of persisting vascular disease or superficial ulceration

</td></tr>
</table>

Example 4-18
10% to 39% Impairment of the Upper Extremity

Subject: 58-year-old man.

History: Gangrenous second finger of right hand. Arteriovenous fistula for chronic hemodialysis due to renal failure secondary to diabetes mellitus.

Current Symptoms: Performs most daily activities.

Physical Exam: Gangrenous second finger.

Clinical Studies: Angiography: tight stenosis distal to AV fistula. Stenosis treated with percutaneous transluminal coronary angioplasty (PTCA), but digit required amputation.

Diagnosis: Gangrene of the finger secondary to PVD.

Impairment Rating: 35% to 39% impairment of the upper extremity.

Comment: Gangrene of a single digit with evidence of persistent PVD. Higher impairment if additional amputated digits or if he experiences symptoms. Additional impairment may be assigned due to degree of renal failure requiring dialysis and evidence of end-organ damage from diabetes mellitus.

Example 4-19
40% to 69% Impairment of the Upper Extremity

Subject: 45-year-old woman.

History: Raynaud's phenomenon from scleroderma for 9 years.

Current Symptoms: Ulcerations on tips of index and ring fingers of both hands, which completely healed with conservative measures and prazosin.

Physical Exam: Autoamputation of the distal half of the distal phalanges of the index and ring fingers of the left hand.

Clinical Studies: A finger/brachial ratio of 0.6 and laser Doppler signals consistent with microcirculatory impairment.

Diagnosis: Scleroderma with Raynaud's phenomenon and multiple digital ulcerations and partial amputation of two digits.

Impairment Rating: 55% impairment of the upper extremity due to vascular disease, combined with 25% impairment of the index and ring fingers due to amputation. Combining these values yields an impairment of 66% of the left upper extremity, or 40% whole person impairment. The right upper extremity is in the middle range of class 2, or 25% of the upper right extremity, or 15% of the body as a whole. Combining these values yields 49% of the body as a whole.

Comment: This woman has experienced Raynaud's phenomenon secondary to obstructive physiology but has also suffered autoamputation of portions of two digits. The left upper extremity was put in the midrange of class 3 because she has loss of only the distal portion of two digits. The right upper extremity was put in the middle range of class 2 because of the presence of ulcerations without amputation.

Chapter 4

Class 5
90%-100% Impairment of the Upper Extremity
Severe and constant pain at rest
or
vascular damage evidenced by signs such as amputation at or above the wrists of both extremities, or amputation of all digits of both extremities with evidence of persistent, widespread, or deep ulceration involving both upper extremities

Example 4-20
90% to 100% Impairment of the Upper Extremity

Subject: 48-year-old man.

History: Traumatic amputation of both hands in construction accident. Constant phantom pain in both extremities.

Current Symptoms: Phantom pain bilaterally.

Physical Exam: Healed amputations of both wrists in upper extremities; no ulcerations noted.

Clinical Studies: None.

Diagnosis: Traumatic amputation with phantom pain.

Impairment Rating: 100% impairment of the upper extremity.

Table 4-5 Criteria for Rating Permanent Impairment of the Lower Extremity Due to Peripheral Vascular Disease

Class 1 0%-9% Impairment of the Lower Extremity	Class 2 10%-39% Impairment of the Lower Extremity	Class 3 40%-69% Impairment of the Lower Extremity	Class 4 70%-89% Impairment of the Lower Extremity	Class 5 90%-100% Impairment the Lower Extremity
Neither intermittent claudication nor pain at rest *or* only transient edema *and* on physical examination, not more than the following findings are present: loss of pulses; minimal loss of subcutaneous tissue; calcification of arteries as detected by radiographic examination; asymptomatic dilation of arteries or of veins, not requiring surgery and not resulting in curtailment of activity	Intermittent claudication on severe usage of the lower extremity *or* persistent edema of a moderate degree, controlled by elastic supports *or* vascular damage evidenced by a sign such as a healed, painless stump of an amputated digit showing evidence of persistent vascular disease, or a healed ulcer	Intermittent claudication on walking as few as 25 yards and no more than 100 yards at average pace *or* marked edema that is only partially controlled by elastic supports *and* vascular damage evidenced by a sign such as healed amputation of two or more digits of one extremity, with evidence of persisting vascular disease or superficial ulceration	Intermittent claudication on walking less than 25 yards, or intermittent pain at rest *or* marked edema that cannot be controlled by elastic supports *or* vascular damage as evidenced by signs such as an amputation at or above an ankle, or amputation of two or more digits of two extremities with evidence of persistent vascular disease; or persistent widespread or deep ulceration involving one extremity	Severe and constant pain at rest *or* vascular damage evidenced by signs such as amputation at or above the ankles of two extremities, or amputation of all digits of two or more extremities with evidence of persistent, widespread, or deep ulceration involving two or more extremities

Class 1
0%-9% Impairment of the Lower Extremity
Neither intermittent claudication nor pain at rest
or
only transient edema
and
on physical examination, not more than the following findings are present: loss of pulses; minimal loss of subcutaneous tissue; calcification of arteries as detected by radiographic examination; asymptomatic dilation of arteries or of veins, not requiring surgery and not resulting in curtailment of activity

Example 4-21
0% to 9% impairment of the Lower Extremity

Subject: 48-year-old man.

History: Left leg edema after coronary artery bypass graft (CABG) surgery. No DVT or lower extremity cellulitis. Compression stocking; no further symptoms. Mild edema 1 year ago when he forgot stocking.

Physical Exam: Normal.

Clinical Studies: Noninvasive venous plethysmography; mild incompetence of left lower extremity veins.

Diagnosis: Mild incompetence of the left lower extremity venous system.

Impairment Rating: 0% to 9% impairment of the lower extremity.

Comment: Mild incompetence of deep venous system following vein harvesting for CABG surgery. Symptoms controlled by compression stocking. Has no limitations. Higher impairment if (*a*) more symptoms, (*b*) venous compression stocking not controlling symptoms on intermittent basis, or (*c*) signs of venous stasis dermatitis or other signs of chronic venous incompetence.

Class 2
10%–39% Impairment of the Lower Extremity

Intermittent claudication on severe usage of the lower extremity

or

persistent edema of a moderate degree, controlled by elastic supports

or

vascular damage evidenced by a sign such as a healed, painless stump of an amputated digit showing evidence of persistent vascular disease, or a healed ulcer

---

Example 4-22
10% to 39% Impairment of the Lower Extremity

Subject: 36-year-old man.

History: Progressive swelling of both lower extremities for 8 years; edema did not recede overnight. Four to eight episodes a year of acute malaise with chills and fever that required treatment of the dermatophytosis and monthly injections of long-acting penicillin.

Current Symptoms: Leg edema receded incompletely with elevation for 3 days; incompletely controlled with heavy-duty, fitted leotard.

Physical Exam: Firm edema of both legs, feet, and toes. Bilateral interdigital fissuring (typical of dermatophytosis).

Clinical Studies: None.

Diagnosis: Lymphedema of both legs secondary to recurring lymphangitis.

Impairment Rating: 20% impairment of the lower extremity.

Comment: Moderate edema incompletely controlled by elastic support.

Example 4-23
10% to 39% Impairment of the Lower Extremity

Subject: 48-year-old woman.

History: Diabetic. Amputation of gangrenous fourth toe 1 year ago. Completed physical rehabilitation; ambulates normally. Returned to teaching.

Current Symptoms: Denies further trouble with lower extremity ulcers.

Physical Exam: Well-healed amputation site; no additional abnormalities. Gait essentially normal.

Clinical Studies: Glucose level: slighty elevated.

Diagnosis: Amputation of left fourth toe for gangrene, now resolved.

Impairment Rating: 20% to 30% impairment of the lower extremity.

Comment: Complete recovery from amputation. Higher impairment if additional digits amputated or if ambulation limited from surgery.

Class 3
40%–69% Impairment of the Lower Extremity

intermittent claudication on walking as few as 25 yards and no more than 100 yards at average pace

or

marked edema that is only partially controlled by elastic supports

and

vascular damage evidenced by a sign such as healed amputation of two or more digits of one extremity, with evidence of persisting vascular disease or superficial ulceration

---

Example 4-24
40% to 69% Impairment of the Lower Extremity

Subject: 54-year-old man.

History: PVD complication: ulcerated left great toe. Conservative treatment failed; toe gangrenous. Toe amputated; returned to work but could not perform duties on foot. Ulcerated then gangrenous right fifth toe 6 months later; toe amputated. Individual recovered; asymptomatic. Gait returned to preoperative level for short distances.

Current Symptoms: Difficulty standing or walking for long periods.

Physical Exam: Well-healed amputation sites; no ulcerations.

Clinical Studies: None.

Diagnosis: Amputation of two digits secondary to PVD.

Impairment Rating: 60% to 69% impairment of the lower extremity.

Comment: Encourage excellent foot hygiene.

Class 4
70%-89% Impairment of the Lower Extremity

Intermittent claudication on walking less than 25 yards, or intermittent pain at rest

or

marked edema that cannot be controlled by elastic supports

or

vascular damage as evidenced by signs such as an amputation at or above an ankle, or amputation of two or more digits of two extremities with evidence of persistent vascular disease; or persistent widespread or deep ulceration involving one extremity

---

Example 4-25
70% to 89% Impairment of the Lower Extremity

Subject: 24-year-old man.

History: 3 years' recurrent thrombophlebitis in lower extremities. Venous stasis ulceration of right ankle 1 year ago; bed rest, skin grafting to effect healing. Long-term oral anticoagulant therapy to prevent further thrombosis.

Current Symptoms: Difficulty with prolonged standing and ambulation.

Physical Exam: Marked standing bilateral leg and ankle edema despite full-length fitted elastic stockings.

Clinical Studies: Noninvasive venous plethysmography: recurrent thrombophlebitis; deep venous insufficiency.

Diagnosis: Recurrent thrombophlebitis with bilateral chronic postphlebitic deep venous insufficiency.

Impairment Rating: 80% impairment of the lower extremity.

Comment: Marked, postphlebitic deep venous insufficiency caused venous stasis ulceration; dependent leg edema poorly controlled by elastic support.

Example 4-26
70% to 89% Impairment of the Lower Extremity

Subject: 62-year-old man.

History: Diabetic.

Current Symptoms: Painful extremity ulcers; tenderness in foot. Claudication when walking short distances.

Physical Exam: Painful ulcers on third, fourth, and fifth toes of left foot.

Clinical Studies: Peripheral angiography: diffuse distal arterial disease. Transcutaneous oximetry: limited amputation unlikely to effect healing.

Diagnosis: Severe claudication with painful ulcers.

Impairment Rating: 80% to 89% impairment of the lower extremity.

Comment: May need BKA to resolve ulcers. Needs excellent control of diabetes.

Class 5
90%-100% Impairment of the Lower Extremity

Severe and constant pain at rest

or

vascular damage evidenced by signs such as amputation at or above the ankles of two extremities, or amputation of all digits of two or more extremities with evidence of persistent, widespread, or deep ulceration involving two or more extremities

---

Example 4-27
90% to 100% Impairment of the Lower Extremity

Subject: 56-year-old man.

History: Myocardial infarction; category III angina pectoris. Type 1 diabetic. Symptomatic arteriosclerosis obliterans in lower extremities for 9 years. Walking capacity < 25 feet; calf pain.

Current Symptoms: Pain worse at night. Progressing renal insufficiency; creatinine 407 mmol/L (4.6 mg/dL).

Physical Exam: Cool extremity. Painful, nonhealing ulcers right great toe and heel.

Clinical Studies: Ankle brachial indices < 0.3.

Diagnosis: Arteriosclerosis obliterans with ischemic ulceration and ischemic rest pain in diabetic man with severe CAD and moderate renal insufficiency.

Impairment Rating: 95% impairment of the lower extremity.

Comment: Severe occlusive peripheral arterial disease warrants procedure to restore pulsatile flow to right leg. Arteriography hazardous due to renal insufficiency; coronary disease markedly increases surgical risk. Consider renal transplant.

4.4 Diseases of the Pulmonary Arteries

Primary pulmonary hypertension is a consequence of obliterative and plexiform changes of unknown etiology in the pulmonary arteriolar bed. Many other causes of pulmonary hypertension include pulmonary parenchymal disease, left-sided HF, CHF, and PVD (either from pulmonary emboli or systemic disease). Pulmonary venous and capillary system disorders can also produce pulmonary hypertension. All of these disorders are classified disorders of the pulmonary circulation for impairment assessment.

The physician should take a careful history of functional impairment and symptoms for individuals with pulmonary hypertension. Classic findings include a right ventricular (RV) lift and an increased intensity of the S_2 pulmonic component. Pulmonary hypertension is often diagnosed by chest roentgenogram changes, RV hypertrophy, or ECG strain. The definitive

assessment of pulmonary hypertension is made by PAP assessment with an echocardiogram or right heart catheterization.[17-20]

4.4a Criteria for Rating Permanent Impairment Due to Pulmonary Hypertension

The degree of pulmonary hypertension can be classified by the measurement of PAP or PA resistance. Impairment classification should be based on more than the observed PAP; also consider the presence or absence of signs and symptoms of right HF. Dyspnea is the most limiting symptom of pulmonary hypertension. Cyanosis may occur from right to left shunting, especially in individuals with pulmonary hypertension associated with CHF.

Table 4-6 lists the impairment criteria for disorders of the pulmonary circulation. (The *Guides* follows the new World Health Organization [WHO] criteria for pulmonary hypertension classification.[21])

Table 4-6 Criteria for Rating Permanent Impairment Due to Pulmonary Hypertension

Class 1 0%-9% Impairment of the Whole Person	Class 2 10%-29% Impairment of the Whole Person	Class 3 30%-49% Impairment of the Whole Person	Class 4 50%-100% Impairment of the Whole Person
No symptoms or signs of right HF and mild pulmonary hypertension (PAP 40-50 mm Hg) or a Doppler echocardiography–derived peak tricuspid velocity of 3.0-3.5 m/sec	No symptoms or signs of right HF and moderate PA hypertension (PAP 51-75 mm Hg)	Moderate pulmonary hypertension (PAP > 75 mm Hg) *and* signs and symptoms of right HF *or* symptoms of mild limitation (class 2) with any degree of pulmonary hypertension	Severe pulmonary hypertension (PAP > 75 mm Hg) *or* symptoms of severe limitation (class 3 or 4) with any degree of pulmonary hypertension

Class 1 0%-9% Impairment of the Whole Person
No symptoms or signs of right HF and mild pulmonary hypertension (PAP 40-50 mm Hg) or a Doppler echocardiography–derived peak tricuspid velocity of 3.0-3.5 m/sec

Example 4-28
0% to 9% Impairment Due to Pulmonary Hypertension

Subject: 43-year-old man.

History: Moderate obesity (body mass index 29). No diet pill or illicit drug use.

Current Symptoms: No symptoms.

Physical Exam: Systolic ejection murmur.

Clinical Studies: Chest roentgenogram: normal. ECG: normal. Echocardiogram: normal ventricular function. Mild pulmonary hypertension; estimated PAP 45 mm Hg. Heart valves: normal.

Diagnosis: Mild pulmonary hypertension.

Impairment Rating: 0% to 5% impairment of the whole person.

Comment: Counsel individual to exercise regularly and lose weight. Higher impairment if right HF symptoms.

Example 4-29
0% to 9% Impairment Due to Pulmonary Hypertension

Subject: 48-year-old woman.

History: Smoker for 35 years.

Current Symptoms: Dyspnea with slight exertion. No angina or peripheral edema.

Physical Exam: Prolonged expiration otherwise normal.

Clinical Studies: Echocardiogram: normal LV size and function, valvular function, right heart size and function. Mild PA hypertension; estimated PAP: 45 mm Hg; systemic pressure: 120 mm Hg. Pulmonary function testing: moderate chronic obstructive pulmonary disease (COPD); FEV_1 55%. Counseled to stop smoking.

Diagnosis: Mild pulmonary hypertension secondary to COPD.

Impairment Rating: 5% impairment of the whole person

Comment: Combine impairment from PA hypertension with respiratory impairment to determine whole person impairment.

Class 2
10%-29% Impairment of the Whole Person
No symptoms or signs of right HF and moderate PA hypertension (PAP 51-75 mm Hg)

Example 4-30
10% to 29% Impairment Due to Pulmonary Hypertension

Subject: 58-year-old woman.

History: Fully recovered from pulmonary embolism 5 years ago.

Current Symptoms: None. Exercises regularly

Physical Exam: Normal; soft, 1/6 holosystolic heart murmur, intensifies with inspiration.

Clinical Studies: Echocardiogram: PAP: 55 mm Hg. Mildly enlarged RV; moderate pulmonary valve regurgitation.

Diagnosis: Moderate pulmonary hypertension secondary to possible pulmonary embolism.

Impairment Rating: 10% to 15% of the whole person.

Comment: Higher impairment if any signs of right HF. Identify potential underlying cause, particularly chronic pulmonary thromboembolic disease.

Example 4-31
10% to 29% Impairment Due to Pulmonary Hypertension

Subject: 38-year-old woman.

History: Heart murmur. Exercises regularly; lost 24.7 kg (55 lbs).

Current Symptoms: Denies right HF symptoms.

Physical Exam: Normal; jugular pressure normal.

Clinical Studies: Echocardiogram: mild tricuspid and pulmonary regurgitation. Mild RV enlargement. Normal systolic function; estimated PAP: 60 mm Hg. Systemic pressure: 110 mm Hg.

Diagnosis: Moderate pulmonary artery hypertension with mild RV enlargement. No signs of HF.

Impairment Rating: 15% to 20% impairment of the whole person.

Comment: Moderate pulmonary hypertension. No evidence of right HF. Evaluate regularly; treat possible causes of pulmonary hypertension to prevent progression. If persistent, consider vasodilator therapy.

Class 3
30%-49% Impairment of the Whole Person
Moderate pulmonary hypertension (PAP > 75 mm Hg)
and
signs and symptoms of right HF
or
symptoms of mild limitation (class 2) with any degree of pulmonary hypertension

Example 4-32
30% to 49% Impairment Due to Pulmonary Hypertension

Subject: 38-year-old woman.

History: Abnormal ECG. 2 years' moderate dyspnea while walking up two flights of stairs.

Current Symptoms: External dyspnea.

Physical Exam: Right ventricular heave; increased P_2.

Clinical Studies: Echocardiogram: estimated PAP: 70 mm Hg. Normal LV, RV function; no significant valvular disease. Systemic pressure 120 mm Hg.

Diagnosis: Primary pulmonary hypertension with symptoms of mild limitation (class 2).

Impairment Rating: 30% to 40% impairment of the whole person.

Comment: Evaluation included cardiac catheterization and pulmonary angiography. Diagnosis made after other causes excluded. Initiate appropriate treatment.

Example 4-33
30% to 49% Impairment Due to Pulmonary Hypertension

Subject: 58-year-old man.

History: Pulmonary embolism after arthroscopic knee surgery 5 years ago.

Current Symptoms: Exertional dyspnea during doubles tennis; moderate (2+) pitting edema at end of workday.

Physical Exam: Parasternal heave left and right lower sternal border; tricuspid regurgitation.

Clinical Studies: Echocardiogram: pulmonary hypertension. PAP: 55 mm Hg; systemic BP: 140 mm Hg. Moderate RV enlargement; moderately severe grade 3 out of 4 tricuspid regurgitation. Started on nitrates, digitalis, and diuretics. After 3 months, dyspnea present; less peripheral edema.

Diagnosis: Moderate pulmonary hypertension and RV failure possibly secondary to pulmonary embolism.

Impairment Rating: 40% to 49% impairment of the whole person.

Comment: Moderate pulmonary hypertension and right HF that improved slightly on medical therapy. Higher impairment if symptoms progress. Directed evaluation and treatment are warranted.

| **Class 4** |
| **50%-100% Impairment of the Whole Person** |
| Severe pulmonary hypertension (PAP > 75 mm Hg) |
| *or* |
| symptoms of severe limitation (class 3 or 4) with any degree of pulmonary hypertension |

Example 4-34
50% to 100% Impairment Due to Pulmonary Hypertension

Subject: 42-year-old woman.

History: Primary pulmonary hypertension. PAP: 80 mm Hg; systemic pressure: 120 mm Hg. Mild shortness of breath when pulling luggage at airport. Denies edema, other symptoms; lips turn blue with exertion.

Current Symptoms: Perform some daily activities without dyspnea; symptomatic with moderately severe exertion.

Phyical Exam: Increased right ventricular heave; increased P_2.

Clinical Studies: Echocardiagram: increased pulmonary pressure estimated at 70 mm Hg.

Diagnosis: Primary pulmonary hypertension with mild symptoms.

Impairment Rating: 50% to 70% impairment of the whole person.

Comment: Higher impairment if greater difficulty performing activities of daily living.

Example 4-35
50% to 100% Impairment Due to Pulmonary Hypertension

Subject: 37-year-old man.

History: Scleroderma; CREST syndrome. Treatment: diuretics, nitrates, and digitalis.

Current Symtoms: Exertional dyspnea with mild to moderate exertion. Daily morning peripheral edema. Very tired by midmorning.

Physical Exam: Changes of scleroderma; systolic heart murmur along lower left sternal border.

Clinical Studies: Echocardiogram: large RV with severely depressed function. Estimated PAP: 58 mm Hg. Normal LV, left-sided heart valve function. Exercise stress test: significant functional impairment; 3.5 minutes on Bruce protocol before stopping with severe dyspnea. Peak HR: 115 BPM.

Diagnosis: Pulmonary hypertension with associated scleroderma and symptoms of moderate to severe functional limitation.

Impairment Rating: 70% to 90% impairment due to cardiovascular disease; combine with impairment due to muskuloskeletal disorders to determine whole person impairment.

Comment: Moderate pulmonary hypertension; significant functional limitation and comorbid disease.

4.5 Cardiovascular Impairment Evaluation Summary

See Table 4.7 for an evaluation summary for the assessment of systemic and pulmonary artery cardiovascular impairment.

Table 4-7 Cardiac Impairment Evaluation Summary

Disorder	History, Including Major Relevant Symptoms	Examination Record	Assessment of Cardiac Function
General	Determine degree of functional impairment with regard to activities of daily living	Jugular venous pressure; comment on carotid and peripheral vascular pulses; heart and lung exam; abdominal exam; fundoscopic exam; blood pressure taken in supine, sitting, and standing positions	Data derived from relevant studies (eg, ECG, echocardiogram, stress tests, cardiac catheterization)
Hypertensive Cardiovascular Disease	Determine symptoms that document cardiac, renal, and cerebrovascular limitation	Comprehensive; note end-organ conditions	ECG, echocardiogram, stress testing, catheterization; serum BUN and creatinine, urinalysis and urinary protein excretion, creatinine clearance or GFR assessment; renal ultrasound; head CT or MRI scan; angiography
Aortic Disease	Determine impairment of daily activities and of cardiac and peripheral vascular function	Comprehensive examination	Transthoracic and transesophageal echocardiography; CT and/or MRI imaging; aortic angiography
Peripheral Vascular Disease	Full history, including degree of limitation of activities of daily living	Comprehensive examination	Stress testing; ankle-brachial pressure indices and transcutaneous oximetry; peripheral angiography; venous imaging with dye or ultrasound/Doppler Lymphatic assessment with contrast or tagged markers
Pulmonary Circulation Disease	Detailed history with regard to functional impairment and prior medical issues, medication usage, and occupational exposure	Comprehensive examination	Echocardiography; pulmonary angiography; CT or MRI imaging

Chapter 4

End-Organ Damage	Diagnosis(es)	Degree of Impairment
Include assessment of sequelae, including end-organ damage and impairment	Record all pertinent diagnosis(es); note if they are at maximal medical improvement; if not, discuss under what conditions and when stability is expected	Criteria outlined in this chapter
Heart; eyes; kidney; brain; monitor for proteinuria, elevated creatinine, reduced creatinine clearance, and abnormal urinary sediment; funduscopic changes including silver-wiring and arterio-venous crossing changes	Hypertension; left ventricular hypertrophy; hypertensive hypertrophic cardiomyopathy; hypertension-related systolic heart failure; hypertension-related diastolic heart failure; hypertensive nephrosclerosis; hypertensive encephalopathy; stroke; TIA	See Table 4-2
Heart; aorta	Aortic aneurysm—thoracic or abdominal; aortic dissection; aortic coarctation; aortic atherosclerosis See also aortic valvular regurgitation	See Table 4-3
Upper and lower extremities	Raynaud's phenomenon; arterial and venous ulceration; claudication; arterial aneurysms excluding the aorta; ischemic digital amputation, gangrene, and thromboangiitis obliterans Venous disorders, including edema, induration, stasis dermatitis, cellulitis, ulceration, and thrombosis Lymphatic disorders, including lymphedema, lymphangitis, and cellulitis	See Tables 4-4 and 4-5
Assess cardiac and pulmonary damage	Primary and secondary pulmonary hypertension; pulmonary embolism; pulmonary veno-occlusive disease; pulmonary vein stenosis	See Table 4-6

Chapter 4

References

1. The sixth report of the Joint National Committee on prevention, detection, evaluation, and treatment of high blood pressure [published erratum appears in *Arch Intern Med*. 1998; 158: 573]. *Arch Intern Med*. 1997;157:2413-2446.

   Guidelines for management and treatment of hypertension provided for racial and ethnic minorities, children, women, and elders as well as patients with LVH, CAD, HF, renal insufficiency, and diabetes. Hypertension may coexist with various other conditions and may be induced by various pressure agents. Clinicians should be aware of these management challenges and take social, cultural, and preexisting conditions into account.

2. Burt VL, Cutler JA, Higgins M, et al. Trends in the prevalence, awareness, treatment, and control of hypertension in the adult US population. Data from the health examination surveys, 1960 to 1991 [published erratum appears in *Hypertension*. 1996;27:1192]. *Hypertension*. 1995;26:60-69.

   Describes secular trends in the distribution of blood pressure and prevalence of hypertension in US adults and changes in rates of awareness, treatment, and control of hypertension.

3. Hall WD, Ferrario CM, Moore MA, et al. Hypertension-related morbidity and mortality in the southeastern United States. *Am J Med Sci*. 1997;313:195-206.

   Highlights the differential regional impact of hypertension within the United States and summarizes the data that document the problem, the consequences, and possible causative factors.

4. Levy D, Larson MG, Vasan RS, Kannel WB, Ho KK. The progression from hypertension to congestive heart failure. *JAMA*. 1996;275:1557-1562.

   Studies the relative and population-attributable risks of hypertension for the development of congestive heart failure (CHF) to assess factors that contribute to the development of overt heart failure in hypertensive subjects. Hypertension is the most common risk factor for CHF and contributes to a large proportion of heart failure cases in this population-based sample. Preventive strategies directed toward earlier and more aggressive blood pressure control are likely to offer the greatest promise for reducing the incidence of CHF and its associated mortality.

5. Glynn RJ, Brock DB, Harris T, et al. Use of antihypertensive drugs and trends in blood pressure in the elderly. *Arch Intern Med*. 1995;155:1855-1860.

   Examines the benefits of treatment for hypertension in the elderly. In the United States, the ongoing therapeutic efforts to lower elevated blood pressure in elderly populations may be contributing to the continuing decline in cardiovascular and stroke mortality.

6. Levy D, Salomon M, D'Agostino RB, Belanger AJ, Kannel WB. Prognostic implications of baseline electrocardiographic features and their serial changes in subjects with left ventricular hypertrophy. *Circulation*. 1994;90:1786-1793.

   Summarizes the prognostic importance of ECG changes associated with hypertension-related ventricular hypertrophy. Persons with ECG evidence of left ventricular hypertrophy are at increased risk for the development of cardiovascular disease.

7. Frohlich ED. Pathophysiology of systemic arterial hypertension. In: Schlant RC, Alexander RW, O'Rourke RA, Roberts R, Sonnenblick EH, eds. *Hurst's The Heart*. 8th ed. New York, NY: McGraw-Hill; 1993:1391-1401.

   Nicely outlines the pathophysiological implications of hypertension.

8. Isselbacher EM, Eagle KA, DeSanctis RW. Diseases of the aorta. In: *Heart Disease by Braunwald*. 5th ed. Philadelphia, Pa: WB Saunders; 1997:1546.

   This chapter provides an excellent summary of contemporary management of diseases of the aorta.

9. Heinemann M, Laas J, Karck M, Borst HG. Thoracic aortic aneurysms after acute type A aortic dissection: necessity for follow-up. *Ann Thorac Surg*. 1990;49:580-584.

   Discusses the long-term prognosis of thoracic aortic aneurysms and underscores the importance of close follow-up of patients having operations for acute type A aortic dissection. Early recognition of progressive downstream aortic pathology permits effective prevention of aortic rupture and timely reoperation.

10. Karalis DG, Chandrasekaran K, Victor MF, Ross JJ Jr, Mintz GS. Recognition and embolic potential of intraaortic atherosclerotic debris. *J Am Coll Cardiol*. 1991;17:73-78.

    Highlights the potential for embolic complications in patients with thoracic aortic atherosclerosis. In a patient with an embolic event, the thoracic aorta should be considered as a potential source. Transesophageal echocardiography can reliably detect intra-aortic atherosclerotic debris, and when it is identified, an invasive aortic procedure should be avoided if possible.

11. Bickerstaff LK, Pairolero PC, Hollier LH, et al. Thoracic aortic aneurysms: a population-based study. *Surgery.* 1982;92:1103-1108.

A population-based perspective on the prevalence of thoracic aortic aneurysms. Actuarial 5-year survival for all 72 patients in study was 13%; for patients with aortic dissection, 7%; and for patients without dissection, 19.2%.

12. Bengtsson H, Bergqvist D, Sternby NH. Increasing prevalence of abdominal aortic aneurysms: necroscopy study. *Eur J Surg.* 1992;158:19-23.

Analyzes the prevalence of abdominal aortic aneurysms in the city of Malmo. Prevalence increased during the last three decades and is age- and sex-dependent.

13. Bickerstaff LK, Hollier LH, Van Peenen HJ, Melton LJ III, Pairolero PC, Cherry KJ. Abdominal aortic aneurysms: the changing natural history. *J Vasc Surg.* 1984;1:6-12.

Provides a contemporary perspective on abdominal aortic aneurysms. Evaluation of data (records, including autopsy reports, of all patients with abdominal aortic aneurysms in a Midwest city with a stable population over a 30-year period) by decade reveals an absolute increase in the incidence of abdominal aortic aneurysms.

14. Widlus DM, Osterman FA Jr. Evaluation and percutaneous management of atherosclerotic peripheral vascular disease. *JAMA.* 1989;261:3148-3154.

Review article. This review provides a contemporary assessment of atherosclerotic peripheral vascular disease including current treatment strategies and outcome data.

15. Coffman JD. Intermittent claudication—be conservative. *N Engl J Med.* 1991;325:577-578.

This editorial summarizes contemporary issues surrounding percutaneous transluminal angioplasty and peripheral vascular revascularization.

16. Schabauer AMA, Rooke TW. Cutaneous laser Doppler flowmetry: applications and findings. *Mayo Clinic Proc.* 1994;69:564-574.

17. McGoon MD, et al. Pulmonary hypertension. In: Giuliani ER, Gersh, BL, McGoon MD, Hayes DL, Schaff HV, eds. *Mayo Clinic Practice of Cardiology.* 3rd ed. St Louis, Mo: Mosby; 1996.

Provides an excellent framework for understanding the pathophysiology of pulmonary hypertension.

18. Rubin LJ. Primary pulmonary hypertension. *Chest.* 1993;104:236-250.

Summarizes the consensus opinion of the American College of Chest Physicians.

19. D'Alonzo GE, Barst RJ, Ayres SM, et al. Survival in patients with primary pulmonary hypertension: results from a national prospective registry. *Ann Intern Med.* 1991;115:343-349.

Characterizes mortality in persons diagnosed with primary pulmonary hypertension and investigates factors associated with survival. Mortality most closely associated with right ventricular hemodynamic function and characterized by means of an equation that uses three variables: mean pulmonary artery pressure, mean right atrial pressure, and cardiac index. The equation, validated prospectively, can be used as an adjunct in planning treatment strategies and allocating medical response.

20. Burrows B, Kettel LJ, Niden AH, Rabinowitz M, Diener CF. Patterns of cardiovascular dysfunction in chronic obstructive lung disease. *N Engl J Med.* 1972;286:912-918.

Provides insight into the interaction between chronic obstructive airway disease and cardiovascular disease.

21. Fishman AP, McGoon MD, Chazova IE, Fedullo PF, Kneussl M, Peacock AJ, et al. Diagnosis and assessment of pulmonary hypertension. In: Rich S, ed. *Primary Pulmonary Hypertension: Executive Summary from the World Symposium: Primary Pulmonary Hypertension 1998.*

This is the most recent update on primary pulmonary hypertension and provides the latest WHO definitions for pulmonary hypertension severity. It is accessible on the Internet: http://www.who.int/ncd/cvd/pph.html.

Chapter 4

Chapter 5

The Respiratory System

Introduction

This chapter provides criteria for evaluating permanent impairment of the respiratory system as it affects overall lung function and the ability to perform the activities of daily living. The respiratory system includes the tracheobronchial tree, pulmonary parenchyma, and ribcage.

The following sections have been revised for the fifth edition: (1) criteria for asthma impairment were updated to incorporate guidelines recently published by the American Thoracic Society (ATS)[1]; (2) respiratory impairment criteria now incorporate the lower limits of normal[2] for forced vital capacity (FVC), forced expiratory volume in the first second (FEV_1), and diffusing capacity for carbon monoxide (Dco); and (3) the section on sleep apnea has been updated to reflect current assessment and practice.

5.1 Principles of Assessment

Before using the information in this chapter, the *Guides* user should become familiar with Chapters 1 and 2 and the Glossary. Chapters 1 and 2 discuss the *Guides'* purpose, applications, and methods for performing and reporting impairment evaluations. The Glossary provides definitions of common terms used by many specialties in impairment evaluations.

The purpose of respiratory impairment assessment is to determine if a permanent respiratory impairment exists, quantify its severity, assess its impact on the ability to perform activities of daily living, and, if possible, identify the cause of the abnormality and recommend measures to prevent further impairment and ensure optimum function.

An impairment, as stated in Chapter 1, is "a loss, loss of use, or derangement of any body part, organ system, or organ function" (Table 1-1). Not all impairments result in a functional loss or affect the ability to perform activities of daily living. Respiratory impairments that produce a decrement of lung function and affect the ability to perform activities of daily living are assigned an impairment rating. For example, an anatomic change such as a circumscribed pleural plaque would be an impairment based on an abnormality in anatomic structure. However, if there were no abnormality in lung function and no decrease in the ability to perform activities of daily living, the individual would be assigned a 0% impairment rating.

Changes in organ function are the primary criteria for determining the impairment class. To establish the specific impairment percentage, consider both the severity and prognosis of the condition and how the impairment affects the individual's ability to perform the activities of daily living listed in Table 1-2. Table 5-13 is provided at the end of the chapter to ensure all pertinent information is included in the respiratory assessment.

Begin the evaluation with an inquiry into specific symptoms and their severity, duration, and manner of onset. Since environmental exposure frequently leads to symptomatic complaints, it is important to determine if the individual's personal habits or surroundings, such as cigarette smoking and workplace exposures, explain or contribute to the symptoms. A thorough history enables the examiner to direct the physical examination to areas of concern and then identify the most useful diagnostic and evaluative studies. For instance, structural and movement disorders of the chest wall or diaphragm found on physical examination would prompt different investigations than an observation of wheezing. Radiographic techniques such as chest roentgenograms or computed tomography (CT) scans help elucidate anatomic abnormalities that are sometimes diagnostic of specific disease processes. To assess impairment, weigh both subjective and objective information derived from thorough history-taking, physical examination, imaging and laboratory studies, and pulmonary function tests. These complementary evaluation techniques enable the examiner to obtain an accurate and thorough view of the impairment's nature, as well as the individual's limitations and ability to perform activities of daily living.

5.1a Interpretation of Symptoms and Signs

Symptomatic assessment of individuals with respiratory disease is diagnostically useful, but it provides limited quantitative information and should not serve as the sole criterion upon which to make decisions about impairment. Rather, the examiner should obtain objective data about the extent of the limitation and integrate those findings with the subjective data to estimate the degree of permanent impairment.

5.1b Description of Clinical Studies

Clinical studies used to assess pulmonary impairment include radiographs; other imaging studies, including CT scans and MR images; pulmonary function tests; and exercise testing. **Pulmonary function tests** are the most useful in assessing functional changes.

5.2 Symptoms Associated With Respiratory Disease

The major symptoms of pulmonary disease include dyspnea; cough, sputum production, and hemoptysis; wheezing; and chest pain or tightness. The examiner needs to document these symptoms and their course over time, and correlate the symptoms with objective studies to assess their importance and implications. The significance of respiratory symptoms is better understood when integrated with findings from more objective measures such as the physical examination, radiography, lung function, and laboratory studies.

5.2a Dyspnea

Dyspnea is the most common symptom noted on initial examination of individuals with any type of pulmonary impairment. Despite its importance, dyspnea is nonspecific; it is often caused by cardiac, hematologic, metabolic, or neurologic disease, or by anxiety or physical deconditioning.

Dyspnea can be evaluated and quantitated using several systems. The most widely used classification system, developed with the ATS, (Table 5-1), is based on the American Thoracic Society/Division of Lung Diseases Respiratory Symptom questionnaire.[3] The ATS classification is best used in conjunction with more objective respiratory function measurements. If a disparity is found between subjective complaints of dyspnea and findings on respiratory testing, consider a nonrespiratory dyspnea component.[4]

Table 5-1 Impairment Classification of Dyspnea*

Severity	Definition and Question
Mild	Do you have to walk more slowly on the level than people of your age because of breathlessness?
Moderate	Do you have to stop for breath when walking at your own pace on the level?
Severe	Do you ever have to stop for breath after walking about 100 yards or for a few minutes on the level?
Very severe	Are you too breathless to leave the house, or breathless on dressing or undressing?

* The person's lowest level of physical activity and exertion that produces breathlessness denotes the severity of dyspnea.[3]

5.2b Cough, Sputum Production, and Hemoptysis

Coughing can be an important indicator of respiratory tract disease, although it is difficult to quantify and not easily measured. Document its presence or absence, whether it is productive or nonproductive of sputum, its relationship to work or other activities, its duration, its association with hemoptysis, and whether further investigation is warranted.

An acute, self-limited cough is most commonly due to infection or irritation. A subacute or recurrent, nonproductive cough may be a manifestation of asthma and should be investigated with pulmonary function testing. A chronic, productive cough may indicate bronchitis. According to ATS criteria, the term *chronic bronchitis* may be used to describe a sputum-producing cough that occurs on most days for at least 3 consecutive months a year for at least 2 consecutive years.[4]

Hemoptysis frequently accompanies bronchitis and pneumonia, usually as blood-streaked sputum. Serious conditions that often manifest with hemoptysis include bronchogenic carcinoma, pulmonary emboli, bronchiectasis, tuberculosis, aspergilloma, and arteriovenous malformations. At a minimum, hemoptysis requires radiologic evaluation that may uncover respiratory or other impairment-producing types of diseases.

5.2c Wheezing

Subjects with partial airway obstruction often report high-pitched, musical sounds, or wheezing. These sounds can be generated at any point along the respiratory tract from the glottis to the bronchioles. Inspiratory wheezing, or stridor, suggests laryngeal disease; expiratory wheezing indicates bronchospasm or localized bronchial narrowing. Information about seasonal wheezing is also diagnostically significant. Wheezing and/or cough occurring primarily in the workplace or having a definite temporal relationship to work suggests occupational asthma; wheezing that follows several minutes of exercise suggests exercise-induced asthma; and wheezing that usually accompanies respiratory tract infections is classified as asthmatic bronchitis. While these different varieties of asthma are commonly described as separate entities, there is substantial overlap among the syndromes. This is due to the underlying commonalities of airway hyperresponsiveness in all types of asthma.

5.2d Thoracic Cage Abnormalities

Osseous spine abnormalities may produce respiratory impairment due to mechanical factors involving the size of the chest cavity and restriction of rib motion. Kyphoscoliosis, the most common of these abnormalities, is characterized by curvature of the vertebral column from side to side in the frontal plane (scoliosis) and from the dorsal to the ventral aspect of the sagittal plane (kyphosis). The Cobb method is the most common measurement tool for curvature severity. With this method, posteroanterior and lateral spinal radiographs measure the curvature angles. Only severe curvature angles—that is, Cobb angles that are greater than 100°—are likely to lead to respiratory failure. Even when there are severe spinal deformities, respiratory decompensation usually does not occur until middle age or later.

With severe spinal abnormalities, respiratory compromise is produced by the combined effects of restricted lung volume, decreased cross-sectional area of the vascular bed, and age-related decrease in chest wall compliance. Progressive stiffness of the chest wall with advancing age increases the work of breathing and leads to hypoventilation, which produces hypoxia and hypercapnia. Hypoxia is a powerful pulmonary vasoconstrictor and further decreases the vascular cross-sectional area, eventually leading to cor pulmonale. Judge the severity of respiratory impairment on the criteria described in the sections on forced respiratory maneuvers (5.4d), diffusing capacity for carbon monoxide (5.4e), and the criteria for rating impairment due to respiratory disease (5.4g) in this chapter.

5.3 Tobacco Use and Environmental Exposure Associated With Respiratory Disease

5.3a Tobacco Use

Exposure to tobacco smoke is a common cause of respiratory impairment. Although susceptibility to the adverse effects of cigarette smoke varies, there is a discernible dose-response relationship. The examiner should ask the individual's current age; the age at which he or she started smoking; the average number of packs smoked per day if the smoking has continued; and, if the person quit smoking at any time, the age and date he or she quit smoking.

Multiply the number of years of smoking by the number of packs smoked per day to produce the standard measure of pack-years of cigarette smoking. Use this information to assess the impact of personal habits on respiratory impairment. Cigarette smoking is the most frequent causative factor in the development of chronic bronchitis, emphysema, and lung cancer, and it can exacerbate asthma. Chronic exposure to environmental tobacco smoke may also be a factor in the origin of lung cancer, and it can also exacerbate asthma. Smoking cessation should be noted since it often benefits respiratory status. Although the anatomic abnormalities of emphysema are irreversible, both bronchospasm and productive cough can be favorably affected by the discontinuation of cigarette use. In addition, risk of bronchogenic carcinoma decreases progressively in the first 10 to 15 years after quitting smoking. After that time, the risk stabilizes at a point slightly higher than that of someone who has never smoked.[5]

5.3b Environmental Exposure

Environmental exposures in the workplace often are cited as causative or contributory factors in the development of respiratory impairment. It is important to obtain a complete **occupational history** from the individual to evaluate the possible effect of these exposures. A chief component of the history contains a chronological description of work activities beginning with the first year of employment and includes names of employers, the specific types of work performed, the materials used by the person, and the potentially toxic materials present in the workplace. Employers are required to maintain a list (made available to the employee and the treating physician in the form of Material Safety Data Sheets) of potentially toxic materials used in the workplace, their chemical descriptions, and their physical and health hazards. This information can be quite helpful to the examiner to direct the diagnostic and evaluative process. To assess its significance, ask the individual to estimate the frequency and intensity of exposure to each substance, as well as information about the use of respiratory protective devices.

Respiratory injuries in the workplace can occur in several different patterns, depending on the nature of the inhaled material and the circumstances of exposure. Acute lung injury may be the result of inhalation of a highly irritative gas, fume, mist, or vapor that results in noncardiogenic pulmonary edema or acute respiratory distress syndrome. If the individual survives the acute lung injury, the healing process may produce diffuse pulmonary fibrosis or obliterative bronchiolitis, which may lead to functional impairment. Depending on the nature, duration, and intensity of exposure, inhalation of irritative substances can cause subsequent persistent problems such as chronic bronchitis and airway hyperreactivity. Allergic pulmonary reactions can result from inhalation of organic material or certain types of reactive chemical molecules, causing asthma or hypersensitivity pneumonitis. Inhalation of fibrogenic dust can cause pneumoconiosis over a prolonged period. Workplace exposures can also exacerbate underlying conditions such as asthma, chronic bronchitis, or emphysema.

In addition to information on workplace exposure, inquire about home and environmental exposure (including hobbies or leisure time activities) to organic and inorganic agents such as allergens, bioaerosols, paints, glues, or pesticides. In the home, exposure to pets and use of cool-mist vaporizers, humidifiers, and indoor hot tubs also may be associated with respiratory disease.

5.4 Examinations, Clinical Studies, and Other Tests for Evaluating Respiratory Disease

5.4a Physical Examination
Although a thorough physical examination is mandatory to reach valid conclusions about an individual's impairment, certain portions of the examination are particularly pertinent in evaluating the respiratory system. Observe and record respiratory rate, use of accessory muscles, and body habitus. Noisy breath sounds are a physical finding that may indicate airflow obstruction. A breathing pattern characterized by pursed lip breathing during expiration suggests chronic obstructive pulmonary disease (COPD). Inspect the thoracic cage for vertebral or rib cage deformity and movement of the ribs with inspiration and expiration. A barrel-shaped chest may indicate hyperinflation. Percuss the chest to ascertain hyperresonance or consolidation and assess diaphragmatic motion.

Chest auscultation detects decreased breath sounds, crackles, wheezes, or rhonchi. Describe the intensity, quality, and location of these, as well as whether they are heard during inspiration, expiration, or both. Inspiratory crackles, heard in two thirds of people with chronic interstitial lung disease, may be associated with restrictive respiratory impairment. Wheezes and rhonchi are indicative of bronchial abnormalities and are often accompanied by obstructive airway disease. Auscultate during both quiet breathing and forced expiration before excluding wheezing. Diffuse, bilateral, expiratory wheezing indicates generalized bronchospasm, while unilateral or localized wheezing may be caused by partial bronchial obstruction due to an endobronchial tumor or mucus plugging. Early inspiratory crackles or opening snaps may be heard in diseases of airflow obstruction and particularly in bronchiolitis obliterans.

Cyanosis, indicated by a bluish tint of the lips and nail beds, is a striking but unreliable indicator of severe pulmonary impairment. Poor lighting in the examination room, anemia, and skin pigmentation can interfere with assessment of severity. Suspicion of cyanosis calls for pulse oximetry or arterial blood gas analysis.

Digital clubbing is characterized by loss of the angle at the junction of the cuticle and the nail, softening of the nail bed, increased curvature of the nails, and widening of the distal portions of the fingers and toes. Chest diseases associated with clubbing include pulmonary fibrosis, bronchiectasis, bronchogenic carcinoma, pleural tumors, lung abscess, empyema, and cyanotic congenital heart disease.

Chapter 5

5.4b Chest Roentgenograms

The initial radiographic examination should include posteroanterior and lateral views of the chest taken in full inspiration. Chest radiographic findings often correlate poorly with physiologic findings in diseases with airflow limitation, such as asthma and emphysema. Chronic radiographic abnormalities of the chest may be classified as parenchymal, bronchovascular, cardiovascular, pleural, or osseous. Mediastinal or tracheal changes may be observed. Terms used to describe parenchymal changes can be classified as hyperinflation, fibrosis, cavitary, or cystic.

Hyperinflation is characteristic of airway obstruction. Radiographic findings of hyperinflation are seen in airway obstruction, while volume restriction is associated with fibrosis, loss of chest wall compliance, or severe neuromuscular weakness. Severe chronic obstructive pulmonary disease is manifested radiographically by diaphragm flattening, attenuation of pulmonary vasculature within the parenchyma, increased anteroposterior diameter of the chest, and increased retrosternal air space. An individual with an acute asthmatic attack can have radiographic evidence of hyperinflation without parenchymal vascular attenuation; when the asthmatic attack dissipates, the radiographic appearance reverts to normal.

Diffuse fibrotic changes in the pulmonary parenchyma may appear linear (streaky) and/or nodular (rounded). Specific diagnostic information is obtained by noting both the type and the predominant location of fibrotic changes and whether they are focal or diffuse. For example, silicosis is manifested by nodular opacities that predominate in the upper portions of the chest, while asbestosis is manifested by linear opacities that typically are most marked in lower portions of the lungs. Pleural changes such as pleural plaques may also be present in individuals with asbestosis or may be the sole manifestation of past asbestos exposure.

The International Labor Organization (ILO) adopted a standardized method of classifying radiographic abnormalities associated with fibrotic changes caused by pneumoconiosis.[6] The National Institute for Occupational Safety and Health (NIOSH) regularly administers a course and examination to certify knowledge and proficiency in the use of this method. Information on courses and programs can be obtained from the NIOSH Division of Respiratory Disease Studies, Morgantown, WVa, or by calling 800 35-NIOSH.

Evidence of cardiovascular abnormalities associated with chronic pulmonary disease is suggested when chest films show evidence of pulmonary hypertension and/or cor pulmonale. Pulmonary hypertension is indicated by enlargement of pulmonary arteries in the hila and rapid tapering of the peripheral vessels. Cor pulmonale presents as an enlargement of the right ventricle and the radiographic indicators of pulmonary hypertension. The presence of pulmonary hypertension and/or cor pulmonale and the severity of those processes may need to be confirmed by additional clinical and laboratory tests.

5.4c Computed Tomography

Computed tomography (CT) and high-resolution computed tomography (HRCT) are radiographic techniques than can augment the standard chest radiograph and are more sensitive in evaluating certain pulmonary diseases such as asbestosis. Conventional CT is obtained using 10-mm-thick slices through various lung fields. This technique is good for evaluating nodules with high radiographic attenuation. The HRCT, which consists of 1- to 2-mm thick slices every 10 mm, is useful for evaluating changes with low radiographic attenuation such as early interstitial lung disease. The standard CT and/or HRCT can provide greater accuracy as part of a thorough assessment of the pulmonary parenchyma. It should be noted that, in general, the HRCT delivers significantly less whole body effective dose radiation than the standard CT.

With regard to airway disease, HRCT can detect early changes in the lung consistent with focal emphysema; regional air trapping associated with small airway disease, such as obliterative bronchiolitis; and large airway abnormalities, such as bronchiectasis. For example, air trapping of the type seen with obliterative bronchiolitis is best demonstrated by comparing full inspiratory and full expiratory scans. Prone and supine position scans also are helpful in distinguishing hydrostatic changes related to blood volume that are transient and can occur in the dependent position of the lungs from fixed parenchymal abnormalities.[7,8]

5.4d Forced Expiratory Maneuvers (Simple Spirometry)

Pulmonary function tests, performed on standardized equipment with validated administration techniques, provide the framework for evaluation of respiratory system impairment. Spirometric testing equipment, calibration, and administration techniques must conform to the guidelines of the 1994 ATS Statement on Standardization of Spirometry.[9–15]

If tolerated by the individual, remove pulmonary medications up to 24 hours before **spirometry** or methacholine challenge testing to assess pulmonary function without the effects of medication.

Forced expiratory maneuver measurements are made from at least three acceptable spirometric tracings that demonstrate uniformity pertaining to both the expiratory flow pattern and concordance of at least two of the test results within 5% of each other. Measurements include the following: forced vital capacity (FVC), forced expiratory volume in the first second (FEV_1), and the ratio of these measurements (FEV_1/FVC). Use the tracings with the highest FVC and FEV_1 to calculate the FEV_1/FVC ratio, even if these measurements occur on different expiratory efforts.[12-14,16]

Repeat spirometry after bronchodilator administration if FEV_1/FVC is below 0.70 or if there is wheezing on physical examination. Use the spirogram indicating the best effort, before or after administration of a bronchodilator, to determine FVC and FEV_1 for impairment assessment. Postbronchodilator FEV_1 and FVC are important in understanding potential medication responsiveness and prognosis.[12,14,17,18]

Figure 5-1 Lung Capacities and Volumes in the Normal State and in Three Abnormal Conditions*

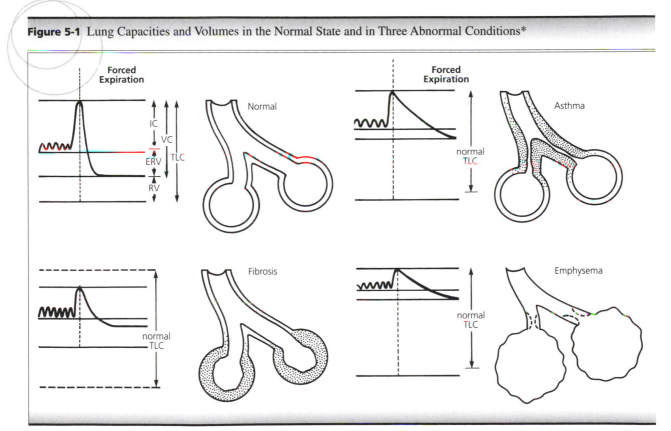

IC = inspiratory capacity; **VC** = vital capacity; **TLC** = total lung capacity; **RV** = residual volume; **ERV** = expiratory reserve volume.

*Residual volume, and therefore total lung capacity, cannot be measured by spirometry alone.

To use pulmonary function measures, obtain measurements of the FVC, FEV, and Dco and compare these to the predicted normal values as presented in Tables 5-2a through 5-7a. For the average or mean predicted normal value, find the individual's age in the left-hand column and height along the top row; the predicted value lies at the intersection of the appropriate row and column. In addition, identify the lower limit of normal for the measure of interest by using Tables 5-2b through 5-7b. The lower limit of normal has been calculated based upon the standard convention of the lower limit of normal lying at the fifth percentile, below the upper 95% of the reference population, according to recommendations from the ATS.[13,14] The lower limits of normal are used to distinguish between class 1 and class 2 respiratory impairment in Table 5-12.

North American whites have larger spirometric values for a given age, height, and gender than North American blacks, with a similar tendency noted for Hispanics, Native Americans, and Asians. Population values of normal lung function have been identified for blacks. The ATS Task Force for Interpretation of Pulmonary Function recommends an adjustment on a population basis for predicted lung function in blacks. Multiply values for predicted normal FVC (Tables 5-2a and 5-3a) by 0.88; for predicted normal FEV_1 (Tables 5-4a and 5-5a) by 0.88; and for normal single-breath Dco (Tables 5-6a and 5-7a) by 0.93. In cases where the correction value may not apply, the examiner may choose not to use this correction and instead may provide an explanation why it is inappropriate. Reliable population data are not yet available for other ethnic groups, such as Hispanics, Native Americans, and Asians. For these ethnic groups, the values for North American whites may be used.[16,19–21]

The FEV_1/FVC ratio helps diagnose obstructive airway disease. However, according to the most recent ATS statement on pulmonary function testing interpretation, the absolute volume or the percentage of predicted value of FEV_1 is the primary parameter for assessing severity of obstruction, although the FEV_1/FVC may be helpful.[13] Rather, judge severity on the absolute value or the percentage of predicted value of FEV_1.

5.4e Diffusing Capacity for Carbon Monoxide (Dco)

Use single-breath Dco to evaluate all levels of impairment. The single-breath Dco testing method is described in a 1995 ATS statement.[14,22] The Dco measurement provides information about gas transfer efficiency across the lungs.[23] Several physiologic factors affect the gas transfer process, including alveolar-capillary membrane thickness, available gas exchange surface area, gas solubility, pulmonary capillary blood volume, hematocrit, test gas concentration gradient across the alveolar-capillary membrane, and hemoglobin-binding site availability.

Mechanical factors that affect Dco results include test gas inhalation speed, inspiration depth, period of breath holding, and expiration speed. While mechanical factors generally are controlled by Dco test automation, extrapulmonary factors are important to ascertain proper interpretation. For example, cigarette smoking can elevate the blood's carbon monoxide levels, causing as much as 10% to 12% hemoglobin saturation and decreasing Dco. Instruct the individual not to smoke for at least 8 hours before the test.

See Tables 5-6a and 5-7a for reference values for population-based predicted normal **diffusing capacity.** Use these tables in a manner similar to the spirometry tables. A laboratory that tests Dco under conditions or with procedures different than that recommended by the ATS should either develop and verify its own prediction equations or use an accepted and verified equation.

See Table 5-12 for classification of respiratory impairment based on the testing results of FVC, FEV_1, FEV_1/FVC, and Dco. Also consider the possible contribution of extrapulmonary factors to respiratory system impairment. For example, morbid obesity may decrease FVC, and anemia may decrease Dco. Evaluate other organ system impairments according to the criteria given in other *Guides* chapters and combine those impairment ratings with the respiratory system impairment rating (see the Combined Values Chart, p. 604).

Table 5-2a Predicted Normal Forced Vital Capacity (FVC) in Liters for Men (BTPS)*

Age	Height (cm)																								
	146	148	150	152	154	156	158	160	162	164	166	168	170	172	174	176	178	180	182	184	186	188	190	192	194
18	3.72	3.84	3.96	4.08	4.20	4.32	4.44	4.56	4.68	4.80	4.92	5.04	5.16	5.28	5.40	5.52	5.64	5.76	5.88	6.00	6.12	6.24	6.36	6.48	6.60
20	3.68	3.80	3.92	4.04	4.16	4.28	4.40	4.52	4.64	4.76	4.88	5.00	5.12	5.24	5.36	5.48	5.60	5.72	5.84	5.96	6.08	6.20	6.32	6.44	6.56
22	3.64	3.76	3.88	4.00	4.12	4.24	4.36	4.48	4.60	4.72	4.84	4.96	5.08	5.20	5.32	5.44	5.56	5.68	5.80	5.92	6.04	6.16	6.28	6.40	6.52
24	3.60	3.72	3.84	3.95	4.08	4.20	4.32	4.44	4.56	4.68	4.80	4.92	5.04	5.16	5.28	5.40	5.52	5.64	5.76	5.88	6.00	6.12	6.24	6.36	6.48
26	3.55	3.67	3.79	3.91	4.03	4.15	4.27	4.39	4.51	4.63	4.75	4.87	4.99	5.11	5.23	5.35	5.47	5.59	5.71	5.83	5.95	6.07	6.19	6.31	6.43
28	3.51	3.63	3.75	3.87	3.99	4.11	4.23	4.35	4.47	4.59	4.71	4.83	4.95	5.07	5.19	5.31	5.43	5.55	5.67	5.79	5.91	6.03	6.15	6.27	6.39
30	3.47	3.59	3.71	3.83	3.95	4.07	4.19	4.31	4.43	4.55	4.67	4.79	4.91	5.03	5.15	5.27	5.39	5.51	5.63	5.75	5.87	5.99	6.11	6.23	6.35
32	3.43	3.55	3.67	3.79	3.91	4.03	4.15	4.27	4.39	4.51	4.63	4.75	4.87	4.99	5.11	5.23	5.35	5.47	5.59	5.71	5.83	5.95	6.07	6.19	6.31
34	3.38	3.50	3.62	3.74	3.86	3.98	4.10	4.22	4.34	4.46	4.58	4.70	4.82	4.94	5.06	5.18	5.30	5.42	5.54	5.66	5.78	5.90	6.02	6.14	6.26
36	3.34	3.46	3.58	3.70	3.82	3.94	4.06	4.18	4.30	4.42	4.54	4.66	4.78	4.90	5.02	5.14	5.26	5.38	5.50	5.62	5.74	5.86	5.98	6.10	6.22
38	3.30	3.42	3.54	3.66	3.78	3.90	4.02	4.14	4.26	4.38	4.50	4.62	4.74	4.86	4.98	5.10	5.22	5.34	5.46	5.58	5.70	5.82	5.94	6.06	6.18
40	3.25	3.37	3.49	3.61	3.73	3.85	3.97	4.09	4.21	4.33	4.45	4.57	4.69	4.81	4.93	5.05	5.17	5.29	5.41	5.53	5.65	5.77	5.89	6.01	6.13
42	3.21	3.33	3.45	3.57	3.69	3.81	3.93	4.05	4.17	4.29	4.41	4.53	4.65	4.77	4.89	5.01	5.13	5.25	5.37	5.49	5.61	5.73	5.85	5.97	6.09
44	3.17	3.29	3.41	3.53	3.65	3.77	3.89	4.01	4.13	4.25	4.37	4.49	4.61	4.73	4.85	4.97	5.09	5.21	5.33	5.45	5.57	5.69	5.81	5.93	6.05
46	3.13	3.25	3.37	3.49	3.61	3.73	3.85	3.97	4.09	4.21	4.33	4.45	4.57	4.69	4.81	4.93	5.05	5.17	5.29	5.41	5.53	5.65	5.77	5.89	6.01
48	3.08	3.20	3.32	3.44	3.56	3.68	3.80	3.92	4.04	4.16	4.28	4.40	4.52	4.64	4.76	4.88	5.00	5.12	5.24	5.36	5.48	5.60	5.72	5.84	5.96
50	3.04	3.16	3.28	3.40	3.52	3.64	3.76	3.88	4.00	4.12	4.24	4.36	4.48	4.60	4.72	4.84	4.96	5.08	5.20	5.32	5.44	5.56	5.68	5.80	5.92
52	3.00	3.12	3.24	3.36	3.48	3.60	3.72	3.84	3.96	4.08	4.20	4.32	4.44	4.56	4.68	4.80	4.92	5.04	5.16	5.28	5.40	5.52	5.64	5.76	5.88
54	2.95	3.07	3.19	3.31	3.43	3.55	3.67	3.79	3.91	4.03	4.15	4.27	4.39	4.51	4.63	4.75	4.87	4.99	5.11	5.23	5.35	5.47	5.59	5.71	5.83
56	2.91	3.03	3.15	3.27	3.39	3.51	3.63	3.75	3.87	3.99	4.11	4.23	4.35	4.47	4.59	4.71	4.83	4.95	5.07	5.19	5.31	5.43	5.55	5.67	5.79
58	2.87	2.99	3.11	3.23	3.35	3.47	3.59	3.71	3.83	3.95	4.07	4.19	4.31	4.43	4.55	4.67	4.79	4.91	5.03	5.15	5.27	5.39	5.51	5.63	5.75
60	2.83	2.95	3.07	3.19	3.31	3.43	3.55	3.67	3.79	3.91	4.03	4.15	4.27	4.39	4.51	4.63	4.75	4.87	4.99	5.11	5.23	5.35	5.47	5.59	5.71
62	2.78	2.90	3.02	3.14	3.26	3.38	3.50	3.62	3.74	3.86	3.98	4.10	4.22	3.34	4.46	4.58	4.70	4.82	4.94	5.06	5.18	5.30	5.42	5.54	5.66
64	2.74	2.86	2.98	3.10	3.22	3.34	3.46	3.58	3.70	3.82	3.94	4.06	4.18	4.30	4.42	4.54	4.66	4.78	4.90	5.02	5.14	5.26	5.38	5.50	5.62
66	2.70	2.82	2.94	3.06	3.18	3.30	3.42	3.54	3.66	3.78	3.90	4.02	4.14	4.26	4.38	4.50	4.62	4.74	4.86	4.98	5.10	5.22	5.34	5.46	5.58
68	2.65	2.77	2.89	3.01	3.13	3.25	3.37	3.49	3.61	3.73	3.85	3.97	4.09	4.21	4.33	4.45	4.57	4.69	4.81	4.93	5.05	5.17	5.29	5.41	5.53
70	2.61	2.73	2.85	2.97	3.09	3.21	3.33	3.45	3.57	3.69	3.81	3.93	4.05	4.17	4.29	4.41	4.53	4.65	4.77	4.89	5.01	5.13	5.25	5.37	5.49
72	2.57	2.69	2.81	2.93	3.05	3.17	3.29	3.41	3.53	3.65	3.77	3.89	4.01	4.13	4.25	4.37	4.49	4.61	4.73	4.85	4.97	5.09	5.21	5.33	5.45
74	2.53	2.65	2.77	2.89	3.01	3.13	3.25	3.37	3.49	3.61	3.73	3.85	3.97	4.09	4.21	4.33	4.45	4.57	4.69	4.81	4.93	5.05	5.17	5.29	5.41

*FVC in liters = 0.0600 H – 0.0214 A – 4.650. R^2 = 0.54; SEE = 0.644; 95% confidence level = 1.115. Definitions of abbreviations: R^2 = coefficient of determination; SEE = standard error of estimate; H = height in cm; A = age in years. BTPS = body temperature, ambient pressure, and saturated with water vapor at these conditions. Adapted from Crapo et al.[2]

Table 5-2b Predicted Lower Limit of Normal Forced Vital Capacity (FVC) for Men*

Age	Height (cm)																								
	146	148	150	152	154	156	158	160	162	164	166	168	170	172	174	176	178	180	182	184	186	188	190	192	194
18	2.605	2.725	2.845	2.965	3.085	3.205	3.325	3.445	3.565	3.685	3.805	3.925	4.045	4.165	4.285	4.405	4.525	4.645	4.765	4.885	5.005	5.125	5.245	5.365	5.485
20	2.565	2.685	2.805	2.925	3.045	3.165	3.285	3.405	3.525	3.645	3.765	3.885	4.005	4.125	4.245	4.365	4.485	4.605	4.725	4.845	4.965	5.085	5.205	5.325	5.445
22	2.525	2.645	2.765	2.885	3.005	3.125	3.245	3.365	3.485	3.605	3.725	3.845	3.965	4.085	4.205	4.325	4.445	4.565	4.685	4.805	4.925	5.045	5.165	5.285	5.405
24	2.485	2.605	2.725	2.835	2.965	3.085	3.205	3.325	3.445	3.565	3.685	3.805	3.925	4.045	4.165	4.285	4.405	4.525	4.645	4.765	4.885	5.005	5.125	5.245	5.365
26	2.435	2.555	2.675	2.795	2.915	3.035	3.155	3.275	3.395	3.515	3.635	3.755	3.875	3.995	4.115	4.235	4.355	4.475	4.595	4.715	4.835	4.955	5.075	5.195	5.315
28	2.395	2.515	2.635	2.755	2.875	2.995	3.115	3.235	3.355	3.475	3.595	3.715	3.835	3.955	4.075	4.195	4.315	4.435	4.555	4.675	4.795	4.915	5.035	5.155	5.275
30	2.355	2.475	2.595	2.715	2.835	2.955	3.075	3.195	3.315	3.435	3.555	3.675	3.795	3.915	4.035	4.155	4.275	4.395	4.515	4.635	4.755	4.875	4.995	5.115	5.235
32	2.315	2.435	2.555	2.675	2.795	2.915	3.035	3.155	3.275	3.395	3.515	3.635	3.755	3.875	3.995	4.115	4.235	4.355	4.475	4.595	4.715	4.835	4.955	5.075	5.195
34	2.265	2.385	2.505	2.625	2.745	2.865	2.985	3.105	3.225	3.345	3.465	3.585	3.705	3.825	3.945	4.065	4.185	4.305	4.425	4.545	4.665	4.785	4.905	5.025	5.145
36	2.225	2.345	2.465	2.585	2.705	2.825	2.945	3.065	3.185	3.305	3.425	3.545	3.665	3.785	3.905	4.025	4.145	4.265	4.385	4.505	4.625	4.745	4.865	4.985	5.105
38	2.185	2.305	2.425	2.545	2.665	2.785	2.905	3.025	3.145	3.265	3.385	3.505	3.625	3.745	3.865	3.985	4.105	4.225	4.345	4.465	4.585	4.705	4.825	4.945	5.065
40	2.135	2.255	2.375	2.495	2.615	2.735	2.855	2.975	3.095	3.215	3.335	3.455	3.575	3.695	3.815	3.935	4.055	4.175	4.295	4.415	4.535	4.655	4.775	4.895	5.015
42	2.095	2.215	2.335	2.455	2.575	2.695	2.815	2.935	3.055	3.175	3.295	3.415	3.535	3.655	3.775	3.895	4.015	4.135	4.255	4.375	4.495	4.615	4.735	4.855	4.975
44	2.055	2.175	2.295	2.415	2.535	2.655	2.775	2.895	3.015	3.135	3.255	3.375	3.495	3.615	3.735	3.855	3.975	4.095	4.215	4.335	4.455	4.575	4.695	4.815	4.935
46	2.015	2.135	2.255	2.375	2.495	2.615	2.735	2.855	2.975	3.095	3.215	3.335	3.455	3.575	3.695	3.815	3.935	4.055	4.175	4.295	4.415	4.535	4.655	4.775	4.895
48	1.965	2.085	2.205	2.325	2.445	2.565	2.685	2.805	2.925	3.045	3.165	3.285	3.405	3.525	3.645	3.765	3.885	4.005	4.125	4.245	4.365	4.485	4.605	4.725	4.845
50	1.925	2.045	2.165	2.285	2.405	2.525	2.645	2.765	2.885	3.005	3.125	3.245	3.365	3.485	3.605	3.725	3.845	3.965	4.085	4.205	4.325	4.445	4.565	4.685	4.805
52	1.885	2.005	2.125	2.245	2.365	2.485	2.605	2.725	2.845	2.965	3.085	3.205	3.325	3.445	3.565	3.685	3.805	3.925	4.045	4.165	4.285	4.405	4.525	4.645	4.765
54	1.835	1.955	2.075	2.195	2.315	2.435	2.555	2.675	2.795	2.915	3.035	3.155	3.275	3.395	3.515	3.635	3.755	3.875	3.995	4.115	4.235	4.355	4.475	4.595	4.715
56	1.795	1.915	2.035	2.155	2.275	2.395	2.515	2.635	2.755	2.875	2.995	3.115	3.235	3.355	3.475	3.595	3.715	3.835	3.955	4.075	4.195	4.315	4.435	4.555	4.675
58	1.755	1.875	1.995	2.115	2.235	2.355	2.475	2.595	2.715	2.835	2.955	3.075	3.195	3.315	3.435	3.555	3.675	3.795	3.915	4.035	4.155	4.275	4.395	4.515	4.635
60	1.715	1.835	1.955	2.075	2.195	2.315	2.435	2.555	2.675	2.795	2.915	3.035	3.155	3.275	3.395	3.515	3.635	3.755	3.875	3.995	4.115	4.235	4.355	4.475	4.595
62	1.665	1.785	1.905	2.025	2.145	2.265	2.385	2.505	2.625	2.745	2.865	2.985	3.105	2.225	3.345	3.465	3.585	3.705	3.825	3.945	4.065	4.185	4.305	4.425	4.545
64	1.625	1.745	1.865	1.985	2.105	2.225	2.345	2.465	2.585	2.705	2.825	2.945	3.065	3.185	3.305	3.425	3.545	3.665	3.785	3.905	4.025	4.145	4.265	4.385	4.505
66	1.585	1.705	1.825	1.945	2.065	2.185	2.305	2.425	2.545	2.665	2.785	2.905	3.025	3.145	3.265	3.385	3.505	3.625	3.745	3.865	3.985	4.105	4.225	4.345	4.465
68	1.535	1.655	1.775	1.895	2.015	2.135	2.255	2.375	2.495	2.615	2.735	2.855	2.975	3.095	3.215	3.335	3.455	3.575	3.695	3.815	3.935	4.055	4.175	4.295	4.415
70	1.495	1.615	1.735	1.855	1.975	2.095	2.215	2.335	2.455	2.575	2.695	2.815	2.935	3.055	3.175	3.295	3.415	3.535	3.655	3.775	3.895	4.015	4.135	4.255	4.375
72	1.455	1.575	1.695	1.815	1.935	2.055	2.175	2.295	2.415	2.535	2.655	2.775	2.895	3.015	3.135	3.255	3.375	3.495	3.615	3.735	3.855	3.975	4.095	4.215	4.335
74	1.415	1.535	1.655	1.775	1.895	2.015	2.135	2.255	2.375	2.495	2.615	2.735	2.855	2.975	3.095	3.215	3.335	3.455	3.575	3.695	3.815	3.935	4.055	4.175	3.180

*FVC values are given in liters. The values listed here reflect the FVC as listed in Table 5–2a minus 1.115 L (95% confidence interval). Adapted from Crapo et al.[2]

Table 5-3a Predicted Normal Forced Vital Capacity (FVC) in Liters for Women (BTPS)*

Age	Height (cm)																								
	146	148	150	152	154	156	158	160	162	164	166	168	170	172	174	176	178	180	182	184	186	188	190	192	194
18	3.19	3.29	3.39	3.48	3.58	3.68	3.78	3.88	3.98	4.07	4.17	4.27	4.37	4.47	4.56	4.66	4.76	4.86	4.96	5.06	5.15	5.25	5.35	5.45	5.55
20	3.15	3.24	3.34	3.44	3.54	3.64	3.74	3.83	3.93	4.03	4.13	4.23	4.32	4.42	4.52	4.62	4.72	4.82	4.91	5.01	5.11	5.21	5.31	5.41	5.50
22	3.10	3.20	3.30	3.40	3.50	3.59	3.69	3.79	3.89	3.99	4.09	4.18	4.28	4.38	4.48	4.58	4.67	4.77	4.87	4.97	5.07	5.17	5.26	5.36	5.46
24	3.06	3.16	3.26	3.35	3.45	3.55	3.65	3.75	3.85	3.94	4.04	4.14	4.24	4.34	4.43	4.53	4.63	4.73	4.83	4.93	5.02	5.12	5.22	5.32	5.42
26	3.02	3.12	3.21	3.31	3.41	3.51	3.61	3.70	3.80	3.90	4.00	4.10	4.20	4.29	4.39	4.49	4.59	4.69	4.78	4.88	4.98	5.08	5.18	5.28	5.37
28	2.97	3.07	3.17	3.27	3.37	3.46	3.56	3.66	3.76	3.86	3.96	4.05	4.15	4.25	4.35	4.45	4.54	4.64	4.74	4.84	4.94	5.04	5.13	5.23	5.33
30	2.93	3.03	3.13	3.23	3.32	3.42	3.52	3.62	3.72	3.81	3.91	4.01	4.11	4.21	4.31	4.40	4.50	4.60	4.70	4.80	4.89	4.99	5.09	5.19	5.29
32	2.89	2.99	3.08	3.18	3.28	3.38	3.48	3.57	3.67	3.77	3.87	3.97	4.07	4.16	4.26	4.36	4.46	4.56	4.65	4.75	4.85	4.95	5.05	5.15	5.24
34	2.84	2.94	3.04	3.14	3.24	3.34	3.43	3.53	3.63	3.73	3.83	3.92	4.02	4.12	4.22	4.32	4.42	4.51	4.61	4.71	4.81	4.91	5.00	5.10	5.20
36	2.80	2.90	3.00	3.10	3.19	3.29	3.39	3.49	3.59	3.68	3.78	3.88	3.98	4.08	4.18	4.27	4.37	4.47	4.57	4.67	4.76	4.86	4.96	5.06	5.16
38	2.76	2.86	2.95	3.05	3.15	3.25	3.35	3.45	3.54	3.64	3.74	3.84	3.94	4.03	4.13	4.23	4.33	4.43	4.53	4.62	4.72	4.82	4.92	5.02	5.11
40	2.71	2.81	2.91	3.01	3.11	3.21	3.30	3.40	3.50	3.60	3.70	3.79	3.89	3.99	4.09	4.19	4.29	4.38	4.48	4.58	4.68	4.78	4.87	4.97	5.07
42	2.67	2.77	2.87	2.97	3.06	3.16	3.26	3.36	3.46	3.56	3.65	3.75	3.85	3.95	4.05	4.14	4.24	4.34	4.44	4.54	4.64	4.73	4.83	4.93	5.03
44	2.63	2.73	2.82	2.92	3.02	3.12	3.22	3.32	3.41	3.51	3.61	3.71	3.81	3.90	4.00	4.10	4.20	4.30	4.40	4.49	4.59	4.69	4.79	4.89	4.98
46	2.58	2.68	2.78	2.88	2.98	3.08	3.17	3.27	3.37	3.47	3.57	3.67	3.76	3.86	3.96	4.06	4.16	4.25	4.35	4.45	4.55	4.65	4.75	4.84	4.94
48	2.54	2.64	2.74	2.84	2.93	3.03	3.13	3.23	3.33	3.43	3.52	3.62	3.72	3.82	3.92	4.01	4.11	4.21	4.31	4.41	4.51	4.60	4.70	4.80	4.90
50	2.50	2.60	2.69	2.79	2.89	2.99	3.09	3.19	3.28	3.38	3.48	3.58	3.68	3.78	3.87	3.97	4.07	4.17	4.27	4.36	4.46	4.56	4.66	4.76	4.86
52	2.46	2.55	2.65	2.75	2.85	2.95	3.04	3.14	3.24	3.34	3.44	3.54	3.63	3.73	3.83	3.93	4.03	4.12	4.22	4.32	4.42	4.52	4.62	4.71	4.81
54	2.41	2.51	2.61	2.71	2.80	2.90	3.00	3.10	3.20	3.30	3.39	3.49	3.59	3.69	3.79	3.89	3.98	4.08	4.18	4.28	4.38	4.47	4.57	4.67	4.77
56	2.37	2.47	2.57	2.66	2.76	2.86	2.96	3.06	3.15	3.25	3.35	3.45	3.55	3.65	3.74	3.84	3.94	4.04	4.14	4.23	4.33	4.43	4.53	4.63	4.73
58	2.33	2.42	2.52	2.62	2.72	2.82	2.91	3.01	3.11	3.21	3.31	3.41	3.50	3.60	3.70	3.80	3.90	4.00	4.09	4.19	4.29	4.39	4.49	4.58	4.68
60	2.28	2.38	2.48	2.58	2.68	2.77	2.87	2.97	3.07	3.17	3.26	3.36	3.46	3.56	3.66	2.76	3.85	3.95	4.05	4.15	4.25	4.34	4.44	4.54	4.64
62	2.24	2.34	2.44	2.53	2.63	2.73	2.83	2.93	3.02	3.12	3.22	3.32	3.42	3.52	3.61	3.71	3.81	3.91	4.01	4.11	4.20	4.30	4.40	4.50	4.60
64	2.20	2.29	2.39	2.49	2.59	2.69	2.79	2.88	2.98	3.08	3.18	3.28	3.37	3.47	3.57	3.67	3.77	3.87	3.96	4.06	4.16	4.26	4.36	4.45	4.55
66	2.15	2.25	2.35	2.45	2.55	2.64	2.74	2.84	2.94	3.04	3.14	3.23	3.33	3.43	3.53	3.63	3.72	3.82	3.92	4.02	4.12	4.22	4.31	4.41	4.51
68	2.11	2.21	2.31	2.40	2.50	2.60	2.70	2.80	2.90	2.99	3.09	3.19	3.29	3.39	3.48	3.58	3.68	3.78	3.88	3.98	4.07	4.17	4.27	4.37	4.47
70	2.07	2.16	2.26	2.36	2.46	2.56	2.66	2.75	2.85	2.95	3.05	3.15	3.24	3.34	3.44	3.54	3.64	3.74	3.83	3.93	4.03	4.13	4.23	4.33	4.42
72	2.02	2.12	2.22	2.32	2.42	2.51	2.61	2.71	2.81	2.91	3.01	3.10	3.20	3.30	3.40	3.50	3.59	3.69	3.79	3.89	3.99	4.09	4.18	4.28	4.38
74	1.98	2.08	2.18	2.27	2.37	2.47	2.57	2.67	2.77	2.86	2.96	3.06	3.16	3.26	3.36	3.45	3.55	3.65	3.75	3.85	3.94	4.04	4.14	4.24	4.34

*FVC in liters = 0.0491 H – 0.0216 A – 3.590. $R^2 = 0.74$; SEE = 0.393; 95% confidence interval = 0.676. Definitions of abbreviations: R^2 = coefficient of determination; SEE = standard error of estimate; H = height in cm; A = age in years. BTPS = body temperature, ambient pressure, and saturated with water vapor at these conditions. Adapted from Crapo et al.[2]

Table 5-3b Predicted Lower Limit of Normal Forced Vital Capacity (FVC) for Women*

Age	Height (cm)																								
	146	148	150	152	154	156	158	160	162	164	166	168	170	172	174	176	178	180	182	184	186	188	190	192	194
18	2.514	2.614	2.714	2.804	2.904	3.004	3.104	3.204	3.304	3.394	3.494	3.594	3.694	3.794	3.884	3.984	4.084	4.184	4.284	4.384	4.474	4.574	4.674	4.774	4.874
20	2.474	2.564	2.664	2.764	2.864	2.964	3.064	3.154	3.254	3.354	3.454	3.554	3.644	3.744	3.844	3.944	4.044	4.144	4.234	4.334	4.434	4.534	4.634	4.734	4.824
22	2.424	2.524	2.624	2.724	2.824	2.914	3.014	3.114	3.214	3.314	3.414	3.504	3.604	3.704	3.804	3.904	3.994	4.094	4.194	4.294	4.394	4.494	4.584	4.684	4.784
24	2.384	2.484	2.584	2.674	2.774	2.874	2.974	3.074	3.174	3.264	3.364	3.464	3.564	3.664	3.754	3.854	3.954	4.054	4.154	4.254	4.344	4.444	4.544	4.644	4.744
26	2.344	2.444	2.534	2.634	2.734	2.834	2.934	3.024	3.124	3.224	3.324	3.424	3.524	3.614	3.714	3.814	3.914	4.014	4.104	4.204	4.304	4.404	4.504	4.604	4.694
28	2.294	2.394	2.494	2.594	2.694	2.784	2.884	2.984	3.084	3.184	3.284	3.374	3.474	3.574	3.674	3.774	3.864	3.964	4.064	4.164	4.264	4.364	4.454	4.554	4.654
30	2.254	2.354	2.454	2.554	2.644	2.744	2.844	2.944	3.044	3.134	3.234	3.334	3.434	3.534	3.634	3.724	3.824	3.924	4.024	4.124	4.214	4.314	4.414	4.514	4.614
32	2.214	2.314	2.404	2.504	2.604	2.704	2.804	2.894	2.994	3.094	3.194	3.294	3.394	3.484	3.584	3.684	3.784	3.884	3.974	4.074	4.174	4.274	4.374	4.474	4.564
34	2.164	2.264	2.364	2.464	2.564	2.664	2.754	2.854	2.954	3.054	3.154	3.244	3.344	3.444	3.544	3.644	3.744	3.834	3.934	4.034	4.134	4.234	4.324	4.424	4.524
36	2.124	2.224	2.324	2.424	2.514	2.614	2.714	2.814	2.914	3.004	3.104	3.204	3.304	3.404	3.504	3.594	3.694	3.794	3.894	3.994	4.084	4.184	4.284	4.384	4.484
38	2.084	2.184	2.274	2.374	2.474	2.574	2.674	2.774	2.864	2.964	3.064	3.164	3.264	3.354	3.454	3.554	3.654	3.754	3.854	3.944	4.044	4.144	4.244	4.344	4.434
40	2.034	2.134	2.234	2.334	2.434	2.534	2.624	2.724	2.824	2.924	3.024	3.114	3.214	3.314	3.414	3.514	3.614	3.704	3.804	3.904	4.004	4.104	4.194	4.294	4.394
42	1.994	2.094	2.194	2.294	2.384	2.484	2.584	2.684	2.784	2.884	2.974	3.074	3.174	3.274	3.374	3.464	3.564	3.664	3.764	3.864	3.964	4.054	4.154	4.254	4.354
44	1.954	2.054	2.144	2.244	2.344	2.444	2.544	2.644	2.734	2.834	2.934	3.034	3.134	3.224	3.324	3.424	3.524	3.624	3.724	3.814	3.914	4.014	4.114	4.214	4.304
46	1.904	2.004	2.104	2.204	2.304	2.404	2.494	2.594	2.694	2.794	2.894	2.994	3.084	3.184	3.284	3.384	3.484	3.574	3.674	3.774	3.874	3.974	4.074	4.164	4.264
48	1.864	1.964	2.064	2.164	2.254	2.354	2.454	2.554	2.654	2.754	2.844	2.944	3.044	3.144	3.244	3.334	3.434	3.534	3.634	3.734	3.834	3.924	4.024	4.124	4.224
50	1.824	1.924	2.014	2.114	2.214	2.314	2.414	2.514	2.604	2.704	2.804	2.904	3.004	3.104	3.194	3.294	3.394	3.494	3.594	3.684	3.784	3.884	3.984	4.084	4.184
52	1.784	1.874	1.974	2.074	2.174	2.274	2.364	2.464	2.564	2.664	2.764	2.864	2.954	3.054	3.154	3.254	3.354	3.444	3.544	3.644	3.744	3.844	3.944	4.034	4.134
54	1.734	1.834	1.934	2.034	2.124	2.224	2.324	2.424	2.524	2.624	2.714	2.814	2.914	3.014	3.114	3.214	3.304	3.404	3.504	3.604	3.704	3.794	3.894	3.994	4.094
56	1.694	1.794	1.894	1.984	2.084	2.184	2.284	2.384	2.474	2.574	2.674	2.774	2.874	2.974	3.064	3.164	3.264	3.364	3.464	3.554	3.654	3.754	3.854	3.954	4.054
58	1.654	1.744	1.844	1.944	2.044	2.144	2.234	2.334	2.434	2.534	2.634	2.734	2.824	2.924	3.024	3.124	3.224	3.324	3.414	3.514	3.614	3.714	3.814	3.904	4.004
60	1.604	1.704	1.804	1.904	2.004	2.094	2.194	2.294	2.394	2.494	2.584	2.684	2.784	2.884	2.984	2.084	3.174	3.274	3.374	3.474	3.574	3.664	3.764	3.864	3.964
62	1.564	1.664	1.764	1.854	1.954	2.054	2.154	2.254	2.344	2.444	2.544	2.644	2.744	2.844	2.934	3.034	3.134	3.234	3.334	3.434	3.524	3.624	3.724	3.824	3.924
64	1.524	1.614	1.714	1.814	1.914	2.014	2.114	2.204	2.304	2.404	2.504	2.604	2.694	2.794	2.894	2.994	3.094	3.194	3.284	3.384	3.484	3.584	3.684	3.774	3.874
66	1.474	1.574	1.674	1.774	1.874	1.964	2.064	2.164	2.264	2.364	2.464	2.554	2.654	2.754	2.854	2.954	3.044	3.144	3.244	3.344	3.444	3.544	3.634	3.734	3.834
68	1.434	1.534	1.634	1.724	1.824	1.924	2.024	2.124	2.224	2.314	2.414	2.514	2.614	2.714	2.804	2.904	3.004	3.104	3.204	3.304	3.394	3.494	3.594	3.694	3.794
70	1.394	1.484	1.584	1.684	1.784	1.884	1.984	2.074	2.174	2.274	2.374	2.474	2.564	2.664	2.764	2.864	2.964	3.064	3.154	3.254	3.354	3.454	3.554	3.654	3.744
72	1.344	1.444	1.544	1.644	1.744	1.834	1.934	2.034	2.134	2.234	2.334	2.424	2.524	2.624	2.724	2.824	2.914	3.014	3.114	3.214	3.314	3.414	3.504	3.604	3.704
74	1.304	1.404	1.504	1.594	1.694	1.794	1.894	1.994	2.094	2.184	2.284	2.384	2.484	2.584	2.684	2.774	2.874	2.974	3.074	3.174	3.264	3.364	3.464	3.564	3.664

*FVC values are given in liters. The values listed here reflect the FVC as listed in Table 5–3a minus 0.676 L (95% confidence interval). Adapted from Crapo et al.[2]

Table 5-4a Predicted Normal Forced Expiratory Volume in the First Second (FEV_1) in Liters for Men*

Age	Height (cm) 146	148	150	152	154	156	158	160	162	164	166	168	170	172	174	176	178	180	182	184	186	188	190	192	194
18	3.42	3.50	3.58	3.66	3.75	3.83	3.91	3.99	4.08	4.16	4.24	4.33	4.41	4.49	4.57	4.66	4.74	4.82	4.91	4.99	5..07	5.15	5.24	5.32	5.40
20	3.37	3.45	3.53	3.61	3.70	3.78	3.86	3.95	4.03	4.11	4.19	4.28	4.36	4.44	4.53	4.61	4.69	4.77	4.86	4.94	5.02	5.11	5.19	5.27	5.35
22	3.32	3.40	3.48	3.57	3.65	3.73	3.81	3.90	3.98	4.06	4.15	4.23	4.31	4.39	4.48	4.56	4.64	4.73	4.81	4.89	4.97	5.05	5.14	5.22	5.30
24	3.27	3.35	3.43	3.52	3.60	3.68	3.77	3.85	3.93	4.01	4.10	4.18	4.26	4.35	4.43	4.51	4.59	4.68	4.76	4.84	4.92	5.01	5.09	5.17	5.26
26	3.22	3.30	3.39	3.47	3.55	3.63	3.72	3.80	3.88	3.97	4.05	4.13	4.21	4.30	4.38	4.46	4.54	4.63	4.71	4.79	4.88	4.90	5.04	5.12	5.21
28	3.17	3.25	3.34	3.42	3.50	3.59	3.67	3.75	3.83	3.92	4.00	4.08	4.16	4.25	4.33	4.41	4.50	4.58	4.66	4.74	4.83	4.91	4.99	5.08	5.16
30	3.12	3.21	3.29	3.37	3.45	3.54	3.62	3.70	3.78	3.87	3.95	4.03	4.12	4.20	4.28	4.36	4.45	4.53	4.61	4.70	4.78	4.86	4.94	5.03	5.11
32	3.07	3.16	3.24	3.32	3.40	3.49	3.57	3.65	3.74	3.82	3.90	3.98	4.07	4.15	4.23	4.32	4.40	4.48	4.56	4.65	4.73	4.81	4.90	4.98	5.06
34	3.02	3.11	3.19	3.27	3.36	3.44	3.52	3.60	3.69	3.77	3.85	3.94	4.02	4.10	4.18	4.27	4.35	4.43	4.52	4.60	4.68	4.76	4.85	4.93	5.01
36	2.98	3.06	3.14	3.22	3.31	3.39	3.47	3.56	3.64	3.72	3.80	3.89	3.97	4.05	4.14	4.22	4.30	4.38	4.47	4.55	4.63	4.71	4.80	4.88	4.96
38	2.93	3.01	3.09	3.18	3.26	3.34	3.42	3.51	3.59	3.67	3.76	3.84	3.92	4.00	4.09	4.17	4.25	4.33	4.42	4.50	4.58	4.67	4.75	4.83	4.91
40	2.88	2.96	3.04	3.13	3.21	3.29	3.38	3.46	3.54	3.62	3.71	3.79	3.87	3.95	4.04	4.12	4.20	4.29	4.37	4.45	4.53	4.62	4.70	4.78	4.87
42	2.83	2.91	3.00	3.08	3.16	3.24	3.33	3.41	3.49	3.57	3.66	3.74	3.82	3.91	3.99	4.07	4.15	4.24	4.32	4.40	4.49	4.57	4.65	4.73	4.82
44	2.78	2.86	2.95	3.03	3.11	3.19	3.28	3.36	3.44	3.53	3.61	3.69	3.77	3.86	3.94	4.02	4.11	4.19	4.27	4.35	4.44	4.52	4.60	4.69	4.77
46	2.73	2.81	2.90	2.98	3.06	3.15	3.23	3.31	3.39	3.48	3.56	3.64	3.73	3.81	3.89	3.97	4.06	4.14	4.22	4.31	4.39	4.47	4.55	4.64	4.72
48	2.68	2.77	2.85	2.93	3.01	3.10	3.18	3.26	3.35	3.43	3.51	3.59	3.68	3.76	3.84	3.93	4.01	4.09	4.17	4.25	4.34	4.42	4.50	4.59	4.67
50	2.63	2.72	2.80	2.88	2.97	3.05	3.13	3.21	3.30	3.38	3.46	3.55	3.63	3.71	3.79	3.88	3.96	4.04	4.12	4.21	4.29	4.37	4.46	4.54	4.62
52	2.59	2.67	2.75	2.83	2.92	3.00	3.08	3.17	3.25	3.33	3.41	3.50	3.58	3.66	3.74	3.83	3.91	3.99	4.08	4.16	4.24	4.32	4.41	4.49	4.57
54	2.54	2.62	2.70	2.79	2.87	2.95	3.03	3.12	3.20	3.28	3.36	3.45	3.53	3.61	3.70	3.78	3.86	3.94	4.03	4.11	4.19	4.28	4.36	4.44	4.52
56	2.49	2.57	2.65	2.74	2.82	2.90	2.98	3.07	3.15	3.23	3.32	3.40	3.48	3.56	3.65	3.73	3.81	3.90	3.98	4.06	4.14	4.23	4.31	4.39	4.48
58	2.44	2.52	2.60	2.69	2.77	2.85	2.94	3.02	3.10	3.18	3.27	3.35	3.43	3.52	3.60	3.68	3.76	3.85	3.93	4.01	4.10	4.18	4.26	4.34	4.43
60	2.39	2.47	2.55	2.64	2.72	2.80	2.89	2.97	3.05	3.14	3.22	3.30	3.38	3.47	3.55	3.63	3.72	3.80	3.88	3.96	4.05	4.13	4.21	4.29	4.38
62	2.34	2.42	2.51	2.59	2.67	2.76	2.84	2.92	3.00	3.09	3.17	3.25	3.34	3.42	3.50	3.58	3.67	3.75	3.83	3.91	4.00	4.08	4.16	4.25	4.33
64	2.29	2.38	2.46	2.54	2.62	2.71	2.79	2.87	2.96	3.04	3.12	3.20	3.29	3.37	3.45	3.53	3.62	3.70	3.78	3.87	3.95	4.03	4.11	4.20	4.28
66	2.24	2.33	2.41	2.49	2.58	2.66	2.74	2.82	2.91	2.99	3.07	3.15	3.24	3.32	3.40	3.49	3.57	3.65	3.73	3.82	3.90	3.98	4.07	4.15	4.23
68	2.20	2.28	2.36	2.44	2.53	2.61	2.69	2.77	2.86	2.94	3.02	3.11	3.19	3.27	3.35	3.44	3.52	3.60	3.69	3.77	3.85	3.93	4.02	4.10	4.18
70	2.15	2.23	2.31	2.39	2.48	2.56	2.64	2.73	2.81	2.89	2.97	3.06	3.14	3.22	3.31	3.39	3.47	3.55	3.64	3.72	3.80	3.89	3.97	4.05	4.13
72	2.10	2.18	2.26	2.35	2.43	2.51	2.59	2.68	2.76	2.84	2.93	3.01	3.09	3.17	3.26	3.34	3.42	3.51	3.59	3.67	3.75	3.84	3.92	4.00	4.08
74	2.05	2.13	2.21	2.30	2.38	2.46	2.55	2.63	2.71	2.79	2.88	2.96	3.04	3.13	3.21	3.29	3.37	3.46	3.54	3.62	3.70	3.79	3.87	3.95	4.04

*FEV_1 in liters = 0.0414 H – 0.0244 A – 2.190. R^2 = 0.64; SEE = 0.486; 95% confidence interval = 0.842. Definitions of abbreviations: R^2 = coefficient of determination; SEE = standard error of estimate; H = height in cm; A = age in years. BTPS = body temperature, ambient pressure, and saturated with water vapor at these conditions. Adapted from Crapo et al.[2]

Table 5-4b Predicted Lower Limit of Normal Forced Expiratory Volume in the First Second (FEV_1) for Men*

Age	Height (cm) 146	148	150	152	154	156	158	160	162	164	166	168	170	172	174	176	178	180	182	184	186	188	190	192	194
18	2.578	2.658	2.738	2.818	2.908	2.988	3.068	3.148	3.238	3.318	3.398	3.488	3.568	3.648	3.728	3.818	3.898	3.978	4.068	4.148	4.228	4.308	4.398	4.478	4.558
20	2.528	2.608	2.688	2.768	2.858	2.938	3.018	3.108	3.188	3.268	3.348	3.438	3.518	3.598	3.688	3.768	3.848	3.928	4.018	4.098	4.178	4.268	4.348	4.428	4.508
22	2.478	2.558	2.638	2.728	2.808	2.888	2.968	3.058	3.138	3.218	3.308	3.388	3.468	3.548	3.638	3.718	3.798	3.888	3.968	4.048	4.128	4.208	4.298	4.378	4.458
24	2.428	2.508	2.588	2.678	2.758	2.838	2.928	3.008	3.088	3.168	3.258	3.338	3.418	3.508	3.588	3.668	3.748	3.838	3.918	3.998	4.078	4.168	4.248	4.328	4.418
26	2.378	2.458	2.548	2.628	2.708	2.788	2.878	2.958	3.038	3.128	3.208	3.288	3.368	3.458	3.538	3.618	3.698	3.788	3.868	3.948	4.038	4.058	4.198	4.278	4.368
28	2.328	2.408	2.498	2.578	2.658	2.748	2.828	2.908	2.988	3.078	3.158	3.238	3.318	3.408	3.488	3.568	3.658	3.738	3.818	3.898	3.988	4.068	4.148	4.238	4.318
30	2.278	2.368	2.448	2.528	2.608	2.698	2.778	2.858	2.938	3.028	3.108	3.188	3.278	3.358	3.438	3.518	3.608	3.688	3.768	3.858	3.938	4.018	4.098	4.188	4.268
32	2.228	2.318	2.398	2.478	2.558	2.648	2.728	2.808	2.898	2.978	3.058	3.138	3.228	3.308	3.388	3.478	3.558	3.638	3.718	3.808	3.888	3.968	4.058	4.138	4.218
34	2.178	2.268	2.348	2.428	2.518	2.598	2.678	2.758	2.848	2.928	3.008	3.098	3.178	3.258	3.338	3.428	3.508	3.588	3.678	3.758	3.838	3.918	4.008	4.088	4.168
36	2.138	2.218	2.298	2.378	2.468	2.548	2.628	2.718	2.798	2.878	2.958	3.048	3.128	3.208	3.298	3.378	3.458	3.538	3.628	3.708	3.788	3.868	3.958	4.038	4.118
38	2.088	2.168	2.248	2.338	2.418	2.498	2.578	2.668	2.748	2.828	2.918	2.998	3.078	3.158	3.248	3.328	3.408	3.488	3.578	3.658	3.738	3.828	3.908	3.988	4.068
40	2.038	2.118	2.198	2.288	2.368	2.448	2.538	2.618	2.698	2.778	2.868	2.948	3.028	3.108	3.198	3.278	3.358	3.448	3.528	3.608	3.688	3.778	3.858	3.938	4.028
42	1.988	2.068	2.158	2.238	2.318	2.398	2.488	2.568	2.648	2.728	2.818	2.898	2.978	3.068	3.148	3.228	3.308	3.398	3.478	3.558	3.648	3.728	3.808	3.888	3.978
44	1.938	2.018	2.108	2.188	2.268	2.348	2.438	2.518	2.598	2.688	2.768	2.848	2.928	3.018	3.098	3.178	3.268	3.348	3.428	3.508	3.598	3.678	3.758	3.848	3.928
46	1.888	1.968	2.058	2.138	2.218	2.308	2.388	2.468	2.548	2.638	2.718	2.798	2.888	2.968	3.048	3.128	3.218	3.298	3.378	3.468	3.548	3.628	3.708	3.798	3.878
48	1.838	1.928	2.008	2.088	2.168	2.258	2.338	2.418	2.508	2.588	2.668	2.748	2.838	2.918	2.998	3.088	3.168	3.248	3.328	3.408	3.498	3.578	3.658	3.748	3.828
50	1.788	1.878	1.958	2.038	2.128	2.208	2.288	2.368	2.458	2.538	2.618	2.708	2.788	2.868	2.948	3.038	3.118	3.198	3.278	3.368	3.448	3.528	3.618	3.698	3.778
52	1.748	1.828	1.908	1.988	2.078	2.158	2.238	2.328	2.408	2.488	2.568	2.658	2.738	2.818	2.898	2.988	3.068	3.148	3.238	3.318	3.398	3.478	3.568	3.648	3.728
54	1.698	1.778	1.858	1.948	2.028	2.108	2.188	2.278	2.358	2.438	2.518	2.608	2.688	2.768	2.858	2.938	3.018	3.098	3.188	3.268	3.348	3.438	3.518	3.598	3.678
56	1.648	1.728	1.808	1.898	1.978	2.058	2.138	2.228	2.308	2.388	2.478	2.558	2.638	2.718	2.808	2.888	2.968	3.058	3.138	3.218	3.298	3.388	3.468	3.548	3.638
58	1.598	1.678	1.758	1.848	1.928	2.008	2.098	2.178	2.258	2.338	2.428	2.508	2.588	2.678	2.758	2.838	2.918	3.008	3.088	3.168	3.258	3.338	3.418	3.498	3.588
60	1.548	1.628	1.708	1.798	1.878	1.958	2.048	2.128	2.208	2.298	2.378	2.458	2.538	2.628	2.708	2.788	2.878	2.958	3.038	3.118	3.208	3.288	3.368	3.448	3.538
62	1.498	1.578	1.668	1.748	1.828	1.918	1.998	2.078	2.158	2.248	2.328	2.408	2.498	2.578	2.658	2.738	2.828	2.908	2.988	3.068	3.158	3.238	3.318	3.408	3.488
64	1.448	1.538	1.618	1.698	1.778	1.868	1.948	2.028	2.118	2.198	2.278	2.358	2.448	2.528	2.608	2.688	2.778	2.858	2.938	3.028	3.108	3.188	3.268	3.358	3.438
66	1.398	1.488	1.568	1.648	1.738	1.818	1.898	1.978	2.068	2.148	2.228	2.308	2.398	2.478	2.558	2.648	2.728	2.808	2.888	2.978	3.058	3.138	3.228	3.308	3.388
68	1.358	1.438	1.518	1.598	1.688	1.768	1.848	1.928	2.018	2.098	2.178	2.268	2.348	2.428	2.508	2.598	2.678	2.758	2.848	2.928	3.008	3.088	3.178	3.258	3.338
70	1.308	1.388	1.468	1.548	1.638	1.718	1.798	1.888	1.968	2.048	2.128	2.218	2.298	2.378	2.468	2.548	2.628	2.708	2.798	2.878	2.958	3.048	3.128	3.208	3.288
72	1.258	1.338	1.418	1.508	1.588	1.668	1.748	1.838	1.918	1.998	2.088	2.168	2.248	2.328	2.418	2.498	2.578	2.668	2.748	2.828	2.908	2.998	3.078	3.158	3.238
74	1.208	1.288	1.368	1.458	1.538	1.618	1.708	1.788	1.868	1.948	2.038	2.118	2.198	2.288	2.368	2.448	2.528	2.618	2.698	2.778	2.858	2.948	3.028	3.108	3.198

*FEV_1 values are given in liters. The values listed here reflect the FEV_1 as listed in Table 5–4a minus 0.842 L (95% confidence interval). Adapted from Crapo et al.[2]

Chapter 5

Table 5-5a Predicted Normal Forced Expiratory Volume in the First Second (FEV_1) in Liters for Women*

Age	Height (cm) 146	148	150	152	154	156	158	160	162	164	166	168	170	172	174	176	178	180	182	184	186	188	190	192	194
18	2.96	3.02	3.09	3.16	3.23	3.30	3.37	3.43	3.50	3.57	3.64	3.71	3.78	3.85	3.91	3.98	4.05	4.12	4.19	4.26	4.32	4.39	4.46	4.53	4.60
20	2.91	2.97	3.04	3.11	3.18	3.25	3.32	3.38	3.45	3.52	3.59	3.66	3.73	3.79	3.86	3.93	4.00	4.07	4.14	4.20	4.27	4.34	4.41	4.48	4.55
22	2.85	2.92	2.99	3.06	3.13	3.20	3.26	3.33	3.40	3.47	3.54	3.61	3.67	3.74	3.81	3.88	3.95	4.02	4.09	4.15	4.22	4.29	4.36	4.43	4.50
24	2.80	2.87	2.94	3.01	3.08	3.15	3.21	3.28	3.35	3.42	3.49	3.56	3.62	3.69	3.76	3.83	3.90	3.97	4.03	4.10	4.17	4.24	4.31	4.38	4.44
26	2.75	2.82	2.89	2.96	3.03	3.09	3.16	3.23	3.30	3.37	3.44	3.50	3.57	3.64	3.71	3.78	3.85	3.91	3.98	4.05	4.12	4.19	4.26	4.33	4.39
28	2.70	2.77	2.84	2.91	2.97	3.04	3.11	3.18	3.25	3.32	3.39	3.45	3.52	3.59	3.66	3.73	3.80	3.86	3.93	4.00	4.07	4.14	4.21	4.27	4.34
30	2.65	2.72	2.79	2.86	2.92	2.99	3.06	3.13	3.20	3.27	3.33	3.40	3.47	3.54	3.61	3.68	3.74	3.81	3.88	3.95	4.02	4.09	4.15	4.22	4.29
32	2.60	2.67	2.74	2.80	2.87	2.94	3.01	3.08	3.15	3.21	3.28	3.35	3.42	3.49	3.56	3.63	3.69	3.76	3.83	3.90	3.97	4.04	4.10	4.17	4.24
34	2.55	2.62	2.68	2.75	2.82	2.89	2.96	3.03	3.10	3.16	3.23	3.30	3.37	3.44	3.51	3.57	3.64	3.71	3.78	3.85	3.92	3.98	4.05	4.12	4.19
36	2.50	2.57	2.63	2.70	2.77	2.84	2.91	2.98	3.04	3.11	3.18	3.25	3.32	3.39	3.45	3.52	3.59	3.66	3.73	3.80	3.87	3.93	4.00	4.07	4.14
38	2.45	2.51	2.58	2.65	2.72	2.79	2.86	2.92	2.99	3.06	3.13	3.20	3.27	3.34	3.40	3.47	3.54	3.61	3.68	3.75	3.81	3.88	3.95	4.02	4.09
40	2.40	2.46	2.53	2.60	2.67	2.74	2.81	2.87	2.94	3.01	3.08	3.15	3.22	3.28	3.35	3.42	3.49	3.56	3.63	3.69	3.76	3.83	3.90	3.97	4.04
42	2.34	2.41	2.48	2.55	2.62	2.69	2.75	2.82	2.89	2.96	3.03	3.10	3.17	3.23	3.30	3.37	3.44	3.51	3.58	3.64	3.71	3.78	3.85	3.92	3.99
44	2.29	2.36	2.43	2.50	2.57	2.64	2.70	2.77	2.84	2.91	2.98	3.05	3.11	3.18	3.25	3.32	3.39	3.46	3.52	3.59	3.66	3.73	3.80	3.87	3.93
46	2.24	2.31	2.38	2.45	2.52	2.58	2.65	2.72	2.79	2.86	2.93	2.99	3.06	3.13	3.20	3.27	3.34	3.41	3.47	3.54	3.61	3.68	3.75	3.82	3.88
48	2.19	2.26	2.33	2.40	2.46	2.53	2.60	2.67	2.74	2.81	2.88	2.94	3.01	3.08	3.15	3.22	3.29	3.35	3.42	3.49	3.56	3.63	3.70	3.76	3.83
50	2.14	2.21	2.28	2.35	2.41	2.48	2.55	2.62	2.69	2.76	2.82	2.89	2.96	3.03	3.10	3.17	3.23	3.30	3.37	3.44	3.51	3.58	3.65	3.71	3.78
52	2.09	2.16	2.23	2.29	2.36	2.43	2.50	2.57	2.64	2.70	2.77	2.84	2.91	2.98	3.05	3.12	3.18	3.25	3.32	3.39	3.46	3.53	3.59	3.66	3.73
54	2.04	2.11	2.18	2.24	2.31	2.38	2.45	2.52	2.59	2.65	2.72	2.79	3.86	2.93	3.00	3.06	3.13	3.20	3.27	3.34	3.41	3.47	3.54	3.61	3.68
56	1.99	2.06	2.12	2.19	2.26	2.33	2.40	2.47	2.53	2.60	2.67	2.74	2.81	2.88	2.94	3.01	3.08	3.15	3.22	3.29	3.36	3.42	3.49	3.56	3.63
58	1.94	2.00	2.07	2.14	2.21	2.28	2.35	2.42	2.48	2.55	2.62	2.69	2.76	2.83	2.89	2.96	3.03	3.10	3.17	3.24	3.30	3.37	3.44	3.51	3.58
60	1.89	1.95	2.02	2.09	2.16	2.23	2.30	2.36	2.43	2.50	2.57	2.64	2.71	2.77	2.84	2.91	2.98	3.05	3.12	3.18	3.25	3.32	3.39	3.46	3.53
62	1.83	1.90	1.97	2.04	2.11	2.18	2.24	2.31	2.38	2.45	2.52	2.59	2.66	2.72	2.79	2.86	2.93	3.00	3.07	3.13	3.20	3.27	3.34	3.41	3.48
64	1.78	1.85	1.92	1.99	2.06	2.13	2.19	2.26	2.33	2.40	2.47	2.54	2.60	2.67	2.74	2.81	2.88	2.95	3.01	3.08	3.15	3.22	3.29	3.36	3.42
66	1.73	1.80	1.87	1.94	2.01	2.07	2.14	2.21	2.28	2.35	2.42	2.48	2.55	2.62	2.69	2.76	2.83	2.90	2.96	3.03	3.10	3.17	3.24	3.31	3.37
68	1.68	1.75	1.82	1.89	1.95	2.02	2.09	2.16	2.23	2.30	2.37	2.43	2.50	2.57	2.64	2.71	2.78	2.84	2.91	2.98	3.05	3.12	3.19	3.25	3.32
70	1.63	1.70	1.77	1.84	1.90	1.97	2.04	2.11	2.18	2.25	2.31	2.38	2.45	2.52	2.59	2.66	2.72	2.79	2.86	2.93	3.00	3.07	3.14	3.20	3.27
72	1.58	1.65	1.72	1.78	1.85	1.92	1.99	2.06	2.13	2.19	2.26	2.33	2.40	2.47	2.54	2.61	2.67	2.74	2.81	2.88	2.95	3.02	3.08	3.15	3.22
74	1.53	1.60	1.67	1.73	1.80	1.87	1.94	2.01	2.08	2.14	2.21	2.28	2.35	2.42	2.49	2.55	2.62	2.69	2.76	2.83	2.90	2.96	3.03	3.10	3.17

*FEV_1 in liters = 0.0342 H – 0.0225 A – 1.578. R^2 = 0.80; SEE = 0.326; 95% confidence interval = 0.561. Definitions of abbreviations: R^2 = coefficient of determination; SEE = standard error of estimate; H = height in cm; A = age in years. BTPS = body temperature, ambient pressure, and saturated with water vapor at these conditions. Adapted from Crapo et al.[2]

Table 5-5b Predicted Lower Limit of Normal Forced Expiratory Volume in the First Second (FEV_1) for Women*

Age	Height (cm) 146	148	150	152	154	156	158	160	162	164	166	168	170	172	174	176	178	180	182	184	186	188	190	192	194
18	2.399	2.459	2.529	2.599	2.669	2.739	2.809	2.869	2.939	3.009	3.079	3.149	3.219	3.289	3.349	3.419	3.489	3.559	3.629	3.699	3.759	3.829	3.899	3.969	4.039
20	2.349	2.409	2.479	2.549	2.619	2.689	2.759	2.819	2.889	2.959	3.029	3.099	3.169	3.229	3.299	3.369	3.439	3.509	3.579	3.639	3.709	3.779	3.849	3.919	3.989
22	2.289	2.359	2.429	2.499	2.569	2.639	2.699	2.769	2.839	2.909	2.979	3.049	3.109	3.179	3.249	3.319	3.389	3.459	3.529	3.589	3.659	3.729	3.799	3.869	3.939
24	2.239	2.309	2.379	2.449	2.519	2.589	2.649	2.719	2.789	2.859	2.929	2.999	3.059	3.129	3.199	3.269	3.339	3.409	3.469	3.539	3.609	3.679	3.749	3.819	3.879
26	2.189	2.259	2.329	2.399	2.469	2.529	2.599	2.669	2.739	2.809	2.879	2.939	3.009	3.079	3.149	3.219	3.289	3.349	3.419	3.489	3.559	3.629	3.699	3.769	3.829
28	2.139	2.209	2.279	2.349	2.409	2.479	2.549	2.619	2.689	2.759	2.829	2.889	2.959	3.029	3.099	3.169	3.239	3.299	3.369	3.439	3.509	3.579	3.649	3.709	3.779
30	2.089	2.159	2.229	2.299	2.359	2.429	2.499	2.569	2.639	2.709	2.769	2.839	2.909	2.979	3.049	3.119	3.179	3.249	3.319	3.389	3.459	3.529	3.589	3.659	3.729
32	2.039	2.109	2.179	2.239	2.309	2.379	2.449	2.519	2.589	2.649	2.719	2.789	2.859	2.929	2.999	3.069	3.129	3.199	3.269	3.339	3.409	3.479	3.539	3.609	3.679
34	1.989	2.059	2.119	2.189	2.259	2.329	2.399	2.469	2.539	2.599	2.669	2.739	2.809	2.879	2.949	3.009	3.079	3.149	3.219	3.289	3.359	3.419	3.489	3.559	3.629
36	1.939	2.009	2.069	2.139	2.209	2.279	2.349	2.419	2.479	2.549	2.619	2.689	2.759	2.829	2.889	2.959	3.029	3.099	3.169	3.239	3.309	3.369	3.439	3.509	3.579
38	1.889	1.949	2.019	2.089	2.159	2.229	2.299	2.359	2.429	2.499	2.569	2.639	2.709	2.779	2.839	2.909	2.979	3.049	3.119	3.189	3.249	3.319	3.389	3.459	3.529
40	1.839	1.899	1.969	2.039	2.109	2.179	2.249	2.309	2.379	2.449	2.519	2.589	2.659	2.719	2.789	2.859	2.929	2.999	3.069	3.129	3.199	3.269	3.339	3.409	3.479
42	1.779	1.849	1.919	1.989	2.059	2.129	2.189	2.259	2.329	2.399	2.469	2.539	2.609	2.669	2.739	2.809	2.879	2.949	3.019	3.079	3.149	3.219	3.289	3.359	3.429
44	1.729	1.799	1.869	1.939	2.009	2.079	2.139	2.209	2.279	2.349	2.419	2.489	2.549	2.619	2.689	2.759	2.829	2.899	2.959	3.029	3.099	3.169	3.239	3.309	3.369
46	1.679	1.749	1.819	1.889	1.959	2.019	2.089	2.159	2.229	2.299	2.369	2.429	2.499	2.569	2.639	2.709	2.779	2.849	2.909	2.979	3.049	3.119	3.189	3.259	3.319
48	1.629	1.699	1.769	1.839	1.899	1.969	2.039	2.109	2.179	2.249	2.319	2.379	2.449	2.519	2.589	2.659	2.729	2.789	2.859	2.929	2.999	3.069	3.139	3.199	3.269
50	1.579	1.649	1.719	1.789	1.849	1.919	1.989	2.059	2.129	2.199	2.259	2.329	2.399	2.469	2.539	2.609	2.669	2.739	2.809	2.879	2.949	3.019	3.089	3.149	3.219
52	1.529	1.599	1.669	1.729	1.799	1.869	1.939	2.009	2.079	2.139	2.209	2.279	2.349	2.419	2.489	2.559	2.619	2.689	2.759	2.829	2.899	2.969	3.029	3.099	3.169
54	1.479	1.549	1.619	1.679	1.749	1.819	1.889	1.959	2.029	2.089	2.159	2.229	3.299	2.369	2.439	2.499	2.569	2.639	2.709	2.779	2.849	2.909	2.979	3.049	3.119
56	1.429	1.499	1.559	1.629	1.699	1.769	1.839	1.909	1.969	2.039	2.109	2.179	2.249	2.319	2.379	2.449	2.519	2.589	2.659	2.729	2.799	2.859	2.929	2.999	3.069
58	1.379	1.439	1.509	1.579	1.649	1.719	1.789	1.859	1.919	1.989	2.059	2.129	2.199	2.269	2.329	2.399	2.469	2.539	2.609	2.679	2.739	2.809	2.879	2.949	3.019
60	1.329	1.389	1.459	1.529	1.599	1.669	1.739	1.799	1.869	1.939	2.009	2.079	2.149	2.209	2.279	2.349	2.419	2.489	2.559	2.619	2.689	2.759	2.829	2.899	2.969
62	1.269	1.339	1.409	1.479	1.549	1.619	1.679	1.749	1.819	1.889	1.959	2.029	2.099	2.159	2.229	2.299	2.369	2.439	2.509	2.569	2.639	2.709	2.779	2.849	2.919
64	1.219	1.289	1.359	1.429	1.499	1.569	1.629	1.699	1.769	1.839	1.909	1.979	2.039	2.109	2.179	2.249	2.319	2.389	2.449	2.519	2.589	2.659	2.729	2.799	2.859
66	1.169	1.239	1.309	1.379	1.449	1.509	1.579	1.649	1.719	1.789	1.859	1.919	1.989	2.059	2.129	2.199	2.269	2.339	2.399	2.469	2.539	2.609	2.679	2.749	2.809
68	1.119	1.189	1.259	1.329	1.389	1.459	1.529	1.599	1.669	1.739	1.809	1.869	1.939	2.009	2.079	2.149	2.219	2.279	2.349	2.419	2.489	2.559	2.629	2.689	2.759
70	1.069	1.139	1.209	1.279	1.339	1.409	1.479	1.549	1.619	1.689	1.749	1.819	1.889	1.959	2.029	2.099	2.159	2.229	2.299	2.369	2.439	2.509	2.579	2.639	2.709
72	1.019	1.089	1.159	1.219	1.289	1.359	1.429	1.499	1.569	1.629	1.699	1.769	1.839	1.909	1.979	2.049	2.109	2.179	2.249	2.319	2.389	2.459	2.519	2.589	2.659
74	0.969	1.039	1.109	1.169	1.239	1.309	1.379	1.449	1.519	1.579	1.649	1.719	1.789	1.859	1.929	1.989	2.059	2.129	2.199	2.269	2.339	2.399	2.469	2.539	2.609

*FEV_1 values are given in liters. The values listed here reflect the FEV_1 as listed in Table 5–5a minus 0.561 L (95% confidence interval). Adapted from Crapo et al.[2]

Table 5-6a Predicted Normal Diffusing Capacity for Carbon Monoxide (Dco) for Men (STPD)*

Age	146	148	150	152	154	156	158	160	162	164	166	168	170	172	174	176	178	180	182	184	186	188	190	192	194
18	29.8	30.6	31.4	32.2	33.1	33.9	34.7	35.5	36.3	37.1	38.0	38.8	39.6	40.4	41.2	42.1	42.9	43.7	44.5	45.4	46.2	47.0	47.8	48.6	49.4
20	29.3	30.2	31.0	31.8	32.6	33.4	34.3	35.1	35.9	36.7	37.5	38.4	39.2	40.0	40.8	41.6	42.5	43.3	44.1	44.9	45.7	46.6	47.4	48.2	49.0
22	28.9	29.7	30.6	31.4	32.2	33.0	33.8	34.7	35.5	36.3	37.1	37.9	38.8	39.6	40.4	41.2	42.0	42.9	43.7	44.5	45.3	46.1	47.0	47.8	48.6
24	28.5	29.3	30.1	31.0	31.8	32.6	33.4	34.2	35.1	35.9	36.7	37.5	38.3	39.2	40.0	40.8	41.6	42.4	43.3	44.1	44.9	45.7	46.5	47.4	48.2
26	28.1	28.9	29.7	30.5	31.4	32.2	33.0	33.8	34.6	35.5	36.3	37.1	37.9	38.7	39.6	40.4	41.2	42.0	42.8	43.7	44.5	45.3	46.1	46.9	47.8
28	27.7	28.5	29.3	30.1	30.9	31.8	32.6	33.4	34.2	35.0	35.9	36.7	37.5	38.3	39.1	40.0	40.8	41.6	42.4	43.2	44.1	44.9	45.7	46.5	47.3
30	27.2	28.1	28.9	29.7	30.5	31.3	32.2	33.0	33.8	34.6	35.4	36.3	37.1	37.9	38.7	39.6	40.4	41.2	42.0	42.8	43.6	44.5	45.3	46.1	46.9
32	26.8	27.6	28.5	29.3	30.1	30.9	31.7	32.6	33.4	34.2	35.0	35.8	36.7	37.5	38.3	39.1	39.9	40.8	41.6	42.4	43.2	44.1	44.9	45.7	46.5
34	26.4	27.2	28.1	28.9	29.7	30.5	31.3	32.1	33.0	33.8	34.6	35.4	36.2	37.1	37.9	38.7	39.5	40.4	41.2	42.0	42.8	43.6	44.4	45.3	46.1
36	26.0	26.8	27.6	28.4	29.3	30.1	30.9	31.7	32.5	33.4	34.2	35.0	35.8	36.6	37.5	38.3	39.1	39.9	40.7	41.6	42.4	43.2	44.0	44.8	45.7
38	25.6	26.4	27.2	28.0	28.8	29.7	30.5	31.3	32.1	32.9	33.8	34.6	35.4	36.2	37.0	37.9	38.7	39.5	40.3	41.1	42.0	42.8	43.6	44.4	45.2
40	25.1	26.0	26.8	27.6	28.4	29.2	30.1	30.9	31.7	32.5	33.3	34.2	35.0	35.8	36.6	37.4	38.3	39.1	39.9	40.7	41.5	42.4	43.2	44.0	44.8
42	24.7	25.5	26.4	27.2	28.0	28.8	29.6	30.5	31.3	32.1	32.9	33.7	34.6	35.4	36.2	37.0	37.8	38.7	39.5	40.3	41.1	41.9	42.8	43.6	44.4
44	24.3	25.1	25.9	26.8	27.6	28.4	29.2	30.0	30.9	31.7	32.5	33.3	34.1	35.0	35.8	36.6	37.4	38.2	39.1	39.9	40.7	41.5	42.3	43.2	44.0
46	23.9	24.7	25.5	26.3	27.2	28.0	28.8	29.6	30.4	31.3	32.1	32.9	33.7	34.6	35.4	36.2	37.0	37.8	38.6	39.5	40.3	41.1	41.9	42.7	43.6
48	23.5	24.3	25.1	25.9	26.7	27.6	28.4	29.2	30.0	30.8	31.7	32.5	33.3	34.1	34.9	35.8	36.6	37.4	38.2	39.1	39.9	40.7	41.5	42.3	43.1
50	23.1	23.9	24.7	25.5	26.3	27.1	28.0	28.8	29.6	30.4	31.2	32.1	32.9	33.7	34.5	35.4	36.2	37.0	37.8	38.6	39.4	40.3	41.1	41.9	42.7
52	22.6	23.4	24.3	25.1	25.9	26.7	27.6	28.4	29.2	30.0	30.8	31.6	32.5	33.3	34.1	34.9	35.7	36.6	37.4	38.2	39.0	39.9	40.7	41.6	42.3
54	22.2	23.0	23.8	24.7	25.5	26.3	27.1	27.9	28.8	29.6	30.4	31.2	32.0	32.9	33.7	34.5	35.3	36.1	37.0	37.8	38.6	39.4	40.2	41.1	41.9
56	21.8	22.6	23.4	24.2	25.1	25.9	26.7	27.5	28.3	29.2	30.0	30.8	31.6	32.4	33.3	34.1	34.9	35.7	36.5	37.4	38.2	39.0	39.8	40.6	41.5
58	21.4	22.2	23.0	23.8	24.6	25.5	26.3	27.1	27.9	28.7	29.6	30.4	31.2	32.0	32.8	33.7	34.5	35.3	36.1	36.9	37.8	38.6	39.4	40.2	41.0
60	20.9	21.8	22.6	23.4	24.2	25.0	25.9	26.7	27.5	28.3	29.1	30.0	30.8	31.6	32.4	33.2	34.1	34.9	35.7	36.5	37.3	38.2	39.0	39.8	40.6
62	20.5	21.3	22.2	23.0	23.8	24.6	25.4	26.3	27.1	27.9	28.7	29.5	30.4	31.2	32.0	32.8	33.6	34.5	35.3	36.1	36.9	37.7	38.6	39.4	40.2
64	20.1	20.9	21.7	22.6	23.4	24.2	25.0	25.8	26.7	27.5	28.3	29.1	29.9	30.8	31.6	32.4	33.2	34.1	34.9	35.7	36.5	37.3	38.1	39.0	39.8
66	19.7	20.5	21.3	22.1	23.0	23.8	24.6	25.4	26.2	27.1	27.9	28.7	29.5	30.4	31.2	32.0	32.8	33.6	34.4	35.3	36.1	36.9	37.7	38.6	39.4
68	19.3	20.1	20.9	21.7	22.6	23.4	24.2	25.0	25.8	26.6	27.5	28.3	29.1	29.9	30.7	31.6	32.4	33.2	34.0	34.9	35.7	36.5	37.3	38.1	38.9
70	18.8	19.7	20.5	21.3	22.1	22.9	23.8	24.6	25.4	26.2	27.0	27.9	28.7	29.5	30.3	31.1	32.0	32.8	33.6	34.4	35.2	36.1	36.9	37.7	38.5
72	18.4	19.2	20.1	20.9	21.7	22.5	23.3	24.2	25.0	25.8	26.6	27.4	28.3	29.1	29.9	30.7	31.5	32.4	33.2	34.0	34.8	35.6	36.5	37.3	38.1
74	18.0	18.8	19.6	20.5	21.3	22.1	22.9	23.7	24.6	25.4	26.2	27.0	27.8	28.7	29.5	30.3	31.1	31.9	32.8	33.6	34.4	35.2	36.0	36.9	37.7

*Dco in mL/min/mm Hg = 0.410 H − 0.210 A − 26.31. R^2 = 0.60; SEE = 4.82; 95% confidence interval = 8.2. Definitions of abbreviations: R^2 = coefficient of determination; SEE = standard error of estimate; H = height in cm; A = age in years. STPD = temperature 0°C, pressure 760 mm Hg, and dry (0 water vapor). The regression analysis has been normalized to a standard hemoglobin of 146 g/L by means of Cotes' modification of the relationship described by Roughton and Forster. Adapted from Crapo and Morris.[9]

Table 5-6b Predicted Lower Limit of Normal Diffusing Capacity for Carbon Monoxide (Dco) for Men*

Age	146	148	150	152	154	156	158	160	162	164	166	168	170	172	174	176	178	180	182	184	186	188	190	192	194
18	21.6	22.4	23.2	24.0	24.9	25.7	26.5	27.3	28.1	28.9	29.8	30.6	31.4	32.2	33.0	33.9	34.7	35.5	36.3	37.2	38.0	38.8	39.6	40.4	41.2
20	21.1	22.0	22.8	23.6	24.4	25.2	26.1	26.9	27.7	28.5	29.3	30.2	31.0	31.8	32.6	33.4	34.3	35.1	35.9	36.7	37.5	38.4	39.2	40.0	40.8
22	20.7	21.5	22.4	23.2	24.0	24.8	25.6	26.5	27.3	28.1	28.9	29.7	30.6	31.4	32.2	33.0	33.8	34.7	35.5	36.3	37.1	37.9	38.8	39.6	40.4
24	20.3	21.1	21.9	22.8	23.6	24.4	25.2	26.0	26.9	27.7	28.5	29.3	30.1	31.0	31.8	32.6	33.4	34.2	35.1	35.9	36.7	37.5	38.3	39.2	40.0
26	19.9	20.7	21.5	22.3	23.2	24.0	24.8	25.6	26.4	27.3	28.1	28.9	29.7	30.5	31.4	32.2	33.0	33.8	34.6	35.5	36.3	37.1	37.9	38.7	39.6
28	19.5	20.3	21.1	21.9	22.7	23.6	24.4	25.2	26.0	26.8	27.7	28.5	29.3	30.1	30.9	31.8	32.6	33.4	34.2	35.0	35.9	36.7	37.5	38.3	39.1
30	19.0	19.9	20.7	21.5	22.3	23.1	24.0	24.8	25.6	26.4	27.2	28.1	28.9	29.7	30.5	31.4	32.2	33.0	33.8	34.6	35.4	36.3	37.1	37.9	38.7
32	18.6	19.4	20.3	21.1	21.9	22.7	23.5	24.4	25.2	26.0	26.8	27.6	28.5	29.3	30.1	30.9	31.7	32.6	33.4	34.2	35.0	35.9	36.7	37.5	38.3
34	18.2	19.0	19.9	20.7	21.5	22.3	23.1	23.9	24.8	25.6	26.4	27.2	28.0	28.9	29.7	30.5	31.3	32.2	33.0	33.8	34.6	35.4	36.2	37.1	37.9
36	17.8	18.6	19.4	20.2	21.1	21.9	22.7	23.5	24.3	25.2	26.0	26.8	27.6	28.4	29.3	30.1	30.9	31.7	32.5	33.4	34.2	35.0	35.8	36.6	37.5
38	17.4	18.2	19.0	19.8	20.6	21.5	22.3	23.1	23.9	24.7	25.6	26.4	27.2	28.0	28.8	29.7	30.5	31.3	32.1	32.9	33.8	34.6	35.4	36.2	37.0
40	16.9	17.8	18.6	19.4	20.2	21.0	21.9	22.7	23.5	24.3	25.1	26.0	26.8	27.6	28.4	29.2	30.1	30.9	31.7	32.5	33.3	34.2	35.0	35.8	36.6
42	16.5	17.3	18.2	19.0	19.8	20.6	21.4	22.3	23.1	23.9	24.7	25.5	26.4	27.2	28.0	28.8	29.6	30.5	31.3	32.1	32.9	33.7	34.6	35.4	36.2
44	16.1	16.9	17.7	18.6	19.4	20.2	21.0	21.8	22.7	23.5	24.3	25.1	25.9	26.8	27.6	28.4	29.2	30.0	30.9	31.7	32.5	33.3	34.1	35.0	35.8
46	15.7	16.5	17.3	18.1	19.0	19.8	20.6	21.4	22.2	23.1	23.9	24.7	25.5	26.4	27.2	28.0	28.8	29.6	30.4	31.3	32.1	32.9	33.7	34.5	35.4
48	15.3	16.1	16.9	17.7	18.5	19.4	20.2	21.0	21.8	22.6	23.5	24.3	25.1	25.9	26.7	27.6	28.4	29.2	30.0	30.9	31.7	32.5	33.3	34.1	34.9
50	14.9	15.7	16.5	17.3	18.1	18.9	19.8	20.6	21.4	22.2	23.0	23.9	24.7	25.5	26.3	27.2	28.0	28.8	29.6	30.4	31.2	32.1	32.9	33.7	34.5
52	14.4	15.2	16.1	16.9	17.7	18.5	19.4	20.2	21.0	21.8	22.6	23.4	24.3	25.1	25.9	26.7	27.5	28.4	29.2	30.0	30.8	31.7	32.5	33.4	34.1
54	14.0	14.8	15.6	16.5	17.3	18.1	18.9	19.7	20.6	21.4	22.2	23.0	23.8	24.7	25.5	26.3	27.1	27.9	28.8	29.6	30.4	31.2	32.0	32.9	33.7
56	13.6	14.4	15.2	16.0	16.9	17.7	18.5	19.3	20.1	21.0	21.8	22.6	23.4	24.2	25.1	25.9	26.7	27.5	28.3	29.2	30.0	30.8	31.6	32.4	33.3
58	13.2	14.0	14.8	15.6	16.4	17.3	18.1	18.9	19.7	20.5	21.4	22.2	23.0	23.8	24.6	25.5	26.3	27.1	27.9	28.7	29.6	30.4	31.2	32.0	32.8
60	12.7	13.6	14.4	15.2	16.0	16.8	17.7	18.5	19.3	20.1	20.9	21.8	22.6	23.4	24.2	25.0	25.9	26.7	27.5	28.3	29.1	30.0	30.8	31.6	32.4
62	12.3	13.1	14.0	14.8	15.6	16.4	17.2	18.1	18.9	19.7	20.5	21.3	22.2	23.0	23.8	24.6	25.4	26.3	27.1	27.9	28.7	29.5	30.4	31.2	32.0
64	11.9	12.7	13.5	14.4	15.2	16.0	16.8	17.6	18.5	19.3	20.1	20.9	21.7	22.6	23.4	24.2	25.0	25.9	26.7	27.5	28.3	29.1	29.9	30.8	31.6
66	11.5	12.3	13.1	13.9	14.8	15.6	16.4	17.2	18.0	18.9	19.7	20.5	21.3	22.2	23.0	23.8	24.6	25.4	26.2	27.1	27.9	28.7	29.5	30.4	31.2
68	11.1	11.9	12.7	13.5	14.4	15.2	16.0	16.8	17.6	18.4	19.3	20.1	20.9	21.7	22.5	23.4	24.2	25.0	25.8	26.7	27.5	28.3	29.1	29.9	30.7
70	10.6	11.5	12.3	13.1	13.9	14.7	15.6	16.4	17.2	18.0	18.8	19.7	20.5	21.3	22.1	22.9	23.8	24.6	25.4	26.2	27.0	27.9	28.7	29.5	30.3
72	10.2	11.0	11.9	12.7	13.5	14.3	15.1	16.0	16.8	17.6	18.4	19.2	20.1	20.9	21.7	22.5	23.3	24.2	25.0	25.8	26.6	27.4	28.3	29.1	29.9
74	9.8	10.6	11.4	12.3	13.1	13.9	14.7	15.5	16.4	17.2	18.0	18.8	19.6	20.5	21.3	22.1	22.9	23.7	24.6	25.4	26.2	27.0	27.8	28.7	29.5

*Dco values are given in mL/min/mm Hg. The values listed here reflect the Dco as listed in Table 5–6a minus 8.2 (95% confidence interval). Adapted from Crapo and Morris.[9]

Table 5-7a Predicted Normal Diffusing Capacity for Carbon Monoxide (Dco) for Women (STPD)*

Age	Height (cm)																								
	146	148	150	152	154	156	158	160	162	164	166	168	170	172	174	176	178	180	182	184	186	188	190	192	194
18	26.0	26.5	27.0	27.6	28.1	28.6	29.2	29.7	30.2	30.8	31.3	31.9	32.4	32.9	33.5	34.0	34.5	35.1	35.6	36.1	36.7	37.2	37.7	38.3	38.8
20	25.7	26.2	26.7	27.3	27.8	28.4	28.9	29.4	30.0	30.5	31.0	31.6	32.1	32.6	33.2	33.7	34.2	34.8	35.3	35.8	36.4	36.9	37.4	38.0	38.5
22	25.4	25.9	26.5	27.0	27.5	28.1	28.6	29.1	29.7	30.2	30.7	31.3	31.8	32.3	32.9	33.4	33.9	34.5	35.0	35.5	36.1	36.6	37.1	37.7	38.2
24	25.1	25.6	26.2	26.7	27.2	27.8	28.3	28.8	29.4	29.9	30.4	31.0	31.5	32.0	32.6	33.1	33.6	34.2	34.7	35.2	35.8	36.3	36.8	37.4	37.9
26	24.8	25.3	25.9	26.4	26.9	27.5	28.0	28.5	29.1	29.6	30.1	30.7	31.2	31.7	32.3	32.8	33.3	33.9	34.4	34.9	35.5	36.0	36.5	37.1	37.6
28	24.5	25.0	25.6	26.1	26.6	27.2	27.7	28.2	28.8	29.3	29.8	30.4	30.9	31.4	32.0	32.5	33.0	33.6	34.1	34.6	35.2	35.7	36.2	36.8	37.3
30	24.2	24.7	25.3	25.8	26.3	26.9	27.4	27.9	28.5	29.0	29.5	30.1	30.6	31.1	31.7	32.2	32.7	33.3	33.8	34.3	34.9	35.4	35.9	36.5	37.0
32	23.9	24.4	25.0	25.5	26.0	26.6	27.1	27.6	28.2	28.7	29.2	29.8	30.3	30.8	31.4	31.9	32.4	33.0	33.5	34.1	34.6	35.1	35.7	36.2	36.7
34	23.6	24.1	24.7	25.2	25.7	26.3	26.8	27.3	27.9	28.4	28.9	29.5	30.0	30.6	31.1	31.6	33.2	32.7	33.2	33.8	34.3	34.8	35.4	35.9	36.4
36	23.3	23.8	24.4	24.9	25.4	26.0	26.5	27.1	27.6	28.1	28.7	29.2	29.7	30.3	30.8	31.3	31.9	32.4	32.9	33.5	34.0	34.5	35.1	35.6	36.1
38	23.0	23.6	24.1	24.6	25.2	25.7	26.2	26.8	27.3	27.8	28.4	28.9	29.4	30.0	30.5	31.0	31.6	32.1	32.6	33.2	33.7	34.2	34.8	35.3	35.8
40	22.7	23.3	23.8	24.3	24.9	25.4	25.9	26.5	27.0	27.5	28.1	28.6	29.1	29.7	30.2	30.7	31.3	31.8	32.3	32.9	33.4	33.9	34.5	35.0	35.5
42	22.4	23.0	23.5	24.0	24.6	25.1	25.6	26.2	26.7	27.2	27.8	28.3	28.8	29.4	29.9	30.4	31.0	31.5	32.0	32.6	33.1	33.6	34.2	34.7	35.2
44	22.1	22.7	23.2	23.7	24.3	24.3	25.3	25.9	26.4	26.9	27.5	28.0	28.5	29.1	29.6	30.1	30.7	31.2	31.7	32.3	32.8	33.3	33.9	34.4	34.9
46	21.8	22.4	22.9	23.4	24.0	24.5	25.0	25.6	26.1	26.6	27.2	27.7	28.2	28.8	29.3	29.8	30.4	30.9	31.4	32.0	32.5	33.0	33.6	34.1	34.6
48	21.5	22.1	22.6	23.1	23.7	24.2	24.7	25.3	25.8	26.3	26.9	27.4	27.9	28.5	29.0	29.5	30.1	30.6	31.1	31.7	32.2	32.8	33.3	33.8	34.4
50	21.2	21.8	22.3	22.8	23.4	23.9	24.4	25.0	25.5	26.0	26.6	27.1	27.6	28.2	28.7	29.3	29.8	30.3	30.9	31.4	31.9	32.5	33.0	33.5	34.1
52	20.9	21.5	22.0	22.5	23.1	23.5	24.1	24.7	25.2	25.8	26.3	26.8	27.4	27.9	28.4	29.0	29.5	30.0	30.6	31.1	31.6	32.2	32.7	33.2	33.8
54	20.6	21.2	21.7	22.3	22.8	23.3	23.9	24.4	24.9	25.5	26.0	26.5	27.1	27.6	28.1	28.7	29.2	29.7	30.3	30.8	31.3	31.9	32.4	32.9	33.5
56	20.4	20.9	21.4	22.0	22.5	23.0	23.6	24.1	24.6	25.2	25.7	26.2	26.8	27.3	27.8	28.4	28.9	29.4	30.0	30.5	31.0	31.6	32.1	32.6	33.2
58	20.1	20.6	21.1	21.7	22.2	22.7	23.3	23.8	24.3	24.9	25.4	25.9	26.5	27.0	27.5	28.1	28.6	29.1	29.7	30.2	30.7	31.3	31.8	32.3	32.9
60	19.8	20.3	20.8	21.4	21.9	22.4	23.0	23.5	24.0	24.6	25.1	25.6	26.2	26.7	27.2	27.8	28.3	28.8	29.4	29.9	30.4	31.0	31.5	32.0	32.6
62	19.5	20.0	20.5	21.1	21.6	22.1	22.7	23.2	23.7	24.3	24.8	25.3	25.9	26.4	26.9	27.5	28.0	28.5	29.1	29.6	30.1	30.7	31.2	31.7	32.3
64	19.2	19.7	20.2	20.8	21.3	21.8	22.4	22.9	23.4	24.0	24.5	25.0	25.6	26.1	26.6	27.2	27.7	28.2	28.8	29.3	29.8	30.4	30.9	31.5	32.0
66	18.9	19.4	19.9	20.5	21.0	21.5	22.1	22.6	23.1	23.7	24.2	24.1	25.3	25.8	26.3	26.9	27.4	28.0	28.5	29.0	29.6	30.1	30.6	31.2	31.7
68	18.6	19.1	19.6	20.2	20.7	21.2	21.8	22.3	22.8	23.4	23.9	24.5	25.0	25.5	26.1	26.6	27.1	27.7	28.2	28.7	29.3	29.8	30.3	30.9	31.4
70	18.3	18.8	19.3	19.9	20.4	21.0	21.5	22.0	22.6	23.1	23.5	24.2	24.7	25.2	25.8	26.3	26.8	27.4	27.9	28.4	29.0	29.5	30.0	30.6	31.1
72	18.0	18.5	19.1	19.6	20.1	20.7	21.2	21.1	22.3	22.8	23.3	23.9	24.4	24.9	25.5	26.0	26.5	27.1	27.6	28.1	28.7	29.2	29.7	30.3	30.8
74	17.7	18.2	18.8	19.3	19.8	20.4	20.9	21.4	22.0	22.5	23.0	23.6	24.1	24.6	25.2	25.7	26.2	26.8	27.3	27.8	28.4	28.9	29.4	30.0	30.5

*Dco is mL/min/mm Hg = 0.267 H – 0.148 A – 10.34. R^2 = 0.60; SEE = 3.40; 95% confidence interval = 5.74. Definitions of abbreviations: R^2 = coefficient of determination; SEE = standard error of estimate; H = height in cm; A = age in years. STPD = temperature 0°C, pressure 760 mm Hg, and dry (0 water vapor). The regression analysis has been normalized to a standard hemoglobin of 125 g/L (the original equation was normalized to a standard hemoglobin of 146 g/L) by means of Cotes' modification of the relationship described in Roughton and Forster. Adapted from Crapo and Morris.[9]

Table 5-7b Predicted Lower Limit of Normal Diffusing Capacity for Carbon Monoxide (Dco) for Women*

Age	Height(cm)																								
	146	148	150	152	154	156	158	160	162	164	166	168	170	172	174	176	178	180	182	184	186	188	190	192	194
18	20.26	20.76	21.26	21.86	22.36	22.86	23.46	23.96	24.46	25.06	25.56	26.16	26.66	27.16	27.76	28.26	28.76	29.36	29.86	30.36	30.96	31.46	31.96	32.56	33.06
20	19.96	20.46	20.96	21.56	22.06	22.66	23.16	23.66	24.26	24.76	25.26	25.86	26.36	26.86	27.46	27.96	28.46	29.06	29.56	30.06	30.66	31.16	31.66	32.26	32.76
22	19.66	20.16	20.76	21.26	21.76	22.36	22.86	23.36	23.96	24.46	24.96	25.56	26.06	26.56	27.16	27.66	28.16	28.76	29.26	29.76	30.36	30.86	31.36	31.96	32.46
24	19.36	19.86	20.46	20.96	21.46	22.06	22.56	23.06	23.66	24.16	24.66	25.26	25.76	26.26	26.86	27.36	27.86	28.46	28.96	29.46	30.06	30.56	31.06	31.66	32.16
26	19.06	19.56	20.16	20.66	21.16	21.76	22.26	22.76	23.36	23.86	24.36	24.96	25.46	25.96	26.56	27.06	27.56	28.16	28.66	29.16	29.76	30.26	30.76	31.36	31.86
28	18.76	19.26	19.86	20.36	20.86	21.46	21.96	22.46	23.06	23.56	24.06	24.66	25.16	25.66	26.26	26.76	27.26	27.86	28.36	28.86	29.46	29.96	30.46	31.06	31.56
30	18.46	18.96	19.56	20.06	20.56	21.16	21.66	22.16	22.76	23.26	23.76	24.36	24.86	25.36	25.96	26.46	26.96	27.56	28.06	28.56	29.16	29.66	30.16	30.76	31.26
32	18.16	18.66	19.26	19.76	20.26	20.86	21.36	21.86	22.46	22.96	23.46	24.06	24.56	25.06	25.66	26.16	26.66	27.26	27.76	28.36	28.86	29.36	29.96	30.46	30.96
34	17.86	18.36	18.96	19.46	19.96	20.56	21.06	21.56	22.16	22.66	23.16	23.76	24.26	24.86	25.36	25.86	27.46	26.96	27.46	28.06	28.56	29.06	29.66	30.16	30.66
36	17.56	18.06	18.66	19.16	19.66	20.26	20.76	21.36	21.86	22.36	22.96	23.46	23.96	24.56	25.06	25.56	26.16	26.66	27.16	27.76	28.26	28.76	29.36	29.86	30.36
38	17.26	17.86	18.36	18.86	19.46	19.96	20.46	21.06	21.56	22.06	22.66	23.16	23.66	24.26	24.76	25.26	25.86	26.36	26.86	27.46	27.96	28.46	29.06	29.56	30.06
40	16.96	17.56	18.06	18.56	19.16	19.66	20.16	20.76	21.26	21.76	22.36	22.86	23.36	23.96	24.46	24.96	25.56	26.06	26.56	27.16	27.66	28.16	28.76	29.26	29.76
42	16.66	17.26	17.76	18.26	18.86	19.36	19.86	20.46	20.96	21.46	22.06	22.56	23.06	23.66	24.16	24.66	25.26	25.76	26.26	26.86	27.36	27.86	28.46	28.96	29.46
44	16.36	16.96	17.46	17.96	18.56	18.56	19.56	20.16	20.66	21.16	21.76	22.26	22.76	23.36	23.86	24.36	24.96	25.46	25.96	26.56	27.06	27.56	28.16	28.66	29.16
46	16.06	16.66	17.16	17.66	18.26	18.76	19.26	19.86	20.36	20.86	21.46	21.96	22.46	23.06	23.56	24.06	24.66	25.16	25.66	26.26	26.76	27.26	27.86	28.36	28.86
48	15.76	16.36	16.86	17.36	17.96	18.46	18.96	19.56	20.06	20.56	21.16	21.66	22.16	22.76	23.26	23.76	24.36	24.86	25.36	25.96	26.46	27.06	27.56	28.06	28.66
50	15.46	16.06	16.56	17.06	17.66	18.16	18.66	19.26	19.76	20.26	20.86	21.36	21.86	22.46	22.96	23.56	24.06	24.56	25.16	25.66	26.16	26.76	27.26	27.76	28.36
52	15.16	15.76	16.26	16.76	17.36	17.76	18.36	18.96	19.46	20.06	20.56	21.06	21.66	22.16	22.66	23.26	23.76	24.26	24.86	25.36	25.86	26.46	26.96	27.46	28.06
54	14.86	15.46	15.96	16.56	17.06	17.56	18.16	18.66	19.16	19.76	20.26	20.76	21.36	21.86	22.36	22.96	23.46	23.96	24.56	25.06	25.56	26.16	26.66	27.16	27.76
56	14.66	15.16	15.66	16.26	16.76	17.26	17.86	18.36	18.86	19.46	19.96	20.46	21.06	21.56	22.06	22.66	23.16	23.66	24.26	24.76	25.26	25.86	26.36	26.86	27.46
58	14.36	14.86	15.36	15.96	16.46	16.96	17.56	18.06	18.56	19.16	19.66	20.16	20.76	21.26	21.76	22.36	22.86	23.36	23.96	24.46	24.96	25.56	26.06	26.56	27.16
60	14.06	14.56	15.06	15.66	16.16	16.66	17.26	17.76	18.26	18.86	19.36	19.86	20.46	20.96	21.46	22.06	22.56	23.06	23.66	24.16	24.66	25.26	25.76	26.26	26.86
62	13.76	14.26	14.76	15.36	15.86	16.36	16.96	17.46	17.96	18.56	19.06	19.56	20.16	20.66	21.16	21.76	22.26	22.76	23.36	23.86	24.36	24.96	25.46	25.96	26.56
64	13.46	13.96	14.46	15.06	15.56	16.06	16.66	17.16	17.66	18.26	18.76	19.26	19.86	20.36	20.86	21.46	21.96	22.46	23.06	23.56	24.06	24.66	25.16	25.76	26.26
66	13.16	13.66	14.16	14.76	15.26	15.76	16.36	16.86	17.36	17.96	18.46	18.36	19.56	20.06	20.56	21.16	21.66	22.26	22.76	23.26	23.86	24.36	24.86	25.46	25.96
68	12.86	13.36	13.86	14.46	14.96	15.46	16.06	16.56	17.06	17.66	18.16	18.76	19.26	19.76	20.36	20.86	21.36	21.96	22.46	22.96	23.56	24.06	24.56	25.16	25.66
70	12.56	13.06	13.56	14.16	14.66	15.26	15.76	16.26	16.86	17.36	17.76	18.46	18.96	19.46	20.06	20.56	21.06	21.66	22.16	22.66	23.26	23.76	24.26	24.86	25.36
72	12.26	12.76	13.36	13.86	14.36	14.96	15.46	15.36	16.56	17.06	17.56	18.16	18.66	19.16	19.76	20.26	20.76	21.36	21.86	22.36	22.96	23.46	23.96	24.56	25.06
74	11.96	12.46	13.06	13.56	14.06	14.66	15.16	15.66	16.26	16.76	17.26	17.86	18.36	18.86	19.46	19.96	20.46	21.06	21.56	22.06	22.66	23.16	23.66	24.26	24.76

*Dco values are given in mL/min/mm Hg. The values listed here reflect the Dco as listed in Table 5–7a minus 5.74 (95% confidence interval). Adapted from Crapo and Morris.[9]

Chapter 5

5.4f Cardiopulmonary Exercise Testing

Cardiopulmonary exercise testing is sometimes useful in assessing whether an individual's complaint of dyspnea (see Table 5-1) is a result of respiratory or other conditions. A person's cardiac and conditioning status must be considered in performing the test and in interpreting the results.

The cardiopulmonary exercise gas-exchange measurement can be an additional means of assessing the severity and cause of exercise intolerance. Simultaneous measurement of carbon dioxide (CO_2) production, minute ventilation, and heart rate allows determination of whether exercise capacity limitation is due to cardiac, pulmonary, or coexisting impairments. When properly performed and interpreted, these tests can help differentiate pulmonary impairment from cardiac impairment or physical deconditioning effects.[24]

Exercise capacity is measured by oxygen consumption per unit time ($\dot{V}o_2$) in milliliters per kilogram multiplied by minutes (mL/[kg•min]) or in metabolic equivalents (METS), a unit of expended energy equal to 3.5 mL/(kg•min) oxygen consumption. MET is discussed in Chapter 3 in the sections on the heart and aorta. Generally, an individual can sustain a work level equal to 40% of his or her measured maximum $\dot{V}o_2$ for an 8-hour period.[25] Table 5-8 shows the relationship between work intensity and oxygen consumption.

Table 5-8 Impairment Classification for Prolonged Physical Work Intensity by Oxygen Consumption*

Work Intensity for 70-kg Person*	Oxygen Consumption	Excess Energy Expenditure
Light work	7 mL/kg; 0.5 L/min	< 2 METS
Moderate work	8-15 mL/kg; 0.6-1.0 L/min	2-4 METS
Heavy work	16-20 mL/kg; 1.1-1.5 L/min	5-6 METS
Very heavy work	21-30 mL/kg; 1.6-2.0 L/min	7-8 METS
Arduous work	> 30 mL/kg; > 2.0 L/min	> 8 METS

*Adapted from Astrand and Rodahl.[26] mL/kg indicates milliliter per kilogram; L/min, liter per minute; and METS, metabolic equivalents (multiples of resting oxygen uptake).

Use cardiopulmonary exercise testing judiciously since these studies can be difficult to perform, are more expensive, and are sometimes more invasive than conventional tests. Ordinarily, exercise capacity measurements are not used to study individuals with normal results on routine pulmonary function tests. However, they can be helpful when the results of pulmonary function tests do not correlate with the individual's symptoms or when additional information is needed to clarify the nature and severity of an impairment.[27] Do not use exercise capacity measurements to study individuals with medical contraindications such as unstable cardiac disease.

Arterial Blood Gas Analysis

Because of its invasive nature, use arterial blood gas analysis only when necessary to evaluate pulmonary impairment. Arterial blood gas analysis results may be outside the normal range for reasons other than pulmonary disease. For most individuals with obstructive lung disease, exercise capacity correlates better with FEV_1 than arterial partial pressure of oxygen (Po_2). For purposes of evaluating permanent impairment, hypoxia must be measured on two separate occasions at least 4 weeks apart.

Pulse oximetry, which is less invasive than arterial blood gas, often provides an adequate estimate of hypoxia. Arterial blood gases, although more invasive, provide a more accurate measurement of hypoxia. Physicians should use their clinical judgment as to which measurement is needed, based on individual assessment.

An arterial blood gas determination may indicate the presence of severe impairment even when a person's condition is stable and he or she is receiving optimal therapy. An arterial Po_2 of less than 55 mm Hg is evidence of severe impairment when an individual is examined at rest while breathing room air at sea level. Severe impairment may also be diagnosed with an arterial Po_2 of less than 60 mm Hg if the person also has one or more of the following conditions: pulmonary hypertension, cor pulmonale, increasingly severe hypoxia during exercise testing, or erythrocytosis.

5.4g Criteria for Rating Impairment Due to Respiratory Disease

Table 5-12 presents criteria for estimating the permanent impairment rating for different respiratory conditions, discussed below. Perform spirometry and Dco on each person being evaluated.[3] $\dot{V}o_2$max may provide additional information in selected individuals when indicated. The person must meet all of the listed criteria except for $\dot{V}o_2$max in order to be considered nonimpaired. At least one of the listed criteria must be fulfilled to place an individual in any class with an impairment rating. As discussed in Chapter 1, in individuals where the preinjury or preillness values differ from the population-listed values, the examiner may depart from the population-listed normal values for determining an impairment rating, using the preinjury and preillness "normal" value, and explain the reason for the departure.

5.5 Asthma

Asthma is an airway inflammatory disease characterized by episodic and variable airflow limitation and airway hyperresponsiveness. A diagnosis of asthma requires relevant symptoms (eg, cough, sputum, wheeze, chest tightness, or breathlessness) and *either* evidence of airflow obstruction that is partially or completely reversible (either spontaneously or after treatment) or airway reactivity to methacholine *or* histamine in the absence of airflow limitation.[10]

Variable airflow obstruction can be detected with pulmonary function testing, which shows a reversible obstructive airway pattern. Airway hyperresponsiveness is detected by bronchial challenge testing with methacholine or histamine.[28] Airway hyperresponsiveness is defined as a positive methacholine or histamine challenge, as reflected by a decrease in FEV_1 of 20% (PC_{20}) from baseline, upon provocation with less than or equal to 8 mg/mL of methacholine or histamine using the tidal breathing method or its equivalent.[1,18] The results from methacholine testing should be expressed as the provocation concentration to cause a fall in FEV_1 of 20% (PC_{20}).

While different varieties of asthma exist, they all share an underlying commonality of airway hyperresponsiveness. Occupational asthma represents a special subset of asthma subjects. This abnormality has now surpassed pneumoconiosis as the most commonly reported occupational lung disease linked to a particular occupational environment or agent. Besides directly causing occupational asthma, work exposures can acutely exacerbate an underlying asthmatic condition, which can subsequently return to preexposure baseline status with removal from exposure. Work exposures can also cause a more permanent change in an underlying asthmatic condition, which can persist even after removal from exposure. If an individual's asthma is worsening at work, it is important to remove the individual from exposure or, at a minimum, reduce exposure and reevaluate his or her condition when it has stabilized. Although prevention is optimal, medication can substantially modify symptoms and the clinical course of asthma.

Occupational asthma can be caused by sensitizers or irritants. Sensitizers are classified as either high molecular weight or low molecular weight. High-molecular-weight sensitizers of animal or plant origin include animal dander or grain dust. Low-molecular-weight sensitizers, typically organic or inorganic chemicals, include diisocyanates. Sensitizers generally require a latency period for the development of immunologic responsiveness. This latency period may last from a few weeks to several years after first exposure.[29]

In the case of sensitizer-induced asthma (such as toluene diisocyanate or latex), there is a potential for severe exacerbation or fatality upon reexposure. Although many individuals with occupational asthma improve after removal from exposure to either low-molecular-weight or high-molecular-weight sensitizers, more than half fail to recover completely, even after 2 or more years since the last exposure. Those who are sensitized to occupational agents ideally should discontinue further exposure. Both the individual and his or her physician need to monitor the course of asthmatic symptoms, especially if ongoing exposure occurs. Many can be identified as having a particular type of asthma. For those who have allergic asthma, exercise-induced and irritant-induced components may be identified as well.

Irritant-induced asthma, known as reactive airways dysfunction syndrome (RADS), may result from a single high-level exposure to a highly irritating gas, fume, mist, or vapor. The diagnosis of RADS requires (1) inhalation exposure to an acutely irritating concentration of a substance, (2) onset of symptoms (cough, wheezing cough, or dyspnea) within 24 hours after exposure with persistent respiratory symptoms, and (3) functional abnormalities (airway hyperresponsiveness) for more than 3 months, with no preexisting respiratory disease.[30]

Irritant-induced asthma often improves with time; some people may resume their former employment. However, some individuals experience persistent respiratory impairment. Individual assessment is important because reducing the degree and duration of exposure may control symptoms in some people, but complete removal from exposure may be necessary to control symptoms in others.

Occupational and nonoccupational asthma impairment evaluations follow the same guidelines. Both require a thorough review of current occupational and home environments and the likelihood of similar exposures in subsequent workplaces. When assessing impairment due to asthma, information is needed from both clinical and physiologic parameters. The AMA recommends that the examiner follow ATS guidelines when assessing asthma impairment and include measurements of pulmonary mechanics, airway hyperresponsiveness, and medication requirements.[1] Table 5-9 lists the criteria for impairment evaluation for asthma severity. The examiner evaluates the indices listed, including the minimum medication needed to control the individual's asthma.

Before performing an impairment rating for asthma, the examiner needs to determine that the pattern of asthma is clinically stable and well treated, based upon fulfilling the objectives of treatment as detailed by the expert panel report of the National Asthma Education Program.[18,31] The objectives of treatment are: (1) to achieve control or the best overall results (least symptoms, least need for ß-adrenergic agonists when taken only if required, best expiratory flow rates, least diurnal variation of flow rates, and least side effects from medication); (2) to use the minimum amount of medication to maintain control or the best overall results; and (3) to treat exacerbations early to prevent them from becoming severe.

In 1993, the ATS developed guidelines for the evaluation of impairment and/or disability in individuals with asthma.[1] According to the ATS statement, asthma necessitated special guidelines because of its distinct features, including: (1) variable airflow obstruction and change in clinical status over time; (2) partial or complete reversibility of airflow obstruction with therapy; (3) nonspecific airway hyperresponsiveness to irritants such as dusts, gases, fumes, or smoke; and (4) sensitization to occupational agents producing airway inflammation that with repeated exposure may become chronic and irreversible.

In assessing an individual with suspected asthma, if the prebronchodilator FEV_1 is above the lower limit of normal, use methacholine challenge to assess airway responsiveness. The degree of airway hyperresponsiveness and scoring are illustrated in Table 5-9. If the prebronchodilator FEV_1 is below the lower limit of normal, the degree of reversibility is assessed with inhaled bronchodilators (see Table 5-9 for scoring).

To perform the evaluation at a state of maximal medical improvement, choose the optimal drug treatment to minimize symptoms. The type and extent of necessary medication is one measure of impairment severity (see Table 5-9 for scoring). Use of medication, as a score for impairment, is only used in individuals who have a diagnosis of asthma.

The scores for postbronchodilator FEV_1, reversibility of FEV_1 (or PC_{20}), and medication use are added to obtain a summary score for respiratory impairment (see Table 5-10). ATS criteria do not assign impairment percentages. If an impairment percentage is needed, refer to Table 5-10, which assigns impairment classes and percentages to an asthma score. The authors of this chapter have assigned these impairment percentages according to the ATS criteria, based on their clinical judgment. In determining the percent impairment for a particular class, the examiner needs to consider how the person's asthma affects the ability to perform activities of daily living.

Chapter 5

Table 5-9 Impairment Classification for Asthma Severity*

Score	Postbronchodilator FEV₁	% of FEV₁ Change (Reversibility) *or*	PC₂₀ mg/mL or Equivalent (Degree of Airway Hyperresponsiveness)†	Minimum Medication‡
0	≥ lower limit of normal	<10%	> 8 mg/mL	No medication
1	≥ 70% of predicted	10%-19%	8 mg/mL to > 0.6 mg/mL	Occasional but not daily bronchodilator and/or occasional but not daily cromolyn
2	60%-69% of predicted	20%-29%	0.6 mg/mL to > 0.125mg/mL	Daily bronchodilator and/or daily cromolyn and/or daily low-dose inhaled corticosteroid (≤ 800 µg of beclomethasone or equivalent)
3	50%-59% of predicted	≥ 30%	≤ 0.125 mg/mL	Bronchodilator on demand and daily high-dose inhaled corticosteroid (>800 µg of beclomethasone or equivalent) or occasional course (one to three courses a year) of systemic corticosteroid
4	<50% of predicted	. . .	. . .	Bronchodilator on demand and daily high-dose inhaled corticosteroid (>1000 µg of beclomethasone or equivalent) and daily or every other day systemic corticosteroid

*FEV₁ indicates forced expiratory volume in the first second; PC₂₀ is the provocative concentration that causes a 20% fall in FEV₁. Add the scores for postbronchodilator FEV₁, reversibility of FEV₁ (or PC₂₀), and medication use to obtain a summary severity score for rating respiratory impairment.

†When FEV₁ is greater than the lower limit of normal, PC₂₀ should be determined and used for rating of impairment; when FEV₁ is less than 70% of the predicted, the degree of reversibility should be used; and when FEV₁ is between 70% of the predicted and the lower limit of normal, either reversibility or PC₂₀ can be used. The score for minimum medication use is added to the appropriate measurement criteria outlined above.

‡Need for minimum medication should be demonstrated by the treating physician, for example, through previous records of exacerbation when medications have been reduced. Adapted from ATS guidelines.[1]

Table 5-10 Impairment Rating for Asthma*

Total Asthma Score	% Impairment Class	Impairment of the Whole Person
0	1	0%
1-5	2	10%-25%
6-9	3	26%-50%
10-11 or asthma not controlled despite maximal treatment, ie, FEV₁ remaining <50% despite use of > 20 mg/day of prednisone	4	51%-100%

*The impairment rating is calculated as the sum of the individual's scores from Table 5-9. FEV₁ indicates forced expiratory volume in the first second.

5.6 Obstructive Sleep Apnea

Individuals with obstructive sleep apnea experience intermittent, repetitive occlusions of the upper airway during sleep, when the pharyngeal muscles are relaxed. These occlusion periods produce airflow cessation at the nose and mouth that leads to progressive hypoxia, which then causes arousal from sleep. The affected person awakens briefly and reestablishes airway patency, resuming airflow with a loud snore or snorting sound. Because of recurrent awakenings during the night, there is disrupted sleep architecture, without restful sleep. Symptoms of sleep apnea include a history of loud snoring, unsatisfactory sleep pattern, daytime somnolence, cognitive dysfunction, and hypertension. Between 60% and 90% are obese and may have a large neck circumference. When the disorder is severe, erythrocytosis, pulmonary hypertension, and cor pulmonale may result.

Even if total occlusion of the upper airway does not occur during sleep, partial obstruction can lead to significant reduction in airflow and produce obstructive hypopnea, which causes oxyhemoglobin saturation reduction and similar clinical and physiologic abnormalities as seen in obstructive sleep apnea.

A variant of obstructive sleep apnea is the obesity hypoventilation syndrome. The weight of the chest wall in morbidly obese individuals may limit respiratory movements during sleep and wakefulness. As a result, both hypoxia and hypercapnia persist throughout the day as well as during sleep. The same physiologic consequences occur in these individuals as in those with obstructive sleep apnea. In fact, obstructive sleep apnea and obesity hypoventilation syndrome may coexist in the same person.

People affected by obstructive sleep apnea are at significantly increased risk of being involved in motor vehicle collisions. Severe daytime somnolence may prevent them from functioning adequately. Subtle changes in neuropsychological function include memory abnormalities and worsened motor coordination and mood that may affect the person's daily life.

A diagnosis of obstructive sleep apnea is confirmed by nocturnal polysomnography in an accredited sleep laboratory. Once the diagnosis has been established, prescribe continuous positive airway pressure (CPAP) through a nasal device for use during sleep to maintain upper airway patency. Weight loss is the most effective means of long-term management and a possible cure for obstructive sleep apnea if a lower body mass index can be maintained.[32]

Grading obstructive sleep apnea severity depends on the number of apnea/hypopnea episodes observed in polysomnography and the severity of hypoxia caused by these episodes. There are no standard, well-documented criteria for determining the level of impairment based on the results of polysomnography. For purposes of impairment rating as discussed in this chapter, refer to the judgment of a sleep specialist.

5.7 Hypersensitivity Pneumonitis

Hypersensitivity pneumonitis, also known as extrinsic allergic alveolitis, is a granulomatous interstitial and bronchiolar lung disease caused by immune sensitization to organic dusts and some low-molecular-weight chemical antigens. A wide variety of antigenic substances are known to cause this disease. The acute disease is characterized by the onset of respiratory and constitutional symptoms beginning 4 to 8 hours after exposure to the offending material. Symptoms include chest tightness, cough, dyspnea, fever, chills, malaise, and myalgias. Pulmonary function tests in the acute phase of the disease show volume restriction and decreased diffusing capacity. Hypoxia may be demonstrated by pulse oximetry or arterial blood gas testing. Chest radiographs may be normal but often show diffuse micronodular changes in the pulmonary parenchyma. When the person is removed from exposure, the symptoms, physiologic changes, and chest radiographic abnormalities begin to resolve within 1 to 2 days, although they may take 4 to 6 weeks for complete resolution.

In the subacute and chronic presentations of hypersensitivity pneumonitis, the predominant symptoms include exertional dyspnea and cough; some report sputum production, anorexia, fatigue, and weight loss. Pulmonary function studies often show mixed restriction and obstruction with isolated obstructive changes in some individuals. With repeated exposures, pulmonary fibrotic changes may occur as the abnormalities become chronic and irreversible.[33]

Permanently restrict individuals with hypersensitivity pneumonitis from exposure to the sensitizing agent. If pulmonary fibrosis has not supervened, normal pulmonary function may be reestablished. However, the onset of pulmonary fibrosis is likely to produce respiratory impairment and may limit other types of employment. Once the acute episode has resolved and the condition is stable, the examiner may rate the degree of permanent impairment according to the criteria given in Table 5-12.

Asthma, pneumoconiosis, and hypersensitivity pneumonitis may require that the person refrain from working in a specific occupational setting where he or she is exposed to the offending agent. If reassigned where no ongoing exposure occurs, the individual may not have a permanent respiratory impairment.

5.8 Pneumoconiosis

Pneumoconiosis is a term used to describe diseases resulting from the inhalation of mineral dusts such as silica, coal, and asbestos, and metals such as cobalt and beryllium. The radiologic and pathologic patterns of pneumoconiosis from these dusts are usually quite distinct and beyond the scope of this chapter. Latency between exposure to these dusts and development of disease varies, but disease can occur anywhere from 10 up to 30 years after initial exposure.[34]

The severity of impairment related to pneumoconiosis depends on the characteristics of the specific dust inhaled, the dust burden retained in the lungs, the susceptibility of the individual, and the length of time since first exposure. Under some circumstances, the parenchymal changes on chest radiograph may be progressive even after removal from exposure and may or may not be associated with physiologic impairment. Persons who develop pneumoconiosis should limit further exposure to the offending agent, particularly if radiographic changes have occurred at a relatively young age or if there is associated physiologic impairment. However, these individuals may be capable of working at other jobs where the offending dust is not present. See Table 5-12 for criteria for assessment of impairment due to pneumoconiosis.

5.9 Lung Cancer

All persons with lung cancer are severely impaired at diagnosis. At reevaluation 1 year after the diagnosis is established, if the person is found to be free of all evidence of tumor recurrence, then he or she is evaluated according to criteria listed in Table 5-12. If there is still evidence of tumor, the he or she is considered to be severely impaired (class 4 impairment); if the tumor recurs, the person will also be considered to be severely impaired (class 4 impairment). Table 5-11 (the Karnofsky scale), specifically developed to describe the capabilities of individuals with cancer, may be used to further describe the capabilities of a person with lung cancer and enable categorization within a particular class.

Table 5-11 Scale for Judging Capabilities of Subjects With Cancer*

Grade	Description
0	Fully active; able to carry on all predisease activities without restrictions
1	Restricted in physically strenuous activity but ambulatory and able to carry out light tasks, such as light work in home or office
2	Requires occasional to considerable care for most needs and frequent medical care
3	Capable only of limited self-care and confined to bed or chair at least half of waking hours
4	Almost totally impaired; cannot care for self, and totally confined to bed or chair

Adapted from Moossa et al.[35]

5.10 Permanent Impairment Due to Respiratory Disorders

Table 5-12 lists criteria for estimating the permanent impairment rating due to respiratory disorders, using pulmonary function and exercise test results. Perform spirometry and Dco on each person being evaluated.[3] $\dot{V}o_2$max may provide additional information in selected individuals when indicated. Determine the predicted values for FVC, FEV_1, and Dco using Tables 5-2a through 5-7a, and calculate the percent predicted (observed/predicted value). Determine the lower limit of normal for FVC, FEV_1, and Dco using Tables 5-2b through 5-7b. The person must meet all of the listed criteria except for $\dot{V}o_2$max in order to be considered nonimpaired. At least one of the listed criteria must be fulfilled to place an individual in any class with an impairment rating. As discussed in Chapter 1, in individuals where the preinjury or preillness values differ from the population-listed values, the examiner may depart from the population-listed normal values for determining an impairment rating, using the preinjury and preillness "normal" value, and explain the reason for the departure.

The classification system in Table 5-12 considers only pulmonary function measurements for an impairment rating. It is recognized that pulmonary impairment can occur that does not significantly impact pulmonary function and exercise test results but that does impact the ability to perform activities of daily living, such as with bronchiectasis.

In these limited cases, the physician may assign an impairment rating based on the extent and severity of pulmonary dysfunction and the inability to perform activities of daily living (see Table 1-2). Measured losses of pulmonary function, and corresponding impairment classes, result in a loss in the ability to perform some activities of daily living. The physician can use these associations as a reference. A detailed description with supporting, objective documentation of the type of pulmonary impairment and its impact on the ability to perform activities of daily living is required.

Table 5-12 Impairment Classification for Respiratory Disorders, Using Pulmonary Function and Exercise Test Results*

Pulmonary Function Test	Class 1 0% Impairment of the Whole Person	Class 2 10%-25% Impairment of the Whole Person	Class 3 26%-50% Impairment of the Whole Person	Class 4 51%-100% Impairment of the Whole Person
FVC	Measured FVC ≥ lower limit of normal (see Tables 5-2b and 5-3b) **and**	≥ 60% of predicted and < lower limit of normal **or**	≥ 51% and ≤ 59% of predicted **or**	≤ 50% of predicted **or**
FEV_1	Measured FEV_1 ≥ lower limit of normal (see Tables 5-4b and 5-5b) **and**	≥ 60% of predicted and < lower limit of normal **or**	≥ 41% and ≤ 59% of predicted **or**	≤ 40% of predicted **or**
FEV_1/FVC	FEV_1/FVC ≥ lower limit of normal† **and**			
Dco	Dco ≥ lower limit of normal (see Tables 5-6b and 5-7b) **or**	≥ 60% of predicted and < lower limit of normal **or**	≥ 41% and ≤ 59% of predicted **or**	≤ 40% of predicted **or**
$\dot{V}o_2$max	$\dot{V}o_2$max ≥ 25 mL/(kg•min) **or** > 7.1 METS	≥ 20 and < 25 mL/(kg•min) **or** 5.7-7.1 METS	≥ 15 and < 20 mL/(kg•min) **or** 4.3 to < 5.7 METS	< 15 mL/(kg•min) **or** < 1.05 L/min **or** < 4.3 METS

*FVC indicates forced vital capacity; FEV_1, forced expiratory volume in the first second; Dco, diffusing capacity for carbon monoxide; $\dot{V}o_2$max, maximum oxygen consumption; and METS, metabolic equivalents (multiples of resting oxygen uptake). Dco is primarily of value for persons with restrictive lung disease. In classes 2 and 3, if FVC, FEV_1, and FEV_1/FVC are normal and Dco is between 41% and 79%, then an exercise test is required to determine level of impairment.

†Refer to Crapo RO, Morris AH, Gardner RM for the lower limit of normal for FEV_1/FVC.[2]

| Class 1 |
| 0% Respiratory Impairment |
| **Measured FVC:** ≥ lower limit of normal (see Tables 5-2b and 5-3b) |
| *and* |
| **Measured FEV₁:** ≥ lower limit of normal (see Tables 5-4b and 5-5b) |
| *and* |
| **FEV₁/FVC:** ≥ lower limit of normal |
| *and* |
| **Dco:** ≥ lower limit of normal (see Tables 5-6b and 5-7b) |
| *or* |
| **V̇o₂max:** ≥ 25 mL/(kg•min) *or* 7.1 METS |

Example 5-1
0% Impairment Due to Chronic Bronchitis

Subject: 40-year-old man.

History: Foundry worker for 21 years; nonsmoker.

Current Symptoms: Daily productive cough for several years; on most days for 3 consecutive months; no dyspnea on exertion.

Physical Exam: Height: 188 cm (6 ft 2 in); weight 95.3 kg (210 lb).

Clinical Studies: Scattered rhonchi in both lungs. Chest radiograph: normal. FVC (L): observed 5.67; predicted 5.77; observed/predicted 98%. FEV₁ (L): observed 4.51; predicted 4.62; observed/predicted 98%. FEV₁/FVC: observed 79.5%. Dco: observed/predicted 91%.

Diagnosis: Chronic bronchitis.

Impairment Rating: 0% impairment of the whole person.

Comment: Pulmonary function tests normal. If earlier pulmonary function tests available, comparison with current results recommended.

Example 5-2
0% Impairment Due to Respiratory Disease

Subject: 50-year-old man.

History: Delivery truck driver for 25 years; hospitalized for anteroseptal myocardial infarction 3 months earlier; returned to work. Progressive exercise program. Smoker: 35 pack-year history.

Current Symptoms: Shortness of breath carrying three boxes up a flight of stairs. Allowed to return to work after beginning a progressive exercise program.

Physical Exam: Height: 188 cm (6 ft 2 in); weight 86.4 kg (190 lb). Normal breath sounds and cardiac examination.

Clinical Studies: Chest radiograph: left ventricle enlargement; normal lungs. FVC (L): observed 5.28; predicted 5.56; observed/predicted 95%. FEV₁ (L): observed 3.85; predicted 4.37; observed/predicted 88%. FEV₁/FVC: observed 73%. Dco: 91%. V̇o₂: 18 mL/kg.

Diagnosis: Inadequate cardiac output resulting from myocardial infarction.

Impairment Rating: 0% impairment of the whole person based on respiratory function alone.

Comment: Pulmonary function studies indicate class 1 and no respiratory impairment. See *Guides* Chapters 3 and 4 to determine cardiovascular system impairment.

| Class 2 |
| 10%-25% Respiratory Impairment |
| **Measured FVC:** ≥ 60% of predicted and < lower limit of normal |
| *or* |
| **Measured FEV₁:** ≥ 60% of predicted and < lower limit of normal |
| *or* |
| **Dco:** ≥ 60% of predicted and < lower limit of normal |
| *or* |
| **V̇o₂max:** ≥ 20 and < 25 mL/(kg•min) *or* 5.7-7.1 METS |

Example 5-3
10% to 25% Impairment Due to Respiratory Disease

Subject: 54-year-old man.

History: Retired power plant mechanic; routine asbestos exposure from ages 18 to 37. Currently 10-year nonsmoker; previous 24 pack-year history of smoking.

Current Symptoms: Dyspnea when walking on level ground with others his age.

Physical Exam: Height 175 cm (5 ft 9 in); weight 115 kg (253 lb). Auscultation: shortened expiratory phase; no crackles or wheezes. Diminished posterior breath sounds at both lung bases.

Clinical Studies: On radiograph: moderately extensive focal pleural thickening; diffuse pleural thickening of left lateral chest wall extending into left costophrenic angle. Calcified pleural plaque in left hemidiaphragm. No interstitial changes. FVC (L): observed 3.00; predicted 4.69; observed/predicted 64%. FEV₁ (L): observed 2.43; predicted 3.74; observed/predicted 65%. FEV₁/FVC: observed 81%. Dco: observed/predicted 78%.

Diagnosis: Diffuse asbestos-related pleural changes with restrictive physiology. No evidence of parenchymal asbestosis.

Impairment Rating: 10% to 25% impairment of the whole person.

Comment: Diffuse pleural fibrosis may cause permanent restrictive impairment.

Example 5-4
10% to 25% Impairment Due to Respiratory Disease

Subject: 58-year-old woman.

History: Teacher; several years' daily cough with morning sputum production. Smoked 1.5 packs per day from ages 16 to 58. No asthma, pneumonia, or exposure to hazardous dusts, chemicals, or fumes.

Current Symptoms: Some wheezing, especially with colds. No dyspnea, chest pain, or hemoptysis.

Physical Exam: Height: 168 cm (5 ft 6 in); weight: 61 kg (135 lb). Forced exhalation expiratory wheeze.

Clinical Studies: Chest radiograph: normal. FVC (L): observed 2.73; predicted 3.41; observed/predicted 80%. FEV_1 (L): observed 1.83; predicted 2.69; observed/predicted 68%. FEV_1/FVC: observed 67%. Dco: observed/predicted 73%. $\dot{V}o_2$max: 20 mL/kg/min.

Diagnosis: Chronic bronchitis with mild airflow obstruction.

Impairment Rating: 10% to 25% impairment of the whole person.

Comment: Mild airflow obstruction caused by cigarette smoking.

Example 5-5
10% to 25% Impairment Due to Respiratory Disease

Subject: 48-year-old man.

History: Dairy farmer; various hospitalizations for pneumonia. No cardiovascular disease, asthma, or cigarette smoking. Works with hay stored in barn; particularly dusty during winter.

Current Symptoms: Persistent nonproductive cough; short of breath on exertion.

Physical Exam: Height: 177 cm (5 ft 10 in); weight: 77 kg (170 lb). Persistent bilateral end-inspiratory crackles in posterior and lateral bases.

Clinical Studies: Chest radiograph: diffuse fibrotic process throughout both lung fields. Prior radiographs: no change over 5 years. FVC (L): observed 3.47; predicted 4.99; observed/predicted 70%. FEV_1 (L): observed 2.69; predicted 4.00; observed/predicted 67%. FEV_1/FVC: observed 78%. Dco: observed/predicted 64%. $\dot{V}o_2$max: 20 mL/kg/min.

Diagnosis: Hypersensitivity pneumonitis.

Impairment Rating: 10% to 25% impairment of the whole person.

Comment: Pulmonary function impairment; permanently restrict exposure to moldy hay.

Example 5-6
10% to 25% Impairment Due to Respiratory Disease

Subject: 25-year-old man.

History: Self-employed auto body worker; no previous history of asthma. Had been spray painting for 5 years with paints containing hexamethylene diisocyanate (HDI), one of the asthma-causing diisocyanates. Admitted to the hospital with wheezing; a diagnosis of asthma was made; was started on asthma medications. After 2 years of avoidance of HDI, while compliantly following medication regimen of high-dose inhaled corticosteroids and, as needed, beta-agonist bronchodilator, minimum medication need score was 3.

Current Symptoms: Exercise-related and nocturnal coughing and wheezing.

Physical Exam: Normal.

Clinical Studies: Spirometry without bronchodilators and diffusing capacity: normal, but a methacholine challenge test showed airway hyperreactivity with PC_{20} methacholine of 5 mg/mL (score 1).

Diagnosis: Occupational asthma due to HDI.

Impairment Rating: Asthma score (Table 5-9): 4; 10% to 25% impairment of the whole person (Table 5-10).

Comment: No further exposure to diisocyanates is recommended.

Chapter 5

Class 3
26%-50% Respiratory Impairment
Measured FVC: ≥ 51% and ≤ 59% of predicted
or
Measured FEV₁: ≥ 41% and ≤ 59% of predicted
or
Dco: ≥ 41% and ≤ 59% of predicted
or
V̇o₂max: ≥ 15 and < 20 mL/(kg·min) *or* 4.3 to < 5.7 METS

Example 5-7
26% to 50% Impairment Due to Respiratory Disease

Subject: 60-year-old man.

History: Insulator for 40 years; mixed powdered asbestos with water and applied it to pipes and steel beams for first 20 years. Denies cough, wheezing, or chest pain. Nonsmoker. No asthma, pneumonia, or other medical disorders. No medications.

Current Symptoms: Increasing dyspnea for 5 years; difficulty keeping up with others the same age. Unable to walk upstairs past second flight.

Physical Exam: Height: 170 cm (5 ft 7 in); weight: 70.5 kg (155 lb). Questionable finger clubbing; bilateral end-inspiratory crackles at lung bases. Cardiac examination: normal.

Clinical Studies: Chest radiograph: moderately pronounced, small, linear, irregular opacities at lung bases; small, bilateral pleural plaques. FVC (L): observed 2.35; predicted 4.27; observed/predicted 55%. FEV_1 (L): observed 2.10; predicted 3.38; observed/predicted 62%. FEV_1/FVC: observed 89%. Dco: observed 16.0; predicted 30.8; observed/predicted 52%. V̇o₂max: 16 mL/kg/min.

Diagnosis: Asbestosis and asbestos-related pleural plaques.

Impairment Rating: 26% to 50% impairment of the whole person.

Comment: Interstitial lung disease with crackles, decreased vital capacity, and decreased gas exchange. Decreased oxygen uptake probably due to pulmonary dysfunction.

Example 5-8
26% to 50% Impairment Due to Asthma

Subject: 33-year-old woman.

History: Natural rubber latex glove inspector for 7 years; no prior history of asthma, but history of eczema. When away from work, symptoms persisted, exacerbated by weather changes, anxiety, or moderate exercise. Symptoms were less severe than when working with latex.

Current Symptoms: Episodic cough, shortness of breath, chest tightness, and occasional wheezing, with symptom onset within 10 minutes of onset of work and persistent throughout the day. Job involved testing surgical latex gloves for leaks by inflating with compressed air, which released cornstarch glove powder into the air. Symptoms improved, but did not resolve, while on a 12-day vacation.

Physical Exam: Diffuse wheezing.

Clinical Studies: Chest x-ray: normal. Spirometry: showed postbronchodilator FEV_1 68% (score 2), with a 20% change in FEV_1 (score 2). During follow-up 3 months later, she was still on daily low-dose inhaled corticosteroids, with daily bronchodilator use (score 2).

Diagnosis: Latex-induced occupational asthma.

Impairment Rating: Asthma impairment score: 6 based on spirometry results and medication use; 26%-50% impairment of the whole person.

Comment: Individual was given a work restriction to avoid all future exposure to natural rubber latex because of latex allergy and asthma.

Class 4
51%-100% Respiratory Impairment
Measured FVC: ≤ 50% of predicted
or
Measured FEV₁: ≤ 40% of predicted
or
Dco: ≤ 40% of predicted
or
V̇o₂max: < 15 mL/(kg•min) *or* < 1.05 L/min *or* < 4.3 METS

Example 5-9
51% to 100% Impairment Due to Asthma

Subject: 40-year-old man.

History: Golf course groundskeeper for 15 years; lifelong asthma. 2 years' increasing dyspnea with mild exertion; intermittent cough. Nonsmoker. No symptom improvement over weekends. Has been on at least 20 mg of prednisone per day for past year (score 4).

Physical Exam: Height: 180 cm (5 ft 11 in); weight: 70 kg (154 lb). Diffuse expiratory wheezing over entire chest. No clubbing, cyanosis, or lower extremity edema. Cardiac examination: no air trapping.

Clinical Studies: Chest radiograph: no cardiopulmonary disease. Post bronchodilator FVC (L): observed 2.94; predicted 5.2 observed/predicted 57%; post bronchodilator FEV_1 (L): observed 1.16; predicted 4.29 observed/predicted 27% (score 4); change post bronchodilator 22% (score 2). FEV_1/FVC: observed 39%. Methacholine challenge test: not performed; severe baseline obstruction.

Impairment Rating: Asthma score: 10 (Tables 5-9 and 5-10); 51% to 100% impairment of the whole person.

Comment: Pulmonary function studies demonstrate a significant response to bronchodilators but persistent severe airway obstruction. The persistent FEV_1 percentage ≤ 50% of predicted with prolonged use of daily oral prednisone would in itself result in class 4 impairment rating for asthma. Severe symptoms require frequent oral steroids.

Example 5-10
51% to 100% Impairment Due to Emphysema

Subject: 62-year-old man.

History: Bookkeeper in vegetable-processing plant for 38 years; 10 years' gradual shortness of breath: smoked 2.5 packs of cigarettes per day for 50 years (125 pack-years); quit 6 months ago. No other disorders or exposure to hazardous dusts, chemicals, or fumes.

Current Symptoms: Severe dyspnea; unable to perform activities of daily living (driving to/from work, walking on level ground, self-dress). Occasional nonproductive cough; no wheezing, chest pain, or hemoptysis.

Physical Exam: Height: 180 cm (5 ft 11 in); weight: 69.5 kg (153 lb). Distant breath sounds; no crackles or wheezes.

Clinical Studies: Chest radiograph: hyperinflated lungs; pulmonary parenchyma vascular attenuation. FVC (L): observed 2.94; predicted 4.82; observed/predicted 61%. FEV_1 (L): observed 1.16; predicted 3.75; observed/predicted 31%. FEV_1/FVC: 39%. Dco: observed 12.87; predicted 34.5; observed/predicted 37%. V̇o₂max: 10 mL/kg/min.

Diagnosis: Emphysema.

Impairment Rating: 51% to 100% impairment of the whole person.

Comment: Severe emphysema; unlikely to perform any significant exertion without hypoxia.

Chapter 5

5.11 Respiratory Impairment Evaluation Summary

See Table 5–13 for an evaluation summary for the assessment of permanent impairment due to repiratory disorders.

Table 5-13 Repiratory Impairment Evaluation Summary

Disorder	History, Including Selected Relevant Symptoms	Examination Record	Assessment of Respiratory Function
General	Respiratory symptoms (eg, cough); general symptoms Impact of symptoms on function and ability to do daily activities; prognosis if change anticipated Review medical history	Comprehensive physical examination; detailed respiratory system assessment	Data derived from relevant studies (eg, pulmonary function tests)
Obstructive Disorders	Dyspnea; cough; sputum production; infections; medication use; exercise tolerance	Note breath sounds, wheeze, loud P_2, jugular vein distention, right heart prominence	Pulmonary function: spirometry, lung volumes, diffusing capacity, methacholine challenge, radiographs
Restrictive Disorders	Dyspnea; cough; fatigue; sputum; exercise tolerance	Chest wall excursion; crackles; clubbing	Pulmonary function: spirometry, lung volumes, diffusing capacity, imaging studies
Cancer	Exercise tolerance; dyspnea; chest pain; fatigue; weight loss; tobacco use; environmental exposures	Chest wall excursion; crackles; clubbing; adenopathy	Bronchoscopy; pulmonary function tests; biopsy

References

1. Guidelines for the evaluation of impairment/disability in patients with asthma. *Am Rev Respir Dis.* 1993;14:1056-1061.

   A detailed review of the approach to evaluating impairment and disability in patients with asthma.

2. Crapo RO, Morris AH, Gardner RM. Reference spirometric values using techniques and equipment that meet ATS recommendations. *Am Rev Respir Dis.* 1981;123:659-664.

   Reference spirometric values measures in 251 healthy nonsmoking men and women using techniques and equipment that meet ATS recommendations.

3. Ferris BG. Epidemiology standardization project: American Thoracic Society. *Am Rev Respir Dis.* 1978;118(6, pt 2):1-120.

4. Hajiro T, Nishimura K, Tsukino M, Ikeda A, Oga T, Izumi T. A comparison of the level of dyspnea vs disease severity in indicating the health-related quality of life of patients with COPD. *Chest.* 1999;116:1632-1637.

5. US Public Health Service. *The Health Consequences of Smoking: Cancer.* Washington, DC: Office of the Surgeon General, US Dept of Health and Human Services; 1982.

   A detailed monograph on the health effects of smoking.

6. Guidelines for the Use of ILO International Classification of Radiographs of Pneumoconioses. Geneva, Switzerland: International Labour Office; 1980. Occupational Safety and Health Series 22, Rev 80.

   A detailed review of the procedure, use, and interpretation of radiographs using the ILO classification system.

7. Müller NL, Miller RR. Diseases of the bronchioles: CT and histopathologic findings. *Radiology.* 1995;196:3-12.

8. McLoud TC, guest ed. *Clinics in Chest Medicine: Imaging.* Philadelphia, Pa: WB Saunders Co; 1999;20:697-874.

Chapter 5

End-Organ Damage	Diagnosis	Degree of Impairment
Include assessment of sequelae, including end-organ damage and impairment	Record all pertinent diagnosis(es); note if they are at maximal medical improvement; if not, discuss under what conditions and when stability is expected	Criteria outlined in this chapter See Table 5-12
Assess relevant organs (eg, cardiac function, cor pulmonale)	Asthma; chronic bronchitis and emphysema; other obstructive diseases	See Table 5-12 for asthma See Tables 5-9 and 5-10
Assess cardiac function	Idiopathic pulmonary fibrosis; asbestosis; pneumoconiosis; chest wall disorders; others	See Table 5-12
Assess other organ function; signs of metastases	Squamous, adeno, small cell, etc	See Table 5-11

Chapter 5

9. Crapo RO, Morris AH. Standardized single breath normal values for carbon monoxide diffusing capacity. *Am Rev Respir Dis.* 1981;123:185-190.

   Generates prediction equations for DLco and diffusing capacity per unit of lung volume (DL/VA) from 245 normal subjects (122 women and 123 men) using a standardized technique for measuring DLco.

10. American Thoracic Society Ad Hoc Committee on Impairment/Disability Criteria. Evaluation of impairment/disability secondary to respiratory disorders. *Am Rev Respir Dis.* 1986;134:1205-1209.

    A thoughtful review and recommendations from the American Thoracic Society (ATS) on the assessment of impairment and disability due to respiratory disorders.

11. American Thoracic Society: ATS statement—snowbird workshop on standardization of spirometry. *Am Rev Respir Dis.* 1979;119:831-838.

    Classic, early reference on the performance and use of spirometry to assess lung function.

12. American Thoracic Society. Standardization of spirometry—1987 update. *Am Rev Respir Dis.* 1987;136:1285-1298.

    Update to earlier references by ATS on spirometry.

13. American Thoracic Society. Lung function testing: selection of reference values and interpretational strategies. *Am Rev Respir Dis.* 1991;144:1202-1218.

    Reviews respiratory function test methods and interpretation questions.

14. American Thoracic Society. Standardization of spirometry, 1994 update. *Am J Respir Crit Care Med.* 1995;152:1107-1136.

    Summary of the most recent guidelines by ATS on standardizing spirometry testing and interpretation issues.

15. Morris AH, Kanner RE, Crapo RO, Gardner RM. *Clinical Pulmonary Function Testing: A Manual of Uniform Laboratory Procedure.* 2nd ed. Salt Lake City, Utah: Inter-Mountain Thoracic Society; 1984.

Classic reference detailing procedures used for standardized pulmonary function tests.

16. Coultas DB, Gong H Jr, Grad R, et al. State of the art: respiratory diseases in minorities of the United States. *Am J Respir Crit Care Med.* 1993;149:S93-S131.

Discusses the diagnosis, risk factors, and management of respiratory diseases in minorities.

17. Coultas DB, Gong H Jr, Grad R, et al. Respiratory diseases in minorities of the United States [published erratum appears in *Am J Respir Crit Care Med.* 1994; 150:290]. *Am J Respir Crit Care Med.* 1994;149 (3, pt 2):S93-S131.

18. *Guidelines for the Diagnosis and Management of Asthma.* Expert panel report. National Asthma Education Program. Bethesda, Md: National Heart, Lung, and Blood Institute; 1991. National Institutes of Health publication 92-3042A.

A review of evidence-based and consensus criteria for the diagnosis and management of asthma.

19. Crapo RO, Morris AH, Clayton PD, Nixon CR. Lung volumes in healthy nonsmoking adults. *Bull Eur Physiopathol Respir.* 1982;18:419-425.

Total lung capacity (TLC), functional residual capacity, residual volume, and corresponding 95% confidence intervals measured in 245 healthy nonsmoking persons (122 women, 123 men) using a single-breath helium technique.

20. Hankinson JL, Bang KM. Acceptability and reproducibility criteria of the American Thoracic Society as observed in a sample of the general population. *Am Rev Respir Dis.* 1991;143:516-521.

Conducts analysis of spirograms of 6486 subjects from the general population, ages 8 to 90, to determine ability to satisfy the ATS' acceptability and reproducibility criteria. Both older and younger subjects had more difficulty satisfying ATS acceptability and reproducibility criteria, in part associated (particularly in younger subjects) with smaller heights and lung volumes.

21. Hankinson JL, Odencrantz JR, Fedan KB. Spirometric reference values from a sample of the US general population. *Am J Respir Crit Care Med.* 1999;159:179-187.

The latest and most comprehensive-to-date listing of spirometric reference values from a large sample of the United States. Includes new information on spirometric values of various ethnic groups.

22. American Thoracic Society. Single-breath carbon monoxide diffusing capacity (transfer factor). Recommendations for a standard technique—1995 update. *Am J Respir Crit Care Med.* 1995;152(6, pt 1): 2185-2198.

Appropriate use and interpretation of Dco is discussed.

23. Owens GR, Rogers RM, Pennock BF, Levin D. The diffusing capacity as a predictor of arterial oxygen desaturation during exercise in patients with chronic obstructive pulmonary disease. *N Engl J Med.* 1984;310:1218-1221.

Evaluates 48 patients with chronic obstructive pulmonary disease by means of pulmonary-function and exercise testing to determine whether any tests of pulmonary function could predict development of arterial desaturation during exercise. Only two indexes—diffusing capacity and forced expiratory volume in the first second (FEV_1)—were predictive of desaturation.

24. Gallagher CG. Exercise limitation and clinical exercise testing in chronic obstructive pulmonary disease. *Clin Chest Med.* 1994;15:305-326.

Clinical exercise testing is an important tool in assessment of exercise limitation in COPD patients, in assessment of physiologic and psychological factors that contribute to exercise limitation, and in the differential diagnosis of cardiorespiratory disease. Further studies that examine the clinical utility of exercise testing are needed because there are currently insufficient data regarding the utility of many exercise variables.

25. Cotes JE, Zejda J, King B. Lung function impairment as a guide to exercise limitation in work-related lung disorders. *Am Rev Respir Dis.* 1988;137:1089-1093.

The hypothesis that exercise limitation of respiratory origin can be predicted accurately from the lung function impairment is tested using maximal oxygen uptake ($\dot{V}O_2$max) as the dependent variable in a multiple regression analysis.

Chapter 5

26. Astrand P, Rodahl K. *Textbook of Work Physiology.* New York, NY: McGraw-Hill Book Co; 1977:462.

27. Marciniuk DD, Gallagher CG. Clinical exercise testing in interstitial lung disease. *Clin Chest Med.* 1994;15:287-303.

Clinical exercise testing has become an essential tool used in early diagnosis, in the monitoring of treatment effectiveness, and in the assessment of impairment owing to ILD. Despite the assorted causes, the responses to exercise demonstrated by these diseases are generally similar.

28. Braman SS, Corrao WM. Bronchoprovocation testing. *Clin Chest Med.* 1989;10:165-176.

Lists a number of easy and safe techniques that are available to detect nonspecific bronchial hyperresponsiveness.

29. Chan-Yeung M, Malo JL. Occupational asthma. *New Engl J Med.* 1995;333:107-112.

Classic review on the presentations and characteristics of types of occupational asthma.

30. Brooks SM, Weiss MA, Bernstein IL. Reactive airways dysfunction syndrome (RADS): persistent asthma syndrome after high level irritant exposurs. *Chest.* 1985;88:376-384.

Acute, high-level, uncontrolled irritant exposures may cause an asthmalike syndrome that is different from typical occupational asthma in some individuals. It can lead to long-term sequelae and chronic airway disease. Nonimmunologic mechanisms seem operative in the pathogenesis of this syndrome.

31. *Expert Panel Report 2: Guidelines for the Diagnosis and Management of Asthma.* Bethesda, Md: National Institutes of Health; April 1997. NIH publication 97-405.

Latest update for the physician on the diagnosis and treatment of asthma.

32. Hudgel DW. Treatment of obstructive sleep apnea: a review. *Chest.* 1996;109:1346-1358.

An algorithm for the approach to treatment recommendations is presented. Basic to this algorithm is an objective presentation of therapeutic options to the patient with obstructive sleep apnea (OSA) and respecting the patient's preferences.

33. Rose C. Hypersensitivity pneumonitis. In: Harber P, Schenker MA, Balmes J, eds. *Occupational and Environmental Respiratory Disease.* St Louis, Mo: Mosby-Year Book; 1996:201-215.

Review of the diagnosis, presentation, and management of hypersensitivity pneumonitis.

34. American Thoracic Society. The diagnosis of nonmalignant diseases related to asbestos. *Am Rev Respir Dis.* 1986;134:363-368.

Discussion of the nonmalignant manifestations of asbestos disease.

35. Moossa AR, Robson MC, Schimpff SC, eds. *Comprehensive Textbook of Oncology.* Baltimore, Md: Williams & Wilkins; 1986:67.

Bibliography

Jones NL. *Clinical Exercise Testing.* 3rd ed. Philadelphia, Pa: WB Saunders Co; 1987.

Wasserman K, Hansen JE, Sue DY, Whipp BJ. *Principles of Exercise Testing and Interpretation.* Philadelphia, Pa: Lea & Febiger; 1987.

Chapter 5

Chapter 6

The Digestive System

Introduction

This chapter provides criteria for evaluating permanent impairment of the digestive system, consisting of the alimentary canal, liver, biliary tract, and pancreas. The criteria for assigning permanent impairment ratings of digestive system disease include clinically established or objectively determined deviations from normal in the transport and assimilation of ingested food, nutrition metabolism, waste product excretion, and the effect of these problems on individuals' performance of activities of daily living.

The following sections have been revised from the fourth edition: (1) impairment from ulcer disease has been revised since most duodenal and gastric ulcer disease cases can be eradicated with treatment of *H. pylori* infection, and bleeding ulcer treatment has improved with injection or heat therapy, in some cases avoiding gastric resection; (2) orthotopic liver transplantation has reclaimed the lives of many end-stage liver disease patients and significantly reduced the degree of permanent impairment; (3) parenteral nutrition and, in particular, home nutrition programs have completely rehabilitated some and improved the daily lives of many individuals with intestinal failure from a variety of causes; (4) new techniques for improving biliary drainage prevent or delay irreversible liver damage; (5) continued experience with intestinal anastomosis and stomas provides a greater sense of security and self-esteem, improves overall function, and reduces the degree of permanent impairment in some people. Impairments of similar gravity, which have similar impact on the ability to perform activities of daily living for the small and large intestine, have been given the same impairment ratings for comparable classes.

6.1 Principles of Assessment

Before using the information in this chapter, the *Guides* user should become familiar with Chapters 1 and 2 and the Glossary. Chapters 1 and 2 discuss the *Guides'* purpose, applications, and methods for performing and reporting impairment evaluations. The Glossary provides definitions of common terms used by many specialties in impairment evaluation.

6.1a Interpretation of Symptoms and Signs

Some impairment classes refer to symptoms that limit the ability to perform daily activities. When this information is subjective and possible to misinterpret, it should not serve as the sole criterion for assigning impairment ratings. Rather, the examiner should obtain objective data about the limitation's extent and integrate those findings with the subjective data to estimate the degree of permanent impairment.

Esophageal impairment signs and symptoms include dysphagia, pyrosis or heartburn, retrosternal pain, regurgitation, bleeding, and weight loss. Note that occasional, minor dyspepsia, gas, and belching are within the experience of all individuals.

Stomach and duodenum impairment symptoms and signs include nausea, vomiting, pain, bleeding, obstruction, diarrhea, weight loss, and certain types of malabsorption. Some impairments may produce nutritional deficiencies that lead to hematologic and neurologic manifestations, which would be rated separately and combined with digestive system impairments.

Small intestine impairment symptoms and signs include abdominal pain, diarrhea, steatorrhea, bleeding, obstruction, and weight loss, which often are associated with general debility and other extra-intestinal manifestations.

Pancreatic function impairment symptoms and signs include, but are not limited to, pain, anorexia, nausea, vomiting, diarrhea, steatorrhea, weight loss, muscle wasting, jaundice, diabetes mellitus, and debility. Impairment due to endocrine disturbance related to the pancreas is considered in the *Guides* chapter on the endocrine system (Chapter 10).

Colon, rectum, and anus impairment symptoms and signs include abdominal, pelvic, or perineal pain; disordered bowel action; tenesmus; fecal incontinence; bleeding; suppuration; and the appearance of hemorrhoids, fissures, and fistulas. Systemic manifestations may include fever, weight loss, debility, and anemia.

Hepatobiliary impairment symptoms and signs include pain, nausea, vomiting, anorexia, loss of strength and stamina, reduced resistance to infection, altered immune response, jaundice, and pruritus. Advanced liver disease complications include edema and generalized ascites, portal hypertension leading to esophageal varices and hemorrhage, and metabolic disturbances leading to hepatic encephalopathy and renal failure.

Abdominal wall impairment symptoms and signs include typically intermittent discomfort or pain at or near the herniation site, often associated with postural changes or increased abdominal pressure; visible or palpable protrusion or swelling at the herniation site, often appearing and disappearing with abdominal pressure; and more acute and intense pain due to complications, especially incarceration and strangulation of contained bowel or omentum.

Incisional **hernias** may be unsightly and annoying; other symptoms, if any, tend to be related to the incisional hernia size. Inguinal and femoral hernias typically are painful and entail a greater risk of incarceration or strangulation. Most abdominal wall hernias are amenable to surgical correction.

6.1b Description of Clinical Studies

Objective procedures useful in establishing esophageal impairment include, but are not limited to: (1) imaging procedures, such as fluoroscopy and radiography employing contrast media, and computed tomography (CT); (2) peroral endoscopy, including cytologic study or biopsy; and (3) functional tests, such as manometry or intraesophageal pH measurement.

Objective procedures useful in establishing stomach and duodenum impairment include, but are not limited to: (1) imaging techniques, such as fluoroscopy and roentgenography with contrast media, scintigraphy, and CT; (2) peroral endoscopy, with biopsy and cytologic study; (3) gastric secretory tests; (4) malabsorption tests; (5) stool examination; and (6) urea breath test for *H. pylori*.

Objective procedures useful in establishing impairment of the small intestine include, but are not limited to: (1) fluoroscopy and roentgenography employing contrast media; (2) peroral endoscopy and mucosal biopsy; and (3) intestinal malabsorption testing measures such as fecal fat content and urinary d-xylose excretion tests, carbon 14 breath test, and Schilling test.

Objective procedures useful in establishing impairment of pancreatic function include, but are not limited to: (1) ultrasonography; (2) radiography, including plain or scout films of the abdomen, CT, and endoscopic pancreatography; (3) guided, fine-needle aspiration; (4) determination of plasma glucose level and glucose tolerance; (5) assay of pancreatic enzyme activity in blood, urine, and feces; (6) sweat electrolyte test; and (7) procedures such as the secretin test.

Objective procedures useful in establishing colon, rectum, and anus impairment include, but are not limited to: (1) digital and endoscopic examination, including anoscopy, proctoscopy, sigmoidoscopy, and colonoscopy; (2) biopsy; (3) fecal microscopy and culture; and (4) fluoroscopy and roentgenography employing contrast media.

Objective procedures useful in establishing hepatobiliary impairment include, but are not limited to: (1) ultrasonography; (2) contrast radiography, such as percutaneous and endoscopic cholangiography; (3) CT and magnetic resonance imaging (MRI); (4) nucleide scintigraphy; (5) angiography; (6) liver biopsy and fine-needle aspiration; and (7) laboratory tests to assess the bile ducts and various liver functions.

Objective procedures useful in establishing impairment by hernias include, but are not limited to: (1) abdominal wall physical examination and (2) imaging by roentgenography or CT scan with or without contrast media.

6.1c Desirable Weight

Weight loss is an essential criterion for evaluating the severity and consequences of gastrointestinal disorders. To determine impairment resulting from digestive disorders, **desirable weight** may be defined as follows:

1. If possible, the examiner should determine by history or from previous medical records a weight that predates the individual's digestive disorder that is considered usual and customary. The examiner should use that weight as the desirable weight from which any deviation is measured.

2. If the examiner is not able to determine by history or previous medical records a usual and customary weight that predates the disorder, then the examiner should refer to a table of desirable weights and calculate deviations from the lower end of the table's range that corresponds to the individual's gender, height, and body build.

Table 6-1 Desirable Weights for Men by Height and Body Build (indoor clothing weighing 2.3 kg [5 lb] and shoes with 2.5-cm [1-in] heels)*

Height, in (cm)	Weight, lb (kg)		
	Small Frame	Medium Frame	Large Frame
62 (157)	128-134 (58.0-60.7)	131-141 (59.2-63.9)	138-150 (62.5-67.8)
63 (160)	130-136 (59.0-61.7)	133-143 (60.3-64.9)	140-153 (63.5-69.4)
64 (163)	132-138 (60.0-62.7)	135-145 (61.3-66.0)	142-156 (64.5-71.1)
65 (165)	134-140 (60.8-63.5)	137-148 (62.1-67.0)	144-160 (65.3-72.5)
66 (168)	136-142 (61.8-64.6)	139-151 (63.2-68.7)	146-164 (66.4-74.7)
67 (170)	138-145 (62.5-65.7)	142-154 (64.3-69.8)	149-168 (67.5-76.1)
68 (173)	140-148 (63.6-67.3)	145-157 (65.9-71.4)	152-172 (69.1-78.2)
69 (175)	142-151 (64.3-68.3)	148-160 (66.9-72.4)	155-176 (70.1-79.6)
70 (178)	144-154 (65.4-70.0)	151-163 (68.6-74.0)	158-180 (71.8-81.8)
71 (180)	146-157 (66.1-71.0)	154-166 (69.7-75.1)	161-184 (72.8-83.3)
72 (183)	149-160 (67.7-72.7)	157-170 (71.3-77.2)	164-188 (74.5-85.4)
73 (185)	152-164 (68.7-74.1)	160-174 (72.4-78.6)	168-192 (75.9-86.8)
74 (188)	155-168 (70.3-76.2)	164-178 (74.4-80.7)	172-197 (78.0-89.4)
75 (190)	158-172 (71.4-77.6)	167-182 (75.4-82.2)	176-202 (79.4-91.2)
76 (193)	162-176 (73.5-79.8)	171-187 (77.6-84.8)	181-207 (82.1-93.9)

*Copyright © 1996, 1999, The Metropolitan Life Insurance Company.
Courtesy Statistical Bulletin, Metropolitan Life Insurance Company.

Table 6-2 Desirable Weights for Women by Height and Body Build (indoor clothing weighing 1.4 kg [3 lb] and shoes with 2.5-cm [1-in] heels)*

Height, in (cm)	Weight, lb (kg)		
	Small Frame	Medium Frame	Large Frame
58 (147)	102-111 (46.2-50.2)	109-121 (49.3-54.7)	118-131 (53.3-59.3)
59 (150)	103-113 (46.7-51.3)	111-123 (50.3-55.9)	120-134 (54.4-60.9)
60 (152)	104-115 (47.1-52.1)	113-126 (51.1-57.0)	122-137 (55.2-61.9)
61 (155)	106-118 (48.1-53.6)	115-129 (52.2-58.6)	125-140 (56.8-63.6)
62 (157)	108-121 (48.8-54.6)	118-132 (53.2-59.6)	128-143 (57.8-64.6)
63 (160)	111-124 (50.3-56.2)	121-135 (54.9-61.2)	131-147 (59.4-66.7)
64 (163)	114-127 (51.9-57.8)	124-138 (56.4-62.8)	134-151 (61.0-68.8)
65 (165)	117-130 (53.0-58.9)	127-141 (57.5-63.9)	137-155 (62.0-70.2)
66 (168)	120-133 (54.6-60.5)	130-144 (59.2-65.5)	140-159 (63.7-72.4)
67 (170)	123-136 (55.7-61.6)	133-147 (60.2-66.6)	143-163 (64.8-73.8)
68 (173)	126-139 (57.3-63.2)	136-150 (61.8-68.2)	146-167 (66.4-75.9)
69 (175)	129-142 (58.3-64.2)	139-153 (62.8-69.2)	149-170 (67.4-76.9)
70 (178)	132-145 (60.0-65.9)	142-156 (64.5-70.9)	152-173 (69.0-78.6)
71 (180)	135-148 (61.0-66.9)	145-159 (65.6-71.9)	155-176 (70.1-79.6)
72 (183)	138-151 (62.6-68.4)	148-162 (67.0-73.4)	158-179 (71.6-81.2)

*Copyright © 1996, 1999, The Metropolitan Life Insurance Company.
Courtesy Statistical Bulletin, Metropolitan Life Insurance Company.

Tables 6-1 and 6-2 present desirable weights according to height for men and women, respectively. For an obese person, the usual preimpairment weight may not be as physiologically desirable as the current weight. Thus, the examiner should use his or her clinical judgment when assessing the relative importance of weight loss.

6.1d Impairment Determination

Impairment classes, as listed in Tables 6-3 through 6-9, are organ- and system-specific. The impairment classes and percentage ratings reflect anatomic, physiological, and functional abnormalities at the organ and system level and the ability to perform activities of daily living (see Table 1-2). A gastrointestinal system impairment evaluation falling within normal range reflects an individual who performs all activities of daily living with only normal, occasional gastrointestinal symptoms; no limitation of activities; no special diet; and no required medication, with adequate reserve capacity that allows the body to obtain the required nutrition and maintain normal weight.

For the purposes of impairment ratings, the upper digestive tract has been defined to include the esophagus, stomach and duodenum, small intestine, and pancreas. Impairment criteria and classes have been combined for the colon and rectum; anal; liver and biliary impairments; and hernia impairments.

6.2 Upper Digestive Tract (Esophagus, Stomach and Duodenum, Small Intestine, and Pancreas)

6.2a Criteria for Rating Permanent Impairment Due to Upper Digestive Tract Disease

Criteria for evaluating impairments related to upper digestive tract disease are given in Table 6-3.

Chapter 6

Table 6-3 Criteria for Rating Permanent Impairment Due to Upper Digestive Tract (Esophagus, Stomach and Duodenum, Small Intestine, and Pancreas) Disease

Class 1 0%-9% Impairment of the Whole Person	Class 2 10%-24% Impairment of the Whole Person	Class 3 25%-49% Impairment of the Whole Person	Class 4 50%-75% Impairment of the Whole Person
Symptoms or signs of upper digestive tract disease, or anatomic loss or alteration *and* continuous treatment not required *and* maintains weight at desirable level* *or* no sequelae after surgical procedures	Symptoms and signs of upper digestive tract disease, or anatomic loss or alteration *and* requires appropriate dietary restrictions and drugs for control of symptoms, signs, or nutritional deficiency *and* weight loss below desirable weight but does not exceed 10%*	Symptoms and signs of upper digestive tract disease, or anatomic loss or alteration *and* appropriate dietary restrictions and drugs do not completely control symptoms, signs, or nutritional state *or* 10%-20% weight loss below desirable weight due to upper digestive tract disorder*	Symptoms and signs of upper digestive tract disease, or anatomic loss or alteration *and* symptoms uncontrolled by treatment *or* greater than 20% weight loss below the desirable weight due to upper digestive tract disorder*

*Refer to Tables 6-1 and 6-2.

Class 1 0%-9% Impairment of the Whole Person
Symptoms or signs of upper digestive tract disease, or anatomic loss or alteration *and* continuous treatment not required *and* maintains weight at desirable level *or* no sequelae after surgical procedures

Example 6-1
0% to 9% Impairment Due to Upper Digestive Tract Disease

Subject: 44-year-old man.

History: Machinist; transient difficulty swallowing; first occurrence 9 months ago while eating broiled lobster.

Current Symptoms: No symptoms of esophageal disease.

Physical Exam: Within normal limits. Weight: 68.1 kg (150 lb); height: 1.78 m (5 ft 10 in); within desirable limits. Healthy appearance; vital signs normal.

Clinical Studies: Chest roentgenogram, ECG: normal. Barium swallow: small, sliding hiatal hernia. Endoscopy: no mucosal defect.

Diagnosis: Hiatal hernia, uncomplicated.

Impairment Rating: 0% impairment of the whole person.

Comment: The original hiatal hernia and motility disorder have neither interfered with normal nutrition nor impaired ability to perform usual daily activities.[1]

Example 6-2
0% to 9% Impairment Due to Stomach or Duodenum Disease or Injury

Subject: 28-year-old man.

History: 5 years' epigastric pain and burning. Minimal weight loss.

Current Symptoms: Denied nausea, vomiting, hematemesis, or melena. Painful episodes last up to 2 weeks, wake him at night, and require antacids, food, and over-the-counter (OTC) H$_2$ blockers for relief. Avoided all ulcerogenic drugs.

Physical Exam: Height: 1.8 m (5 ft 11 in); weight: 72.6 kg (160 lb).

Clinical Studies: Barium meal: deformed duodenal bulb. No gastric retention or pyloric stenosis. Peroral endoscopy: scar of healed ulcer on posterior wall on first portion of duodenum. Endoscopy: 1-cm duodenum ulcer-crater; considerable surrounding deformity. Antral biopsies: positive for *H. pylori;* full-course triple-therapy (omeprazole, clarithromycin, and metronidazole) relieved symptoms. Complete healing at follow-up endoscopy 8 weeks later. Repeat antrum and body biopsies: no *H. pylori.*

Chapter 6

Diagnosis: Resolved peptic duodenal ulcer disease associated with *H. pylori* infection.

Impairment Rating: 0% if remission continues.

Comment: *H. pylori* can be found in 95% to 100% of duodenal ulcer and 70% to 80% of peptic stomach ulcer patients. Successful eradication of infection induces a long remission.[2]

Example 6-3
0% to 9% Impairment Due to Small Intestine Disease

Subject: 35-year-old man.

History: Abdominal operation because of recurrent and protracted fever, abdominal pain, and distention 10 years ago. Approximately 30-cm resection of terminal ileum and ileoascending colostomy construction. Resected specimen histologic findings consistent with regional enteritis (Crohn's disease).

Current Symptoms: Asymptomatic. Has two or three soft stools daily. Performs all activities of daily living without difficulty.

Physical Exam: Weight: 70.3 kg (155 lb) on unrestricted diet; usual preillness weight: 72.6 kg (160 lb).

Clinical Studies: Hemogram and blood chemistry panel: normal. Roentgenograms of remaining small intestine and the ileocolic anastomosis: unremarkable.

Diagnosis: Partial, distal ileal resection (Crohn's disease).

Impairment Rating: 0% impairment of the whole person.

Comment: No symptoms to suggest intestinal disease recurrence; required no therapy for 10 years after operation. Maintained nearly desirable weight; easily performed usual activities. Resected ileum length influences postoperative morbidity. Diarrhea, some malabsorption more likely when 100 cm or more resected; may necessitate reduced fat intake and regular vitamin B_{12} injections, increasing impairment to 10% or more.

Example 6-4
0% to 9% Impairment Due to Pancreatic Disease

Subject: 40-year-old woman.

History: Bartender; episodic epigastric pain associated with elevated serum amylase activity, two to three episodes per year for 3 years. Cholecystectomy for gallstones removal 2 years ago. Reduced-calorie diet corrected exogenous obesity; weight did not fall below desirable level.

Current Symptoms: Pain attacks, especially after large meals or immoderate alcoholic beverage consumption.

Physical Exam: Normal.

Clinical Studies: No clinical or laboratory evidence of pancreatic insufficiency.

Diagnosis: Recurrent acute pancreatitis.

Impairment Rating: 5% impairment of the whole person.

Comment: Preexisting disease appropriately documented and treated. No evidence of residual pancreatic impairment. Individual able to perform normal daily activities despite occasional recurring symptoms.[3]

<table>
<tr><td>**Class 2**
10%-24% Impairment of the Whole Person</td></tr>
<tr><td>Symptoms and signs of upper digestive tract disease, or anatomic loss or alteration
and
requires appropriate dietary restrictions and drugs for control of symptoms, signs, or nutritional deficiency
and
weight loss below desirable weight but does not exceed 10%</td></tr>
</table>

Example 6-5
10% to 24% Impairment Due to Upper Digestive Tract Disease

Subject: 59-year-old woman.

History: 5 years' almost daily retrosternal pain associated with difficulty swallowing.

Current Symptoms: Symptoms less severe when diet limited to soft foods; symptoms aggravated when upset, particularly when worried.

Physical Exam: Height: 1.7 m (5 ft 7 in), medium frame; weight: 53.6 kg (118 lb), within 10% of usual weight of 58 kg (128 lb). BP: 145/90 mm Hg. Appears older than stated age.

Clinical Studies: Chest roentgenogram, ECG: normal; uncoordinated contractions in lower esophagus resulting in "corkscrew" configuration, indicative of diffuse spasm. Esophageal manometry: prolonged high amplitude, irregular synchronous contractions with water swallowing consistent with diffuse spasm. Endoscopy: no mucosal defect.

Diagnosis: Diffuse spasm of the esophagus.

Impairment Rating: 15% impairment of the whole person.

Comment: Persistent symptoms obligated woman to restrict diet. Weight loss did not exceed 10% of desirable level. Daily activities restrained only slightly. Symptomatic management with agents such as nifedepine and diltiazem may be helpful and sufficient; if not, surgical myotomy reported beneficial in 70% to 80% of cases.[4]

Example 6-6
10% to 24% Impairment Due to Gastroesophageal Reflux Disease

Subject: 43-year-old man.

History: Burning retrosternal chest distress increasing in severity and frequency over the last 18 months. Occurred after meals; wakened with occasional sour regurgitation into mouth and coughing episodes. Antacids helped very briefly; improvement noted with OTC histamine receptor blockers. Excellent relief with intensive doses of omeprazole. Long-term medical therapy instituted.

Current Symptoms: Above symptoms recurred when medication stopped after 8 weeks.

Physical Exam: Unremarkable; minimal weight loss.

Clinical Studies: Blood studies: normal. X-rays of esophagus and stomach: suggest lower esophagus ulceration. Endoscopy: moderately severe esophagitis; longitudinal ridging, denuded mucosa in between. Biopsy: inflamed squamous epithelium.

Diagnosis: Moderately severe gastroesophageal reflux disease without stricture.

Impairment Rating: 15% impairment of the whole person.

Comment: Persistent untreated gastroesophageal reflux may result in stricture formation necessitating repeated dilatations, medical therapy resumption. Possible antireflux surgery. Reflux may induce premalignant changes in lower esophagus; regular surveillance and possible surgical treatment increase impairment rating.[5,6]

Example 6-7
10% to 24% Impairment Due to Duodenum Disease

Subject: 40-year-old man.

History: 10 years' intermittent ulcer symptoms. Three bleeding episodes; twice required blood replacement. One transient pyloric obstruction episode.

Current Symptoms: Performance of daily activities repeatedly interrupted. Refuses to consider surgical remedy; requires continuing medical therapy to maintain any degree of symptomatic remission.

Physical Exam: Height: 1.78 m (5 ft 8 in); weight: 59 kg (130 lb), 7% below desirable.

Clinical Studies: Upper GI tract roentgenograms: marked duodenal bulb cloverleaf deformity with 3-mm ulcer fleck.

Diagnosis: Active duodenal ulcer with a history of recurring complications.

Impairment Rating: 15% impairment of the whole person.

Comment: Complicated disease; recurrent symptoms despite medical therapy. *H. pylori* may be factor in chronic complicated duodenal ulcer disease; should be sought and treated. Other ulcer complications, ie, bleeding, respond to injection or thermal/laser therapy; results equal to surgical treatment. Current surgical treatment reserved for ulcers intractable to intensive acid suppression therapy and extremely large duodenal or stomach ulcers.[7]

Example 6-8
10% to 24% Impairment Due to Small Intestine Disease

Subject: 64-year-old woman.

History: Commercial artist; 5 years' diarrhea, weight loss, and vague abdominal distress. All symptoms cleared with oral tetracycline and parenteral cyanocobalamin (vitamin B$_{12}$). Mild diarrhea for several weeks 2 years ago; subsided with tetracycline.

Current Symptoms: Normal nutritional state. No untoward symptoms; relatively unrestricted diet. Periodic intramuscular cyanocobalamin injections.

Physical Exam: Weight: 49.9 kg (110 lb); preillness weight: 54.4 kg (120 lb). Height: 1.55 m (5 ft 1 in).

Clinical Studies: Macrocytic anemia; barium meal examination: extensive small intestine diverticulosis. Roentgenographic examination: persistence of numerous diverticula in small intestine, even more prominent in jejunum.

Diagnosis: Diverticulosis of the small intestine; overgrowth of enteric bacterial flora.

Impairment Rating: 15% impairment due to diverticulosis of the small intestine; combine with appropriate impairment estimate for anemia (see *Guides* Chapter 9, The Hematopoietic System) to determine whole person impairment.

Comment: Performs activities of daily living; unimpaired weight, but dependent on continuing therapy. Diffuse intestinal motility disorder possibly associated with small intestine diverticulosis may produce a progressively disabling condition, "intestinal pseudo-obstruction," with abdominal distention, diarrhea, and malnutrition and with little or no response to usual therapy. Possible longterm parenteral feeding; impairment would advance to class 3 or 4.

Example 6-9
10% to 24% Impairment Due to Pancreatic Disease or Injury

Subject: 35-year-old man.

History: Thrown against steering wheel of truck when it slid off a road. Increasing abdominal pain and distention a few weeks later. Serial ultrasonography: expanding pancreatic cyst. Subtotal pancreatectomy; cyst removed, and associated inflammatory reaction allayed.

Current Symptoms: Intermittent diarrhea, steatorrhea, and diminished stamina 15 months later, despite pancreatic enzyme supplements. Occasional epigastric and back pain.

Physical Exam: Height: 1.9 m (6 ft 3 in); weight: 74.5 kg (164 lb); preillness weight: 81.7 kg (180 lb). No evidence of impaired glucose tolerance or diabetes.

Clinical Studies: Blood studies: normal; modest steatorrhea.

Diagnosis: Status post-subtotal pancreatectomy consequent to trauma, residual chronic pancreatitis and exocrine pancreatic insufficiency.

Impairment Rating: 20% impairment of the whole person.

Comment: Impaired pancreatic exocrine function; weight maintained within 10% of desirable level. Reduced capacity to perform activities of daily living.[3]

Class 3
25%-49% Impairment of the Whole Person
Symptoms and signs of upper digestive tract disease, or anatomic loss or alteration
and
appropriate dietary restrictions and drugs do not completely control symptoms, signs, or nutritional state
or
10%-20% weight loss below desirable weight due to upper digestive tract disorder

Example 6-10
25% to 49% Impairment Due to Upper Digestive Tract Disease

Subject: 49-year-old man.

History: 5 years' intermittent retrosternal pain, dysphagia, and nocturnal regurgitation with occasional and partial remission.

Current Symptoms: Pain less prominent; dysphagia more troublesome. Swallows solid foods only with large volumes of liquids.

Physical Exam: Weight: 70.4 kg (155 lb); preillness weight: 81.7 kg (180 lb). Height: 1.88 m (6 ft 2 in); lanky and gaunt. Normal vital signs.

Clinical Studies: Chest roentgenogram: mediastinum widening; no lung field densities that might indicate aspiration. Barium swallow: markedly dilated and tortuous esophagus terminating in filiform constriction. Endoscopy: no mucosal defect. Successful pneumatic dilation of lower esophageal sphincter after repeated attempts.

Diagnosis: Achalasia of the esophagus.

Impairment Rating: 30% impairment of the whole person.

Comment: Symptoms persistent and progressive despite dietary limitation and esophageal dilation; weight loss exceeded 10% of desirable level. Esophagomyotomy highly recommended due to individual's age and possible combination of antireflux procedure. Basic defect in achalasia, loss of ganglion cells and nerve fibers, cannot be corrected; therapy goal to prevent progressive proximal esophageal dilation. Successful treatment could reduce impairment to class 2. Progressive proximal esophageal dilation with failure or omission of treatment may result in class 4 rating.[5]

Example 6-11
25% to 49% Impairment Due to Stomach or Duodenum Disease or Injury

Subject: 50-year-old woman.

History: Librarian; partial gastrectomy 2 years ago to remove focus of multiple, dysplastic, adenomatous polyps.

Current Symptoms: Lightheadedness, sweating, and palpitation 15 minutes after meals. Symptoms modified by dietary restriction and lying down. Weight dropped since operation to approximately 15% below desirable.

Physical Exam: Weight: 45.4 kg (100 lb); height: 1.6 m (5 ft 3 in). Well-healed scar on upper abdomen; physical examination otherwise unremarkable.

Clinical Studies: Upper GI tract roentgenograms: 70% gastric resection, patent, undistorted gastrojejunostomy.

Diagnosis: Postgastrectomy dumping syndrome.

Impairment Rating: 30% impairment of the whole person.

Comment: Symptoms interfered with performance of normal daily activities despite dietary restriction. Unable to maintain weight within 10% of desirable level.

Example 6-12
25% to 49% Impairment Due to Regional Enteritis

Subject: 38-year-old man.

History: Diarrhea and stamina loss. Partial resection of the distal ileum 3 years ago; evidence of regional enteritis. Several bouts of partial intestinal obstruction, each subsiding with supportive therapy. Required no surgical reintervention. Dietary restriction, vitamin supplements, antidiarrheal agents, and occasional corticosteroid therapy needed to help sustain adequate health state.

Current Symptoms: Episode diarrhea and abdominal cramps.

Physical Exam: Height: 1.6 m (5 ft 3 in); weight: 49.9 kg (110 lb); preillness weight: 59 kg (130 lb).

Clinical Studies: Small intestine roentgenogram: segmental distortion consistent with recurrent inflammation and edema.

Diagnosis: Recurrent regional enteritis, with intestinal malabsorption and recurring obstruction after ileal resection.

Impairment Rating: 40% impairment of the whole person.

Comment: Only marginal function; impaired nutritional state, and weight deficit exceeds 10% of desirable level despite dietary adjustment and medication. Parenteral nutrition therapy (home treatment program), administered characteristically at night while person is asleep, significantly reduces degree of impairment of many individuals. Length and function of remaining normal bowel is an important consideration when assessing severity of impairment.[8]

Example 6-13
25% to 49% Impairment Due to Pancreatic Disease

Subject: 45-year-old woman.

History: Chronic abdominal pain secondary to chronic pancreatitis. Reported a 10-year excessive alcohol intake and repeated acute pancreatitis. Opioid drugs required for some relief. Diabetes mellitus; requires small but multiple daily insulin doses. Diarrhea with steatorrhea over last year helped by pancreatic enzymes.

Current Symptoms: Unable to maintain weight; 15% below ideal. Currently abstaining from alcohol.

Physical Exam: Significant weight loss; abdominal burn marks from heating pads.

Clinical Studies: Abdomen CT scan: calcification throughout pancreas. Endoscopic retrograde cholangiopancreatography: normal biliary ductal system. Main pancreatic duct very distorted with abnormal side branches and small pseudocyst. No evidence of malignancy.

Diagnosis: Chronic pancreatitis with intractable pain; exocrine and endocrine insufficiency.

Impairment Rating: 40% impairment due to chronic pancreatitis. Combine (see the Combined Values Chart, p. 604) with appropriate impairment estimate for diabetes to determine whole person impairment. See Chapter 10, The Endocrine System, for impairment related to diabetes mellitus.

Comment: Impaired exocrine and endocrine pancreatic functions; continuing treatment necessary. Despite treatment, individual unable to bring weight to within 10% of desirable level. Total pancreatectomy may be indicated for pain relief attempt. Continuing alcohol use greatly increases mortality.[3] Offered surgery for duct and pseudocyst drainage and possible pain management. No surgical benefit for diabetes and malabsorption.

Class 4
50%-75% Impairment of the Whole Person
Symptoms and signs of upper digestive tract disease, or anatomic loss or alteration
and
symptoms uncontrolled by treatment
or
greater than 20% weight loss below the desirable weight due to upper digestive tract disorder

Example 6-14
50% to 75% Impairment Due to Upper Digestive Tract Disease

Subject: 62-year-old man.

History: Total gastrectomy 3 years ago for stomach cancer. Esophagoenterostomy (Hunt-Lawrence pouch) constructed.

Current Symptoms: Postoperative anorexia and early satiety; unrelenting weight loss and signs of nutritional deficiency. Marked fatigue, weakness, and inability to read or write except for brief periods.

Physical Exam: Height: 1.75 m (5 ft 9 in); weight: 52.7 kg (116 lb). Malnourished; appears older than stated age. Tongue smooth and glistening. No palpated masses in vicinity of healed upper abdominal scar. Slight pedal edema.

Clinical Studies: Laboratory tests: anemia and hypoproteinemia. Roentgenography: intact esophagojejunostomy; no mucosal defect.

Diagnosis: Postoperative absence of the stomach with esophagojejunal anastomosis; secondary nutritional deficiency.

Impairment Rating: 60% impairment due to total gastrectomy; combine with appropriate anemia impairment estimate (see Chapter 9, The Hematopoietic System) to determine whole person impairment.

Comment: Weight loss exceeds 20% of desirable level; evidence of marked nutritional deficiency. Individual unable to perform many activities of daily living. If he continues to be free of recurrent cancer, consider supplemental parenteral nutrition therapy (home treatment program).

Example 6-15
50% to 75% Impairment Due to Upper Digestive Tract Disease

Subject: 58-year-old man.

History: Almost complete esophageal obstruction. Extensive lower esophagus and proximal stomach resection due to cancer 5 years ago. No evidence of tumor recurrence. Early satiety severely restricts eating ability.

Current Symptoms: Gastrostomy tube for feeding. Dilation of strictured esophagus required once a month to accommodate saliva secretion.

Physical Exam: Height: 1.78 m (5 ft 10 in); weight: 49.9 kg (110 lb); preillness weight: 68.1 kg (150 lb).

Clinical Studies: Endoscopy: unsuccessful surgical correction.

Diagnosis: Stenosing esophagitis.

Impairment Rating: 65% impairment due to stenosing esophagitis and 15% impairment due to gastrostomy; combined 70% impairment of the whole person (see the Combined Values Chart, p. 604). Combine impairments due to cancer and other medical conditions with this impairment percentage.

Comment: Disease symptoms and signs progressed despite exhaustive treatment; further therapy only palliative. Weight loss exceeds 20% of desirable level. Poor prognosis. Esophageal stent may provide palliation and avoidance of dilations.

Example 6-16
50% to 75% Impairment Due to Pancreatic Disease

Subject: 47-year-old man.

History: Manufacturer's representative; 13 months prior onset of vague abdominal pain, weight loss, and uncharacteristic depression, followed by gradually deepening jaundice. Cystic adenocarcinoma occupying most of the pancreas. Surgical eradication of lesion required total pancreatectomy and duodenectomy (Whipple operation). Malabsorption syndrome with steatorrhea only partially relieved by pancreatic enzyme supplements. Brittle diabetes mellitus after operation despite close monitoring and repeated daily insulin injections.

Current Symptoms: Barely able to perform essential activities of daily living.

Physical Exam: Cachectic. Weight declined since operation to 25% below desirable level.

Clinical Studies: Glucose levels: highly variable.

Diagnosis: Pancreatic insufficiency consequent to total pancreatectomy.

Impairment Rating: 70% impairment due to total pancreatic insufficiency; combine with appropriate impairment estimate for diabetes mellitus (see Combined Values Chart, p. 604) to determine whole person impairment (refer to Chapter 10, The Endocrine System).

Comment: Capacity to perform normal activities of daily living seriously impaired by total pancreatic loss; intensive treatment only partially alleviated debility.[3]

Example 6-17
50% to 75% Impairment Due to Small Intestine Disease

Subject: 35-year-old woman.

History: Department store salesperson; life-threatening volvulus 1 year ago. Major small bowel portion entrapped in adhesions from previous operation required extensive resection of incarcerated and strangulated intestine. Dehydration and electrolyte depletion necessitated repeated hospitalization.

Current Symptoms: Dependent on continuous dietary control and nutritional supplements. Takes frequent medication to alleviate abdominal pain and diarrhea. Diminished stamina; needs assistance with essential activities of daily living.

Physical Exam: Height: 1.65 m (5 ft 5 in); weight: 39.5 kg (87 lb), relatively stable; should be at least 57.6 kg (127 lb) for medium frame. Sharply reduced intestinal absorptive capacity. Otherwise normal.

Clinical Studies: Hematologic studies: consistent with malabsorption.

Diagnosis: Intestinal malabsorption due to extensive small bowel resection.

Impairment Rating: 75% impairment of the whole person.

Comment: Nutritional status severely impaired by irreversible small intestine defect. Weight loss exceeds 20% of desirable level; needs assistance with performance of daily living activities.

6.3 Colon, Rectum, and Anus

6.3a Criteria for Rating Permanent Impairment Due to Colonic or Rectal Disease

Criteria for evaluating impairments in function of the colon and rectum are listed in Table 6-4.

Table 6-4 Criteria for Rating Permanent Impairment Due to Colonic and Rectal Disorders

Class 1 0%-9% Impairment of the Whole Person	Class 2 10%-24% Impairment of the Whole Person	Class 3 25%-49% Impairment of the Whole Person	Class 4 50%-75% Impairment of the Whole Person
Signs and symptoms of colonic or rectal disease infrequent and of brief duration *and* limitation of activities, special diet, or medication not required *and* no systemic manifestations present, and weight and nutritional state can be maintained at desirable level *or* no sequelae after surgical procedures	Objective evidence of colonic or rectal disease or anatomic loss or alteration *and* mild gastrointestinal symptoms with occasional disturbances of bowel function, accompanied by moderate pain *and* minimal restriction of diet or mild symptomatic therapy may be necessary *and* no impairment of nutrition results	Objective evidence of colonic or rectal disease or anatomic loss or alteration *and* moderate to severe exacerbations with disturbance of bowel habit, accompanied by periodic or continual pain *and* restriction of activity, special diet, and drugs required during attacks *and* constitutional manifestations (fever, anemia, or weight loss)	Objective evidence of colonic or rectal disease or anatomic loss or alteration *and* persistent disturbances of bowel function present at rest with severe persistent pain *and* complete limitation of activity, continued restriction of diet, and medication do not entirely control symptoms *and* constitutional manifestations (fever, weight loss, or anemia) present *or* no prolonged remission

Class 1 0%-9% Impairment of the Whole Person
Signs and symptoms of colonic or rectal disease infrequent and of brief duration *and* limitation of activities, special diet, or medication not required *and* no systemic manifestations present, and weight and nutritional state can be maintained at desirable level *or* no sequelae after surgical procedures

Example 6-18
0% to 9% Impairment Due to Colonic or Rectal Disease

Subject: 50-year-old woman.

History: Part-time social worker; general good health. Several years' tendency of mildly erratic bowel action with alternating constipation and diarrhea. Stools of varied consistency never contained abnormal materials.

Current Symptoms: Episodes of cramping bowel movements; alternating diarrhea and constipation.

Physical Exam: Normal.

Clinical Studies: Proctosigmoidoscopy: clear mucosa; barium enema: normal colon with several sigmoid diverticula; no evidence of diverticulitis.

Diagnosis: Irritable bowel syndrome and diverticulosis coli.

Impairment Rating: 0% impairment of the whole person.

Comment: Symptoms, while occasionally annoying, do not interfere with performance of daily activities. Needs only minor dietary adjustment.

Class 2	Class 3
10%-24% Impairment of the Whole Person	**25%-49% Impairment of the Whole Person**
Objective evidence of colonic or rectal disease or anatomic loss or alteration	Objective evidence of colonic or rectal disease or anatomic loss or alteration
and	*and*
mild gastrointestinal symptoms with occasional disturbances of bowel function, accompanied by moderate pain	moderate to severe exacerbations with disturbance of bowel habit, accompanied by periodic or continual pain
and	*and*
minimal restriction of diet or mild symptomatic therapy may be necessary	restriction of activity, special diet, and drugs required during attacks
and	*and*
no impairment of nutrition results	constitutional manifestations (fever, anemia, or weight loss)

Example 6-19
10% to 24% Impairment Due to Colonic or Rectal Disease

Subject: 28-year-old woman.

History: Graduate student; part-time teaching assistant; 10 years' recurring ulcerative colitis. Exacerbations produced moderate abdominal distress, diarrhea, and passage of blood-tinged stools. No fever, anemia, or hospitalization. Symptoms responded to moderately restricted diet, antidiarrheal medication, and avoidance of unduly strenuous activity.

Current Symptoms: Episodic diarrhea.

Physical Exam: Guaiac-positive stools.

Clinical Studies: Colonoscopy: varying degrees of granularity and punctate friability in rectosigmoid mucosa; endoscopy: colon remainder appeared normal.

Diagnosis: Idiopathic ulcerative colitis; mild; limited to the rectosigmoid segment.

Impairment Rating: 15% impairment of the whole person.

Comment: Remittent disease; symptoms only occasionally interfere with performance of necessary daily activities. Symptomatic, supportive therapy adequately controls disease.[7]

Example 6-20
25% to 49% Impairment Due to Colonic or Rectal Disease

Subject: 35-year-old man.

History: Computer programmer; Crohn's disease since age 19. Several hospitalizations that required intensive therapy and transfusion of packed red blood cells to correct anemia.

Current Symptoms: Recurring diarrhea associated with cramping abdominal pain and occasional perianal suppuration with draining fistulas. Elective proctocolectomy declined.

Physical Exam: Weight remains 20% or more below desirable level. Guaiac-positive stools.

Clinical Studies: Crohn's disease lesions affecting the perineum, rectum, several colon segments, and the terminal ileum.

Diagnosis: Chronic, recurrent enterocolitis (Crohn's disease).

Impairment Rating: 45% impairment due to enterocolitis; combine with appropriate anemia impairment estimate to determine whole person impairment (see Combined Values Chart, p. 604).

Comment: Chronic inflammatory bowel disease, while remitting occasionally, interferes with performance of daily activities. Requires continuing close observation and treatment. Impaired nutritional status. Continuing Crohn's disease activity mostly in colon with only distal ileum involvement; proctocolectomy and Brooke ileostomy may significantly improve the general condition, perhaps with less impairment.

Class 4
50%-75% Impairment of the Whole Person
Objective evidence of colonic or rectal disease or anatomic loss or alteration
and
persistent disturbances of bowel function present at rest with severe persistent pain
and
complete limitation of activity, continued restriction of diet, and medication do not entirely control symptoms
and
constitutional manifestations (fever, weight loss, or anemia) present
or
no prolonged remission

Example 6-21
50% to 75% Impairment Due to Colonic or Rectal Disease

Subject: 42-year-old woman.

History: 15 years' chronic ulcerative colitis. Activity limited; required intensive treatment, including occasional blood transfusion. Persistent fever, anemia, and jaundice.

Current Symptoms: Increasing debility; nutritional deficiency. Further complications of inflammatory bowel disease.

Physical Exam: Cachectic; jaundice and hepatomegaly.

Clinical Studies: Barium enema, colonoscopy: extensive and severe colon involvement. Liver function tests: severely abnormal; liver biopsy: nonsuppurative cholangitic cirrhosis.

Diagnosis: Chronic ulcerative colitis, severe; sclerosing cholangitis with cirrhosis.

Impairment Rating: 60% impairment due to ulcerative colitis; combine with appropriate impairment estimates for the liver disorder and anemia (see Combined Values Chart, p. 604) to determine the whole person impairment.

Comment: Declined liver transplantation option. Physician does not consider colectomy as a therapeutic option due to general debility and advanced, complicated disease. Proctocolectomy has no beneficial effect on sclerosing cholangitis.[9] Increased acceptability of new anastomosis such as ileal-pouch anal anastomosis provides greater security and privacy and may lead to earlier surgery in severe ulcerative colitis.

6.3b Criteria for Rating Permanent Impairment Due to Anal Disease

Criteria for evaluating permanent impairments of the anus are listed in Table 6-5.

Table 6-5 Criteria for Rating Permanent Impairment Due to Anal Disease

Class 1 0%-9% Impairment of the Whole Person	Class 2 10%-19% Impairment of the Whole Person	Class 3 20%-35% Impairment of the Whole Person
Signs of organic anal disease or anatomic loss or alteration	Signs of organic anal disease or anatomic loss or alteration	Signs of organic anal disease and anatomic loss or alteration
or	*and*	*and*
mild incontinence involving gas or liquid stool	moderate but partial fecal incontinence requiring continual treatment	complete fecal incontinence
or	*or*	*or*
anal symptoms mild, intermittent, and controlled by treatment	continual anal symptoms incompletely controlled by treatment	signs of organic anal disease and severe anal symptoms unresponsive or amenable to therapy

Example 6-22
0% to 9% Impairment Due to Anal Disease

Subject: 45-year-old man.

History: Acute pararectal abscess surgically drained 5 years ago. Anal fistula; recurrent acute infection and intermittent drainage. Fistulectomy 1 year ago.

Current Symptoms: No further infection or drainage; regular bowel activity.

Physical Exam: Well-healed anal scar with slight anal orifice distortion; no anal sphincter weakness.

Clinical Studies: Proctosigmoidoscopy: normal except for anal scarring.

Diagnosis: Healed anal fistula.

Impairment Rating: 0% to 5% impairment of the whole person.

Comment: Documented anal disease appropriately and successfully treated. Performance of daily activities unimpaired.

Example 6-23
10% to 19% Impairment Due to Anal Disease

Subject: 32-year-old woman.

History: 14 years' Crohn's colitis, usually well controlled by medical therapy. During one exacerbation, developed pararectal abscess that ruptured spontaneously and led to development of chronically draining anal fistula. Later developed small rectovaginal fistula. Anal dysfunction symptoms occasionally recurred; usually tolerably controlled by treatment. Anal fistula surgery attempt inadvisable because of disease extent elsewhere in the rectum and colon.

Current Symptoms: Episodic fecal incontinence.

Physical Exam: Inactive perianal disease.

Clinical Studies: Colonoscopy: Crohn's disease throughout colon and rectum.

Diagnosis: Chronic anal fistula with moderate impairment of anal function, associated with Crohn's disease of the colon.

Impairment Rating: 10% impairment due to anal disorder; combine with colonic disease and gynecologic impairment ratings to determine whole person impairment (see the Combined Values Chart, p. 604).

Comment: Impaired anal function, but symptoms responsive to treatment when required. Slightly impaired ability to perform activities of daily living.

Chapter 6

Class 3
20%-35% Impairment of the Whole Person
Signs of organic anal disease and anatomic loss or alteration
and
complete fecal incontinence
or
signs of organic anal disease and severe anal symptoms unresponsive or amenable to therapy

Example 6-24
20% to 35% Impairment Due to Anal Disease

Subject: 56-year-old man.

History: Pararectal abscess that drained sponta-neously; 3 years' recurrent infection; fistulous tracts opened four other areas surrounding anus. Two-stage surgical repair; incision and excision of substantial portions of the anal sphincter muscle. Recovery delayed by wound infections.

Current Symptoms: Perineum eventually healed; no fecal control. Despite daily rectal irrigation, soils himself occasionally.

Physical Exam: Complete functional loss of anal sphincter mechanism.

Clinical Studies: None.

Diagnosis: Anal incontinence due to complete loss of sphincter function.

Impairment Rating: 25% impairment of the whole person.

Comment: Uncontrollable fecal incontinence not amenable to further therapy. Sigmoid colostomy might provide greater comfort and security with less impairment (see Table 6-6).

Table 6-6 Impairments from Surgically Created Stomas

Created Stoma	% Impairment of the Whole Person
Esophagostomy	10%-15%
Gastrostomy	10%-15%
Jejunostomy	15%-20%
Ileostomy	15%-20%
Ileal pouch-anal anastomosis	15%-20%
Colostomy	5%-10%

6.4 Enterocutaneous Fistulas

Evaluate permanent enterocutaneous fistulas of the gastrointestinal tract, biliary tract, or pancreas that are associated with diseases of these structures or their treatment as part of the primarily involved organ system. Permanent, **surgically created stomas** usually are provided to compensate for anatomic losses and to allow either ingress to or egress from the alimentary tract.

If an individual has a permanent, surgically created stoma, combine a percentage based on Table 6-6 with an estimate based on criteria related to the involved organ (see the Combined Values Chart, p. 604).

Many people with well-functioning, long-standing stomas such as Brooke ileostomy or descending colostomy lead full and active lives with few limita-tions in overall performance of daily activities.

Chapter 6

6.5 Liver and Biliary Tract

6.5a Criteria for Rating Permanent Impairment Due to Liver or Biliary Tract Disease

Criteria for evaluating permanent impairment of the liver and biliary tract are listed in Tables 6-7 and 6-8.

Table 6-7 Criteria for Rating Permanent Impairment Due to Liver Disease

Class 1 0%-14% Impairment of the Whole Person	Class 2 15%-29% Impairment of the Whole Person	Class 3 30%-49% Impairment of the Whole Person	Class 4 50%-95% Impairment of the Whole Person
Persistent liver disease objective evidence; no symptoms of liver disease and no history of ascites, jaundice, or bleeding esophageal varices within 3 years *and* good nutrition and strength *and* biochemical studies indicate minimal disturbance in function *or* primary disorders of bilirubin metabolism	Chronic liver disease objective evidence; no liver disease symptoms and no history of ascites, jaundice, or bleeding esophageal varices within 3 years *and* good nutrition and strength *and* biochemical studies indicate more severe liver damage than class 1	Progressive chronic liver disease objective evidence or history of jaundice, ascites, or bleeding esophageal or gastric varices within past year *and* possibly affected nutrition and strength *or* intermittent hepatic encephalopathy	Progressive chronic liver disease objective evidence or persistent jaundice or bleeding esophageal or gastric varices, with central nervous system manifestations of hepatic insufficiency *and* poor nutritional state

Table 6-8 Criteria for Rating Permanent Impairment Due to Biliary Tract Disease

Class 1 0%-14% Impairment of the Whole Person	Class 2 15%-29% Impairment of the Whole Person	Class 3 30%-49% Impairment of the Whole Person	Class 4 50%-95% Impairment of the Whole Person
Occasional biliary tract dysfunction episode	Recurrent biliary tract impairment, irrespective of treatment	Irreparable biliary tract obstruction with recurrent cholangitis	Persistent jaundice; progressive liver disease due to common bile duct obstruction

Chapter 6

Class 1
0%-14% Impairment of the Whole Person

Persistent liver disease objective evidence; no symptoms of liver disease and no history of ascites, jaundice, or bleeding esophageal varices within 3 years

and

good nutrition and strength

and

biochemical studies indicate minimal disturbance in function

or

primary disorders of bilirubin metabolism

Class 2
15%-29% Impairment of the Whole Person

Chronic liver disease objective evidence; no liver disease symptoms and history of ascites, jaundice, or bleeding esophageal or gastric varices within past year

and

good nutrition and strength

and

biochemical studies indicate more severe liver damage than class 1

Example 6-25
0% to 14% Impairment Due to Liver Disease

Subject: 30-year-old man.

History: Excessive alcohol consumption. Hospitalized 5 years ago for severe delirium tremens, fever, and jaundice. Liver biopsy specimen: extensive fatty metamorphosis with steatonecrosis, scattered inflammatory cell infiltration, and minimal periportal fibrosis.

Current Symptoms: Since hospital release, abstains from alcohol, feels well, and exhibits normal vigor and appetite.

Physical Exam: Well-developed, muscular man; no jaundice or ascites. Liver edge was palpated 2 cm below right costal margin.

Clinical Studies: Liver function tests: within normal limits; serum aspartate aminotransferase (AST; formerly serum glutamic oxaloacetic transaminase) level: 1.5 times normal.

Diagnosis: History of acute alcoholic hepatitis and steatonecrosis, with residual slight hepatomegaly, without changes in ability to perform activities of daily living.

Impairment Rating: 0% impairment of the whole person.

Comment: Preexisting disease well documented. Satisfactory recovery; only minimal evidence of residual hepatic impairment. Requires no treatment other than continued abstinence from alcohol; engages fully in normal activities of daily living. Most individuals with alcohol abuse history need considerable help from professionals and family to continue abstinence; failure risks recurrent alcoholic hepatitis episodes that, if severe, may be fatal or lead to cirrhosis and class 4 impairment.[10]

Example 6-26
15% to 29% Impairment Due to Liver Disease

Subject: 35-year-old man.

History: Plumber; acute viral hepatitis with a protracted convalescence 10 years ago.

Current Symptoms: Disease quiescent; no visible icterus, ascites, or GI tract bleeding. Satisfactory strength and nutritional state; limited stamina.

Physical Exam: Well nourished and well muscled. Several small telangiectasias on left shoulder. Nontender, firm, rounded liver edge palpated 4 cm below right costal margin; inferior spleen margin palpated 1 cm below left costal margin.

Clinical Studies: Liver function tests: serum bilirubin, 36 mmol/L (2.1 mg/dL); serum albumin, 40 g/L; serum globulin, 40 g/L; and serum AST, 70 U/L. Positive serum hepatitis B surface antigen and core antibodies. Liver biopsy specimen: periportal hepatitis and piecemeal necrosis (now called "interface hepatitis"); early indications of extension between portal tracts and central veins.

Diagnosis: Chronic hepatitis B.

Impairment Rating: 15% impairment of the whole person.

Comment: Documented evidence of chronic active hepatitis; can perform normal activities of daily living, although has reduced stamina. Slight to moderate impaired liver function. Chronic hepatitis implies 6 months or more of inflammation; nomenclature for specific forms reflects etiologic or pathologic mechanisms. Cirrhosis likely; progression to class 3 or 4 impairment. Timing this evolution less predictable; may be influenced by treatment programs. Increased impairment if hepatitis C is present with elevated risk of hepatocellular carcinoma.[11]

Class 3
30%-49% Impairment of the Whole Person
Irreparable biliary tract obstructon with recurrent cholangitis

Class 4
50%-95% Impairment of the Whole Person
Persistent jaundice, progressive liver disease due to common bile duct obstruction

Example 6-27
30% to 49% Impairment Due to Biliary Tract Disese

Subject: 46-year-old woman.

History: Teacher; concerned about increasing pruritus, loss of strength, and decreased stamina. Itch onset 2 years ago; routine blood chemistry: elevated serum alkaline phosphatase. Ingested no drugs known to cause cholestasis; antimitochondrial antibody test positive.

Current Symptoms: Recent significantly increased impairment: unable to complete all daily activities due to increasing debility.

Physical Exam: Generalized hyperpigmentation, scratch marks, mild jaundice, a few xanthomata, and probable splenomegaly.

Clinical Studies: Laboratory studies: alkaline phosphatase 4 times normal levels; serum bilirubin: 5 mg/dL, positive antimitochondrial antibody. Retrograde cholangiogram: normal extrahepatic ducts. Liver biopsy: small bile ducts damaged, interlobular bile ducts damaged; scarring consistent with primary biliary cirrhosis. Discussed liver transplantation as future consideration. Responded only minimally to various treatment protocols. Cholestasis increased to 12 mg serum bilirubin. Individual awaited liver transplant donor availability.

Diagnosis: Primary biliary cirrhosis.

Impairment Rating: 40% at time of confirmed diagnosis; progression to class 4 impairment when put on liver transplant waiting list.

Comment: Primary biliary cirrhosis is a relentlessly progressive liver disease that leads to class 4 impairment. Orthotopic liver transplantation offers significant benefit and should be considered early. Currently, the majority of recipients report a remarkable improvement in quality of life and many enjoy normal lifestyles, although compliance with drug therapies and follow-up visits are required. A successful transplant may ultimately reduce the impairment of the whole person.[12,13]

Example 6-28
50% to 95% Impairment Due to Biliary Tract Disease

Subject: 55-year-old woman.

History: Repeated acute cholecystitis attacks for 5 years. Refused to seek medical care because of religious beliefs.

Current Symptoms: Increasingly frequent and severe bouts of right upper quadrant pain, nausea, vomiting, fever, jaundice, dark urine, and pruritus. Unable to perform many basic activities of daily living for over a year.

Physical Exam: Jaundiced; right upper quadrant pain to palpitation.

Clinical Studies: Laboratory tests: biliary obstruction and advanced liver damage. Liver biopsy specimen: advanced biliary cirrhosis. Declined any consideration of an invasive procedure that might alleviate disease.

Diagnosis: Biliary cirrhosis, secondary to recurrent and progressive obstruction of bile ducts.

Impairment Rating: 85% impairment of the whole person.

Comment: Severe and irreparable impairment of liver and biliary tract function. Needs live-in assistance to perform normal activities of daily living. Laparoscopic removal of calculus containing gallbladder, endoscopic extraction of common bile duct stones, and great variety of billiary drainage procedures may greatly reduce the total impairment rating.[13]

6.6 Hernias

6.6a Criteria for Rating Permanent Impairment Due to Herniation

Criteria for evaluating impairment due to herniation are listed in Table 6-9.

Table 6-9 Criteria for Rating Permanent Impairment Due to Herniation

Class 1 0%-9% Impairment of the Whole Person	Class 2 10%-19% Impairment of the Whole Person	Class 3 20%-30% Impairment of the Whole Person
Palpable defect in supporting structures of abdominal wall *and* slight protrusion at site of defect with increased abdominal pressure; readily reducible *or* occasional mild discomfort at site of defect but not precluding most activities of daily living	Palpable defect in supporting structures of abdominal wall *and* frequent or persistent protrusion at site of defect with increased abdominal pressure; manually reducible *or* frequent discomfort, precluding heavy lifting but not hampering some activities of daily living	Palpable defect in supporting structures of abdominal wall *and* persistent, irreducible, or irreparable protrusion at site of defect *and* limitation in activities of daily living

Class 1 0%-9% Impairment of the Whole Person
Palpable defect in supporting structures of abdominal wall *and* slight protrusion at site of defect with increased abdominal pressure; readily reducible *or* occasional mild discomfort at site of defect but not precluding most activities of daily living

Example 6-29
0% to 9% Impairment Due to Hernia

Subject: 60-year-old woman.

History: Cholecystectomy for calculous biliary tract disease relief 3 years ago. Uneventful postoperative course.

Current Symptoms: No complaints; eating well; no abdominal discomfort.

Physical Exam: Healed oblique, right upper quadrant incision; palpable defect in middle part. Slight, visible protrusion at this site when individual rose from supine position. No pain or discomfort in scar region, which she perceived as unsightly.

Clinical Studies: None.

Diagnosis: Uncomplicated incisional hernia.

Impairment Rating: 0% impairment of the whole person.

Comment: Asymptomatic incisional hernia only mildly annoying. No significant risk of complication. No limit in ability to perform activities of daily living.

Class 2
10%-19% Impairment of the Whole Person
Palpable defect in supporting structures of abdominal wall
and
frequent or persistent protrusion at site of defect with increased abdominal pressure; manually reducible
or
frequent discomfort, precluding heavy lifting but not hampering some activities of daily living

Class 3
20%-30% Impairment of the Whole Person
Palpable defect in supporting structures of abdominal wall
and
persistent, irreducible, or irreparable protrusion at site of defect
and
limitation in activities of daily living

Example 6-30
10% to 19% Impairment Due to Hernia

Subject: 50-year-old man.

History: Several years' recurring protrusion in right inguinal area upon straining or exerting increased intra-abdominal pressure.

Current Symptoms: Protrusion visible with bowel movements; reduces hernia himself; no discomfort.

Physical Exam: Enlarged protrusion entered scrotum base; easily and painlessly reduced. Declined recommended surgical repair; willing to accept heavy lifting preclusion and risk possible complications.

Clinical Studies: None.

Diagnosis: Reducible right indirect inguinal hernia.

Impairment Rating: 10% impairment of the whole person.

Comment: Restricted exertion; chose to live with limitation. Aware of possible consequences of unrepaired inguinal hernia; declined operation. No impairment of normally sedentary activities of daily living.

Example 6-31
20% to 30% Impairment Due to Hernia

Subject: 64-year-old man.

History: Nearing retirement; recurrent, bilateral, inguinal hernias despite three previous attempts at repair: two on the right side and one on the left. Reluctant to submit to further repair attempts.

Current Symptoms: Frequent discomfort. No supervening complications.

Physical Exam: Protrusions only partially reducible.

Clinical Studies: None.

Diagnosis: Recurrent bilateral inguinal hernias after unsuccessful herniorrhaphy.

Impairment Rating: 30% impairment of the whole person.

Comment: Recurrent inguinal hernias only partially reducible despite repeated surgical repair. Individual obliged to wear supporting device. Frequent inguinal discomfort. Restricted in performance of normal activities of daily living, including sports. Possible hazard if supporting device exerts local pressure on partially reduced hernia. Encourage further repair attempts with possible reinforcing mesh use.

Chapter 6

6.7 Digestive System Impairment Evaluation Summary

See Table 6-10 for an evaluation summary for the assessment of permanent impairment due to digestive system disorders.

Table 6-10 Digestive System Impairment Evaluation Summary

Disorder	History, Including Selected Relevant Symptoms	Examination Record	Assessment of Dysfunction
General	Gastrointestional symptoms (eg, change in appetite, pain, diarrhea) and general symptoms; impact of symptoms on function and ability to do daily activities Prognosis if change anticipated Review medical history	Comprehensive physical examination; detailed GI system assessment	Data derived from relevant studies (eg, barium swallow, upper and lower endoscopy)
Esophageal Disease	Dysphagia for solids and/or liquids G-E reflux Previous proximal gastrectomy or interposition surgery Need for dilations and/or medications History of aspiration Limitation of physical activity	Evidence of weight loss Duration of symptoms Evidence of scleroderma or other mesenchymal disease Previous motility studies for achalasia or diffuse spasm	Location and degree of stricture Is proximal esophagus dilated? Endoscopic appearance and biopsy results
Stomach Diseases	Vomiting, weight loss, past gastrectomy dumping symptoms; family history of ulcer or endocrinopathy Persistent ulcer diathesis despite treatment Any history of use of ulcerogenic drugs (NSAIDS, ASA) Limited physical activity	Weight loss; diabetes with neuropathy	Size of gastric pouch Location and function of gastrojejunal amastomosis Endoscopic evaluation of structures Motility studies
Small Intestine Disease	Diarrhea (frequency, nocturnal); abdominal colic and distention History of volvulus Hemorrhage Family history of celiac sprue, motility disorder Weight loss Previous surgery Limited activity	Note weight loss Abdominal distention, masses Perianal disease Arthropathy Presence of dermatitis herpetiformis	Barium studies Possibly enteroclysis study, jejunal cultures, and mucosal biopsy Antigliadin antibody Motility studies Amount of intact small intestine (estimate whether more or less than 200 cm)
Pancreatic Disease	History of acute pancreatitis (documented) Frequency; duration; associated jaundice, nausea, anorexia; alcohol intake; adequacy of pain control GI bleeding (consider splenic vein thrombosis) Associated chronic lung disease (think of cystic fibrosis)	Abdominal masses; fistulae; previous gallstones; evidence of weight loss; jaundice	Ultrasound pancreas and biliary tract Consider transduodenal ultrasonography, CT scan, ERCP, measure of steatorrhea, plain film of abdomen for calcification Sweat Na+ to exclude cystic fibrosis

Assessment of End-Organ Damage	Diagnosis(es)	Degree of Impairment
Include assessment of sequelae, including end-organ damage and impairment	Record all pertinent diagnosis(es); note if they are at maximal medical improvement; if not, discuss under what conditions and when stability is expected	Criteria outlined in this chapter
Motility studies if indicated Response to therapy Need for esophageal stent or interposition surgery Frequency of dilations	GERD with inflammatory stricture Barrett's esophagus with or without malignant change Stricture secondary to scleroderma Achalasia, diffuse spasm, Zenker's diverticulum	See Table 6-3
Response to dietary management Trial of antisecretory drugs, prokinetic agents	Postgastrectomy state Diabetic gastroparesis Possible Zollinger-Ellison syndrome Paraesophageal hernia with gastric volvulus	See Table 6-3
Effects of malabsorption of iron, B_{12}, folate tetany Failure to grow Response to gluten restriction, steroids Parenteral nutrition	Celiac sprue possible lymphoma complication Regional enteritis; Crohn's; ischemic bowel disease Radiation enteritis Chronic pseudo-obstruction; mechanical obstruction (adhesions)	See Table 6-3
Degree of fat maldigestion and malabsorption Presence of diabetes mellitus Need for pain control, including celiac plexus and/or splanchnic block	Alcoholic pancreatitis Chronic relapsing pancreatitis Pancreatitis secondary to biliary tract disease Cystic fibrosis	See Table 6-3

Chapter 6

Table 6-10 Digestive System Impairment Evaluation Summary (continued)

Disorder	History, Including Selected Relevant Symptoms	Examination Record	Assessment of Dysfunction
Large Intestine Disease	History of previous colon surgery (length remaining, nature of anastomoses) Bleeding; need for transfusions Stool frequency, pattern (nocturnal incontinence) Abdominal pain Weight loss Limited activity	Abdominal masses Perianal disease Fistulae arthropathy	Sigmoidoscopy; colonoscopy Possible barium studies; mucosal biopsies Defecation studies; motility; possible EMG of sphincter activity
Liver disease	Alcohol intake (past, present) Previous use of hepatotoxic drugs Presence of ascites, edema, jaundice, iron overload (multiple transfusions) History of GI hemorrhage Pruritus; primary biliary cirrhosis Limited physical activity	Cutaneous and ocular signs of chronic liver disease Ascites; edema; skin pigmentation (hemochromatosis) Evidence of previous surgery in region of liver Keyser-Fleischer rings in eyes Evidence of ulcerative colitis Xanthomata	Nutritional status, including hemoglobin, protein, prothrombin time Platelets Etiologic studies, including complete hepatitis serology markers Renal function HIV studies Diabetes if hemochromatosis (serum iron and ferritin saturation antitrypsin Antimitochondrial antibody; exclude genetic and infiltrative diseases (eg, amyloidosis, sarcoidosis, polycystic disease) Copper studies
Biliary Tract Disease	Previous biliary tract surgery Episodes of cholecystitis, biliary colic, jaundice Family history of bilirubin metabolism disorder Bleeding; pruritus	Previous attempts at dissolution therapy and or lithotripsy Jaundice Presence of scratch marks Splenomegaly Abdominal fistula	Ultrasound studies ERCP Transhepatic cholangiography if needed Prothrombin time
Hernia	Discomfort, pain associated with postural changes Limited physical activity	Abdominal protrusion or swelling	Roentgenography; CT scan

References

1. McCord GS, Staiano A, Clouse RE. Achalasia, diffuse spasm and non-specific disorders. *Baillieres Clin Gastroenterol.* 1991; 5:307-335.

   A categorization method of the manometric abnormalities of diffuse spasm and nonspecific disorders.

2. Trytgat GNJ, et al. The role of infectious agents in peptic ulcer disease. *Gastroenterol Int.* 1993;6:76-89.

3. Banks PA, et al. The spectrum of chronic pancreatitis. *Parenteral Care.* 1989;23(9):163-196.

4. Henderson RD, Ryder D, Marryatt G. Extended esophagal myotomy and short fundoplication hernia repair in diffuse esophageal spasm. *Ann Thorac Surg.* 1987;43:25-31.

   A follow-up study of the surgical management of diffuse esophageal spasm. Result: Good results from surgery achieved in 94% of patients followed 5 to 10.7 years.

5. Pope CE II. Acid reflux disorders. *N Engl J Med.* 1994;331:656-660.

   General review.

6. Lagergren J, Bergstrom R, Lindgren A, Nyren O. Symptomatic gastroesophageal reflux as a risk factor for gastroesophageal adenocarcinoma. *N Engl J Med.* 1999;340:825-831.

   An epidemiologic investigation of the possible association between gastroesophageal reflux and adenocarcinoma, indicating a positive but weak association.

Assessment of End-Organ Damage	Diagnosis(es)	Degree of Impairment
Uncontrollable diarrhea; intractible constipation Megacolon	Inflammatory bowel disease; ulcerative colitis; Crohn's disease; colectomy with ileostomy or ileoanal pouch anastomosis	See Table 6-4
CNS tolerance to hemorrhage Fluid and salt overload Possible pancreatic insufficiency Secondary development of hepatoma Intractable prothrombin time prolongation; platelet deficiency; leukopenia	Alcoholic liver disease; cirrhosis; hepatoma; posthepatitic cirrhosis (previous HBV, HCV); hemochromatosis; Wilson's disease Primary biliary cirrhosis Sclerosing cholangitis	See Table 6-7
Persistent hyperbilirubinemia after obstruction relieved Findings at surgery	Biliary tract stricture; impacted stones; sclerosing cholangitis Primary biliary cirrhosis	See Table 6-8
Possible incarceration or strangulation of bowel or omentum	Abdominal wall hernia; umbilical hernia; incisional hernia; inguinal hernia; femoral hernia	See Table 6-9

7. Lau JYW, et al. Endoscopic retreatment or surgery after initial endoscopic control of bleeding ulcers. *N Engl J Med.* 1999;340:751-756.

   A prospective, randomized study of patients with bleeding peptic ulcers comparing endoscopic retreatment with surgery after initial endoscopy. Result: Endoscopic retreatment reduces the need for surgery with fewer complications.

8. Scolapio JS, Fleming CR, Kelly DG, Wick DM, Zinsmeister AR. Survival of home parenteral nutrition (HPN)-treatment patients: 20 years of experience at the Mayo Clinic. *Mayo Clin Proc.* 1999;74:217-222.

   A retrospective review of medical records of all Mayo Clinic patients treated with HPN between 1975 and 1995. Results: Most deaths during treatment with HPN are a result of the primary disease; HPN-related deaths are uncommon.

9. Cangemi JR, Wiesner RH, Beaver SJ, et al. Effect of proctocolectomy for chronic ulcerative colitis on the natural history of primary sclerosing cholangitis. *Gastroenterology.* 1989;96:790-794.

   A study of the progression of clinical, biochemical, cholangiographic, and hepatic histologic features in 45 patients with both primary sclerosing cholangitis and chronic ulcerative colitis and the benefits of proctocolectomy. Result: Proctocolectomy for chronic ulcerative colitis has no beneficial effect on the primary sclerosing cholangitis in patients with both diseases.

10. Pemberton JH, Phillips SF. In: Sleisinger and Fordtran. *Gastrointestinal and Liver Disease.* Vol 2. 6th ed. 1998:1762-1768.

11. Kiyosawa K, Sodeyama T, Tanaka E, et al. Interrelationships of blood transfusion, non-A, non-B hepatitis and hepatocellular carcinoma: analysis by detection of antibody to hepatitis C virus. *Hepatology.* 1990;12:671-675.

A study to clarify the relationship between hepatitis C virus infection and the development of hepatocellular carcinomas as a sequela of non-A, non-B posttransfusion hepatitis. Result: A causal association between hepatitis C virus and hepatocellular carcinoma was indicated.

12. Munoz SJ. Long term management of the liver transplant recipient. *Med Clin North Am.* 1996;80:1103-1120.

A team approach to the long-term management of liver transplant recipients enables survival in terms of decades, rather than years.

13. Desmet VJ. Current problems in diagnosis of biliary disease and cholestasis. *Semin Liver Dis.* 1986;6:233-245.

Bibliography

Bennett JC, Plum F, eds. *Cecil's Textbook of Medicine.* 20th ed. Philadelphia, Pa: WB Saunders Co; 1996.

Haubrich WS, Schaffner F, Berk JE, eds. *Bockus Gastroenterology.* 5th ed. Philadelphia, Pa: WB Saunders Co; 1994.

Miura S, Shikata J, Hasebe M, Kobayashi K. Long-term outcome of massive small bowel resection. *Am J Gastroenterol.* 1991;86:454-459.

Sherlock S, ed. *Diseases of the Liver and Biliary System.* 8th ed. Oxford, England: Blackwell Scientific Publications; 1989. Out of print.

Chapter 7

The Urinary and Reproductive Systems

Introduction

This chapter provides criteria for evaluating permanent impairments of the urinary and male and female reproductive systems as they affect the body's overall function and an individual's ability to perform activities of daily living.

The following sections have been revised for the fifth edition: (1) the criteria for upper and lower urinary tract impairment have been revised; (2) impairment classes for bladder and urethral dysfunction have been revised to reflect an increased understanding of bladder impairment and to incorporate results from urodynamic studies; (3) the reproductive system sections have been updated to reflect more common cases and approaches; and (4) updated and detailed references are listed for the disorders discussed.

7.1 Principles of Assessment

Before using the information in this chapter, the *Guides* user should become familiar with Chapters 1 and 2 and the Glossary. Chapters 1 and 2 discuss the *Guides'* purpose, applications, and methods for performing and reporting impairment evaluations. The Glossary provides definitions of common terms used by many specialties in impairment evaluation.

The purpose of urinary and reproductive system impairment assessment is to determine whether a permanent impairment in these systems exists, to assess the severity and document the impact of the impairment on the ability to perform activities of daily living, and to prevent further impairment.

Pathologic abnormalities in other systems (eg, the hematologic, endocrine, or neurologic systems) may produce urinary or reproductive system impairment. These abnormalities are combined with urinary or reproductive system impairments to produce a whole person impairment rating. For example, an intracranial brain lesion above the pons will produce some degree of bladder hyperreflexia and an urgent need to urinate. However, an intracranial brain lesion below the pons in the spinal cord will result not only in a hyperreflexic bladder but also in detrusor-sphincter dyssynergia that may result in difficulty urinating, and high intravesical pressures that could lead to vesicoureteral reflux and hydronephrosis. Urinary tract dysfunction is also seen with lumbosacral injury below the T10 vertebra level and would be combined with musculoskeletal dysfunction to determine whole person impairment.

To determine the individual's placement within a particular class range, assess the disease's severity and impact on the ability to perform the activities of daily living as listed in Table 1-2. Impairment ratings are greater for urinary tract or reproductive impairments, which have more of an effect on the ability to perform activities of daily living.

7.1a Interpretation of Symptoms and Signs

Some impairment classes refer to limitations in the ability to perform daily activities because of symptoms. When this information is subjective and possibly misinterpreted, it should not serve as the sole criterion upon which decisions about impairment are made. Rather, obtain objective data about the limitation's

extent and integrate the findings with the subjective data to estimate the degree of permanent impairment.

7.2 The Urinary System

The urinary system consists of the upper urinary tract (the kidneys and ureters), the bladder, and the urethra. The parenchyma of the kidneys produces urine, which is conducted by the renal calices, pelves, and ureters to the bladder and then the urethra.

The kidneys are an important homeostatic regulatory organ. The degree to which kidney and conduit abnormalities may affect the whole person ranges from a clinically undetectable change to marked specific and generalized manifestations of deterioration of the nephron reserves, loss of kidney function, and urine transport abnormalities.

The bladder is a voluntarily controllable urine reservoir that normally permits several hours of urine retention. Bladder dysfunction may be due to pathologic conditions within or outside the urinary system. Within the urinary system, bladder tumors, stones, and inflammatory lesions may produce urinary system impairment.

In women, the urethra is a urinary conduit containing a voluntary sphincter. In men, the urethra possesses a voluntary sphincter and propulsive muscles and is a conduit for urine and seminal ejaculations.

Permanent, surgically created urinary diversions are usually performed to compensate for anatomic losses and to allow for urine outflow. Diversions are evaluated as a part of, and in conjunction with, the assessment of the involved portion of the urinary tract. When evaluating permanent impairment of any segment of the urinary system, impairments of all components of the upper and lower tract must be evaluated and combined to determine renal system impairment (see the Combined Values Chart, p. 604).

7.2a Interpretation of Urinary Symptoms and Signs

Symptoms and signs of upper urinary tract function impairment may include changes in urination; edema; decreased physical stamina; appetite and weight loss; anemia; uremia; loin, abdominal, or costovertebral angle pain; hematuria; chills and fever; hypertension and its complications; abnormalities in the appearance of the urine or its sediment; and biochemical blood changes. Renal disease, especially in early stages, may be made evident only by laboratory findings.

Signs and symptoms of bladder function impairment may include urinary frequency, dysuria, urinary incontinence, urine retention, hematuria, pyuria, passage of urinary calculi, and a suprapubic mass.

Signs and symptoms of urethra function impairment include dysuria, diminished urinary stream, urinary retention, incontinence, extraneous or ectopic urinary openings, periurethral masses, and diminished urethral caliber.

7.2b Description of Clinical Studies

Two clinically useful renal function determinations, serum creatinine and the renal clearance of endogenous creatinine, may serve as criteria for evaluating upper urinary tract function. The serum creatinine level reflects overall renal function. Under normal hydration conditions, the serum creatinine level should be less than 133 µmol/L (1.5 mg/dL).

The glomerular filtration rate, which measures renal clearance of endogenous creatinine, gives a quantitative estimate of the total functioning nephron population. Because longer periods of urine collection improve the reliability of renal function clearance tests, use 24-hour endogenous creatinine clearance measurements. The normal creatinine clearance ranges are 130 to 200 L/24 h (90 to 139 mL/min) for men and 115 to 180 L/24 h (80 to 125 mL/min) for women.

If there are discrepancies in these two test results or additional information is needed, tests—such as metabolic studies, tests of the concentration levels of electrolytes and other chemicals in serum and urine, urine osmolalities, urinalyses, urine cultures, radiologic investigations, isotope renograms, and renal computed tomographic (CT) scans—may be necessary to determine impairment.

Parenchymal disfiguration and conduit abnormality assessment may require diagnostic procedures such as endoscopy, study of one or both kidneys, biopsy, arteriography, radiography of the urinary tract, CAT scan, or magnetic resonance imaging (MRI).

Objective techniques useful in evaluating bladder function include (but are not limited to) cystoscopy, cystography, voiding cystourethrography, cystometry, uroflometry, urinalysis, and urine cultures.

Objective techniques useful in evaluating urethral function include (but are not limited to) urethroscopy, urethrography, cystourethrography, endoscopy, and cystometrography.

7.3 Upper Urinary Tract

7.3a Criteria for Rating Permanent Impairment Due to Upper Urinary Tract Disease

The impairment criteria for evaluating upper urinary tract disease are given in Table 7-1. The **creatinine clearance,** the most accurate reflection of renal function, is an important criterion in each class because it quantifies the degree of upper urinary tract functional impairment.

From a physiologic point of view, the individual with only one functioning kidney may have normal overall renal function because of the efficiency of the remaining kidney. However, with only one kidney, a normal safety factor is lost. Consider the individual with only one functioning kidney as having a 10% whole person impairment because of such an essential organ loss. Combine this percentage with the estimate for any other permanent impairment (see the Combined Values Chart, p. 604).

Renal function deterioration that requires either peritoneal dialysis or hemodialysis indicates severe impairment in the 60% to 95% range, or a class 4 impairment (Table 7-1). Successful renal transplantation may result in marked renal function improvement; the impairment is now in the 15% to 34% range, or a class 2 impairment. However, transplant recipients require continuous observation and medication, which may add to their impairment. For this reason, depending upon the impairment's effect on the activities of daily living (see Table 1-2), one may add 0% to 5% to the final renal function impairment estimate, as discussed in Chapter 1.[1]

Also, evaluate impairment that is related to complications of the disease or therapy, such as cushingoid changes and osteoporosis, as they arise, and combine the appropriate percentages with the final renal impairment estimate (see the Combined Values Chart, p. 604).

Table 7-1 Criteria for Rating Permanent Impairment Due to Upper Urinary Tract Disease

| Class 1
0%-14% Impairment of the Whole Person | Class 2
15%-34% Impairment of the Whole Person | Class 3
35%-59% Impairment of the Whole Person | Class 4
60%-95% Impairment of the Whole Person |
|---|---|---|---|
| Diminution of upper urinary tract function, as evidenced by creatinine clearance of 75-90 L/24 h (52-62.5 mL/min)

or

intermittent symptoms and signs of upper urinary tract dysfunction that do not require continuous treatment or surveillance

or

only one kidney is functioning | Diminution of upper urinary tract function as evidenced by creatinine clearance of 60-75 L/24 h (42-52 mL/min)

or

symptoms and signs of upper urinary tract disease or dysfunction necessitate continuous surveillance and frequent treatment, although creatinine clearance is greater than 75 L/24 h (52 mL/min)

or

successful renal transplantation results in marked renal function improvement | Diminution of upper urinary tract function as evidenced by creatinine clearance of 40-60 L/24 h (28-42 mL/min)

or

symptoms and signs of upper urinary tract disease or dysfunction are incompletely controlled by surgical or continuous medical treatment, although creatinine clearance is 60-75 L/24 h (42-52 mL/min) | Diminution of upper urinary tract function as evidenced by creatinine clearance below 40 L/24 h (28 mL/min)

or

symptoms and signs of upper urinary tract disease or dysfunction persist despite surgical or continuous medical treatment, although creatinine clearance is 40-60 L/24 h (28-42 mL/min)

or

renal function deterioration requires either peritoneal dialysis or hemodialysis |

| Class 1
0%-14% Impairment of the Whole Person |
|---|
| Diminution of upper urinary tract function, as evidenced by creatinine clearance of 75-90 L/24 h (52-62.5 mL/min)

or

intermittent symptoms and signs of upper urinary tract dysfunction that do not require continuous treatment or surveillance

or

only one kidney is functioning |

Example 7-1
0% to 14% Impairment Due to Upper Urinary Tract Disease

Subject: 22-year-old man.

History: Backache, fever, hematuria, headache, and hypertension during attack of hemolytic streptococcal tonsillitis at age 12. Urine: red blood cell, red blood cell casts; 2.4 g protein/24 h. Creatinine clearance: 72 L/24 h (50 mL/min). Creatinine clearance 6 months later: 130 L/24 h (90 mL/min).

Current Symptoms: None.

Physical Exam: Normal.

Clinical Studies: Urinalysis: normal. Creatinine clearance: 158 L/24 h (110 mL/min). Biopsy showed no renal disease.

Diagnosis: Complete recovery from poststreptococcal acute glomerulonephritis.

Impairment Rating: 0% impairment of the whole person.

Comment: Full recovery with no permanent impairment.

Example 7-2
0% to 14% Impairment Due to Upper Urinary Tract Disease

Subject: 40-year-old man.

History: Acute renal colic. Passage of small urinary calculus. Two previous episodes of renal colic. Spontaneous passage of urinary calculi.

Current Symptoms: Occasional flank pain; limited physical activity.

Physical Exam: Normal.

Clinical Studies: Normal excretory urograms with no evidence of metabolic disease. Urine, creatinine clearance, and phenolsulfonphthalein study results: within normal limits.

Diagnosis: Recurrent renal calculi.

Impairment Rating: 5% impairment of the whole person.

Comment: Occasional renal colic, affecting sexual function and activities of daily living.

Class 2
15%-34% Impairment of the Whole Person
Diminution of upper urinary tract function as evidenced by creatinine clearance of 60-75 L/24 h (42-52 mL/min) *or* symptoms and signs of upper urinary tract disease or dysfunction necessitate continuous surveillance and frequent treatment, although creatinine clearance is greater than 75 L/24 h (52 mL/min) *or* successful renal transplantation results in marked renal function improvement

Example 7-3
15% to 34% Impairment Due to Upper Urinary Tract Disease

Subject: 45-year-old man.

History: Childhood nephritis; emergency appendectomy; appendiceal abscess drainage. Adequate postoperative urine output. Serum creatinine: 248 μmol/L (2.8 mg/dL). Prolonged convalescence. Anemia subsided and stamina returned to normal.

Current Symptoms: Feels well 12 months after appendectomy and engages in most usual daily activities. Decreased exercise tolerance for competitive social activities (eg, basketball).

Physical Exam: Unremarkable.

Clinical Studies: Urine: trace protein (0.75 g/24 h). Excretory urograms show no architectural abnormality. Creatinine clearance: 60 to 70 L/24 h (42 to 49 mL/min).

Diagnosis: Persistent proteinuria after childhood nephritis, aggravated by surgery years later.

Impairment Rating: 15% impairment of the whole person.

Comment: Protein restriction.

Example 7-4
15% to 34% Impairment Due to Upper Urinary Tract Disease

Subject: 52-year-old man.

History: Retroperitoneal fibrosis; left lower ureter function severely damaged; ureter surgically reconstructed.

Current Symptoms: Upon discontinuing antibacterial medication, repeated pyelonephritis attacks that disrupt activity.

Physical Exam: Flank tenderness.

Clinical Studies: Excretory urography: vesicoureteral reflux despite apparently normal left kidney architecture and function. Creatinine clearance: 100 L/24 h (69 mL/min).

Diagnosis: Active unilateral chronic pyelonephritis secondary to vesicoureteral reflux.

Impairment Rating: 15% impairment of the whole person.

Comment: Pyelonephritis recurrence. No surgical intervention; left kidney appears normal, with no functional deterioration.

Example 7-5
15% to 34% Impairment Due to Upper Urinary Tract Disease

Subject: 50-year-old woman.

History: Successful operation for parathyroid adenoma. Periodic pyelonephritis attacks from residual calculi in both kidneys with sporadic passage of stones. Continuous medication controls urinary tract infection; antibiotics correct pyelonephritis attacks.

Current Symptoms: Infrequent high fever, chills, and back pain.

Physical Exam: Bilateral flank tenderness.

Clinical Studies: Creatinine clearance: stable 65 L/24 h (45 mL/min). Excretory urography: bilateral pyelocaliceal deformities; kidney size unchanged in 3 years.

Diagnosis: Renal calculi and bilateral chronic pyelonephritis.

Impairment Rating: 30% impairment due to upper urinary tract impairment. Combine urinary tract impairment with parathyroid impairment for impairment of the whole person (see the Combined Values Chart, p. 604).

Comment: Prevent complications with increased water and fluid intake and compliancy with daily medications.

Example 7-6
15% to 34% Impairment Due to Upper Urinary Tract Disease

Subject: 28-year-old man.

History: Hemodialysis for marked azotemia and oliguria from progressive chronic glomerulonephritis. Successful renal transplantation of mother's kidney; good renal function. Azathioprine and prednisone maintenance treatment; close observation for osteoporosis development.

Current Symptoms: Asymptomatic.

Physical Exam: Cushingoid features.

Clinical Studies: Creatinine clearance: 108 L/24 h (75 ml/min).

Diagnosis: Functioning renal transplant.

Impairment Rating: 25% impairment of the whole person due to renal disease and the need for continuous medication. Combine any permanent impairment percent related to a complication with the renal impairment estimate (see the Combined Values Chart, p. 604).

Comment: Reevaluate if secondary infection or other complication develops due to immunosuppressive therapy.

Class 3
35%-59% Impairment of the Whole Person
Diminution of upper urinary tract function as evidenced by creatinine clearance of 40-60 L/24 h (28-42 mL/min)
or
symptoms and signs of upper urinary tract disease or dysfunction are incompletely controlled by surgical or continuous medical treatment, although creatinine clearance is 60-75 L/24 h (42-52 mL/min)

Example 7-7
35% to 59% Impairment Due to Upper Urinary Tract Disease

Subject: 48-year-old man.

History: Calculi in minor calices of both kidneys. Multiple endoscopic and open surgical stone removals. Continuous antibacterial medication.

Current Symptoms: Periodic chills, fever, and back pain. Spends several days per month ill at home.

Physical Exam: Bilateral flank tenderness.

Clinical Studies: Notable diminution of a kidney; bilateral pyelographic architectural changes from previous surgeries and recurrent pyelonephritis. Creatinine clearance: 65 L/24 h (45 mL/min). Infected urine.

Diagnosis: Renal calculi with bilateral recurrent pyelonephritis.

Impairment Rating: 50% impairment of the whole person.

Comment: Monitor and treat recurrent infections.

Example 7-8
35% to 59% Impairment Due to Upper Urinary Tract Disease

Subject: 48-year-old man.

History: Hematuria from automobile crash injury. Blood pressure: 150/90 mm Hg. Hospital bed rest for 1 week, then discharged. All other findings within normal limits. Blood pressure later: 240/160 mm Hg. Malignant hypertensive retinopathy. Creatinine clearance: 58 L/24 h (40 mL/min).

Current Symptoms: Severe headaches 16 months later.

Physical Exam: Blood pressure: 170/110 mm Hg (after surgery); 155/95 mm Hg in 6 months. Eyegrounds: group 2 changes (Keith-Wagener-Barker classification). Left kidney removed.

Clinical Studies: Damaged left kidney on radiologic studies. Creatinine clearance: 40 L/24 h (28 mL/min). Definite left renovascular hypertension. Malignant hypertensive changes on right kidney biopsy. Ischemia and juxtaglomerular hypertrophy on left kidney histologic examination.

Diagnosis: Left nephrectomy for malignant hypertensive vascular disease.

Impairment Rating: 55% arteriolar nephrosclerosis impairment and 10% nephrectomy impairment. Combine for 60% urinary system impairment. Combine 60% impairment with appropriate cardiovascular impairment value to determine impairment of the whole person (see the Combined Values Chart, p. 604).

Comment: Monitor renal function; protein restriction check.

Example 7-9
35% to 59% Impairment Due to Upper Urinary Tract Disease

Subject: 52-year-old woman.

History: Needs help with some everyday activities. No clear-cut nephritis history.

Current Symptoms: Chronic fatigue.

Physical Exam: Pale; appears weak.

Clinical Studies: Moderate anemia. Elevated serum creatinine level. Diffuse bilateral glomerulonephritis on renal biopsy. Contracted kidneys and normal pyelocaliceal architecture evident on high-dose excretory urography. Urine culture: negative. Creatinine clearance: 50 L/24 h (35 mL/min).

Diagnosis: Chronic glomerulonephritis with renal atrophy.[2]

Impairment Rating: 59% impairment due to upper urinary tract impairment. Combine with appropriate rating for anemia to determine impairment of the whole person (see the Combined Values Chart, p. 604).

Comment: Monitor renal function.

Class 4
60%-95% Impairment of the Whole Person
Diminution of upper urinary tract function as evidenced by creatinine clearance below 40 L/24 h (28 mL/min)
or
symptoms and signs of upper urinary tract disease or dysfunction persist despite surgical or continuous medical treatment, although creatinine clearance is 40-60 L/24 h (28-42 mL/min)
or
renal function deterioration requires either peritoneal dialysis or hemodialysis

Example 7-10
60% to 95% Impairment Due to Upper Urinary Tract Disease

Subject: 44-year-old man.

History: Family history of polycystic renal disease. Gross hematuria; protein-restricted diet. Until current episode, worked regularly and felt well.

Current Symptoms: Relatively asymptomatic. Sudden flank pain.

Physical Exam: Normal.

Clinical Studies: Serum creatinine: 707 to 884 µmol/L (8 to 10 mg/dL) (increased in 2 years preceding acute episode). Creatinine clearance: 35 L/24 h (24 mL/min). Bilateral deformities characteristic of polycystic renal disease on endoscopy and retrograde urograms.

Diagnosis: Bilateral polycystic renal disease; advanced renal insufficiency.

Impairment Rating: 70% impairment of the whole person.

Example 7-11
60% to 95% Impairment Due to Upper Urinary Tract Disease

Subject: 25-year-old woman.

History: Severe abruptio placentae. Creatinine clearance: 35 L/24 h (24 mL/min). Bilateral deformities characteristic of polycystic renal disease on endoscopy and retrograde urograms. Periodic peritoneal dialysis. Anuria for 49 days, then oliguria, then increased urine output. Serum creatinine level fell without peritoneal dialysis after 60 days. Performed some activities of daily living despite severely compromised renal function 12 months after anuria.

Current Symptoms: Fatigued; requires daily nap.

Physical Exam: Unremarkable.

Clinical Studies: Percutaneous renal biopsy. Renal cortical necrosis. Creatinine clearance: 11.5 L/24 h (8 mL/min).

Diagnosis: Renal cortical necrosis and severe chronic renal failure.

Impairment Rating: 75% impairment of the whole person.

Example 7-12
60% to 95% Impairment Due to Upper Urinary Tract Disease

Subject: 56-year-old woman.

History: Chronic progressive glomerulonephritis. Severe anemia, azotemia, and oliguria. Twice-weekly hemodialysis. Felt well 1 or 2 days after treatment.

Current Symptoms: Nausea, lethargy, and edema before hemodialysis.

Physical Exam: Cachetic; bilateral peripheral edema.

Clinical Studies: Moderate anemia.

Diagnosis: Severe chronic renal failure and refractory anemia.

Impairment Rating: 80% to 90% impairment of the whole person.

Comment: Renal failure and chronic refractory anemia justify high impairment rating.

7.4 Urinary Diversion

7.4a Criteria for Rating Permanent Impairment Due to Urinary Diversion Disorders

The impairment criteria for evaluating urinary diversion disorders are given in Table 7-2.

Table 7-2 Criteria for Rating Permanent Impairment Due to Urinary Diversion Disorders

Diversion Type	% Impairment of the Whole Person
Ureterointestinal	10%
Cutaneous ureterostomy	10%
Nephrostomy	15%

Example 7-13
10% Impairment Due to Ureteroileostomy

Subject: 52-year-old woman.

History: Anterior pelvic exenteration and ureteroileostomy for cervical carcinoma. No recurrent cancer for 7 years. Calculi removed from both kidneys.

Current Symptoms: Periodic pyelonephritis, even with continual medication.

Physical Exam: Flank tenderness.

Clinical Studies: Pyelonephritis on radiologic studies. Creatinine clearance: 60 L/24 h (24 mL/min).

Diagnosis: Ureteroileostomy, urinary diversion, and chronic bilateral pyelonephritis.

Impairment Rating: 65% impairment due to bilateral pyelonephritis and 10% impairment due to ureteroileostomy; combine these with appropriate rating due to pelvic exenteration (ie, bladder, lower ureters, uterus, cervix, vagina, fallopian tubes, and ovaries excision) to determine impairment of the whole person (see the Combined Values Chart, p. 604).

Example 7-14
15% Impairment Due to Nephrostomy

Subject: 56-year-old man.

History: Bilateral nephrostomies. Obliterative, fibrotic, ureteral disease for 5 years. Renal calculi removed. Unsuccessful surgical attempt to reconstitute normal conduit function. Urinary infection unresponsive to treatment. Performed some activities of daily living without assistance.

Current Symptoms: Hematuria with change of nephrostomy tubes. Occasional fever and flank pain.

Physical Exam: Nephrostomy tubes in both flanks.

Clinical Studies: Creatinine clearance: 50 L/24 h (35 mL/min).

Diagnosis: Pyeloureteral disease requiring bilateral nephrostomy diversion.

Impairment Rating: 65% impairment due to pyeloureteral disease and 15% impairment due to bilateral nephrostomies; combine for 70% impairment of the whole person (see the Combined Values Chart, p. 604).

7.5 Bladder

7.5a Criteria for Rating Permanent Impairment Due to Bladder Disease

The impairment criteria for evaluating bladder disease are given in Table 7.3.

Table 7-3 Criteria for Rating Permanent Impairment Due to Bladder Disease

Class 1 0%-15% Impairment of the Whole Person	Class 2 16%-40% Impairment of the Whole Person	Class 3 41%-70% Impairment of the Whole Person
Symptoms and signs of bladder disorder *and* requires intermittent treatment *and* normal function between malfunctioning episodes	Symptoms and signs of bladder disorder, eg, urinary frequency (urinating more than every 2 hours); severe nocturia (urinating more than three times a night) *and* requires continuous treatment	Poor reflex activity (eg, intermittent urine dribbling, loss of control, urinary urgency) *and/or* no voluntary control on micturition; reflex or areflexic bladder on urodynamics

Class 1 0%-15% Impairment of the Whole Person
Symptoms and signs of bladder disorder *and* requires intermittent treatment *and* normal function between malfunctioning episodes

Example 7-15
0% to 15% Impairment Due to Bladder Disease

Subject: 41-year-old woman.

History: Radium treatment for uterine fibroids 20 years previously. Emergency hospitalization and blood vessel fulguration for recent urinary tract bleeding (1 to 2 weeks to 6 months) from postirradiation bladder telangiectasia.

Current Symptoms: Marked frequency of urination.

Physical Exam: Unremarkable.

Clinical Studies: Blood and urine studies between attacks: normal.

Diagnosis: Postirradiation telangiectasia of the bladder.

Impairment Rating: 10% impairment of the whole person.

Comment: Regular cystoscopic monitoring may be required.

Example 7-16
0% to 15% Impairment Due to Bladder Disease

Subject: 42-year-old man.

History: Chronic renal infection resistant to antibiotic therapy. Insignificant relief with anticholinergic medications. Good general physical condition. Refused surgical urinary diversion.

Current Symptoms: Severe cystitis. Emptied bladder less than every 30 minutes. Used urine-collecting device. Could not retain urine long enough to perform usual activities of daily living.

Physical Exam: Bladder tenderness to percussion.

Clinical Studies: Urine: numerous white blood cells; few red blood cells. Small bladder capacity on urodynamics.

Diagnosis: Chronic cystitis.

Impairment Rating: 10% impairment due to cystitis; combine with appropriate rating for upper urinary tract disorder to determine impairment of the whole person (see the Combined Values Chart, p. 604).

Comment: Frequent urine cultures.

Chapter 7

<table>
<tr><td>

Class 2
16%-40% Impairment of the Whole Person

Symptoms and signs of bladder disorder, eg, urinary frequency (urinating more than every 2 hours); severe nocturia (urinating more than three times a night)

and

requires continuous treatment

</td></tr>
</table>

Example 7-17
16% to 40% Impairment Due to Bladder Disease

Subject: 35-year-old woman.

History: Progressive and painful urinary frequency, urinating every 10 to 15 minutes day and night. Interstitial cystitis; ineffective treatment with bladder dilation with various agents. Cystectomy and ureteroileostomy. Resumed most normal activities.

Current Symptoms: Adjusting to changes in bowel movements.

Physical Exam: Ureteroileostomy functioning well.

Clinical Studies: Normal, uninfected upper urinary tract.

Diagnosis: Contracted, fixed bladder requiring urinary diversion.

Impairment Rating: 20% impairment of the whole person due to urinary diversion procedure after bladder removal.

Comment: Monitor.

<table>
<tr><td>

Class 3
41%-70% Impairment of the Whole Person

Poor reflex activity (eg, intermittent urine dribbling, loss of control, urinary urgency)

and/or

no voluntary control on micturition; reflex or areflexic bladder on urodynamics

</td></tr>
</table>

Example 7-18
41% to 70% Impairment Due to Bladder Disease

Subject: 60-year-old man.

History: Cerebrovascular accident. Regained motor function but had residual bladder dysfunction. Urinated every 45 minutes. Urinary incontinence requires protective padding.

Current Symptoms: Urinates six times a night. Anticholinergic medications improve daytime urination frequency to every 1 to 1½ hours, nocturia to four times nightly. Improved urge incontinence.

Physical Exam: Bladder tenderness.

Clinical Studies: Hyperreflexic, hypercontractile bladder on urodynamics. [3-6]

Diagnosis: Urge incontinence, frequency, and nocturia due to neurologic bladder dysfunction.

Impairment Rating: 45% impairment due to urinary incontinence and poor reflex activity.

Comment: Monitor for urinary infections.

Example 7-19
41% to 70% Impairment Due to Bladder Disease

Subject: 25-year-old man.

History: Tetraplegia following auto accident.

Current Symptoms: Lost full bowel and bladder control; paralysis of upper and lower extremities.

Physical Exam: Sphincterotomy. External condom and intermittent catheterization.

Clinical Studies: None.

Diagnosis: Tetraplegia, with bowel and bladder dysfunction.

Impairment Rating: 50% impairment due to total loss of urinary control; combine with appropriate ratings due to bowel and musculoskeletal impairments to determine whole person impairment (see Combined Values Chart, p. 604).

Comment: Monitor renal function and for urinary tract infection.

Example 7-20
41% to 70% Impairment Due to Bladder Disease

Subject: 35-year-old man.

History: Fell from building roof; lumbar spine compression fracture and lumbar spinal cord contusion. Initially paraplegic. Recovered use of lower extremities with surgical debridement and rehabilitation.

Current Symptoms: Perineum and perirectal numbness. Total urinary and bowel incontinence.

Physical Exam: Cauda equina neurologic deficit. External condom catheter.

Clinical Studies: MRI: vertebral compression fracture. Urodynamics: areflexic bladder.

Diagnosis: Neurogenic bladder impairment.[7,8]

Impairment Rating: 60% impairment due to total loss of urinary control; combine with musculoskeletal impairment rating to determine whole person impairment (see Combined Values Chart, p. 604).

7.6 Urethra

7.6a Criteria for Rating Permanent Impairment Due to Urethral Disease

The impairment criteria for evaluating urethral disease are given in Table 7-4.

Table 7-4 Criteria for Rating Permanent Impairment Due to Urethral Disease

Class 1 0%-10% Impairment of the Whole Person	Class 2 11%-20% Impairment of the Whole Person	Class 3 21%-40% Impairment of the Whole Person
Symptoms and signs of a urethral disorder **and** requires intermittent therapy for control	Symptoms and signs of a urethral disorder **and** cannot effectively be controlled by treatment	Urethral dysfunction resulting in intermittent urine dribbling and loss of voluntary urinary control

Class 1
0%-10% Impairment of the Whole Person
Symptoms and signs of a urethral disorder
and
requires intermittent therapy for control

Example 7-21
0% to 10% Impairment Due to Urethral Disease

Subject: 27-year-old man.

History: Urethral stricture; dilation every few weeks. No urinary tract infection.

Current Symptoms: Symptom-free between dilations; symptomatic only as urethra gradually constricted.

Physical Exam: Urethral narrowing.

Clinical Studies: Unremarkable.

Diagnosis: Traumatic urethral stricture.

Impairment Rating: 5% impairment of the whole person.

Comment: Monitor renal function. If urethra closes completely, may need surgical intervention.

Class 2
11%-20% Impairment of the Whole Person
Symptoms and signs of a urethral disorder
and
cannot effectively be controlled by treatment

Example 7-22
11% to 20% Impairment Due to Urethral Disease

Subject: 23-year-old man.

History: Considerable ventral surface penis laceration, which caused a surgically uncorrectable fistula. Performed most activities of daily living and could ejaculate during intercourse but was infertile.

Current Symptoms: Could not urinate normally.

Physical Exam: Fistulous opening on the ventral surface of the penis.

Clinical Studies: Urine cultures: positive for bacteria. Renal function: normal.

Diagnosis: Urethral fistula.

Impairment Rating: 15% impairment due to urethral fistula; combine with impairment for sexual dysfunction (see the Combined Values Chart, p. 604) to determine whole person impairment.

Comment: Monitor kidney function.

Example 7-23
11% to 20% Impairment Due to Urethral Disease

Subject: 31-year-old man.

History: Struck by vehicle. Pelvic fracture, symphysis fracture dislocation, prostatomembranous and bulbomembranous urethral lacerations. Stabilized and healed pelvic fracture. Repaired urethral lacerations. Uncorrectable extensive urethral strictures from postoperative fibrosis. Frequent urethral dilations to urinate 2 years later.

Current Symptoms: Chronic urinary tract infections with ascending pyelonephritis secondary to urethral obstruction and frequent urethral instrumentation.

Physical Exam: Scarred undersurface of urethra with fistulous tracts.

Clinical Studies: Creatinine clearance: 65 L/24 h (45 mL/min).

Diagnosis: Traumatic urethral stricture with chronic pyelonephritis.

Impairment Rating: 20% impairment due to urethral stricture and 25% impairment due to upper urinary tract damage combine for 40% impairment of the whole person (see the Combined Values Chart, p. 604).

Comment: Monitor kidney function. If hydronephrosis, may need urinary diversion.

Class 3
21%-40% Impairment of the Whole Person
Urethral dysfunction resulting in intermittent urine dribbling and loss of voluntary urinary control

Example 7-24
21% to 40% Impairment Due to Urethral Disease

Subject: 35-year-old woman.

History: After delivery of third child, urinary incontinence with coughing, sneezing, lifting, brisk walking, or running. No urinary tract infections.

Current Symptoms: Urinary incontinence.

Physical Exam: Urethra and bladder neck hypermobility; moderate uterine prolapse.

Clinical Studies: No neurologic abnormalities on urodynamics.

Diagnosis: Female stress urinary incontinence due to pelvic relaxation.[9]

Impairment Rating: 25% due to stress urinary incontinence; combine with 10% impairment for uterine prolapse (see Section 7.8c) for 33% impairment of the whole person.

Comment: Urinary incontinence requires protective padding. Stress urinary incontinence due to pelvic relaxation is partly treatable by surgery and may then change the impairment rating.

Example 7-25
21% to 40% Impairment Due to Urethral Disease

Subject: 56-year-old man.

History: Radical prostatectomy; localized prostate carcinoma. Discharged postoperative day 4. Urethral catheter removed 2 weeks postoperatively. Excellent Kegel exercise compliance. Urinary incontinence requires protective padding. Normal sexual function before procedure.

Current Symptoms: Intermittent urine loss with coughing, sneezing, or heavy lifting 6 months postoperatively. No erections 6 months after surgery.

Physical Exam: No anastomotic stricture or obstruction on cystoscopic examination.

Clinical Studies: No neurologic bladder abnormality and poor urinary sphincter tone on urodynamics.

Diagnosis: Stress urinary incontinence after radical prostatectomy.[10]

Impairment Rating: 25% impairment due to stress urinary incontinence; combine with 20% impairment for sexual dysfunction.

Comment: Urinary incontinence requires protective padding. Incontinence may be treatable with the placement of an artificial sphincter around the bulbous urethra, which may change the impairment rating.

Example 7-26
21% to 40% Impairment Due to Urethral Disease

Subject: 21-year-old man.

History: Factory worker crushed between forklift and wall. Fractured bony pelvis; totally severed urethra at prostate apex; severely lacerated perineum. Unsuccessful immediate reconstructive urethral surgery; ureterosigmoidostomy 1 year later. Right kidney hydronephrosis. Diversion converted to ileal conduit.

Current Symptoms: Sporadic renal infections. Impotent. Periodically unable to perform usual daily activities due to occasional urinary tract infections.

Physical Exam: Healed pelvic fracture. No musculoskeletal impairment.

Clinical Studies: Creatinine clearance: 70 L/24 h (49 mL/min).

Diagnosis: Severed urethra; hydronephrosis with recurrent urinary tract infection; impotence.

Impairment Rating: 21% impairment due to severed urethra; combine with 30% impairment due to upper urinary tract impairment, 10% impairment due to ureteroileostomy, and impairment due to sexual dysfunction (see the Combined Values Chart, p. 604) to determine whole person impairment.

Comment: Monitor serum electrolytes and for renal function deterioration.

7.7 Male Reproductive Organs

The male reproductive organs include the penis, scrotum, testicles, epididymides, spermatic cords, prostate, and seminal vesicles. See the following sections for impairment percentages for male reproductive organs for 40- to 65-year-old men. Increase the percentages by 50% for men younger than 40, and decrease the percentages by 50% for men older than 65. For instance, class 3 impairment in a 35-year-old man would be rated at 30% (20% + 0.5[20%]). New treatments, when successful, may decrease the degree of impairment.

7.7a Penis

The penis has the sexual functions of erection and ejaculation. The penis's urinary function is discussed in the first part of this chapter on the urethra (Section 7.6). Penile functional impairment symptoms and signs include erection and sensation abnormalities and partial or complete loss of the penis.

When evaluating penis impairment, consider both sexual and urinary function impairment. Determine sexual function impairment according to the following classifications. To determine impairment of the whole person, combine this estimate with the appropriate percentage for estimated urinary function impairment. This classification also may be used to estimate penile implant use impairment (see the Combined Values Chart, p. 604).

Objective techniques useful in evaluating penis function include (but are not limited to) penile tumescence studies, Doppler ultrasound penile blood flow evaluations, dynamic cavernosometry and cavernosography, and angiography.[10-14]

7.7b Criteria for Rating Permanent Impairment Due to Penile Disease

The impairment criteria for evaluating penile disease are given in Table 7-5.

Table 7-5 Criteria for Rating Permanent Impairment Due to Penile Disease

Class 1 0%-10% Impairment of the Whole Person	Class 2 11%-19% Impairment of the Whole Person	Class 3 20% Impairment of the Whole Person
Sexual function possible but with varying degrees of difficulty of erection, ejaculation, or sensation	Sexual function possible with sufficient erection but with impaired ejaculation and sensation	No sexual function possible

---

Class 1
0%-10% Impairment of the Whole Person

Sexual function possible but with varying degrees of difficulty of erection, ejaculation, or sensation

---

Example 7-27
0% to 10% Impairment Due to Penile Disease

Subject: 32-year-old man.

History: Compressive penile shaft injury.

Current Symptoms: Normal sensation and ejaculation; pain when positions varied.

Physical Exam: Healing with partial cicatrization of left mid-corpus cavernosum. Bowstring left curvature occurred during erections.

Clinical Studies: None.

Diagnosis: Posttraumatic fibrosis of left mid-corpus cavernosum.

Impairment Rating: $5\% + 0.5(5\%) = 8\%$ impairment of the whole person (age of subject considered).

Comment: May need surgical correction.

Class 2
11%-19% Impairment of the Whole Person

Sexual function possible with sufficient erection but with impaired ejaculation and sensation

---

Example 7-28
11% to 19% Impairment Due to Penile Disease

Subject: 28-year-old man.

History: Fractured pelvis; wide symphysis pubis separation; perivesical and periprostatic hematomas; prostatomembranous urethral tear. Injuries corrected with reconstructive surgery; no subsequent urinary difficulty.

Current Symptoms: Erection and intercourse possible; no penile sensation and ejaculation.

Physical Exam: Scarred undersurface of the urethra.

Clinical Studies: Urinary flow: normal.

Diagnosis: Posttraumatic ejaculatory dysfunction and penile anesthesia.[13]

Impairment Rating: $10\% + 0.5(10\%) = 15\%$ impairment of the whole person (age of subject is considered).

Comment: Periodically check urine flow rate and monitor kidney function. Possibility of a urethra stricture. Recurrence likely.

Class 3
21% -35% Impairment of the Whole Person

No sexual function possible

Example 7-29
20% Impairment Due to Penile Disease

Subject: 18-year-old man.

History: Traumatic penile dislocation.

Current Symptoms: Erection not possible.

Physical Exam: Preserved genital appearance; urethral function with corporeal repair and urethroplasty.

Clinical Studies: Doppler flow studies: showed markedly diminished penile arterial blood flow.

Diagnosis: Posttraumatic vascular and neurologic penile insufficiency.

Impairment Rating: $20\% + 0.5(20\%) = 30\%$ of the whole person (age of subject is considered).

Comment: Monitor urinary flow rates to forestall urethral stricture.

7.7c Scrotum

The scrotum covers, protects, and provides a suitable environment for the testicles. Scrotum function impairment symptoms and signs include pain, enlargement, testicular immobility, inappropriate testicle location, and masses. Objective techniques useful in evaluating scrotum function include, but are not limited to, observation, palpation, testicular examination, and scrotal ultrasound.

7.7d Criteria for Rating Permanent Impairment Due to Scrotal Disease

The impairment criteria for evaluating scrotal disease are given in Table 7-6.

Table 7-6 Criteria for Rating Permanent Impairment Due to Scrotal Disease

Class 1 0%-10% Impairment of the Whole Person	Class 2 11%-20% Impairment of the Whole Person	Class 3 21%-35% Impairment of the Whole Person
Partial scrotal loss or symptoms and signs of disease; no evidence of testicular malfunction; possible testicular malpositioning	Architectural alteration or disease symptoms and signs such that testicles must be implanted somewhere other than a scrotal position to preserve testicular function, and pain or discomfort with activity *or* total scrotum loss	Signs and symptoms of scrotal disease uncontrolled by treatment, limiting physical activities

Class 1 0%-10% Impairment of the Whole Person
Partial scrotal loss or symptoms and signs of disease; no evidence of testicular malfunction; possible testicular malpositioning

Example 7-30
0% to 10% Impairment Due to Scrotal Disease

Subject: 38-year-old man.

History: Injury resulting in loss of all scrotal skin. Good cosmetic result with split-thickness skin graft reconstruction.

Current Symptoms: Discomfort during exercise and certain positions.

Physical Exam: Testicular mobility affected.

Clinical Studies: No testicular malfunction.

Diagnosis: Scrotal skin ablation; split-thickness skin graft scrotal reconstruction.

Impairment Rating: 5% impairment of the whole person (age of subject is considered).

Class 2 11%-20% Impairment of the Whole Person
Architectural alteration or disease symptoms and signs such that testicles must be implanted somewhere other than a scrotal position to preserve testicular function, and pain or discomfort with activity *or* total scrotum loss

Example 7-31
11% to 20% Impairment Due to Scrotal Disease

Subject: 50-year-old man.

History: Extensive burns on lower extremities, genitals, and abdomen. Satisfactory skin grafting on abdomen and lower extremities; testicles transplanted to subcutaneous pouches in the thighs to permit adequate scrotal area skin coverage.

Current Symptoms: Self-conscious about grafted regions.

Physical Exam: Testicles palpable in the thighs.

Clinical Studies: Semen analysis: pending.

Diagnosis: Burn ablation of the scrotum.

Impairment Rating: 15% impairment of the whole person, combine with any fertility impairment.

Comment: Rule out infertility with sperm analysis.

> **Class 3**
> **21%-35% Impairment of the Whole Person**
>
> Signs and symptoms of scrotal disease uncontrolled by treatment, limiting physical activities

Example 7-32
21% to 35% Impairment Due to Scrotal Disease

Subject: 55-year-old man.

History: High-dose external beam pelvic radiation therapy for prostate carcinoma. Apparently cured of cancer 5 years later.

Current Symptoms: Large genitals and weeping skin, which severely limit physical activities.

Physical Exam: Penis and scrotum lymphedema.

Clinical Studies: Prostate-specific antigen (PSA): 0

Diagnosis: Postirradiation lymphedema of penile and scrotal skin.

Impairment Rating: 30% impairment of the whole person due to persisting symptoms, lack of effective therapy, and limitation of physical activity.

Comment: No effective treatment.

7.7e Testicles, Epididymides, and Spermatic Cords

The testicles produce spermatozoa and synthesize male steroid hormones. The epididymides and spermatic cords transport the spermatozoa.

Testicular, epididymal, and spermatic cord impairment signs and symptoms include local or referred pain; tenderness and change in size, contour, position, and texture; and testicular hormones and seminal fluid abnormalities.

Objective techniques useful in evaluating testicular, epididymal, and spermatic cord function include (but are not limited to) vasography; ultrasound; lymphangiography; spermatic arteriography and venography; biopsy; semen analysis; and follicle-stimulating, ketosteroid, and hydroxysteroid hormone studies.

7.7f Criteria for Rating Permanent Impairment Due to Testicular, Epididymal, and Spermatic Cord Disease

The impairment criteria for evaluating testicular, epididymal, and spermatic cord disease are given in Table 7-7.

Table 7-7 Criteria for Rating Permanent Impairment Due to Testicular, Epididymal, and Spermatic Cord Disease

Class 1 0%-10% Impairment of the Whole Person	Class 2 11%-15% Impairment of the Whole Person	Class 3 16%-20% Impairment of the Whole Person
Testicular, epididymal, or spermatic cord disease symptoms and signs and anatomic alteration *and* no continuous treatment required *and* no seminal or hormonal function abnormalities *or* solitary testicle	Testicular, epididymal, or spermatic cord disease symptoms and signs and anatomic alteration *and* requires frequent or continuous treatment or treatment is not possible *and* detectable seminal or hormonal abnormalities	Trauma or disease produces bilateral anatomic loss of the primary sex organs *or* no detectable seminal or hormonal function

> **Class 1**
> **0%-10% Impairment of the Whole Person**
>
> Testicular, epididymal, or spermatic cord disease symptoms and signs and anatomic alteration
>
> *and*
>
> no continuous treatment required
>
> *and*
>
> no seminal or hormonal function abnormalities
>
> *or*
>
> solitary testicle

Example 7-33
0% to 10% Impairment Due to Testicular, Epididymal, and Spermatic Cord Disease

Subject: 36-year-old man.

History: Repeated epididymal orchitis from recurrent epididymitis. Turned down vas deferens ligations. Might want to have children.

Current Symptoms: Pain and swelling of testicles.

Physical Exam: Normal prostate; tender testicles.

Clinical Studies: Normal seminal fluid.

Diagnosis: Chronic epididymitis secondary to chronic prostatitis.

Impairment Rating: 5% impairment due to epididymitis and 5% impairment due to prostatitis (age of subject is considered) combine for a 10% whole person impairment (see the Combined Values Chart, p. 604).

Comment: Prostatic massage and urine cultures to effectively treat urinary tract infection.

> **Class 2**
> **11%-15% Impairment of the Whole Person**
>
> Testicular, epididymal, or spermatic cord disease symptoms and signs and anatomic alteration
>
> *and*
>
> requires frequent or continuous treatment or treatment is not possible
>
> *and*
>
> detectable seminal or hormonal abnormalities

Example 7-34
11% to 15% Impairment Due to Testicular, Epididymidal, and Spermatic Cord Disease

Subject: 30-year-old man.

History: Bilateral orchitis caused by mumps 2 years ago; bilateral testicular atrophy. Fathered two children.

Current Symptoms: Currently infertile.

Physical Exam: No abnormality.

Clinical Studies: Notable oligospermia on semen analysis.

Diagnosis: Oligospermia.

Impairment Rating: 15% impairment of the whole person.

> **Class 3**
> **16%-20% Impairment of the Whole Person**
>
> Trauma or disease produces bilateral anatomic loss of the primary sex organs
>
> *or*
>
> no detectable seminal or hormonal function

Example 7-35
16% to 20% Impairment Due to Testicular, Epididymal, and Spermatic Cord Disease

Subject: 18-year-old man.

History: Injury caused by farm machinery; amputation of scrotum and its contents. Examined 2 years later when in stable condition.

Current Symptoms: Normal erections; not sexually active.

Physical Exam: Scarred perineal area.

Clinical Studies: None.

Diagnosis: Traumatic orchiectomy.

Impairment Rating: 20% impairment due to testicle loss; combine with impairments due to scrotal loss and endocrine gland loss for whole person impairment (see the Combined Values Chart, p. 604).

7.7g Prostate and Seminal Vesicles

The prostate and seminal vesicles provide the appropriate nutrition, environment, and transport for spermatozoa and semen. Impairments associated with urinary functions of the parts of the urethra involved with the prostate and seminal vesicles are discussed in the first part of this chapter on the urethra (Section 7.6).

Symptoms and signs of impairment in the prostate and seminal vesicles include local or referred pain; tenderness; size and textural changes; testicular, epididymal, and spermatic cord function disturbances; oligospermia; hemospermia; and urinary tract abnormalities.

Objective techniques useful in evaluating prostate and seminal vesicle function include (but are not limited to) urography, endoscopy, prostatic ultrasonography, vasography, biopsy, prostate secretion examination, and hormone excretion pattern analysis.

7.7h Criteria for Rating Permanent Impairment Due to Prostate and Seminal Vesicle Disease

The impairment criteria for evaluating prostate and seminal vesicle disease are given in Table 7-8.

Table 7-8 Criteria for Rating Permanent Impairment Due to Prostate and Seminal Vesicle Disease

Class 1 0%-10% Impairment of the Whole Person	Class 2 11%-15% Impairment of the Whole Person	Class 3 16%-20% Impairment of the Whole Person
Prostate and seminal vesicle dysfunction signs and symptoms *and* anatomic alteration *and* does not require continuous treatment	Frequent and severe prostate and seminal vesicle dysfunction or disease symptoms and signs *and* anatomic alteration *and* requires continuous treatment	Prostate and seminal vesicle ablation; occurs almost exclusively with extirpative surgery for prostate cancer; combine impairment estimates for prostate and seminal vesicle loss with impairment for sexual dysfunction or urinary incontinence if present (see the Combined Values Chart, p. 604)

Class 1 0%-10% Impairment of the Whole Person
Prostate and seminal vesicle dysfunction signs and symptoms *and* anatomic alteration *and* does not require continuous treatment

Example 7-36
0% to 10% Impairment Due to Prostate and Seminal Vesicle Disease

Subject: 42-year-old man.

History: Acute prostatitis episodes for 10 years.

Current Symptoms: Some mild perineal discomfort requiring pain medication. Fever.

Physical Exam: Tender prostate.

Clinical Studies: Prostatic massage and bacterial cultures.

Diagnosis: Chronic prostatitis with acute febrile episodes.

Impairment Rating: 5% impairment of the whole person (10% − 0.5[10%]).

Comment: May need periodic urine cultures with sensitivity testing to control urinary tract infections.

Class 2
11%-15% Impairment of the Whole Person

Frequent and severe prostate and seminal vesicle dysfunction or disease symptoms and signs

and

anatomic alteration

and

requires continuous treatment

Example 7-37
11% to 15% Impairment Due to Prostate and Seminal Vesicle Disease

Subject: 34-year-old man.

History: Drainage of prostate abscess 15 months ago; continuous prostatitis symptoms and signs tolerated only with constant antibacterial medications.

Current Symptoms: Perineal pain; low-grade fever.

Physical Exam: Tender and enlarged prostate.

Clinical Studies: Hemospermia.

Diagnosis: Recurrent acute and chronic prostatitis.

Impairment Rating: 15% (10% + 0.5[10%]) impairment of the whole person (age of subject is considered).

Comment: If obstructive symptoms, may need cystoscopic examination and possible TURP.

Class 3
16%-20% Impairment of the Whole Person

Prostate and seminal vesicle ablation; occurs almost exclusively with extirpative surgery for prostate cancer; combine impairment estimates for prostate and seminal vesicle loss with impairment for sexual dysfunction or urinary incontinence if present (see the Combined Values Chart, p. 604)

Example 7-38
16% to 20% Impairment Due to Prostate and Seminal Vesicle Disease

Subject: 50-year-old man.

History: Radical prostactectomy for cancer of the prostate.

Current Symptoms: No difficulty in urinating. Occasional nocturnal incontinence. Some impairment of sexual function.

Physical Exam: No anastomotic stricture in the urethra.

Clinical Studies: PSA = 0

Diagnosis: No residual disease after radical prostatectomy.

Impairment Rating: 16% impairment due to prostate and seminal vesicle ablation; combine with impairment for loss of sexual function (see the Combined Values Chart, p. 604).

Comment: Monitor PSA for recurrence of cancer.

7.8 Female Reproductive Organs

The female reproductive organs include the vulva, vagina, cervix, uterus, fallopian tubes, and ovaries. Female reproductive system impairment is influenced by age, especially if the woman is of childbearing age. Consider the physiologic differences between premenopausal and postmenopausal women when evaluating and estimating female reproductive organ impairment.[15]

7.8a Vulva and Vagina

The vulva has cutaneous, sexual, and urinary functions. Urinary function is discussed in the first part of this chapter on the urethra (Section 7.6). The vagina has a sexual function and also serves as a birth passageway. The clitoris is an erectile organ that has an important role in sexual functioning.

Vulval and vaginal function impairment symptoms and signs include sensation alteration or loss; lubrication loss; partial or complete absence; vulvovaginitis; vulvitis; vaginitis; cicatrization; ulceration; stenosis; atrophy or hypertrophy; neoplasia or dysplasia; difficulties with sexual intercourse, urination, or vaginal delivery; and underlying perineal structure support defect.

7.8b Criteria for Rating Permanent Impairment Due to Vulval and Vaginal Disease

The impairment criteria for evaluating vulval and vaginal disease are given in Table 7-9.

Table 7-9 Criteria for Rating Permanent Impairment Due to Vulval and Vaginal Disease

Class 1 0%-15% Impairment of the Whole Person	Class 2 16%-25% Impairment of the Whole Person	Class 3 26%-35% Impairment of the Whole Person
Vulval or vaginal disease or deformity symptoms and signs do not require continuous treatment *and* sexual intercourse possible *and* vagina adequate for childbirth if premenopausal	Vulval or vaginal disease or deformity symptoms and signs require continuous treatment *and* sexual intercourse possible only with some degree of difficulty *and* limited potential for vaginal delivery if premenopausal	Vulval or vaginal disease or deformity symptoms and signs uncontrolled by treatment *and* sexual intercourse not possible *and* vaginal delivery not possible if premenopausal

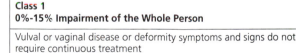

Class 1 0%-15% Impairment of the Whole Person
Vulval or vaginal disease or deformity symptoms and signs do not require continuous treatment *and* sexual intercourse possible *and* vagina adequate for childbirth if premenopausal

Example 7-39
0% to 15% Impairment Due to Vulval and Vaginal Disease

Subject: 38-year-old woman.

History: Obese; vaginal birth to three living children. Recurrent chronic genitocrural dermatitis. Treated for intense pruritus and active dermatitis. Discomfort more marked during warm and humid weather. Symptom remission with control of weight, avoidance of tight clothing, and careful observance of hygienic measures. Satisfying sexual intercourse possible when no excessive vulval irritation.

Current Symptoms: Dermatitis improved. Asymptomatic.

Physical Exam: Slight erythema.

Clinical Studies: Fungal infection culture results: negative. Glucose: normal.

Diagnosis: Dermatitis of the vulva; intertrigo.

Impairment Rating: 5% impairment of the whole person.

Class 2
16%-25% Impairment of the Whole Person
Vulval or vaginal disease or deformity symptoms and signs require continuous treatment
and
sexual intercourse possible only with some degree of difficulty
and
limited potential for vaginal delivery if premenopausal

Class 3
26%-35% Impairment of the Whole Person
Vulval or vaginal disease or deformity symptoms and signs uncontrolled by treatment
and
sexual intercourse not possible
and
vaginal delivery not possible if premenopausal

Example 7-40
16% to 25% Impairment Due to Vulval and Vaginal Disease

Subject: 34-year-old woman.

History: Surgical correction of rectovaginal fistula after vaginal delivery of second child. Severe vaginal stenosis. Intermittent vaginal dilatation under anesthesia; continuous use of vaginal cream. Third pregnancy ended with cesarean section because vaginal delivery deemed hazardous.

Current Symptoms: Sexual intercourse possible, but painful with no sexual sensation or enjoyment.

Physical Exam: Small and shallow vagina; erythematous.

Clinical Studies: None.

Diagnosis: Severe postoperative vaginal stenosis..

Impairment Rating: 25% impairment of the whole person (age of subject is considered).

Example 7-41
25% to 35% Impairment Due to Vulval and Vaginal Disease

Subject: 30-year-old woman.

History: Two children. Invasive squamous cell cervical carcinoma. Radiation treatment. Vesicovaginal fistula, rectovaginal fistula, and severe vaginal stenosis. Pregnancy unlikely.

Current Symptoms: Sexual intercourse impossible.

Physical Exam: Vaginal depth 2 cm; sinus tract 5 mm diameter led to cervix. Mucus, feces, and urine discharged through sinus.

Clinical Studies: None.

Diagnosis: Vesicovaginal fistula, rectovaginal fistula, and severe vaginal stenosis.

Impairment Rating: 25% + 10% for age consideration = 35% impairment of the whole person. Combine with appropriate estimates for bladder and rectal impairments to determine impairment for whole person (see the Combined Values Chart, p. 604).

Comment: May need urinary diversion.

7.8c Cervix and Uterus

The cervix serves as a passageway for spermatozoa and menstrual blood, maintains closure of the uterus during pregnancy, and serves as a portion of the birth canal during vaginal delivery. Hormones, elaborated by the ovaries or administered exogenously, influence the uterus. The uterus serves as the organ of menstruation, a means of spermatozoa transportation, and the container of fertilization products. The uterus supplies the power for the first and third stages of labor and, in part, for the second stage.

Cervical and uterine functional impairment symptoms and signs include abnormalities of menstruation, fertility, pregnancy, or labor; excessive cervical canal size, stenosis, or atresia; cervical incompetence during pregnancy; noncyclic hemorrhage; uterine displacement; dysplasia; and neoplasia.

Objective techniques useful in evaluating cervical and uterine function include (but are not limited to) cervical mucous studies; vaginal, cervical, and intrauterine cytologic smears; biopsy; ultrasound; radiologic studies using radiopaque contrast media; blood and urine hormone studies; basal body temperature recordings; sperm concentration, mobility, and viability studies; uterus dilation and curettage; endometrium microscopic study; gynecography; laparoscopy; computed tomography; magnetic resonance imaging; hysteroscopy; ultrasound placental localization techniques; and saline solution sonohysterography.

7.8d Criteria for Rating Permanent Impairment Due to Cervical and Uterine Disease

The impairment criteria for evaluating cervical and uterine disease are given in Table 7-10.

Table 7-10 Criteria for Rating Permanent Impairment Due to Cervical and Uterine Disease

Class 1 0%-15% Impairment of the Whole Person	Class 2 16%-25% Impairment of the Whole Person	Class 3 26%-35% Impairment of the Whole Person
Cervical or uterine disease or deformity symptoms and signs do not require continuous treatment	Cervical or uterine disease or deformity symptoms and signs require continuous treatment	Cervical or uterine disease or deformity symptoms and signs are not controlled by treatment
or	*or*	*or*
cervical stenosis, if present, requires no treatment	cervical stenosis, if present, requires periodic treatment	complete cervical stenosis
or		*or*
anatomic cervical or uterine loss in the postmenopausal period		anatomic or complete functional cervical or uterine loss in the premenopausal period

Class 1 0%-15% Impairment of the Whole Person
Cervical or uterine disease or deformity symptoms and signs do not require continuous treatment
or
cervical stenosis, if present, requires no treatment
or
anatomic cervical or uterine loss in the postmenopausal period

Example 7-42
0% to 15% Impairment Due to Cervical and Uterine Disease

Subject: 22-year-old woman.

History: Menarche at 14 years. Menstrual periods lasted 3 days, normal volume; no noncyclic bleeding. Pregnant after $1\frac{1}{2}$ years of marriage; no contraceptives. No leiomyoma growth during pregnancy; no pain associated with tumor. Healthy 5 lb 12 oz infant delivered at 38 weeks. Menstrual periods after delivery averaged 32 days between cycles; normal volume and duration.

Current Symptoms: None.

Physical Exam: Slight uterine asymmetry on pelvic examination; interior smooth; nontender mass 4 cm in diameter projected from uterus.

Clinical Studies: Leiomyoma confirmed on ultrasound.

Diagnosis: Asymptomatic subserous uterine leiomyoma.

Impairment Rating: 0% impairment of the whole person.

Example 7-43
0% to 15% Impairment Due to Cervical and Uterine Disease

Subject: 60-year-old woman.

History: Adenomyosis; vaginal hysterectomy 20 years previously; vaginal vault prolapse.

Current Symptoms: Pelvic pressure; large bulge protruding from vulva.

Physical Exam: Vaginal vault prolapse; no significant rectocele, cystocele, or uterine-vaginal angle descent.

Clinical Studies: Discharge: no infection.

Diagnosis: Posthysterectomy vaginal vault prolapse.

Impairment Rating: 15% uterine loss impairment; combine with impairment for vaginal prolapse to determine whole person impairment (see Combined Values Chart, p. 604).

Comment: Preferred nonoperative approach. Doughnut pessary reduced vaginal prolapse; pessary changed twice weekly. Povidone-iodine douche diminished vaginal discharge. Symptoms resolved.

Class 2 16%-25% Impairment of the Whole Person
Cervical or uterine disease or deformity symptoms and signs require continuous treatment
or
cervical stenosis, if present, requires periodic treatment

Example 7-44
16% to 25% Impairment Due to Cervical and Uterine Disease

Subject: 30-year-old woman.

History: Cervical conization. Para 2. Partial cervical stenosis; menstrual blood retention. Cervical dilation necessary at 2- to 4-month intervals due to hematometria and dysmenorrhea. Pregnant 2 years after conization. Infant delivered by cesarean section before labor onset at 38 weeks; abruptio placentae.

Current Symptoms: Requires cervical dilation at 2-month intervals.

Physical Exam: Narrowed cervix.

Clinical Studies: None.

Diagnosis: Incomplete cervical stenosis.

Impairment Rating: 16% impairment of the whole person.

Class 3 26%-35% Impairment of the Whole Person
Cervical or uterine disease or deformity symptoms and signs are not controlled by treatment
or
complete cervical stenosis
or
anatomic or complete functional cervical or uterine loss in the premenopausal period

Example 7-45
26% to 35% Impairment Due to Cervical and Uterine Disease

Subject: 34-year-old woman.

History: Severe uterine prolapse due to vaginal delivery of large infant after long, difficult labor. Surgical anterior and posterior vaginal wall repair, extensive cervical amputation, and posterior uterine fixation by broad ligament plication.

Current Symptoms: Three carefully managed, subsequent pregnancies each ended in spontaneous abortion between 12 and 16 weeks' gestation due to premature cervical dilation.

Physical Exam: Large, prolapsed uterus.

Clinical Studies: Pap smear: pending.

Diagnosis: Partial cervical absence and incompetence; uterine prolapse.

Impairment Rating: 30% impairment due to cervical incompetence.

Comment: Incompetent cervix repair impossible due to partial cervical absence.

Chapter 7

Example 7-46
26% to 35% Impairment Due to Cervical and Uterine Disease

Subject: 28-year-old woman.

History: Gravida 0. Stage IB invasive cervical squamous cell carcinoma. Lymph nodes did not show metastatic disease. Radical hysterectomy with pelvic lymphadenectomy; ovaries conserved.

Current Symptoms: Asymptomatic.

Physical Exam: Normal vagina.

Clinical Studies: None.

Diagnosis: No uterus in a reproductive-age woman secondary to treatment of invasive cervical squamous cell carcinoma.

Impairment Rating: 30% impairment of the whole person.

7.8e Fallopian Tubes and Ovaries

The fallopian tubes transport ova and spermatozoa. The ovaries develop and release ova and secrete sex and reproductive hormones.

Symptoms and signs of fallopian tube and ovarian dysfunction include vaginal bleeding or discharge; fallopian tube stenosis or obstruction; abnormal morphologic characteristics; pelvic masses; neoplasms; absent, infrequent, or abnormal ovulation; abnormal hormone secretion; and menstrual dysfunction.

Objective techniques useful in evaluating fallopian tube and ovarian function include (but are not limited to) cervical and vaginal cytologic smears; pelvic roentgenography; hysterosalpingography; gynecography; ovarian biopsy; blood and urine hormonal assays; ultrasound; computed tomography; magnetic resonance imaging; laparoscopy; and basal body temperature studies.

7.8f Criteria for Rating Permanent Impairment Due to Fallopian Tube and Ovarian Disease

Evaluate any associated endocrine impairment in accordance with the criteria set forth in the *Guides* Chapter 10, The Endocrine System.

The impairment criteria for evaluating fallopian tube and ovarian disease are given in Table 7-11.

Table 7-11 Criteria for Rating Permanent Impairment Due to Fallopian Tube and Ovarian Disease

Class 1 0%-15% Impairment of the Whole Person	Class 2 16%-25% Impairment of the Whole Person	Class 3 26%-35% Impairment of the Whole Person
Fallopian tube or ovarian disease or deformity symptoms and signs do not require continuous treatment *or* only one functioning fallopian tube or ovary in the premenopausal period *or* bilateral fallopian tube or ovarian functional loss in the postmenopausal period	Fallopian tube or ovarian disease or deformity symptoms and signs require continuous treatment, but tubal patency persists and ovulation is possible	Fallopian tube or ovarian disease or deformity symptoms and signs *and* total tubal patency loss or failure to produce ova in the premenopausal period *or* bilateral fallopian tube or ovarian loss in the premenopausal period

Class 1
0%-15% Impairment of the Whole Person
Fallopian tube or ovarian disease or deformity symptoms and signs do not require continuous treatment
or
only one functioning fallopian tube or ovary in the premenopausal period
or
bilateral fallopian tube or ovarian functional loss in the postmenopausal period

Class 2
16%-25% Impairment of the Whole Person
Fallopian tube or ovarian disease or deformity symptoms and signs require continuous treatment, but tubal patency persists and ovulation is possible

Example 7-47
0% to 15% Impairment Due to Fallopian Tube and Ovarian Disease

Subject: 28-year-old woman.

History: No pregnancy after 6 years of marriage. Average frequency of sexual intercourse; no contraceptives. Menstruated every 40 to 60 days since menarche at age 12. Administered clomiphene citrate to induce ovulation; conceived in second cycle. Delivered healthy, full-term infant.

Current Symptoms: Asymptomatic.

Physical Exam: Normal.

Clinical Studies: Bilateral tubal patency on hysterosalpingogram. Normal sperm count on husband's semen analysis.

Diagnosis: Irregular ovulation secondary to hypothalamic-pituitary dysfunction.

Impairment Rating: 5% impairment of the whole person.

Example 7-48
16% to 25% Impairment Due to Fallopian Tube and Ovarian Disease

Subject: 27-year-old woman.

History: Two children. Increasing pain secondary to severe pelvic endometriosis. Laparotomy for bilateral ovarian endometriomas resection, peritoneal implant resection and fulguration; presacral neurectomy. Normal pregnancy resulting in birth of healthy infant. Breast-fed for 14 months. Continuous medical therapy for chronic, recurring pain suppression.

Current Symptoms: Pelvic pain secondary to recurrent endometriosis.

Physical Exam: Tender uterus and adnexae.

Clinical Studies: Cultures: no infection.

Diagnosis: Recurrent pelvic endometriosis.

Impairment Rating: 20% impairment of the whole person.

<table>
<tr><td>

Class 3
26%-35% Impairment of the Whole Person

Fallopian tube or ovarian disease or deformity symptoms and signs

and

total tubal patency loss or failure to produce ova in the premenopausal period

or

bilateral fallopian tube or ovarian loss in the premenopausal period

</td></tr>
</table>

Example 7-49
26% to 35% Impairment Due to Fallopian Tube and Ovarian Disease

Subject: 32-year-old woman.

History: Two children.

Current Symptoms: Severe pelvic infection.

Physical Exam: Uterus: normal size; enlarged tubes bilaterally.

Clinical Studies: Total proximal and distal fallopian tube occlusion; bilateral 6-cm hydrosalpinx. Bilateral salpingectomy.

Diagnosis: Bilateral salpingectomy.

Impairment Rating: 30% impairment of the whole person.

Example 7-50
26% to 35% Impairment Due to Fallopian Tube and Ovarian Disease

Subject: 27-year-old woman.

History: Childhood Wilms tumor; radical nephrectomy; chemotherapy and abdominal radiation.

Current Symptoms: Erratic menstruation. Never pregnant. No pregnancy after 5 years of unprotected intercourse.

Physical Exam: Nephrectomy scar.

Clinical Studies: Normal sperm count on husband's semen analysis. Bilateral tubal patency on hysterosalpingogram. Primary ovarian failure on hormonal studies.

Diagnosis: Infertility due to primary ovarian failure.

Impairment Rating: 30% impairment due to loss of ovarian function (age of subject is considered); combine with appropriate impairment rating for upper urinary tract disorder for impairment of the whole person (see Combined Values Chart, p. 604)

7.9 Urinary and Reproductive Systems Impairment Evaluation Summary

Table 7-12 gives an evaluation summary for the assessment of urinary and reproduction systems impairment.

Table 7-12 Urinary and Reproductive Systems Impairment Evaluation Summary

Disorder	History, Including Selected Relevant Symptoms	Examination Record	Assessment of Function
General Urinary	Urology symptoms (eg, change in frequency of micturition, dysuria, chills, fever, hematuria, infection, loin or abdominal or costovertebral pain, loss of appetite, weight loss, impaired stamina, edema, dry, dusky skin)	Comprehensive physical examination; abdominal palpation for tenderness; scrotal exam; testes and epididymis exam; rectal exam; prostate exam; vaginal and rectal exam; urine: gross for sugar and albumin; microscopic; culture and cell cytology; ultrasound kidney; cystogrde exam with retrograde exam if needed	Blood BUN; creatinine; electrolytes; 24-hr creatinine clearance; fasting blood sugar; renal isotope studies for kidney function; intravenous pyelogram (urogram) for tumors or stone disease or spiral CT; voiding and retrograde cystourethrogram to rule out a stricture; urodynamics; bladder pressure studies for neurogenic bladder dysfunction
Male Reproductive	Sexual history of erections, ejaculation, discharge, scrotal pain, tenderness, reproduction, dysuria, hematuria, nocturia	Genital and rectal examination; prostatic exam	Evaluation of penile blood flow; urinalysis; semen analysis; ultrasound; vasography, hormone levels
Female Reproductive	Abnormalities of menstruation, pain, discharge, change in sensation, altered lubrication	Pelvic examination	Cervical and vaginal smears; ultrasound; hormonal assays; hysterosalpingography; laparoscopy; CT; MRI

References

1. Cassidy MJ, Beck RM. Renal functional reserve in live related kidney donors. *Am J Kidney Dis.* 1988;11:468-472.

   The single kidney responds appropriately to a meat-protein load. There is no evidence from this study to suggest that hyperfiltration damaged the remaining kidney.

2. Schena FP, Cameron JS. Treatment of proteinuric idiopathic glomerulonephritides in adults: a retrospective survey. *Am J Med.* 1988;85:315-326.

   A review of the worldwide medical literature was undertaken to determine whether treatment with currently available drugs has been beneficial in patients with glomerulonephritides.

3. Nitti VW, Adler H, Combs AJ. The role of urodyamics in the evaluation of voiding dysfunction in men after cerebrovascular accident. *J Urol.* 1996;155:263-266.

   The etiology of voiding dysfunction was determined in men who were at risk for obstructive uropathy after a cerebrovascular accident to evaluate whether the cause of voiding dysfunction could be predicted by the type (obstructive or irritative) or by the onset of symptoms.

4. Perkash I. Detrusor-sphincter dyssynergia and detrusor hyperreflexia leading to hydronephrosis during intermittent catheterization. *J Urol.* 1978;120:620-622.

   Two cases of spinal cord injury with detrusor-sphincter dyssynergia and detrusor hyperreflexia are presented. The importance of early diagnosis and appropriate management of detrusor-sphincter dyssynergia associated with detrusor hyperreflexia is discussed.

5. Burney TL, Senapati M, Desai S, Choudhary ST, Badlani GH. Acute cerebrovascular accident and lower urinary tract dysfunction: a prospective correlation of the site of the brain injury with urodynamic findings. *J Urol.* 1996;156:1748-1750.

   Evaluates the effects of an acute cerebrovascular accident on the lower urinary tract and correlates the site of cerebrovascular accident with findings on urodynamic study.

6. Khan Z, Hertanu J, Yang WC, Melman A, Leiter E. Predictive correlation of urodynamic dysfunction and brain injury after cerebrovascular accident. *J Urol.* 1981;126:86-88.

7. Yokoyama O, Hasegawa T, Ishiura Y, Ohkawa M, Sugiyama Y, Izumida S. Morphological and functional factors predicting bladder deterioration after spinal cord injury. J Urol. 1996;155:271-274.

End-Organ Damage	Diagnosis(es)	Degree of Impairment
Renal failure leading to uremia; congestive heart failure; hepatorenal failure; damage due to metastatic disease—spine, prostate, lungs	Cystitis; bladder tumor; testicular tumor; traumatic loss of testes; urethral damage and stricture; enlarged prostate	Criteria outlined in this chapter; Tables 7-1, 7-2, 7-3, and 7-4
	Absent kidney; polycystic kidney disease; malpositioned kidneys; renal stone disease; renal tumors; neurogenic bladder	
	Erection disorders; fertility disorders	
Penile or prostatic; if cancer, distant metastatic sites	Impotence; ejaculatory dysfunction; infertility; prostatitis; benign prostatic hypertrophy; cancer of reproductive organs (penile, testicular, prostatic)	Tables 7-5, 7-6, 7-7, and 7-8
Pelvic area; abdomen	Vaginitis; infection; ulceration; atrophy or hypertrophy; dysplasia; infertility; endometriosis; cancer; strictures; stenosis	Tables 7-9, 7-10, and 7-11

Investigation of factors predictive of morphological and functional deterioration of the bladder in patients with spinal cord injury.

8. Perkash I. Detrusor-sphincter dyssynergia and dyssynergic responses: recognition and rationale for early modified transurethral sphincterotomy in complete spinal cord injury lesions. *J Urol*. 1978;120:469-474.

Some characteristics are described for detrusor-sphincter dyssynergia and the dyssynergic response in spinal injury patients with complete lesions. The urodynamic evaluation and clinical problems are analyzed in 53 patients to identify the importance of early recognition of sphincter dyssynergia.

9. McGuire EJ, Fitzpatrick CC, Wan J, et al. Clinical assessment of urethral sphincter function. *J Urol*. 1993;150(5 Pt 1):1452-1454.

Measurements of urethral pressures, such as maximum urethral pressure, are widely believed to have relevance in the management of urinary incontinence despite evidence to the contrary. In this study, maximum urethral pressure and the abdominal pressure required to cause stress incontinence were measured in 125 women with stress incontinence. In women, the abdominal pressure required to cause stress incontinence was unrelated to maximum urethral pressure.

10. Walsh PC, ed. *Campbell's Urology*. 7th ed. Philadelphia, Pa: WB Saunders Co; 1998.

11. Shabsigh R, Fishman IJ, Quesada ET, Seale-Hawkins CK, Dunn JK. Evaluation of vasculogenic erectile impotence using duplex ultrasonography. *J Urol*. 1989;142:1469-1474.

A total of 140 patients underwent penile vascular evaluation with intracavernous papaverine injection combined with duplex ultrasonography. Of these patients, eight were potent men who were evaluated for reasons other than erectile failure. These potent men were used as controls to obtain normal values. The remaining 132 patients had erectile impotence of various etiologies.

12. American Association of Clinical Endocrinologists. AACE Clinical practice guidelines for the evaluation and treatment of male sexual dysfunction. *Endocr Pract*. 1998;4:4.

13. Kaplan H. Psychosexual dysfunctions. In Cooper, Frances, Sacks, eds. *The Personality Disorders and Neurosis*. Philadelphia, Pa: JB Lippincott Co; 1986:467-479.

14. NIH Consensus Conference. Impotence. NIH consensus development panel on impotence. *JAMA*. 1993;270:83-90.

15. Danforth DN, ed. *Textbook of Obstetrics and Gynecology*. 5th ed. Philadelphia, Pa: JB Lippincott Co; 1986.

Chapter 8

The Skin

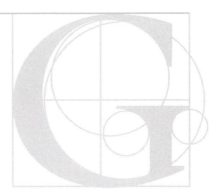

Introduction

This chapter provides criteria for evaluating permanent impairment of the skin and its appendages and estimating the extent to which skin impairments affect the ability to perform activities of daily living (see Table 1-2). Permanent impairment of the skin is any dermatologic abnormality or loss that persists after medical treatment and rehabilitation and that is unlikely to change significantly in the next year, with or without medical **treatment.**

Table 8-1 summarizes skin components, functions, and disorders. Skin functions include: (1) providing a protective covering; (2) participating in sensory perception, temperature regulation, fluid regulation, electrolyte balance, immunobiologic defenses, and trauma resistance; and (3) regenerating the epidermis and its appendages.

Table 8-1 Structure, Functions, and Disorders of the Skin*

Structure or Component	Functions	Disorders
Epidermis		
Stratum corneum	Barrier against microorganisms, chemicals, and water loss	Infection; contact dermatitis; xerosis
Squamous and basal cells	Stratum corneum regeneration; wound repair	Squamous or basal cell carcinoma; ulceration
Melanocytes	Protection from ultraviolet radiation	Vitiligo; sunburn; hyperpigmentation; melanoma
Langerhans cells	Immune surveillance	Allergic contact dermatitis
Dermis		
Blood vessels and mast cells	Nutrition; thermoregulation; vasodilation	Ulceration; heat stroke; urticaria (contact, systemic); hand-arm vibration syndrome
Lymphatics	Immune surveillance; lymphatic circulation	Lymphedema
Nerve tissue	Sensory perception	Neuropathies; pain; itching; sensory changes
Connective tissue	Protection from trauma; wound repair	Hypertrophic and atrophic scars; scleroderma
Eccrine (sweat) glands	Thermoregulation	Heat intolerance
Sebaceous glands	Synthesis of skin surface lipids	Acne; chloracne; xerosis
Hair	Insulation; outward appearance	Folliculitis; alopecia
Nails	Manipulation of small objects	Paronychia; dystrophy; onycholysis; difficulty with grasping

*Modified from Mathias,⁵ Table 10-7, p. 138.

Protective skin functions include barrier defenses against chemical irritant and allergic sensitizer damage, microorganism invasion, and ultraviolet light injuries. Temperature regulation involves proper sweat gland and small blood vessel functioning. The barrier defense against fluid loss is related to the intactness of the stratum corneum.

Revisions from the fourth edition include: (1) new sections on contact dermatitis and natural rubber latex allergy; (2) a new section on cancer; and (3) updated clinical information and references.

8.1 Principles of Assessment

Before using the information in this chapter, the *Guides* user should become familiar with Chapters 1 and 2 and the Glossary. Chapters 1 and 2 discuss the *Guides'* purpose, applications, and methods for performing and reporting impairment evaluations. The Glossary provides definitions of common terms used by many specialties in impairment evaluation.

Skin disorders may develop from exposure to physical, mechanical, biological, and chemical agents. Identification and avoidance of these agents may prevent ongoing skin disorder aggravation. Physicians need to determine the clinical course and permanence

of skin disorders associated with possible intermittent exposures.

Clinical evaluation requires sound clinical judgment based on a detailed medical history, thorough physical examination, and judicious use of diagnostic procedures. Ancillary diagnostic and laboratory procedures include patch, open, prick, intracutaneous, and serologic allergy tests; Wood's light examinations, cultures, and scrapings for bacteria, fungi, and viruses; and biopsies.

To determine the appropriate impairment class (Table 8-2) for an affected individual, evaluate the severity of the skin condition and the impact of the skin condition on the ability to perform activities of daily living (see Table 1-2). Determine the appropriate percentage within any impairment class by considering the frequency, intensity, and complexity of the medical condition and the treatment regimen. In general, the more frequent and intense the symptoms, signs, and medical treatment, the higher the estimated impairment rating within any impairment class. Table 8-2 lists the impairment classes and percents of whole person impairment for *all* dermatologic disorders. A brief overview of those disorders follows.

Impairments of other body systems, such as behavioral problems, restriction of motion or ankylosis of joints, and respiratory, cardiovascular, endocrine, or gastrointestinal tract disorders, may be associated with skin impairments. When there is a permanent impairment of more than one body system, evaluate the extent of whole person impairment related to each system and combine the estimated impairment percentages (see the Combined Values Chart, p. 604) to determine total impairment.

8.1a Interpretation of Symptoms and Signs

In some cases, limitations in the ability to perform daily activities are based on symptoms. This information may be subjective and possibly misinterpreted, and it should not serve as the sole criterion for impairment rating decisions. Rather, obtain objective data about the extent of the limitation and integrate findings with subjective data to estimate the permanent impairment rating.

8.1a.1 Pruritus

Pruritus is a common symptom of dermatologic conditions. Pruritus is a subjective, unpleasant sensation and symptom that provokes the desire to scratch and rub the skin. The itching sensation may be intolerable. Pruritus is closely related to pain and is mediated by pain receptors and fibers when they are weakly stimulated. Like pain, pruritus may be defined as a unique complex of afferent stimuli that interacts with the individual's emotional or affective state of mind.

The pruritus sensation has two elements that are extremely variable in makeup and time. Peripheral neural stimulation varies from the absence of sensation to awareness that stimuli are producing a usual or unusual sensation. Central nervous system reaction is modified by state of attentiveness, experience, motivation at the moment, and such stimuli as exercise, sweat, and temperature change.

When evaluating pruritus associated with skin disorders, consider (1) how the pruritus interferes with performance of the activities of daily living, and (2) to what extent the pruritus description is supported by such objective skin signs as lichenification, excoriation, or hyperpigmentation. Subjective itching complaints that cannot be substantiated objectively may require referral or consultation.

8.1b Description of Procedures

Common clinical investigations for dermatologic conditions include skin testing, biopsy, and relevant laboratory studies.

8.1b.1 Patch Testing, Performance, Interpretation, and Relevance

The sine qua non for the diagnosis of allergic contact dermatitis is a properly performed and interpreted patch test. The information from patch testing complements an appropriate, detailed history. Patch testing may significantly contribute to the diagnosis and management of contact dermatitis.

Be aware that patch testing may yield false-positive and false-negative results. Selecting the proper concentration of the suspected allergen, vehicle, site of application, and type of patch is critical for procedure validity. Making such selections and determining test result relevance require considerable skill and experience.

Interpret a positive or negative **patch test** result in conjunction with the clinical history and a detailed knowledge of testing procedures. Although appropriate test concentrations and vehicles have been established for many sensitizers, there are no established vehicle and concentration standards for the vast number of chemicals in use.

Patch test results require careful interpretation to discern allergic from irritant responses, as well as to appropriately interpret whether the result is relevant to the individual's dermatitis and exposures. Patch tests are only used to detect contact allergy and are only one component in a complete evaluation. Further details about patch testing, its values, and its limitations are discussed in standard texts, some of which are listed at the end of this chapter.

8.2 Disfigurement

Skin **disfigurement** is an altered or abnormal appearance that may be an alteration of color, shape, or structure, or a combination of these. Disfigurement may be a residual of injury or disease, or it may accompany a recurrent or ongoing disorder. Examples of disfigurement include giant pigmented nevi, nevus flammeus, cavernous hemangioma, and pigmentation alteration.

Disfigurement usually has no effect on body function and may have little or no effect on the ability to perform activities of daily living, except if the disfigurement causes social rejection or an unfavorable self-image with self-imposed isolation, lifestyle alteration, or other behavioral changes. If impairment in the ability to perform activities of daily living due to disfigurement does exist, it is usually manifested by a behavior change, such as withdrawal from social contacts. Behavioral changes are evaluated in accordance with the criteria in the *Guides* Chapter 14, Mental and Behavioral Disorders.

Evaluate impairments related to disfigurement or altered pigmentation in accordance with the criteria given in Table 8-2 and described later in this chapter. Enhance disfigurement descriptions with good color photographs that show multiple defect views. Estimate the probable duration and permanency of the disfigurement. Describe in writing the possibility of improving the condition through medical or surgical therapy and the extent to which it can be concealed cosmetically, as with hairpieces, wigs, or cosmetics. Depict with photographs if possible.

Evaluate the effect on the performance of the activities of daily living if a scar involves the loss of sweat gland function, hair growth, nail growth, or pigment formation. Evaluate burns and scars according to the criteria in this chapter; give special consideration to the injury's impact on the individual's ability to perform activities of daily living. When impairment resulting from a burn or scar is based on peripheral nerve dysfunction or loss of range of motion, evaluate the skin impairment separately and combine the impairment rating with that from Chapters 13, The Central and Peripheral Nervous System; 16, The Upper Extremities; or 17, The Lower Extremities. If chest wall excursion is limited or if there are behavioral changes secondary to disfigurement, consult Chapter 5, The Respiratory System, or Chapter 14, Mental and Behavioral Disorders.

8.3 Scars and Skin Grafts

Scars, cutaneous abnormalities that result from the healing of burned, traumatized, or diseased tissue, represent a special type of disfigurement. Give the scars' dimensions in centimeters, and describe their shape, color, anatomic location, and any evidence of ulceration, depression, or elevation. Indicate whether the scar is "atrophic" or "hypertrophic"; soft and pliable or hard and indurated, thin or thick, and smooth or rough; and attachment, if any, to underlying bones, joints, muscles, or other tissue. Good color photographs with multiple views of the defect enhance the scars' description.

Consider the tendency of a scar to disfigure when evaluating whether there is permanent impairment due to scarring. Also consider whether the scar can be changed, made less visible, or concealed. Function may be restored without improving appearance, and appearance may be improved without altering function.

Skin grafts may be used to replace skin losses resulting from trauma or disease. Grafts commonly lack hair, lubrication, pliability, and sensation, and they may demonstrate altered pigmentation. These changes affect the function and appearance of the graft site. The altered lubrication, pliability, and sensation may result in diminished protection against microorganisms and diminished resistance to mechanical, chemical, and thermal trauma. The altered appearance may be significant if the area involves exposed parts, such as the dorsum of the hand, the face, or the neck.

8.4 Contact Dermatitis

Contact **dermatitis** is an inflammatory skin reaction induced by exposure to an external agent and is the most frequent cause of occupational skin disease. Contact dermatitis most often involves the hands, wrists, and forearms, although any area may be affected. Two types of contact dermatitis are generally recognized: irritant (80% of cases), which results from direct tissue damage, and allergic (20% of cases), in which tissue damage is mediated through type IV delayed cellular hypersensitivity. Irritant and allergic contact dermatitis may coexist in the same person and are often difficult to differentiate on physical examination and histologically.

Irritants may be strong (absolute) or weak (marginal). Cumulative exposure to marginal irritants causes most cases of contact dermatitis and may impair the barrier function of the skin, allowing the penetration of potential allergens. Many cutaneous allergens, such as chromates, nickel salts, epoxy resins, and preservatives, are also primary irritants. Allergy can be induced or maintained by chemicals in concentrations insufficient to irritate nonallergic skin. Allergen cross-sensitivity is an important phenomenon in which an individual who is allergic to one chemical (eg, urushiol in poison ivy or poison oak) also will react to structurally related chemicals (eg, in Japanese lacquer, mango, and cashew nutshell oil).

Accurate diagnosis is the key to proper management of contact dermatitis. If the specific agent(s) can be identified (see section on patch testing) and successfully avoided, full recovery usually is anticipated; but if contact continues, the dermatitis may become chronic and disabling, and it may prevent the individual from performing some activities of daily living.

8.5 Natural Rubber Latex Allergy

Latex allergy generally refers to an IgE-mediated immediate hypersensitivity reaction to one or more protein allergens present in natural rubber latex (NRL) devices, especially gloves. Individuals with spina bifida and health care workers are at particular risk; NRL allergy has become a significant medical and occupational health problem. Clinical manifestations range from contact urticaria and angioedema to allergic rhinitis and conjunctivitis, asthma, and anaphylaxis. Contact dermatitis to rubber accelerators and antioxidants added during manufacture has been associated with NRL allergy. A number of NRL-allergic individuals are atopic, with asthma, other environmental type I allergies, and hand eczema. Symptoms and signs of contact urticaria to NRL may be masked by preexisting hand eczema. Also evaluate individuals with NRL allergy for manifestions in other organ systems (eg, respiratory symptoms and asthma). See Chapter 5, The Respiratory System, for an example of NRL-induced asthma.

Allergen avoidance is the current treatment for NRL allergy. When aerosolized, glove powder (an NRL-allergen carrier) can produce respiratory symptoms in susceptible individuals. Affected workers may have to avoid contact with NRL gloves and other NRL-containing products, avoid areas where they might inhale the powder from NRL gloves worn by other workers, and wear a medical alert bracelet.

8.6 Skin Cancer

Skin cancer is the most prevalent of all cancers. Three main types exist: basal cell carcinoma, squamous cell carcinoma, and malignant melanoma.

Basal cell carcinoma (BCC) is the most common form of skin cancer. Predisposing factors include light skin color, inability to tan, sun exposure, blond or red hair, freckling in childhood, therapeutic radiation, and arsenic exposure. Several different clinical and histologic types exist; there is also a much less common, inherited condition called the basal cell nevus or Gorlin syndrome. BCC is usually locally invasive, with a small metastatic potential. The main goal of therapy is complete eradication of the tumor with the highest cure rate and the least amount of disfigurement.

Squamous cell carcinoma (SCC) makes up about one fifth of nonmelanoma skin cancers. SCC is more common in individuals with light skin coloration and can arise from excess sun exposure, leading to precancerous actinic keratoses. Environmental risk factors include arsenic, polycyclic aromatic hydrocarbon, chronic infrared heat, and therapeutic radiation exposure. SCC may also occur in chronic scars from burns, trauma, and inflammatory processes. Several clinical and histologic types exist, but SCC is more likely to metastasize, especially from sites involving the lip, dorsal hand, and temple, as well as in larger, deeper, and more anaplastic lesions. Therapeutic options are the same as for basal cell carcinoma. Sun avoidance and close follow-up are essential in patients with SCC.

Cutaneous malignant melanoma is an increasingly common and lethal malignancy of melanocytes and nevus cells in certain precursor lesions. The increased frequency of melanoma is well documented; rates of incidence are rising more rapidly for this than for any other cancer. The salient challenge for clinicians is to detect and excise melanoma in its earliest stage, as tumor thickness remains the most important prognostic indicator of this malignancy. Early diagnosis and surgical excision of in situ, or early invasive, melanomas are curative in most individuals. Despite advances in chemotherapy and immunotherapy, the efficacy of treatment of advanced melanoma remains limited, and the prognosis of metastatic disease remains guarded.

8.7 Criteria for Rating Permanent Impairment Due to Skin Disorders

The impairment criteria for all dermatologic disorders are given in Table 8-2.

Table 8-2 Criteria for Rating Permanent Impairment Due to Skin Disorders*

Class 1 0%- 9% Impairment of the Whole Person	Class 2 10%-24% Impairment of the Whole Person	Class 3 25%-54% Impairment of the Whole Person	Class 4 55%-84% Impairment of the Whole Person	Class 5 85%-95% Impairment of the Whole Person
Skin disorder signs and symptoms present or intermittently present **and** no or few limitations in performance of activities of daily living; exposure to certain chemical or physical agents may temporarily increase limitation **and** requires no or intermittent treatment	Skin disorder signs and symptoms present or intermittently present **and** limited performance of some activities of daily living **and** may require intermittent to constant treatment	Skin disorder signs and symptoms present or intermittently present **and** limited performance of many activities of daily living **and** may require intermittent to constant treatment	Skin disorder signs and symptoms constantly present **and** limited performance of many activities of daily living, including intermittent confinement at home or other domicile **and** may require intermittent to constant treatment	Skin disorder signs and symptoms constantly present **and** limited performance of most activities of daily living, including occasional to constant confinement at home or other domicile **and** may require intermittent to constant treatment

*The signs and symptoms of disorders in classes 1, 2, and 3 may be intermittent and not present at the time of examination. Consider the impact of the skin disorder on the ability to perform activities of daily living (see Table 1-2) in determining the class of impairment. Consider the frequency and intensity of signs and symptoms (ie, severity) and the frequency and complexity of medical treatment when selecting an appropriate impairment percentage and estimate within any class (see Introduction).

Class 1 0%-9% Impairment of the Whole Person
Skin disorder signs and symptoms present or intermittently present **and** no or few limitations in performance of activities of daily living; exposure to certain chemical or physical agents may temporarily increase limitation **and** requires no or intermittent treatment

Example 8-1
0% to 9% Impairment Due to Allergic Contact Dermatitis

Subject: 27-year-old man.

History: Prepared batches of latex paint for small paint manufacturing company. Related skin disease onset and exacerbation. Despite some accommodations, individual unable to avoid latex paint completely; dermatitis continued. No dermatitis for 1 year after job change.

Current Symptoms: None.

Physical Exam: Hands and arms: no signs of dermatitis.

Clinical Studies: Patch test: strong allergic reaction to 0.1% petrolatum mixture of a nonmercurial preservative, 2-n-4-isothiazolin-3-one, used in company's latex paints. Subsequent evaluation: normal.

Diagnosis: Resolved allergic contact dermatitis caused by preservative.

Impairment Rating: 0% impairment of the whole person.

Comment: While used widely in paint manufacturing, the preservative is not used in other industries where the worker might come into contact with it. No limitation in the performance of daily activities. Latex paint does not contain natural rubber latex (NRL) allergens and does not cause NRL allergy.

Example 8-2
0% to 9% Impairment Due to Thermal Burn Scarring

Subject: 38-year-old woman.

History: Second-degree flame burn to forearm; spontaneously healed.

Current Symptoms: None.

Physical Exam: 7 x 12-cm depigmented area of the arm. Healed skin: normal pliability, lubrication, and sensation.

Clinical Studies: None.

Diagnosis: Scarring caused by thermal burn.

Impairment Rating: 0% impairment of the whole person.

Comment: No interference with activities of daily living.

Example 8-3
0% to 9% Impairment Due to Allergic Contact Dermatitis and Occupational Leukoderma

Subject: 52-year-old man.

History: Janitor; 13 years' transient hand dermatitis from wet work with detergents, including germicidal disinfectant with paratertiary butyl phenol (TBP). Developed depigmentation on sides of most fingers, dorsa of the hands, and distal forearms 10 years ago. Recent depigmentation of upper torso and thighs. Ultraviolet light therapy with oral methoxsalen (PUVA therapy) over 1 year failed to stimulate repigmentation. Cosmetic covering unsatisfactory. Required outdoor maintenance work resulted in frequent sunburn of skin that lacked pigmentation; needs frequent and regular use of protective sunscreen.

Current Symptoms: None; not bothered by skin changes.

Physical Exam: Depigmentation. Early actinic changes with skin wrinkling, bruising, and scaling.

Clinical Studies: Patch test: 2+ reaction to TBP 1% in petrolatum; no other common industrial allergens. Positive patch site depigmented 1 month later.

Diagnosis: Allergic contact dermatitis and occupational leukoderma caused by phenolic chemical, TBP.

Impairment Rating: 5% impairment of the whole person.

Comment: Impairment estimate includes modification of only a few activities of daily living by limiting exposure to sunlight. No effect on self-image or social relationships.

Example 8-4
0% to 9% Impairment Due to Chronic Urticaria

Subject: 35-year-old woman.

History: 10 years' chronic urticaria (hives); no angioedema or ER visits due to related symptoms.

Current Symptoms: Hand lesions; swelling occasionally interferes with driving or grasping objects. Lesions; severe itching rarely interferes with sleep, sexual relations, concentration, and activities of daily living. Asyptomatic with regular nonsedating antihistimine use.

Physical Exam: Without treatment, daily urticarial lesions on 10% to 20% of body surface area (BSA): hands, face, or trunk.

Clinical Studies: Blood smear (200 white blood cells counted): 12% eosinophils.

Diagnosis: Chronic urticaria.

Impairment Rating: 5% impairment of the whole person.

Comment: No limitation in daily activities with current treatment. If sedating antihistamine treatment, ability to perform certain activities—driving or participating in group activities—possibly limited; estimated impairment rating might increase. If change necessary, reevaluate impairment rating. If urticaria uncontrollable, possible 20% impairment estimate.

Example 8-5
0% to 9% Impairment Due to Allergic Contact Dermatitis

Subject: 32-year-old man.

History: Construction worker; blistering dermatitis of hands and feet after work with wet concrete. Severe dermatitis twice treated with oral prednisone. Condition improved away from concrete contact but did not clear completely.

Current Symptoms: Daily chronic dermatitis with occasional exacerbations. Requires intermittent treatment. Performs most but avoids some activities of daily living; avoids contact with water; normal sleep. Handling dry rock or concrete usually aggravates dermatitis.

Physical Exam: Initial severe dermatitis; without exposure, mild dermatitis of fingers, palms, and feet.

Clinical Studies: Patch test: allergic contact dermatitis to chromate, principal allergen in cement and leather shoes.

Diagnosis: Allergic contact dermatitis to chromate from occupational cement exposure.

Impairment Rating: 9% impairment of the whole person.

Comment: Limitation of few activities of daily living, but daily chronic dermatitis requires intermittent treatment.

Class 2
10%-24% Impairment of the Whole Person
Skin disorder signs and symptoms present or intermittently present
and
limited performance of some activities of daily living
and
may require intermittent to constant treatment

Example 8-6
10% to 24% Impairment Due to Chronic Dermatitis

Subject: 28-year-old woman.

History: Eczematous eruption beneath wedding ring on fourth finger of left hand shortly after birth of first child 6 years earlier. Gradually spread to areas on several fingers of both hands despite treatment and avoidance of jewelry use. Eruption persisted for several months, then subsided slowly. Severe hand dermatitis flare-up after birth

of second child 2 years later. No eczema, hay fever, or asthma; no family history of atopy.

Current Symptoms: Good general health. Chronic, low-grade dermatitis despite special precautions. Intermittent treatment required to control dermatitis. Chronic hand dermatitis causes intermittent discomfort and limits some activities of daily living (eg, dishwashing, childcare, and grasping).

Physical Exam: Scarring and lichenification; otherwise normal.

Clinical Studies: Patch test: various food, household, cosmetic, and diagnostic and therapeutic materials nonreactive. Basic labs: normal.

Diagnosis: Chronic dermatitis of the hands due to undetermined factors.

Impairment Rating: 10% impairment of the whole person.

Comment: Chronic dermatitis and impairment of some daily activities indicate class 2. Intermittent nature of symptoms and treatment needed warrant 10% impairment rating.

Example 8-7
10% to 24% Impairment Due to Thermal Burn Hypertrophic Scarring

Subject: 43-year-old man.

History: Healed second-degree burn of anterior part of neck; hypertrophic scar formation involves approximately 1% of body surface area.

Current Symptoms: Scar susceptible to ultraviolet light; wears sun blockers when outdoors. Scar easily irritated and lacks durability; unable to wear clothes that rub neck. Intermittent itching and burning episodes confined to scarred areas stops all activities for 5 to 10 minutes.

Physical Exam: Scar raised, red, hard, and contrasts markedly with adjacent normal skin. Limited neck flexion, extension.

Clinical Studies: None.

Diagnosis: Hypertrophic scar secondary to thermal burn; limitation of neck motion.

Impairment Rating: 10% impairment of the whole person.

Comment: Itching and burning temporarily interrupt some activities of daily living; no treatment is required. Combine skin impairment with the estimated impairment rating for loss of neck motion (see Combined Values Chart, p. 604) to determine total impairment.

Example 8-8
10% to 24% Impairment Due to Latex Allergy and Eczema

Subject: 38-year-old woman.

History: Dental assistant; 18 years' progressively severe chronic hand dermatitis, angioedema of the face, rhinitis, and asthma; flared with powdered natural rubber latex (NRL) gloves. Treatment of topical and systemic corticosteroids. Eczema; jewelry allergy. Some lotions, creams, frequent antibacterial soap hand washing aggravate dermatitis. Nonpowdered NRL gloves cause itching within minutes, hives on wrists and forearms. Visited urgent care center for disseminated urticaria, angioedema, and wheezing.

Current Symptoms: Temporary improvement with hypoallergenic, powder-free NRL gloves. With no NRL exposure, mild hand dermatitis persists; intermittent fingertip fissuring. Occasional difficulty grasping and holding instruments; occasionally uses topical corticosteroids and hand creams. Asthma improved but persists despite use of non-NRL gloves by all office employees.

Physical Exam: Red, swollen, crusted, fissured palms, fingers, and wrists.

Clinical Studies: Patch test: positive reactions to thiuram mix (rubber chemical accelerators in NRL gloves), glutaraldehyde (active ingredient in cold sterilizing solution), and quaternuim-15 (preservative in hand lotions). Latex RAST (Pharmacia CAP): positive (class 3). Prick test: confirmed latex allergy to NRL, bananas, avocado, house dust mites, and various molds.

Diagnosis: Latex allergy and allergic and irritant contact hand eczema.

Impairment Rating: 15% impairment of the whole person.

Comment: Persistent dermatitis limits some activities of daily living; intermittent to constant treatment needed. Allergen avoidance information includes: non-NRL gloves list, methods of avoiding skin and inhalation contact with glutaraldehyde, quaternium-15–free hand lotion, and methods to avoid NRL exposure at both work and home. Prescription for Epi-Pen (auto-injectable epinephrine). Referred to allergist due to worsening rhinitis, asthma, and banana allergy. Determine impairment due to rhinitis and asthma separately and combine with skin impairment rating (see Combined Values Chart, p. 604) to determine total impairment.

Example 8-9
10% to 24% Impairment Due to Atopic Dermatitis

Subject: 25-year-old man.

History: Family history of eczema, hay fever; personal history of infantile eczema with chronic, intermittent, oozing lesions of face, scalp, neck, and upper extremities. Persistent lichenified patches in antecubital, popliteal, and neck areas during remissions. Severe exacerbations during high school; frequency increased during college.

Current Symptoms: Exacerbations once a month for 7 to 10 days; involves shoulders, arms, hands, legs, and trunk. Eczema during exacerbations limits some activities of daily living: difficulty sleeping, washing dishes, and concentrating on complex tasks. Lichenified dermatitis an annoyance but does not significantly limit daily activities. Intermittent application of topical steroid creams during relative remissions. Constant topical steroids, antihistamines, and oatmeal starch baths during flare-ups. Systemic steroids once a year induce remissions.

Physical Exam: Lichenified areas at lateral aspects of neck and arm, leg creases.

Clinical Studies: Basic labs: normal.

Diagnosis: Atopic dermatitis.

Impairment Rating: 15% impairment of the whole person.

Comment: Atopic dermatitis exacerbations precipitated by variety of agents. Estimated impairment based on occasional interference with some activities of daily living, frequency and severity of signs and symptoms, and need for and complexity of medical treatment.

Example 8-10
10% to 24% Impairment Due to Nail Dystrophy and Anonychia

Subject: 40-year-old woman.

History: Swelling, redness of eponychial, paronychial areas of all fingers; severe pain, paresthesia after repeated use of sculptured artificial nail kit consisting of liquid methyl methacrylate monomer and powdered methyl methacrylate polymer. Lost nails on all 10 fingers. Individual observed for several years; no fingernail regrowth.

Current Symptoms: Persistent paresthesia; difficulty grasping small objects such as coins; cold sensitivity, burning, and tingling. Other nonspecialized hand activities aggravate symptoms. Wears adhesive bandages over petroleum jelly on nail beds; wears gloves most waking hours. Woman anxious and depressed; requires occasional psychiatric consultation.

Physical Exam: Exposed and keratinized nail beds; paronychial areas swollen and tender.

Clinical Studies: Patch test: positive; 2% methyl methacrylate monomer in petrolatum.

Diagnosis: Chemically induced nail dystrophy and anonychia.

Impairment Rating: 20% impairment due to chemically induced nail dystrophy.

Comment: Combine with appropriate value for the paresthesia (see Combined Values Chart, p. 604) to determine whole person impairment. Any mental and behavioral impairment would increase the whole person impairment.

Example 8-11
10% to 24% Impairment Due to Zirconium Chloride Burn and Leukoderma

Subject: 30-year-old man.

History: At work splashed with concentrated liquid zirconium chloride over face, scalp, and neck. Despite immediate irrigation, hospitalized for 2 days for chemical burn. Healing and epithelialization occurred without complications; returned to work 22 days after episode. Months later, depigmentation occurred.

Current Symptoms: Depigmented areas sunburn easily, with considerable discomfort, restricting ability to work. Contact with heat (eg, hot showers, extremely warm days, or work as kiln operator) cause marked stinging sensation within affected skin areas, requiring cessation of all activities for 10 to 15 minutes until pain subsides. Occasional muscle twitching and severe discomfort occur within the affected areas, waking individual from sleep once or twice a week. Experiences considerable embarrassment when attempting to explain disfigurement; avoids some social activities previously participated in.

Physical Exam: Pigment loss, hyperesthesia, and intolerance to sunlight and warmth. Well-demarcated areas of depigmentation with borders of hyperpigmentation, surrounding right side of the face (behind right ear to center of face, from midtemple area of scalp to chin, and on left side of neck and behind right ear). Maximum dimensions of depigmented areas on right side of face 16 x 11 cm. Neurologic examination: all depigmented areas hypersensitive to cold, heat, pinprick, and touch.

Clinical Studies: Basic labs: normal.

Diagnosis: Zirconium chloride burn and leukoderma with residual skin dysfunction.

Impairment Rating: 20% impairment of the whole person.

Comment: Percentage of cutaneous impairment reflects decreased ability to perform some activities of daily living. Frequent occurrence of intense signs and symptoms, which precludes the performance of various activities, merits a rating at the upper end of class 2 impairment. If effective medical treatment were available to reduce frequency and intensity of signs and symptoms, estimated impairment percentage could be reduced. Behavioral changes exhibited by individual should be evaluated according to the criteria described in the *Guides* Chapter 14, Mental and Behavioral Disorders; any psychiatric impairment (see Combined Values Chart, p. 604) would be combined with the skin impairment to determine whole person impairment.

Class 3
25%-54% Impairment of the Whole Person

Skin disorder signs and symptoms present or intermittently present

and

limited performance of many activities of daily living

and

may require intermittent to constant treatment

Example 8-12
25% to 54% Impairment Due to Neurodermatitis and Occupational Contact Dermatitis

Subject: 45-year-old man.

History: Nurseryman; exposure to many irritant pesticides. 6 years' persistent, pruritic dermatitis involving ankles, forearms, hands, and occasionally face and neck. Recurrent pyogenic infection with occasional regional lymph node swelling and tenderness. Dermatitis initially responded to topical therapy and irritant avoidance; condition flared up after reexposure. Symptoms continued despite job change, avoidance of incriminated agents. No prior dermatologic problem. Noteworthy: 3 years' headache, memory loss, and anxiety with nausea and vomiting. Intermittent psychological counseling with some relief; little neurodermatitis improvement.

Current Symptoms: Neurodermatitis (itch-scratch syndrome); warm environments, sweating, chemical irritants, and stress provoke severe itching.

Physical Exam: Weeping, excoriated, lichenified plaques and patches of eczema of the face, arms, and hands. Axillary adenopathy.

Clinical Studies: Patch tests: negative to standard tray and work chemicals. Bacterial culture of skin drainage: *Staphylococcus aureus,* coagulase positive.

Diagnosis: Persistent neurodermatitis secondary to occupational contact dermatitis.

Impairment Rating: 30% impairment due to the skin disorder; combine with an estimated mental and behavioral impairment (see Combined Values Chart, p. 604) to determine whole person impairment.

Comment: Unable to fully perform usual activities of daily living or participate in social and recreational activities; difficulty sleeping.

Example 8-13
25% to 54% Impairment Due to Thermal Burn Scarring

Subject: 44-year-old man.

History: Burns to dorsum of both hands and feet; required grafting.

Current Symptoms: Well-healed grafts; residual dryness and cracking, easily injured by minor trauma, noxious chemicals. Bathes, shampoos with gloves on since water and soap irritate hands. Trouble grasping toothbrush, comb, or writing instrument due to cracking, decreased sensation, and skin stiffness. Feet uncomfortable in leather shoes; wears cloth shoes. Intermittent moisturizer use.

Physical Exam: Dry, somewhat atrophic, and stiff grafts on hands and feet.

Clinical Studies: Basic labs: normal.

Diagnosis: Scarring due to thermal burns.

Impairment Rating: 30% impairment of the whole person.

Comment: Many activities of daily living limited. Intermittent treatment and symptoms place him at the lower end of class 3.

Example 8-14
25% to 54% Impairment Due to Follicular Occlusive Triad

Subject: 28-year-old man.

History: 12 years' acne vulgaris, hidradenitis suppurativa, and dissecting cellulitis of the scalp (follicular occlusive triad). Temporary improvement with topical and systemic antibiotics, intralesional corticosteroids, aspiration, marsupialization, zinc sulfate, and two courses of isotretinoin. Last 5 years, developed large cystic lesions, mainly involving posterior scalp, face, neck, upper trunk, axilla, and inguinal area.

Current Symptoms: Lesions accompanied by fever and aching joints. Large lesions on back, chest, and scalp and in the inguinal area make resting difficult in warm weather. Clothing and sweating aggravate disorder. Difficulty sleeping, participating in social and recreational activities, and maintaining regular employment.

Physical Exam: Inflamed cystic lesions located on posterior scalp, face, neck, upper trunk, axilla, and inguinal area. Skin severely scarred.

Clinical Studies: White blood cell count: 22.0×10^9L ($22.0 \times 10^3/\mu$L).

Diagnosis: Acne conglobata; hidradenitis suppurativa; dissecting cellulitis of the scalp; severe scar formation.

Impairment Rating: 30% impairment of the whole person.

Comment: Many activities of daily living limited. Requires frequent systemic antibodies.

Class 4 55%-84% Impairment of the Whole Person
Skin disorder signs and symptoms constantly present ***and*** limited performance of many activities of daily living, including intermittent confinement at home or other domicile ***and*** may require intermittent to constant treatment

Example 8-15
25% to 54% Impairment Due to Pemphigus Vulgaris

Subject: 35-year-old man.

History: 22 months' persistently sore mouth. Vesicles and bullae over face, trunk, and extremities. High doses of oral corticosteroids administered to control disease.

Current Symptoms: Persistent blisters and erosions result in chronic, unremitting pain on swallowing or speaking. Erosions and skin fragility involving mouth, trunk, and genital area; unable to have sexual intercourse, eat solid foods, brush teeth, speak above a whisper, or sleep. Azathioprine therapy added to high-dose corticosteroids; limited disease control. Complex therapy requires frequent physician visits for checkups and laboratory monitoring.

Physical Exam: Many eroded lesions of tongue and oral mucous membranes; lesions over trunk and extremities. Infected bullae of mouth and trunk; increased systolic blood pressure.

Clinical Studies: White blood cell count: leukopenia (secondary to therapy). Biopsy: pemphigus vulgaris.

Diagnosis: Pemphigus vulgaris.

Impairment Rating: 45% impairment of the whole person.

Comment: Interference with many activities of daily living due to lesions and pemphigus pain. Therapy led to leukopenia (see Chapter 9, The Hematopoietic System, for further impairment). Combine impairments of several organ systems (see Combined Values Chart, p. 604) to determine the whole person impairment.

Example 8-16
55% to 84% Impairment Due to Skin Cancer

Subject: 40-year-old man.

History: Laborer; noted to have multiple basal cell carcinomas since age 15 involving both exposed and covered body areas. History of cardiac fibromas.

Current Symptoms: Multiple draining lesions on trunk; reclusive behavior because of inability to go into the sun. Need for continuous surgical removal of skin tumors. Loss of self-esteem.

Physical Exam: Multiple nodular and ulcerated dome-shaped tumors of face and trunk with serosanguineous foul-smelling drainage. Palmar and plantar pits and facial milia.

Clinical Studies: Skin biopsies: basal cell carcinoma. Radiographs: macrocephaly, hypertelorism, frontal bossing, odontogenic keratocysts of the jaws, calcification of the falx cerebri, and bifid ribs.

Diagnosis: Basal cell nevus syndrome with multiple basal cell carcinomas.

Impairment Rating: 55% impairment of the whole person; combine with estimated rating for significant emotional distress from Chapter 14, Mental and Behavorial Disorders (see Combined Values Chart, p. 604), to determine total impairment.

Comment: Basal cell nevus syndrome or Gorlin syndrome is an autosomal dominant disorder with an estimated prevalence of 1 per 56,000. It is characterized by multiple basal cell carcinomas, a range of other tumors, and widespread developmental defects.

Example 8-17
55% to 84% Impairment Due to Skin Disease

Subject: 55-year-old man.

History: Right leg severely injured in crash; deep-vein thrombophlebitis required 6 months' total or partial bed rest in hospital and at home. Right leg swelling increased despite elastic stocking. 4 days after resuming work, spilled can of caustic drain cleaner; second- and third-degree burns over 20% of right lower leg. Burn healed after 12 weeks; scar but no thickening or contracture.

Current Symptoms: Despite elastic support stockings and diuretics, intolerable leg edema. Unable to stay on feet for over 4 hours without significant swelling and discomfort. Periodic treatment, Unna's paste boots; occasional hospital admissions heal ulcers temporarily. Difficulty sleeping; tolerates clothing over leg only 1 or 2 hours. Hospitalized for sepsis and persistent cellulitis.

Physical Exam: Right leg pitting edema below knee. Hypopigmented, atrophic, hyperesthetic scar from midthigh to ankle and from thigh anterior midline to posterior midline. Stasis dermatitis with ulceration. Altered perception of pain and touch; hyperesthesia in scar area. A 4 x 5-cm ulcer with granulating base over right medial malleolus; surrounding skin erythema. Weight-bearing difficulty due to ulcer pain.

Clinical Studies: Ultrasound: chronic phlebitis, right leg.

Diagnosis: Postthrombophlebitis syndrome with stasis dermatitis and ulceration; scar formation secondary to chemical burn.

Impairment Rating: 55% impairment of the whole person.

Comment: Anticipate future episodes of phlebitis, cellulitis, and ulceration. Requires indefinite diligent medical care.

Example 8-18
55% to 84% Impairment Due to Pustular Psoriasis With Psoriatic Arthritis

Subject: 32-year-old man.

History: 2 months' pretibial erythematous, scaly eruption; spread to upper extremities and hand. Pain, swelling, and erythema of knees; sterile urethral discharge. Condition improved only with systemic steroids and cytotoxic agents. Initial possible diagnoses: Reiter's syndrome, keratoderma blennorrhagica, or pustular psoriasis with psoriatic arthritis. Rehospitalized 3 months later with acute, severely exacerbated skin eruption; severe pain, swelling, and deformity of all extremity joints. Oral methotrexate partially controlled disease.

Current Symptoms: Periodic arthritis flare-ups and psoriasis require hospitalization. Exacerbations with generalized pustulation involve trunk, palms, and soles; difficult to care for himself, stand, sit, walk, and drive. Difficulty grasping and tactile discrimination at work; unable to have sexual intercourse.

Physical Exam: Widespread pustular eruption, acute conjunctivitis, and severe arthritis of all hand, wrist, knee, ankle, and toe joints. Hands and feet joints warm, red, and tender; minimal swelling. Flexion deformities in both hands.

Clinical Studies: Radiographs: carpal bones, proximal and distal heads of the metacarpals, and phalanges, marked demineralization. Joint space narrowing and periosteal reactions in metacarpals. Biopsy: exudative psoriasis.

Diagnosis: Pustular psoriasis with psoriatic arthritis.

Impairment Rating: 60% impairment due to psoriasis; combine with appropriate impairment estimates for limitations of joint motion and for any other involved organ system (see Combined Values Chart, p. 604) to determine whole person impairment.

Comment: Reiter's syndrome and pustular psoriasis clinical features may overlap, relapse, and adversely affect the ability to perform activities of daily living.

Example 8-19
55% to 84% Impairment Due to Thermal Burn Scarring and Dyspnea

Subject: 25-year-old man.

History: 3 years' severe burns over 85% of total body surface area; smoke inhalation; some grafts.

Current Symptoms: Unable to work with heavy equipment. Skin fragile, dried, and cracked. Hot, dizzy, and unable to perspire in warm environments. Marked difficulty with writing, walking, and nonspecific hand activities. Scar formation causes pain and decreased range of motion. Feels disfigured. Greatly limited ability to participate in group activities. No sexual relations after injury; short of breath with physical activity.

Physical Exam: Healed atrophic scars over 85% of body; minimally atrophic skin grafts and donor sites. Several depigmented areas, including some on cheeks and backs of hands. Partial destruction of left ear; distorted fingernails. Diminished range of motion of both hands.

Clinical Studies: Basic labs: normal.

Diagnosis: Extensive scarring due to thermal burns and dyspnea.

Impairment Rating: 60% impairment of the whole person.

Comment: Combine the skin (burn) impairment with impairments due to musculoskeletal and pulmonary dysfunction (see Combined Values Chart, p. 604) to determine whole person impairment; adjust to consider any mental and behavioral impairment present.

Example 8-20
55% to 84% Impairment Due to Mycosis Fungoides

Subject: 56-year-old man.

History: 20 years' progressive pruritic rash; pruritic patches on back and extremities. Topical therapy; eruption gradually generalized. Treated with topical nitrogen mustard, PUVA, photophoresis, and electron beam therapy. Eruption uncontrolled with cytotoxic agent or radiation therapy.

Current Symptoms: Confined to home; unable to care for himself, walk, travel, grasp, or participate in sexual activity.

Physical Exam: Diffuse, erythematous, scaly plaques; some quite firm. Many trunk and extremity excoriations; foul-smelling and draining nodular tumors on face, palms, and soles. Palpable axillary and inguinal lymph nodes.

Clinical Studies: Biopsy: skin, lymph node positive for mycosis fungoides. Other labs: normal.

Diagnosis: Mycosis fungoides.

Impairment Rating: 75% impairment of the whole person.

Comment: Tumor-stage, widespread mycosis fungoides requires close medical surveillance. Morbidity is considerable; poor prognosis. Interference with many activities of daily living; most individuals die within 2 to 5 years.

Class 5
85%-95% Impairment of the Whole Person
Skin disorder signs and symptoms constantly present
and
limited performance of most activities of daily living, including occasional to constant confinement at home or other domicile
and
may require intermittent to constant treatment

Example 8-21
85% to 95% Impairment Due to Xeroderma Pigmentosum

Subject: 18-year-old woman.

History: 13 years' photophobia. At 5 years, marked pigmentation of sun-exposed areas of face, chest, arms, and legs. Since then, generalized freckling of skin, several areas of telangiectasia, and multiple basal and squamous cell epitheliomas.

Current Symptoms: Condition progressing in severity; continuous observation and treatment. Confined to home for past year.

Physical Exam: Showed all signs described above.

Clinical Studies: Basic lab findings: normal. Fecal, urinary porphyrin studies: negative.

Diagnosis: Xeroderma pigmentosum.

Impairment Rating: 85% impairment of the whole person.

Comment: Xeroderma pigmentosum is a progressive disease; ultimate impairment approaches 100%, a fatal evolution. May develop metastatic carcinoma from squamous cell carcinomas or malignant melanoma.

Example 8-22
85% to 95% Impairment Due to Epidermolysis Bullosa Dystrophica

Subject: 19-year-old man.

History: Bullous lesions shortly after birth; continuously since then, except for very minor and short remissions. Bullae appeared after slightest trauma; healed with severe scarring and milia.

Current Symptoms: Requires continuous hospitalization.

Physical Exam: Fingers are tapered stumps (mitten deformities for hands). Constant bullae in mouth and pharynx; probably extended to epiglottis. Weight 40% below desirable for height.

Clinical Studies: Roentgenography: esophageal stricture.

Diagnosis: Epidermolysis bullosa dystrophica.

Impairment Rating: 95% impairment due to epidermolysis bullosa dystrophica; combine with impairment estimates for esophagus stricture and fingers (see Combined Values Chart, p. 604) to determine whole person impairment.

Comment: This autosomal recessive disorder is one of the most impairing of all hereditary diseases; impairment approaches 100% and death. Increased risk of aggressive squamous cell carcinoma. Evaluate for any mental and behavioral impairment.

8.8 Skin Impairment Evalution Summary

See Table 8-3 for an evalution summary for the assessment of permanent impairment due to skin disorders.

Table 8-3 Skin Impairment Evaluation Summary

Disorder	History, Including Selected Relevant Symptoms	Examination Record	Assessment of Skin Function
General	Duration, location of rash; itch, redness, welts, eczema, blisters, pimples; nail or pigment change; hair loss; ulcers, scars, growth, grafts Progression, remission, exacerbants Work history, hobbies, etc Associated conditions: atopy, eczema, asthma, rhinitis Impact on activities of daily living	Detailed skin exam: location, symmetry, demarcation Extent, pattern of involvement Sun-exposed or covered area involvement, infection, cellulitis, acute/chronic dermatitis, welts; pigment, hair, or nail changes; scar, grafts, growths Comprehensive physical exam as appropriate	Biopsy Cultures; microscopic scrapings (KOH, etc) Allergy tests (patch, prick, RAST, etc) Specialty; consult as appropriate
Urticaria	Acute; chronic Duration; frequency; location; progression Identify cause: food, infection, allergy, medication, systemic disease, physical agent, familial, etc	Extent; duration (>48-72 hours?) Location, distribution	As appropriate; complete blood count, differential, TSH Complement profile; biopsy if fixed Allergy tests (RAST, open prick, etc)
Dermatitis	Duration, location, itch, redness, nail or pigment change Progression and remission factors Atopy; childhood eczema Work, hobbies, etc	Papules; papulovesicles; erythema; serous discharge; crusting; edema; scale; lichenified or thickened plaques	Clinical presentation and history Biopsy; cultures; allergy tests (see general skin disorders)
Pigmentary Changes	Increased, decreased pigment Congenital; acquired; dermatomal Duration; location; progression Preceding dermatosis Causes: inflammation, chemical contact, occupation, infection, physical, metabolic, endocrine, drugs, neoplasm, etc	Local, disseminated; extent, pattern; Wood's light exam See general skin disorders	Labs as appropriate; biopsy; scrapings (KOH) See general skin disorders
Scars	Burns; trauma; disease grafts; family history (Ehlers-Danlos); other causes Neoplasm; ulcer; dermatitis (x-ray or stats)	Evaluate skin graft function; detail scar dimensions, shape, location, nature; any ulceration, depression, or evaluation	Atrophic or hypertrophic; pliability; changes in underlying structure
Psoriasis	Family history; age at onset; infection; medication Localized; disseminated; pustular Extent of involvement	Extent and location of involvement; type of lesion (plaque, pustular, etc)	Biopsy; lab: streptococcal antibody titers
Bullous Disorders	Congenital; acquired Duration; extent; location; mucosal Family history Pruritus; hand changes; neoplasm	Localized; generalized Vesicles; bullae; hand changes; neoplasm	Biopsy (routine, immunofluorescence); serologic studies (immunofluorescent antibodies), culture; nutritional assessment

End-Organ or System Damage	Diagnosis(es)	Degree of Impairment
Includes assessment of other organs: sinuses, respiratory, systemic components to skin disease Includes assessment of skin damage or sequelae (scars, pigmentation, alopecia, etc)	Record all pertinent diagnoses, medical status, and further treatment plans Prognosis Impact on activities of daily living Date of MMI; list accommodations	Criteria outlined in chapter Description of clinical findings and how these relate to *Guides* criteria Explanation of each estimated impairment List all impairment percentages; estimate whole person impairment percentage (see Table 8-2)
Mucosal angioedema; rhinitis; asthma; anaphylaxis	Acute or chronic urticaria; recurring urticaria; angioedema	See Table 8-2
Exfoliate erythroderma; atopy; rhinitis; asthma	Atopic Contact (allergic irritation) Acute; subacute; chronic Urticaria, photosensitivity, seborrheic; exfoliative, stasis; hand and foot, nummular dermatitis	See general skin disorders, Table 8-2
Systemic changes; deafness; neurologic disorders	Vitiligo, postinflammatory, hyper-hypopigmentation; chemical; scars	See Section 8.2, Disfigurement, and Table 8-2
None for skin unless other organs exposed	Scar; hypertophic scar; keloid graft	See Table 8-2
If urethritis, conjunctivitis, diarrhea, arthritis, consider Reiter's, psoriatic arthritis	Psoriasis vulgaris; pustular; exfoliative (see general skin exam; see table)	See general skin exam and Table 8-2
Psoriatic arthritis Neoplasm; esophageal; neurologic; mental, behavioral; ophthalmologic (conjunctival, symblepharon)	Impetigo; contact dermatitis; insect bites; pemphigoid; pemphigus; dermatitis herpetiformis; epidermolysis; bullosa (congenital, acquired); linear IgA disease	See general skin exam and Table 8-2

References

1. Adams RM. *Occupational Skin Disease.* 3rd ed. Philadelphia, Pa: WB Saunders Co; 1999.

2. *The Cosmetic Benefit Study.* Washington, DC: The Cosmetic, Toiletry and Fragrance Association; 1978.

3. Key MM. Confusing compensation cases. *Cutis.* 1967;3:965-969.

4. Fisher AA. Permanent loss of fingernails from sensitization and reaction to acrylics in a preparation designed to make artificial nails. *J Dermatol Surg Oncol.* 1980;6:70-71.

5. Mathias CGT. The skin. In: Zenz C, ed. *Occupational Medicine.* 2nd ed. Chicago, Ill: Year Book Medical Publishers; 1988.

6. Taylor JS, ed. Occupational dermatoses. *Dermatol Clin North Am.* 1994;12:461-600.

7. Engrav LH, Covey MH, Dutcher KD, et al. Impairment, time out of school, and time off from work after burns. *Plast Reconstr Surg.* 1987;79:927-934.

8. Finlay AY, Khru GK, Luscombe DK, Salek MS. Validation of sickness impact profile and psoriasis disability index in psoriasis. *Br J Dermatol.* 1990;123:751-756.

9. Sherertz EF, Storrs FJ. Occupational contact dermatitis. In: Rosenstock L, Cullen M, eds. *Textbook of Clinical Occupational and Environmental Medicine.* Philadelphia, Pa: WB Saunders Co; 1994.

10. Nethercott JR, Gallant C. Disability due to occupational contact dermatitis. *Occup Med.* 1986;1:199-204.

11. *Preventing Allergic Reaction to Natural Rubber Latex in the Workplace.* Cincinnati, Ohio: National Institute for Occupational Safety and Health; 1997. Publication 97-135.

12. Tarlo SM, Sussman GL, Holness DL. Latex sensitivity in dental students and staff: a cross-sectional study. *J Allergy Clin Immunol.* 1997;99:396-401.

13. Taylor JS, Wattanakrai P, Charous BL, Ownby DR. Year Book focus: latex allergy. In: Thiers BH, Lang PG, eds. *1999 Year Book of Dermatology and Dermatologic Surgery.* St Louis, Mo: Mosby, St Louis University Press; 1999:1-44.

14. Mackey SA, Marks JG. Dermatitis in machinists: a retrospective study. *Am J Contact Derm.* 1993;4:22-26.

15. Hogan DJ, Dannaker CJ, Maibach HI. The prognosis of contact dermatitis. *J Am Acad Dermatol.* 1990;23:300-307.

16. Wigger-Alberti W, Elsner P. Preventive measures in contact dermatitis. *Clin Dermatol.* 1997;15:661-665.

17. Fink JN, ed. Latex allergy. *Immunol Allergy Clin North Am.* 1995;15:1-179.

18. DeGroot H, DeJong N, Duijoter E, VanWyk RG, et al. Prevalence of natural rubber latex allergy (Type I and Type IV) in laboratory workers in the Netherlands. *Contact Dermatitis.* 1993;38:159-163.

19. Agner T, Flyvholm MA, Menne T. Formaldehyde allergy: a follow-up study. *Am J Contact Dermatitis.* 1999;10:12-17.

20. Duarte I, Nakano JT, Lazzarini R. Hand eczema: evaluation of 250 patients. *Am J Contact Dermatitis.* 1998;9:216-223.

21. Drake L, Dorner W, Goltz RW, et al. Guidelines of care for contact dermatitis. *J Amer Acad Dermatol.* 1995;32:109-113.

22. Freedberg IM, Eisen AZ, Wolff K, et al, eds. *Dermatology in General Medicine.* Vol 1. New York, NY: McGraw-Hill; 1999:840-864, 1080-1116.

Chapter 9

The Hematopoietic System

Introduction

This chapter provides criteria for evaluating permanent impairment of the hematopoietic system. The hematopoietic system, including the bone marrow, lymph nodes, and spleen, produces a heterogeneous population of blood-circulating cells (eg, red blood cells, white blood cells, and platelets) and a complex family of proteins critical for blood clotting and immune defenses. Cells from this system also produce proteins that affect daily physiologic responses (eg, granulocyte, granulocyte-macrophage stimulating factors, etc) and respond to many pathologic stimuli (eg, tumor necrosis factor and interleukins). Because the hematopoietic system supports other cells or organs of the body, identifiable defects are assigned impairment ratings only secondarily through altered function of other end organs. For example, very severe anemia can reduce oxygen delivery to the point where the individual suffers a myocardial infarction or stroke. Age and comorbid conditions further complicate the determination of impairment. Most of the products of the hematopoietic system also include remarkable compensatory biologic mechanisms.

Clinical alterations can be **hereditary** or **acquired.** Because of functional adaptation of the young, hereditary defects manifest in childhood are commonly modest in degree of impairment. With age, alterations become more definitive and functional impairment more evident. Abnormalities can be quantitative—production of too many cells (ie, leukemia or polycythemia) or too few cells (ie, anemia or thrombocytopenia)—or they can be qualitative, with production of a defective protein (ie, factor V Leiden or prothrombin 20210A) resulting in an increased propensity for thrombosis.

This edition of the *Guides* has expanded sections on human immunodeficiency virus (HIV) and thrombotic disorders.

9.1 Principles of Assessment

Before using the information in this chapter, the *Guides* user should become familiar with Chapters 1 and 2 and the Glossary. Chapters 1 and 2 discuss the *Guides'* purpose, applications, and methods for performing and reporting impairment evaluations. The Glossary provides definitions of common terms used by many specialties in impairment evaluation.

9.1a Interpretation of Symptoms and Signs

Some impairment classes refer to symptoms that limit the ability to perform daily activities. When this information is subjective and open to misinterpretation, it should not serve as the sole criterion upon which decisions about impairment are made. Rather, the examiner should obtain objective data about the limitations' extent and integrate those findings with the subjective data to estimate the degree of permanent impairment.

Impairment percentages reflect severity of symptoms, physical and laboratory findings, and estimated functional limitations resulting from hematologic abnormality. See Table 9-1 for the functional classifications of hematologic system disease. The activities of daily living are listed in Table 1-2 and the Glossary.

Table 9-1 Functional Classification of Hematologic System Disease

Class	Description
I (none)	No signs or symptoms of disease despite laboratory abnormalities; individual performs the usual activities of daily living (Table 1-2)
II (minimal)	Some signs or symptoms of disease; individual performs the usual activities of daily living with some difficulty
III (moderate)	Signs and symptoms of disease; individual requires varying amounts of assistance from others to perform the usual activities of daily living
IV (marked)	Signs and symptoms of disease; individual requires assistance to perform most or all activities of daily living

9.1b Description of Procedures

Aids to diagnose hematologic impairment vary depending on the suspected diagnosis. Common tests include a complete blood count, bone marrow aspiration and biopsy, hemoglobin electrophoresis, direct and indirect antiglobulin test and cold agglutinin assay, flow cytometry, cytogenetics of peripheral blood and/or bone marrow, immunochemical analysis of immunoglobulins, fat pad biopsy with Congo red stain, and hemostasis studies.

9.2 Anemia

The functional effects of chronic anemia depend on the degree of the cardiovascular system's compensatory response. Regardless of the anemia's pathogenesis, impairment is related to the heart's inability to deliver adequate oxygen to tissues. To compensate for the anemia, the heart increases cardiac output by acceleration of heart rate and also increases oxygen extraction from the tissues (ie, increases arteriovenous difference). Therefore, a person with a mild anemia (hemoglobin level of about 10 g/dL) and a normal cardiovascular system receives a lower impairment rating than a person with underlying dysfunction of the cardiovascular system.

Symptoms of anemia include shortness of breath on exertion, dizziness, throbbing headaches, and fatigue. The speed at which anemia develops at any hemoglobin level correlates to the complexity of symptoms. Greater degrees of anemia may be associated with lack of stamina, fatigue on exertion, fatigue at rest, and dyspnea at rest. Thus, no specific concentrations of hemoglobin determine impairment. Anemia impairment is measured by the limitations of cardiovascular response and may be lessened by a successful blood transfusion.

Many forms of anemia are reversible with specific therapy. Anemias resulting from decreased red cell production due to nutrient deficit (eg, iron-deficiency anemia, megaloblastic anemia secondary to folic acid, vitamin B_{12} deficiency, etc) are correctable with specific nutrient therapy.

A permanent impairment may develop from sequelae of the anemia. In megaloblastic anemia due to B_{12} deficiency, significant neurologic deficit caused by dysmyelinization (particularly of the posterolateral spinal tracks) may occur and result in permanent neurologic impairment. Folic acid deficiency during pregnancy may result in lifelong impairment of the newborn with varying degrees of neural tube defects. In some circumstances of hypoproliferative anemia from chronic renal failure, the anemia is correctable with exogenous erythropoietin even though the renal failure is irreversible. Similarly, many forms of anemia due to increased and, particularly, acquired red cell destruction (ie, hemolytic anemias) are reversible with therapy and therefore do not result in permanent impairment.

Persistent hemolytic anemia may cause a degree of impairment that is related to the anemia's severity. This impairment consideration also applies to aplastic or refractory anemia caused by defective bone marrow function. Persistent refractory anemia may cause impairment regardless of the cause; the degree of impairment is related to the anemia's severity, need for transfusion, and impact on the ability to perform activities of daily living. Additional organ system impairment due to anemia can be combined using the Combined Values Chart (p. 604).

The benefits of red blood cell transfusion normally last 6 to 8 weeks. In individuals with hemolytic anemia caused by serum factors, and in some who have had many transfusions, the survival rate of transfused cells is shortened and transfusions must be repeated every 1 to 5 weeks. Impairment increases as hemolysis becomes more severe.

In **congenital** hemolytic anemias, particularly those related to altered hemoglobin synthesis (eg, hemoglobinopathies and thalassemias), tissue impairment beyond the hematopoietic system results in permanent impairment.[1] Sickle cell diseases, especially sickle cell anemia, are commonly associated with severe, painful vaso-occlusive crisis that can result in functional impairment of varying degrees.[2] These vascular occlusive lesions result in end-organ damage to the bones, heart, kidneys, and liver, compounding the degree of impairment.

9.2a Criteria for Rating Permanent Impairment Due to Anemia

The impairment criteria for anemia are given in Table 9-2.

Table 9-2 Criteria for Rating Permanent Impairment Due to Anemia

Class 1 0%-10% Impairment of the Whole Person	Class 2 11%-30% Impairment of the Whole Person	Class 3 31%-70% Impairment of the Whole Person	Class 4 71%-100% Impairment of the Whole Person
No symptoms *and* hemoglobin 10-12 g/dL *and* no transfusion required	Minimal symptoms *and* hemoglobin 8-10 g/dL *and* no transfusion required	Moderate to marked symptoms *and* hemoglobin 5-8 g/dL* *and* transfusions of 2-3 U required every 4-6 weeks†	Moderate to marked symptoms *and* hemoglobin 5-8 g/dL* *and* transfusions of 2-3 U required every 2 weeks†

*Level before transfusion.

†Implies hemolysis of transfused blood.

Class 1
0%-10% Impairment of the Whole Person
No symptoms
and
hemoglobin 10-12 g/dL
and
no transfusion required

Example 9-1
0% to 10% Impairment Due to Anemia

Subject: 18-year-old man.

History: Seen for medical clearance for regular physical education class.

Current Symptoms: Asymptomatic.

Physical Exam: Normal.

Clinical Studies: Hemoglobin: 120 g/L (12.0 g/dL) with anisocytosis. Hemoglobin electrophoresis: hemoglobin sickle cell type AS.

Diagnosis: Sickle cell trait.

Impairment Rating: 0% impairment of the whole person.

Comment: No impairment in function currently exists or is anticipated during performance of routine sports or daily activities. Ensure that adequate hydration occurs with physical exertion to prevent severe dehydration. The student should avoid prolonged exposure to hypoxia.

Example 9-2
0% to 10% Impairment Due to Anemia With Rheumatoid Arthritis

Subject: 48-year-old woman.

History: More than 10-year history of rheumatoid arthritis, managed with acetylsalicylic acid, nonsteroidal anti-inflammatory drugs, and intermittent corticosteroids.

Current Symptoms: Occasional fatigue, stiffness in hands, and difficulty performing activities of daily living.

Physical Exam: Joint deformities in both hands consistent with rheumatoid arthritis.

Clinical Studies: Hemoglobin: 102 g/L (10.2 g/dL). Hematocrit: 0.31 Proportion of 1.0 (31%). Mean corpuscular volume: 79. Serum ferritin: 110µg/L (110 ng/mL). Remainder of labs normal except for rheumatoid factor.

Diagnosis: Anemia with rheumatoid arthritis.

Impairment Rating: 5% to 10% impairment of the whole person due to anemia; combine with an impairment rating for the rheumatoid arthritis.

Comment: Unlike the rheumatoid arthritis, the anemia is mild. Some people with rheumatoid arthritis or chronic inflammatory lesions develop iron-deficiency anemia due to medication and gastrointestinal blood loss. This woman's normal serum ferritin rules this out. Her anemia is that seen in the anemia of chronic disease.

Class 2
11%-30% Impairment of the Whole Person
Minimal symptoms
and
hemoglobin 8-10 g/dL
and
no transfusion required

Example 9-3
11% to 30% Impairment Due to Autoimmune Hemolytic Anemia

Subject: 59-year-old man.

History: Found to be anemic 2 years after a lung infection.

Current Symptoms: Fatigue; takes naps several days per week; doesn't do vigorous work such as shoveling snow or prolonged yard work.

Physical Exam: Normal; no palpable liver or spleen.

Clinical Studies: Hemoglobin: 95 g/L (9.5 g/dL). Hematocrit: 0.29 Proportion of 1.0 (29%). Serologic evidence of cold agglutinins. Low-grade hemolysis with "laking" on peripheral smear; elevated mean corpuscular volume, which decreased on warming; cold agglutinin, chronic hemolytic disease.

Diagnosis: Autoimmune hemolytic anemia of the cold antibody type.

Impairment Rating: 20% impairment of the whole person.

Comment: Chronicity is established; there is no specific therapy. Anemia limits performance of daily activities. Exposure to colds or viral illnesses carries a risk of abrupt, enhanced red cell destruction with a further anemia. Some individuals, particularly in older age groups, may develop a malignant lymphoma of the large cell type. Regular follow-up is recommended.

Example 9-4
11% to 30% Impairment Due to Sickle Cell Anemia

Subject: 22-year-old woman.

History: Sickle cell anemia since 2 years old. Repeated pain crisis. Hemoglobin 85-95 g/L (8.5-9.5 g/dL) for the last 5 years, without adequate response to hydroxyurea. Pain crises occur four to six times per year. Performance of daily activities limited since vigorous physical work can provoke a pain crisis.

Current Symptoms: Slight fatigue; takes naps when not having a pain crisis. Usually off work several times per year for several days per occurrence due to pain crisis episodes.

Physical Exam: Sickle cell habitus.

Clinical Studies: Hemoglobin: 82 g/L (8.2 g/dL). White blood cell count: 12.0×10^9/L (12,000 × 10^3/µL). Hemoglobin electrophoresis review: confirms sickle cell hemoglobin (SS) with normal fetal and A_2 hemoglobin.

Diagnosis: Sickle cell anemia.

Impairment Rating: 25% impairment of the whole person.

Comment: Decreased risk of other, potential sequelae—avascular necrosis of the femoral heads, cardiomyopathy, renal failure, etc—requires careful monitoring. Transfusions provide transient support and are mainly used for crisis intervention.

Class 3 31%-70% Impairment of the Whole Person
Moderate to marked symptoms
and
hemoglobin 5-8 g/dL
and
transfusions of 2-3 U required every 4-6 weeks

Example 9-5
31% to 70% Impairment Due to Chronic Anemia With Myelodysplastic Syndrome

Subject: 48-year-old woman.

History: Fatigue, decreased appetite, and limited energy 1 year ago led to recognition of a progressive anemia. Erythropoietin has not increased red cell values. Requires transfusions of 1 to 3 U of packed red blood cells every 4 to 5 weeks.

Current Symptoms: Fatigue; decreased energy; needs to rest and take an afternoon nap daily. Can perform light activities of daily living with help. Feels better for 7 to 10 days after transfusions, and then declines in function.

Physical Exam: Signs of anemia; otherwise normal.

Clinical Studies: Bone marrow: myelodysplasia with excess blasts. Hemoglobin: 70 g/L (7.0 g/dL).

Diagnosis: Chronic anemia with myelodysplastic syndrome.

Impairment Rating: 65% impairment of the whole person.

Comment: Condition is likely to progress in terms of the severity of the anemia, with an increase in the frequency of transfusions required since isoimmunization is an inevitable sequela. Individual is at increased risk of transformation to acute leukemia and hemochromatosis due to transfusion requirements.

Example 9-6
31% to 70% Impairment Due to Aplastic Anemia

Subject: 32-year-old woman.

History: Severe aplastic anemia diagnosed 4 years ago. Failed immunosuppressive agents and bone marrow transplantation. Now requires 3 U packed red cells every 4 weeks.

Current Symptoms: Fatigue, especially before transfusions. Very limited exercise tolerance: able to walk for only 5 to 10 minutes before fatigue and shortness of breath occur.

Physical Exam: Signs of anemia.

Clinical Studies: Hemoglobin: 70 g/L (7 g/dL).

Diagnosis: Aplastic anemia.

Impairment Rating: 60% to 69% impairment of the whole person.

Comments: Chronic, severe anemia with continued, significant transfusion needs; ongoing risks of hemochromatosis and comorbid problems likely.[3]

Class 4 71%-100% Impairment of the Whole Person
Moderate to marked symptoms *and* hemoglobin 5-8 g/dL *and* transfusions of 2-3 U required every 2 weeks

Example 9-7
71% to 100% Impairment Due to Anemia

Subject: 36-year-old woman.

History: 2-year history of cerebrovascular accident, with a severe anemia associated with hemolysis and iron deficiency. Developed Budd-Chiari syndrome 4 months ago.

Current Symptoms: Weakness and fatigue; pale skin.

Physical Exam: Pallor; residual left-sided weakness. Pulse: 100 BPM.

Clinical Studies: Hemoglobin: 65 g/L (6.5 g/dL). White blood cell count: 2.5×10^9/L (2500 × 10^3/μL). Platelets: 80×10^9/L (80 × 10^3/μL).

Diagnosis: Severe hemolytic anemia, paroxysmal nocturnal hemoglobinuria, and Budd-Chiari syndrome.

Impairment Rating: 90%+ impairment of the whole person.

Comment: Limited treatment, given the recent Budd-Chiari syndrome.

9.3 Polycythemia and Myelofibrosis

Polycythemia vera is manifested by hematocrit values above 0.52 Proportion of 1.0 (52%) in men and 0.49 Proportion of 1.0 (49%) in women, and by red blood cell volumes above 0.036 L/kg (36 mL/kg) in men and 0.032 L/kg (32 mL/kg) in women. Other frequent symptoms are normal arterial oxygen tension, an enlarged spleen, slight elevation of the white blood cell and platelet counts, and increased leukocyte alkaline phosphatase. An increase in red cell numbers (polycythemia) can be due to cardiopulmonary disease, smoking, or inappropriate secretion of erythropoietin. If the primary cause of polycythemia can be treated and the polycythemia is corrected, there should be no permanent impairment. Phlebotomy to normal hematocrit levels should correct the symptoms of all forms of polycythemia. Polycythemia can lead to other organ system impairments, such as cerebrovascular or cardiovascular occlusions.

Myelofibrosis (bone marrow fibrosis) may also occur in individuals with polycythemia. While some individuals remain relatively asymptomatic for several years, others experience fatigue, weakness, weight loss, perspiration, and low-grade fever, and develop a large spleen. Currently, no therapy exists to relieve the symptoms of myelofibrosis. Transfusions may be needed for severe anemia. Exogenous erythropoietin increases red cell production in some people.

9.3a Criteria for Rating Permanent Impairment Due to Polycythemia and/or Myelofibrosis

Polycythemia can produce end-organ damage to cardiovascular or cerebrovascular areas due to vascular occlusion. Vascular obstruction of the postal venous system similarly can produce end-organ injury to the liver. The impairment rating is based on the end organ involved, degree of injury, and impact on the ability to perform activities of daily living.

The criteria for diagnosis of myelofibrosis, of primary (idiopathic) or secondary (postpolycythemic) etiology, include progressive anemia with red cell changes of anisocytosis and poikilocytosis, a shift to the left of the granulocytic white cell series, and, often, nucleated red blood cells in the peripheral blood. Bone marrow indicates fibrosis with dilated sinusoids and clustering of megakaryocytes. The degree of impairment due to myelofibrosis is reflected by the degree of impairment due to the anemia. Examples are provided in the impairment section on anemia (also see Table 9-2).

Class 3
31%-70% Impairment of the Whole Person

Moderate to marked symptoms

and

hemoglobin 5-8 g/dL

and

transfusions of 2-3 U required every 4-6 weeks

Example 9-8
31% to 70% Impairment Due to Primary Myelofibrosis

Subject: 55-year-old woman.

History: 2-year history of progressive fatigue, abdominal fullness, early satiety, and a 4.5-kg (10-lb) weight loss in the past 6 months.

Current Symptoms: Weakness; night sweats; tender, full feeling in abdomen.

Physical Exam: Evidence of protein wasting. Spleen 8 cm beneath left costal margin.

Clinical Studies: Hemoglobin: 80 g/L (8.0 g/dL). Hematocrit: 0.24 Proportion of 1.0 (24%). White blood cell count: 12.0×10^9/L (12,000 10^3/µL) with shift to left of granulocytes, nucleated red blood cells, and abnormal platelets. Platelet count: 450×10^9/L (450×10^3/µL). Uric acid: 0.54 µmol/L (9.0 mg/dL). Bone marrow: dry aspirate. Myelofibrosis on section.

Diagnosis: Primary myelofibrosis (agnogenic myeloid metaplasia).

Impairment Rating: 50% to 60% impairment of the whole person.

Comment: Clinical symptoms and limitations in function parallel the degree of anemia; the presence of symptomatic splenomegaly and the irreversibility of this condition warrant a higher impairment rating.

9.4 White Blood Cell Diseases or Abnormalities

The primary function of white blood cells (leukocytes) is providing protection against invading microorganisms, foreign proteins, and other materials. Three separate white blood cell "families"—granulocytes, lymphocytes, and monocytes-macrophages—interact to provide this protection. Each white blood cell family has a fixed tissue component that provides the renewal or precursor pool and also functions at fixed sites, including the bone marrow, spleen, and lymph nodes. Abnormalities in white blood cells are expressed as both numbers and alterations in function.

9.4a Granulocytes

Granulocytes protect against infection through the phagocytosis of invading organisms. They function primarily at the site of tissue invasion; the observation or enumeration of granulocytes in the circulation indicates inflammation or infection. Granulocytes have a brief half-life of approximately 6 hours. The granulocyte precursor pool is in the bone marrow, where a very large production capacity exists.

Abnormal granulocyte function is usually congenital, although acquired functional abnormalities may result from drug use or toxin exposure. Frequent infection is an indicator of defective granulocyte function; infection may vary from localized, self-limited infections such as furunculosis to life-threatening infections such as recurring septicemia. Type, frequency, and severity of the recurring infections are the basis for evaluating impairment. An affected individual will have a reasonably consistent infection pattern that facilitates treatment and enables a judgment concerning prognosis.

Two different forms of quantitative granulocyte abnormalities are granulocytopenia and leukemia. Granulocytopenia is characterized by a significant decrease in the total number of granulocytes in the blood. Significant infections due to low numbers are uncommon, unless the granulocyte count is less than 0.50×10^9/L. Irreversible chronic neutropenia with counts below 0.50×10^9/L is associated with a substantially increased risk of infection; the infection defines impairment.

Two types of leukemia, acute granulocytic leukemia and chronic granulocytic leukemia, result in impaired function of the individual and limited life expectancy, even with currently available therapy. Impairment is based on symptoms, physical findings, requirement for and frequency of therapy, and the ability to carry out activities of daily living.

9.4b Lymphocytes

Lymphocytes provide humoral and cellular defense mechanisms. Circulating lymphocytes originate in lymphoid tissues: the bone marrow, spleen, lymph nodes, and thymus. Lymphocytes circulate between the blood and the tissues. Lymphocyte cells have heterogeneous functions.

Of the two major subgroups, the "T," or thymus-derived, lymphocytes are primarily responsible for cellular immunity and are involved in delayed hypersensitivity reactions and transplant rejection. The "B," or bursa-derived, lymphocytes are primarily responsible for humoral immunity related to the production of immunoglobulins and biologically active kinins. Subtypes of both T and B lymphoctyes have distinct functions and abnormalities that produce distinct clinical syndromes.

Lymphocytes can be abnormal in function and/or number, often leading to recurrent infections. Individuals with Hodgkin's disease or connective tissue diseases and those who have been exposed to ionizing radiation all have acquired functional defects. Some "autoimmune" diseases may be a result of functionally altered or numerically predominant subsets of lymphocytes. Impairment ratings due to abnormal numbers of lymphocytes, as with lymphopenia, are based on the severity of the condition, as indicated by recurrent infection, and a limited ability to perform activities of daily living.

The best documentation of defective lymphocyte function or numbers is to determine failure of end functions like generalized immunoglobulin deficiency or delayed hypersensitivity reaction failure. Lymphocyte abnormalities are associated with three forms of neoplastic transformation: (1) leukemias (including chronic lymphatic leukemia, chronic myelogenous leukemia, acute lymphatic leukemia, and hairy cell leukemia)[4]; (2) lymphomas (including Hodgkin's disease, non-Hodgkin's lymphoma, and mycosis fungoides); and (3) multiple myeloma and macroglobulinemia.

Chronic lymphatic leukemia, hairy cell leukemia, and some low-grade lymphomas may be relatively indolent, require no initial therapy unless severe and irreversible, and constitute no impairment for several years. Similarly, multiple myeloma and macroglobulinemia may be asymptomatic initially, manifested only by certain laboratory abnormalities, and constitute no impairment. However, some individuals have a high level of impairment because of recurrent GI tract bleeding. Impairment may be related to developing anemia, the need for chemotherapy or radiation to enlarging lymph nodes, or, in the case of multiple myeloma, bone pain. See Chapters 6, The Digestive System; 16, The Upper Extremities; 17, The Lower Extremities; and 18, Pain, for more information about intestinal bleeding and bone pain.

Human immunodeficiency virus (HIV) infection creates a progressive and ultimately fatal disease process with a complex course and widely variable degrees of functional impairment. HIV can directly destroy CD4T lymphocytes, resulting in impairment of the normal immune response against infection and neoplastic processes. The risk of developing opportunistic infection is, in general, inversely related to the absolute CD4 count.[5, 6]

HIV infection impairment is caused by single- or multiple-organ system involvement from primary HIV infection or the opportunistic infection or neoplastic process from immunologic dysfunction. Essentially, every organ system can be affected, including hematologic, pulmonary, gastrointestinal, neurologic, dermatologic, and renal. Several systems are often simultaneously affected, adding to the complexity of impairment determination.

Acute retroviral syndrome may develop early in HIV infection; symptoms include fever, fatigue, pharyngitis, rash, myalgia, and arthralgia. Quantitative HIV RNA measurements also indicate the extent of HIV infection. Early stages are characterized by a CD4 count greater than 0.50×10^9/L (500 cells/mm^3); individuals are often asymptomatic but may have lymphadenopathy, leukopenia, thrombocytopenia, and dermatologic conditions. Intermediate stages have CD4 counts of 0.20×10^9/L to 0.50×10^9/L (200-500 cells/mm^3); antiretroviral therapy is often initiated to prolong this stage of disease. Individuals may have few or no symptoms or may develop constitutional symptoms, diarrhea, herpes simplex infection, oral or vaginal candidiasis, upper respiratory tract infection, sinusitis, or common bacterial infection. Advanced stages, often defined by CD4 counts less than 0.20×10^9/L (200 cells/mm^3), are associated with an increased incidence of opportunistic infection and meet the Centers for Disease Control and Prevention (CDC) definition for acquired immunodeficiency syndrome (AIDS). At low CD4 level, there is increased incidence of complications, including *Pneumocystis carinii* pneumonia (PCP); *Toxoplasma gondii* encephalitis; tuberculosis; cryptosporidiosis salmonellosis; esophageal candidiasis; neoplasms including Kaposi's sarcoma, lymphoma, and cervical cancer; and neurologic dysfunction, such as mononeuritis multiplex, peripheral neuropathies, cranial nerve palsies, and myelitis. At CD4 levels below 0.10×10^9/L (100 cells mm³), the following are more common: HIV-associated dementia, wasting syndromes, progressive multifocal leukoencephalopathy, cytomegalovirus (CMV) retinitis, disseminated *Mycobacterium avium* complex (MAC), cryptococcal meningitis, disseminated coccidiomycosis, histoplasmosis, and invasive aspergillosis.

The degree of symptomatic involvement and the course of illness in individuals with the same CD4 cell-defined stages varies significantly. Functional impairment can also develop from toxicity responses to antiretroviral treatments, including reverse transcriptase inhibitors; viral protease enzyme inhibitors; and antibacterial, antiviral, antifungal, and antineoplastic therapy. Determine total impairment only after careful assessment of each of the potentially affected organ systems. Also consider the nature and severity of the primary or secondary infections or neoplastic processes. If several organ systems are involved in the HIV infection process, the whole person impairment percentages related to the involved systems are combined using the Combined Values Chart (see p. 604).

9.4c Monocytes-Macrophages

The monocyte-macrophage family ingests foreign proteins, removes cellular debris, particulates material, and modulates immune responses. This functional unit of circulating monocytes and fixed macrophages, "histiocytes," is structurally associated with endothelial cells and fibroblasts in the reticuloendothelial system. This system is recognized primarily by the phagocytic capacity of monocytes and macrophages.

Knowledge about functional defects in the monocyte-macrophage system is limited. The degree of impairment can be associated with the nature, type, and extent of infection. Lipid storage disease is another abnormality in which macrophages become repositories for lipids, and cellular and organ hyperplasia occurs in the spleen, lymph nodes, and

bone marrow. Marrow involvement can produce progressive and massive bone abnormalities and fractures; impairment focuses on the degree of orthopedic deficit.

Neurologic involvement also occurs in some severe forms of lipid storage disease. Enzyme replacement therapy is now available for Gaucher disease, one of the most common types of lipid storage disease. This therapy is incredibly effective at reversing most abnormalities except for neurologic deficit. Impairment depends on the nature of the lipid, rate of deposition, and primarily affected organs.

Neoplastic transformation occurs primarily as acute monocytic leukemia, a relatively rare form of leukemia. Leukemic reticuloendotheliosis is a more chronic variant. The exact cell of origin is not clear, but the condition behaves as a form of chronic neoplastic transformation.

9.4d The Spleen and Splenectomy

A normal spleen cleanses the blood of bacteria and other foreign matter. Splenectomy removes a quarter of the total lymphoid tissue and the major mass of macrophages. As a consequence of splenectomy, some functional abnormalities may develop. These include impaired clearance of certain encapsulated bacteria, such as the pneumococcus. Occasionally, individuals develop overwhelming infections after splenectomy. This occurs in fewer than 2% of people from whom the organ has been removed and is confined mostly to the first 2 years after the operation. The incidence is greatly reduced by prophylactic administration of the polyvalent pneumococcal vaccine. Splenectomy leads to some subtle, albeit clinically silent, morphologic abnormalities of red blood cells and a slight elevation of the platelet count. Splenectomized individuals are not at an increased risk for viral or other infections from nonencapsulated bacteria.

9.4e Criteria for Rating Permanent Impairment Due to White Blood Cell Disease

The impairment criteria for white blood cell disease are given in Table 9-3.

Table 9-3 Criteria for Rating Permanent Impairment Due to White Blood Cell Disease

Class 1 0%-15% Impairment of the Whole Person	Class 2 16%-30% Impairment of the Whole Person	Class 3 31%-55% Impairment of the Whole Person	Class 4 56%-100% Impairment of the Whole Person
Symptoms or signs of leukocyte abnormality *and* needs no or infrequent treatment *and* performs all or most daily activities	Symptoms and signs of leuko-cyte abnormality *and* performs most daily activities, although requires continuous treatment	Requires continuous treatment *and* interference with the ability to perform daily activities; requires occasional assistance from others	Symptoms and signs of leuko-cyte abnormality *and* requires continuous treatment *and* experiences difficulty in perform-ing activities of daily living; requires continuous care from others

---

Class 1
0%-15% Impairment of the Whole Person

Symptoms or signs of leukocyte abnormality

and

needs no or infrequent treatment

and

performs all or most daily activities

Example 9-9
0% to 15% Impairment Due to White Blood Cell Disease

Subject: 21-year-old man.

History: Ruptured spleen in automobile accident. Splenectomy; uneventful postoperative course. Returned to all daily activities in 2 months. Evaluation 8 months after hospital discharge.

Current Symptoms: None.

Physical Exam: Left upper quadrant well-healed scar; otherwise, exam normal.

Clinical Studies: Elevated white blood cell count: $10.0\text{-}18.0 \times 10^9/L$ ($10,000\text{-}18,000 \times 10^3/\mu L$),

Diagnosis: Status postsplenectomy for splenic rupture.

Impairment Rating: 0% impairment of the whole person.

Comment: Postsplenectomy blood changes are not associated with symptoms or any change in the ability to perform activities of daily living. A slight increase in the risk of systemic infection for selected organisms does exist. If the individual experiences repeat infections, the impairment rat-ing should be reevaluated.

Example 9-10
0% to 15% Impairment Due to HIV Infection

Subject: 30-year-old man.

History: Tested for HIV infection because of sexual contact with individual with risk factors for HIV.

Current Symptoms: None.

Physical Exam: Generalized lymphadenopathy.

Clinical Studies: HIV enzyme immunoassay: posi-tive. Western blot: positive. HIV RNA: 5000 copies/mL of plasma. CD4: $0.70 \times 10^9/L$ ($700/mm^3$).

Diagnosis: Asymptomatic HIV infection.

Impairment Rating: 5% to 15% impairment of the whole person.

Comment: Treatment of an asymptomatic HIV-infected individual with a low viral load and high CD4 count is controversial. Current guidelines suggest withholding therapy.

Class 2	Class 3
16%-30% Impairment of the Whole Person	**31%-55% Impairment of the Whole Person**
Symptoms and signs of leukocyte abnormality	Requires continuous treatment
and	*and*
performs most daily activities, although requires continuous treatment	interference with the ability to perform daily activities; requires occasional assistance from others

Example 9-11
16% to 30% Impairment Due to Chronic Granulocytic Leukemia

Subject: 40-year-old man.

History: Pain, tightness in left upper abdominal quadrant. Leukocytes 150.0×10^9/L.

Current Symptoms: None. In remission for 6 months.

Physical Exam: 3.6-kg (8-lb) weight loss. Splenomegaly; spleen extended 12 cm below left costal margin. Posttreatment, spleen extended 4 cm below costal margin.

Clinical Studies: Leukocytes: 150.0×10^9/L (150.0×10^3/μL); many myelocytes and progranulocytes.

Diagnosis: Chronic granulocytic leukemia.

Impairment Rating: 15% impairment of the whole person.

Comment: Remission with daily medication; periodic dosage adjustment.

Example 9-12
16% to 30% Impairment Due to HIV Infection

Subject: 30-year-old man.

History: Known to be HIV infected.

Current Symptoms: Asymptomatic; dismayed about condition and medication regimen; feels well generally.

Physical Exam: Diffuse lymphadenopathy.

Clinical Studies: CD4: 0.35×10^9/L (350/mm³). HIV RNA: 45,000 copies/mL of plasma.

Diagnosis: Asymptomatic, moderately advanced HIV infection.

Impairment Rating: 16% to 30% of the whole person.

Comment: All authorities agree that an individual with CD4 cell counts and viral load in these ranges should receive antiretroviral therapy.

Example 9-13
31% to 55% Impairment Due to White Blood Cell Disease

Subject: 55-year-old woman.

History: Progressive weakness, easily fatigued, dyspnea on exertion for 6 months.

Current Symptoms: Decreased appetite; sleeps often.

Physical Exam: Pallor, lymphadenopathy, and an enlarged spleen.

Clinical Studies: Hemoglobin: 700 g/L (7.0 g/dL); hematocit: 0.21 Proportion of 1.0 (21%); leukocytes: 82.0×10^9/L (82.0×10^3/μL); with 0.96 Proportion of 1.00 (96%) lymphocytes: reticulocytes: 0.130 proportion of red blood cells (13% of red blood cells). Positive direct antiglobulin (Coombs') test.

Diagnosis: Chronic lymphocytic leukemia with autoimmune hemolytic anemia.

Impairment Rating: 40% impairment of the whole person.

Comment: Anemia and some of the related symptoms will respond to steroid therapy. The underlying leukemia can generally be controlled with chemotherapy for 3 to 7 years.

Example 9-14
31% to 55% Impairment Due to Hodgkin's Disease

Subject: 28-year-old man.

History: Initial response to ionizing radiation. Pruritus, chills, and fever.

Current Symptoms: Profound weakness due to anemia that temporarily responded to drug treatment and transfusions.

Physical Exam: Lymphadenopathy below and above diaphragm.

Clinical Studies: Lymph nodes biopsy: showed Hodgkin's disease.

Diagnosis: Recurrent, active Hodgkin's disease.

Impairment Rating: 50% impairment due to advanced Hodgkin's disease.

Comment: Combine with appropriate impairment percentage for anemia (see Combined Values Chart, p. 604) for whole person impairment.

Example 9-15
31% to 55% Impairment Due to Acquired Immunodeficiency Syndrome

Subject: 30-year-old man.

History: Known to be HIV infected. Has consistently refused to take antiretroviral therapy.

Current Symptoms: Complains of weight loss, intermittent temperature elevation, and night sweats.

Physical Exam: Thrush; generalized lymphadenopathy.

Clinical Studies: CD4: 0.11×10^9/L (110/mm³). HIV RNA: 146,000 copies/mL of plasma.

Diagnosis: Acquired immunodeficiency syndrome.

Impairment Rating: 31% to 50% impairment of the whole person.

Comment: Individual should be urged to begin highly active antiretroviral therapy. In addition, prophylaxis to prevent *Pneumocystis carinii* pneumonia should be initiated.

Class 4
56%-100% Impairment of the Whole Person
Symptoms and signs of leukocyte abnormality
and
requires continuous treatment
and
experiences difficulty in performing activities of daily living; requires continuous care from others

Example 9-16
56% to 100% Impairment Due to Acute Leukemia

Subject: 55-year-old man.

History: Profound weakness, chills, night sweats, and fever for 10 months.

Current Symptoms: Relatively stable 6 months later.

Physical Exam: Gingival hypertrophy, nosebleeds. Splenomegaly; spleen extended 4 cm below costal margin; ecchymoses.

Clinical Studies: Hematologic values: hemoglobin 400 g/L (40 g/dL); white blood cell count: 12.0×10^9/L ($12,000 \times 10^3$/μL), 80% blast forms; platelets: 18.0×10^9/L (18.0×10^3/μL).

Diagnosis: Acute leukemia.

Impairment Rating: 90% impairment of the whole person.

Comment: Partial response to treatment. Continuous observation, frequent blood transfusions, and continuing assistance with daily activities required.

Example 9-17
56% to 100% Impairment Due to Acquired Immunodeficiency Syndrome

Subject: 30-year-old man.

History: Has received multiple combinations of antiretroviral therapy over preceding 4 years.

Current Symptoms: Has diarrhea, anorexia, nausea, and persistent oral thrush; very weak.

Physical Exam: Has lost more than 10% of normal body weight; oral thrush; lymphadenopathy.

Clinical Studies: CD4: 0.02×10^9/L (20/mm³). HIV RNA: 1,200,000 copies/mL of plasma.

Diagnosis: Acquired immunodeficiency syndrome.

Impairment Rating: 90% impairment of the whole person.

Comment: Individual has far advanced HIV/AIDS, having failed currently available antiretroviral therapy. Emphasis should be placed upon maintaining prophylaxis against complicating infections. Consideration should be given to entering into a palliative care program for management of terminal illness.

9.5 Hemorrhagic and Platelet Disorders

Hemorrhagic disorders include coagulation disorders and platelet disease. Thrombocytopenia is not rated for impairment unless it is severe, affects function, and is irreversible by steroids, splenectomy, or other therapeutic regimens. Qualitative platelet defects rarely meet criteria for impairment rating unless there is serious bleeding, which also may occur in some rare congenital disorders. Von Willebrand's disease is frequently mild; bleeding occurs only after trauma or surgery. It does not affect function significantly enough to warrant an impairment rating. However, some individuals meet criteria for significant impairment rating because of recurrent GI tract bleeding.[7-10]

Hemorrhagic disorders are either congenital or acquired. In most hereditary disorders, the basic hemostatic defect remains unchanged throughout the individual's life. People with hereditary blood coagulation disorders may require prophylactic therapy to help them perform activities they might otherwise avoid because of the threat of trauma. To control bleeding many may require frequent home treatment, which interferes with daily activity. Impairment ratings vary depending on the frequency of treatment, and the extent of interference with normal activity. (see Table 9-4).

Inherited bleeding disorders may cause complications such as joint dysfunction from recurrent hemorrhaging. Impairment due to this complication is evaluated with criteria found in Chapter 16, The Upper Extremities, and Chapter 17, The Lower Extremities. If several organ systems are impaired, the whole person impairment percents are combined (see Combined Values Chart, p. 604).

Autoimmune thrombocytopenia may require long-term immunosuppressives, which can lead to dysfunction of several organ systems and can hamper daily activity. Complications are evaluated according to the criteria of the affected body system or organ and combined with the impairment percentage for the appropriate blood platelet disorder (see the Combined Values Chart, p. 604).

Acquired blood-clotting defects are usually secondary to severe underlying conditions, such as chronic liver disease. Individuals with venous or arterial thromboembolic disease who receive anticoagulant therapy with a vitamin K antagonist (eg, warfarin sodium) should avoid activities that might lead to trauma. Impairment of the whole person with acquired blood-clotting defects is estimated at 0% to 10%.

9.5a Criteria for Rating Permanent Impairment Due to Hemorrhagic and Platelet Disorders

The impairment criteria for hemorrhagic and platelet disorders are given in Table 9-4.

Table 9-4 Criteria for Rating Permanent Impairment Due to Hemorrhagic and Platelet Disorders

Class 1 0%-15% Impairment of the Whole Person	Class 2 16%-30% Impairment of the Whole Person	Class 3 31%-55% Impairment of the Whole Person	Class 4 56%-100% Impairment of the Whole Person
Symptoms or signs of hemorrhagic and platelet abnormality **and** needs no or infrequent treatment **and** performs all or most daily activities	Symptoms and signs of hemorrhagic and platelet abnormality **and** performs daily activities with continuous treatment	Symptoms and signs of hemorrhagic and platelet abnormality **and** requires continuous treatment **and** interference with daily activities; requires occasional assistance	Symptoms and signs of hemorrhagic and platelet abnormality **and** requires continuous treatment **and** difficulty performing daily activities; requires continuous care

Class 1
0%-15% Impairment of the Whole Person
Symptoms or signs of hemorrhagic and platelet abnormality
and
needs no or infrequent treatment
and
performs all or most daily activities

Class 2
16%-30% Impairment of the Whole Person
Symptoms and signs of hemorrhagic and platelet abnormality
and
performs daily activities with continuous treatment

Example 9-18
0% to 15% Impairment Due to Platelet Disorders

Subject: 49-year-old woman.

History: 5 years' chronic idiopathic autoimmune thrombocytopenia. Splenectomy; corticosteroids and other immunosuppressive drugs for 4 years.

Current Symptoms: No medication. No significant bleeding problem. Chronic low-back pain, which interferes with daily activities.

Physical Exam: Minor bruising. Severe osteoporosis; T12 and L1 compression fractures.

Clinical Studies: Platelets: 30.0×10^9/L (30.0×10^3/μL).

Diagnosis: Chronic idiopathic autoimmune thrombocytopenic purpura.

Impairment Rating: 0% impairment for the underlying bleeding disorder. Combine with appropriate impairment estimate for vertebral fractures and osteoporosis (see Combined Values Chart, p. 604) to determine whole person impairment.

Comment: Current platelet counts are not associated with symptoms. However, she has a slight increased risk of bleeding with surgical procedures. The thrombocytopenia may worsen intermittently (especially with infections) and may require periodic therapeutic intervention.

Example 9-19
16% to 30% Impairment Due to Platelet Disorders

Subject: 18-year-old woman.

History: Lifelong history of low platelets, congenital; requires one to two platelet transfusions per month; on prednisone last several years to reduce transfusion need. Does not participate in vigorous sports for fear of further bruising.

Current Symptoms: Bruises easily; multiple ecchymoses on extremities. Heavy and prolonged menstrual periods.

Physical Exam: Ecchymoses on extremities. Abnormal radii bilaterally; good hand function.

Clinical Studies: Platelets: 8.0×10^9/L (8.0×10^3/μL).

Diagnosis: Amegakaryocytic thrombocytopenic purpura with absent radii syndrome.

Impairment Rating: 30% impairment of the whole person.

Comment: Requirements for prednisone; limitations in performance of vigorous daily activities. Likely future problems as she will probably become resistant to the platelet transfusions.

Class 3
31%-55% Impairment of the Whole Person
Symptoms and signs of hemorrhagic and platelet abnormality
and
requires continuous treatment
and
interference with daily activities; requires occasional assistance

Class 4
56%-95% Impairment of the Whole Person
Symptoms and signs of hemorrhagic and platelet abnormality
and
requires continuous treatment
and
difficulty performing daily activities; requires continuous care

Example 9-20
31% to 55% Impairment Due to Platelet Disorders

Subject: 21-year-old man.

History: Severe factor VIII deficiency (hemophilia A). Frequent spontaneous bleeding into large joints and muscles. Home therapy with intravenous factor VIII concentrate two times per week. Significant chronic dysfunction of left knee, right ankle, and both elbows due to past joint bleeding.

Current Symptoms: Frequent joint, muscle hemorrhages; continuous treatment interferes with performance of usual daily activities.

Physical Exam: Severely restricted range of motion in left knee, right ankle, and both elbows. Joint swelling of knee and ankle.

Clinical Studies: Hemoglobin: 120 g/L (12.0 g/dL). Factor VIII level: 0.001 Proportion of 1.0 (1%); antibodies to factor VIII: not present. aPTT: 120 seconds. X-rays of joints reveal fluid and hypertrophic changes. HIV negative.

Diagnosis: Severe hemophilia A with permanent joint dysfunction secondary to recurrent bleeding.

Impairment Rating: 40% impairment for underlying bleeding disorder; combine with joint impairment (see Combined Values Chart, p. 604) for whole person impairment.

Comment: Control of bleeding episodes with factor VIII replacement will decrease subsequent bony changes. Joint replacement surgery can improve function in specific sites of impairment.

Example 9-21
56% to 95% Impairment Due to Hemorrhagic Disorders

Subject: 58-year-old man.

History: Gastrointestinal bleeding 30 years ago; endoscopy indicated hemorrhagic telangiectasia through the stomach and small intestine. Requires 2 to 6 U packed red blood cells per month; receives IV iron at least once per week.

Current Symptoms: Weakness and fatigue. Black, tarry stools almost daily. Two to three nosebleeds per week.

Physical Exam: Telangiectasias of lips, nasal, and oral mucosa, some of which are friable. Similar but few lesions on the upper trunk.

Clinical Studies: Hemoglobin: 80 g/L (8 g/dL), raised to 100 g/L (10 g/dL) after 3 U of packed red blood cells. Serum iron: 2.1 µmol/L (12 µg/dL), with iron-binding capacity of 75.2 µmol/L (420 µg/dL). Serum ferritin: 5 µg/L (5 ng/mL).

Diagnosis: Hereditary hemorrhagic telangiectasia (Osler-Weber-Rondu syndrome) with severe iron deficiency.

Impairment Rating: 75% impairment of the whole person.

Comment: Significant changes in lifestyle and poor prognosis warrant this impairment rating.

9.5b Myelodysplastic Syndromes

Myelodysplasia of hematopoietic precursors is more frequently recognized after age 50. It occurs as a primary (idiopathic) or secondary form, commonly after exposure to a wide variety of industrial chemicals or after cytoreductive chemotherapy or radiation therapy for neoplastic disease. Causative factors include several drugs, particularly topoisomerase inhibitors and platinum derivatives. The principal primary or secondary hematopoietic changes are defective and decreased cellular proliferation and production. Cell line (red cells, white cells, and platelets) involvement and progression are variable. (For more information, refer to Tables 9-2, 9-3, and 9-4 for rating impairment due to anemia, granulocytopenia, and thrombocytopenia.) Eventually, all cell lines become involved; at least one third of patients progress to a leukemic transformation. For unknown reasons, myelodysplasia sufferers have more constitutional symptoms than expected for peripheral hematologic value levels. Because of its long stable period, myelodysplasia impairment evaluation is combined with the degree of individual component alteration.

9.6 Thrombotic Disorders

Thrombotic disorders involve arteries, veins, or both. Thrombosis may be either primary due to inherited disorder or secondary due to acquired conditions. While each risk factor may contribute to thrombosis, combined factors may lead to a greater risk.[11]

9.6a Inherited Thrombotic Disorders

Known defects include: proteins C, S, and antithrombin III deficiency; defective protein due to mutation associated with venous thrombosis (eg, factor V Leiden and prothrombin 20210A); and increased homocysteine levels due to cystathionine B-synthase deficiency (hyperhomocysteinemia can cause atherosclerosis and thrombosis of the arteries and sometimes of the veins). Seventy percent of individuals with thrombosis have one or more of the above abnormalities; the most common is factor V Leiden mutation.

Clinical indications of congenital thrombotic abnormality include: family history; occurrence at an early age; recurrence; and occurrence at unusual sites (eg, mesenteric, portal, splenic, renal, cerebral, or retinal veins).

9.6b Acquired Thrombotic Disorders

Acquired thrombotic conditions associated with venous thrombosis include: antiphospholipid antibody syndrome (found in some arterial thrombosis, particularly stroke, patients), malignancy, drugs (oral contraceptives), immobility, postoperative phase, multiple trauma, and pregnancy. The acute phase of venous thrombosis is usually treated with heparin, then oral anticoagulation for 3 to 6 months. Individuals with a greater risk of thrombosis require temporary (postsurgery) to lifelong (prophylaxis for inherited thrombotic disorder and recurrent thrombosis) anticoagulation therapy. Hyperhomocysteinemia can be controlled with high doses of folates; arterial thrombosis is treated according to the system involved.

Thrombotic disorder impairment results from systematic complications following thrombosis and anticoagulation regimen. It depends on the type, site, and extent of the organ involvement, as well as the response and complications of anticoagulation. Arterial thrombi may produce ischemic heart disease, stroke, or intermittent claudication. Venous thrombosis usually resolves with no aftereffects. If unresolved, postthrombosis syndrome may develop due to vein lumen narrowing and/or venous valve insufficiency, causing lower extremity edema, venous ulceration, venous thrombosis recurrence, and ambulation limitation.

9.6c Criteria for Rating Permanent Impairment Due to Thrombotic Disorders

Impairment is evaluated according to the affected body system. The impairment rating for a thrombotic disorder is based upon the degree of injury to the end organ, such as the lungs, heart, brain, kidney, extremities, etc, and upon how the disorder affects the individual's capacity to perform activities of daily living. For example, a thrombotic disorder causing a stroke would be rated based on the effects of the stroke, as outlined in the nervous system. Long-term anticoagulation with warfarin or low-molecular-weight heparin increases bleeding risk and constitutes impairment in the 10% range. If there is an impairment rating of several organ systems, whole person impairment ratings for each affected system are combined (see the Combined Values Chart, p. 604).

Example 9-22
Impairment Due to Thrombotic Disorder

Subject: 49-year-old woman.

History: At 40 years of age, five left leg deep vein thromboses; two pulmonary embolisms. Father, brother had multiple venous thromboses. Lifelong Coumadin therapy. Five years' oral anticoagulation. Two hemorrhagic episodes: posttrauma knee hematoma, thigh hematoma; international normalized ratio between 5 and 7. Large hemorrhagic skin necrosis twice when international normalized ratio at 4.

Current Symptoms: Left leg postthrombotic syndrome; severe edema with upright position for over 30 minutes. Frequent thrombotic episodes, therapy-induced hemorrhages, and anticoagulation monitoring interfere with work. Lower extremity swelling requires intermittent wheelchair use.

Physical Exam: Edema of left leg to mid-thigh, which increases when in upright position; ecchymosis (and resolving ecchymosis) of arms and legs.

Clinical Studies: Platelet count and aPTT: normal. INR: 2.8. Protein C antigen: 62% of normal.

Diagnosis: Protein C deficiency with recurrent venous thrombosis and postthrombosis syndrome.

Impairment Rating: 30% from underlying hemorrhagic and thrombotic disorder and anticoagulation complications; 20% from lower extremity condition; combine for whole person impairment (see Combined Values Chart, p. 604).

9.7 Hematologic Impairment Evaluation Summary

Table 9-5 gives an evaluation summary for the assessemnt of hematologic impairment.

Table 9-5 Hematologic Impairment Evaluation Summary

Disorder	History, Including Selected Relevant Symptoms	Examination Record	Assessment of Hematologic Function
General	Symptoms of end-organ impairment, eg, cardiovascular (eg, fatigue, palpitations, chest pain); respiratory (eg, shortness of breath); infections; general symptoms Impact of symptoms on function and ability to do daily activities Prognosis if change anticipated Review medical history	Comprehensive physical examination with focus on affected end-organ systems assessment	Data derived from relevant studies: complete blood counts, serology testing, biopsies of bone, lymph nodes
Red Blood Cell	Symptoms (eg, shortness of breath on exertion, dizziness, throbbing headaches, fatigue) Resulting limitation of physical activity or complications (eg, angina)	Other organ dysfunction (eg, brain, heart, kidneys)	Complete blood count, hemoglobin electrophoresis, etc
White Blood Cell	Fatigue, frequent infections, etc	Detailed history (ie, infections)	Complete blood count, etc
Platelet	Abnormal bleeding from gums, mouth, GI tract, urinary tract Poor hemostasis with trauma Family history of abnormal clotting	Epistaxis; petechiae; purpura; occult fecal blood; splenomegaly; evidence of thrombosis	Complete blood count with platelet count; bleeding time; relevant platelet aggregation studies (prothrombin and partial thromboplastin time to rule out other coagulation disorders)
Bleeding	Excessive bruising Prolonged spontaneous, traumatic bleeding From birth or acquired disorder Family history of bleeding disorder Muscle or joint pain or swelling	Hematoma; joint or muscle swelling; easy bruisability	Complete blood count with platelet count; bleeding time; prothrombin and partial thromboplastin time; fibrinogen factor levels

References

1. Rockey DC. The beta-thalassemias. *N Engl J Med.* 1999;341:99-109.

   Review.

2. Steinberg MH, et al. Management of sickle cell disease. *N Engl J Med.* 1999;340:1021-1030.

   Review.

3. Goodnough LT, et al. The pathophysiology of acquired aplastic anemia. *N Engl J Med.* 1997;336:1365-1372.

   Review.

4. Anaissie EJ, et al. Chronic myelogenous leukemia: biology and therapy. *Ann Intern Med.* 1999;131:207-219.

   Review.

5. Flexner C. Acute human immunodeficiency virus type 1 infection. *N Engl J Med.* 1998;339:33-39.

   Review.

6. Society of General Internal Medicine AIDS Task Force. Optimizing care for persons with HIV infection. *Ann Intern Med.* 1999;131:136-143.

   Review.

End-Organ Damage	Diagnosis(es)	Degree of Impairment
Include assessment of sequelae, including end-organ damage and impairment	Record all pertinent diagnosis(es); note if they are at maximal medical improvement; if not, discuss under what conditions and when stability is expected	Criteria outlined in this chapter
Assess relevant organs (eg, heart, lungs, kidneys) for congestion or dysfunction	Anemias; sickle cell; hemolysis; chronic disease; polycythemias	See Table 9-2
Assess relevant organs (eg, heart, lungs, kidneys, lymph nodes)	Leukemia; lymphoma	See Table 9-3
Due to hemorrhage	Immune thrombocytopenic purpura (ITP); HIV or drug-associated thrombocytopenia; thrombotic thrombocytopenia (TTP); myelodysplasia; leukemia; platelet functional disorder; essential thrombocythemia	See Table 9-4
Due to hemorrhage, hemarthrosis, or nerve impingement	Hemophilia; factor deficiency; Von Willebrand's disease; dysfibinogenimia; disseminated intravascular coagulation	See Table 9-4

7. Therapy for adults with refractory chronic immune thrombocytopenic purpura. *Ann Intern Med.* 1997;126:307-314.

Review.

8. George JN, et al. Chronic idiopathic thrombocytopenic purpura. *N Engl J Med.* 1994;331:1207-1211.

Review. No abstract available.

9. Levi M, et al. Disseminated intravascular coagulation. *N Engl J Med.* 1999;341:586-592.

Review. No abstract available.

10. Hoyer LW. Hemophilia A. *N Engl J Med.* 1994;330:38-47.

Review.

11. Rich S, et al. The hypercoagulable states. *Ann Intern Med.* 1985;102:814-828..

Review.

Bibliography

Colman RW, Hirsh J, Marder VJ, Salzman EW. *Hemostasis and Thrombosis: Basic Principles and Clinical Practice*. 3rd ed. Philadelphia, Pa: JB Lippincott; 1994.

Hoffmann R, Benz EJ Jr, Shattil SJ, Furie B, Cohen HJ, Silberstein LF. *Hematology: Basic Principles and Practice*. 2nd ed. New York, NY: Churchill Livingstone; 1995.

Chapter 10

The Endocrine System

Introduction

This chapter provides criteria for evaluating permanent impairment of the endocrine system. The endocrine system is composed of the hypothalmic-pituitary complex, thyroid, parathyroids, adrenals, islet cell tissue of the pancreas, and gonads. These ductless glands secrete hormones that regulate the activity of organs or tissues of the body. These hormones control growth, bone structure, sexual development and function, metabolism, and electrolyte balance. The various endocrine glands are usually interdependent, and a disorder of one gland may be reflected by dysfunction in one or more of the other endocrine glands, which, in turn, may affect other body systems. Consider multiple system effects when an endocrine permanent impairment is identified.

The following revisions have been made for the fifth edition: (1) the descriptions of endocrine gland function and of disease states have been updated, as well as the techniques for evaluation of these diseases; (2) the nomenclature of test procedures and of disease entities, such as diabetes mellitus, has been updated; and (3) although the criteria for percentage of impairment have remained the same, many more examples of impairment have been included.

10.1 Principles of Assessment

Before using the information in this chapter, the *Guides* user should become familiar with Chapters 1 and 2 and the Glossary. Chapters 1 and 2 discuss the *Guides'* purpose, applications, and methods of performing and reporting impairment evaluations. The Glossary provides definitions of common terms used by many specialties in impairment evaluations.

Dysfunction of an endocrine organ may be the result of an injury to the gland or of disease involving atrophy, hypertrophy, hyperplasia, or neoplasia. An endocrine impairment develops from altered hormone secretion by one or more endocrine glands and the effect of such hormonal aberration on non-endocrine tissue. An impairment rating reflects the severity of the medical condition, the need for medication, and the effects of the impairment on the individual's ability to perform activities of daily living.

When an endocrine disorder results in decreased secretion of a hormone, it is usually possible to replace the hormone by either the oral or the parenteral route, resulting in virtual normalization of body physiology except, of course, for the inability to secrete the hormone. Apart from the need to take the medication on an ongoing basis, decreased secretion alone does not warrant an impairment rating. In cases where the replacement hormone does not completely mimic physiologic hormone secretion, however, the individual may be given an impairment rating to reflect the change in terms of either normal activity or ability to respond to stress.

Endocrine deficiencies may cause or be associated with impairments of other organ systems. Impairment ratings in other body systems are evaluated separately and then combined with the impairment rating from this chapter, using the Combined Values Chart (p. 604) to determine the estimated whole person impairment.

Disorders resulting in increased secretion of a hormone often can be effectively treated. In some cases, treatment may leave the individual with a reduced ability to secrete the hormone. If so, the severity of the resulting condition and the effect on the ability to perform activities of daily living are evaluated to determine the impairment rating.

As stated in Chapter 2, even with appropriate medication, it is debatable whether the individual has regained the previous status of good health. Thus, the examiner may increase the impairment rating by a small percentage (1% to 3%) to account for an incomplete return to a condition of normal health.

10.1a Interpretation of Symptoms and Signs

The endocrine system has a wide array of glands, each with specific symptoms; these symptoms are discussed in each gland section.

10.1b Description of Clinical Studies

Clinical studies for the endocrine system generally assess hyperfunction (increased) or hypofunction (decreased) of a specific gland and are discussed in detail in each section.

10.2 Hypothalamic-Pituitary Axis

The hypothalamus and the pituitary are regarded as a unit because of their interdependent function. The hypothalamus produces chemical factors that either inhibit or enhance production of anterior pituitary **hormones.** The hypothalamus also produces precursors (prohormones) of antidiuretic hormone (ADH) and oxytocin, which travel through neural axons and are stored in the posterior pituitary.

The anterior lobe of the pituitary gland, with modulation by the hypothalamus, produces trophic hormones that control the activity of the thyroid gland (thyrotropin [TSH]), the adrenal gland (corticotropin [ACTH]), and the gonads (luteinizing hormone [LH] and follicle-stimulating hormone [FSH]). The production of growth hormone (GH) and prolactin (PRL) in the anterior lobe of the pituitary gland is also modulated by hypothalamic substances. These two hormones, however, exert their effects directly upon the tissues of the body rather than through stimulation of other hormones. Growth hormone is responsible for growth of the skeleton before epiphyseal closure and, in the adult, maintains normal fat, muscle, glucose, and skeletal metabolism, as well as a sense of well-being. For women, prolactin is necessary for lactation following delivery and for milk production in the suckling process. Its role in the male has not been ascertained.

The posterior lobe of the pituitary is an extension of hypothalamic neurons. It is the location where anti-diuretic hormone (vasopressin) and oxytocin are converted from their prohormone state and released into the blood. Antidiuretic hormone regulates the fluid balance of the body through its ability to influence the excretion of water. The actions of oxytocin may have a role in the process of labor.

Permanent impairments due to altered function of the thyroid gland, adrenal glands, gonads, and growth hormone are discussed in subsequent sections of this chapter.

10.2a Interpretation of Symptoms and Signs

Hypothalamic and pituitary diseases can cause impairments through either structural abnormalities or alterations in hormone production. Structural changes resulting in end-organ impairment are considered in the relevant chapter. Visual field abnormalities are considered in Chapter 12, The Visual System. Temporal lobe seizures, frontal lobe abnormalities, obstructive hydrocephalus, and nonendocrine hypothalamic dysfunction are considered in Chapter 13, The Nervous System.

Hypersecretion by the anterior lobe may be manifested by (1) prolactin hypersecretion resulting from a microadenoma or macroadenoma (prolactinoma), (2) growth hormone hypersecretion caused by a pituitary adenoma, or (3) corticotropin hypersecretion leading to adrenocortical hyperfunction. Prolactin excess results in hypogonadism, which in women may lead to amenorrhea or oligomenorrhea, infertility, varying degrees of estrogen deficiency with its detrimental effect on the vascular and skeletal systems, decreased libido, and galactorrhea. In men, it may result in decreased libido, impotence, or infertility. Impairment from prolactin excess is equivalent to gonadotropic deficiency of the appropriate end organ, that is, secondary ovarian failure in women and testicular failure in men. Gonadal failure is discussed further in Section 10.8 of this chapter.

When growth hormone hypersecretion occurs before epiphyseal closure, gigantism results; when hypersecretion occurs in the adult, acromegaly results. The manifestations of acromegaly include enlargement of the hands and feet, coarseness of facial features, and prognathism. Fatigue and increased perspiration are common symptoms. Acromegaly of long duration leads to morbidity from degenerative arthritis, peripheral neuropathy, and shortened life expectancy resulting from an increased incidence of cardiovascular disease. Growth hormone excess may lead to insulin resistance and glucose intolerance, and it may precipitate or exacerbate diabetes mellitus.

Hyposecretion of a single or of multiple anterior lobe hormones is known as hypopituitarism, and the deficiencies may be either partial or complete. In the adult years, pituitary tumors, infarction (especially postpartum infarction), and surgical or radiotherapeutic interventions are the most common causes, with a lower incidence caused by granulomatous and infiltrative diseases and head trauma.

In adults, hypopituitarism most often results in hypogonadism and a deficiency of growth hormone production. The most common symptoms of hypogonadism in men are impotence, weakness, decreased motivation, and depression. The most common presenting symptom of hypogonadism in women is amenorrhea. Growth hormone deficiency is accompanied most often by muscle weakness and reduced exercise capacity, fat accumulation (especially intra-abdominal), decreased bone density, lack of motivation, a poor sense of well-being, and social isolation. Postpartum pituitary infarction also results in an inability to lactate. Hypopituitarism in a person with diabetes mellitus results in decreasing insulin requirements with an increased incidence of hypoglycemic episodes. Effects of dysfunction of TSH and ACTH secretion will be discussed in Sections 10.3 and 10.5, respectively.

Hyperfunction of the posterior lobe, which causes the syndrome of inappropriate antidiuretic hormone secretion (SIADH), may result from a variety of central nervous system disorders; however, SIADH is rarely permanent. Inability of the kidneys to secrete a water load leads to hyponatremia if water intake is not restricted. Fatigue and lethargy, progressing to confusion, coma, and seizures, may result depending on the degree of hyponatremia.

Hypofunction of the posterior lobe results in ADH deficiency and diabetes insipidus. Hypofunction usually stems from diseases involving the hypothalamus or pituitary stalk and, less commonly, from diseases of the pituitary gland itself. The hypofunction may be hereditary, or it may be related to trauma, surgery, metastatic tumors, craniopharyngioma, histiocytosis X, or other conditions. If thirst response is normal, diabetes insipidus is mostly an inconvenience because of polyuria, polydipsia, and nocturia. If the inability to ingest an adequate amount of fluid ensues or if thirst is impaired because of concomitant hypothalamic disease, severe dehydration and hypernatremia may result, leading to central nervous system changes, eg, mental depression or coma.

10.2b Description of Clinical Studies

Structural abnormalities are evaluated by roentgenograms of the sella turcica, computed tomography (CT), and magnetic resonance imaging (MRI). Angiography occasionally is required. Evaluation of visual fields may be needed; vision impairments are discussed in *Guides* Chapter 12, The Visual System.

Hormonal function must be assessed, and this is often done by stimulation or suppression testing. Growth hormone deficiency is assessed by measuring GH in the blood after stimulation testing with insulin, exercise, levodopa, arginine, or other agents. Corticotropin deficiency is assessed by measuring serum corticotropin and cortisol levels and by stimulation testing with insulin or corticotropin-releasing hormone (CRH).

The diagnosis of secondary hypothyroidism (pituitary and hypothalamic hypothyroidism) is made by demonstrating low concentrations of thyroid hormones without elevation of the thyrotropin level. In this circumstance, CT scanning or MRI and tests of pituitary function, including measurement of thyrotropin secretion after an injection of protirelin (TRH), are needed to determine whether the hypothalamus or the pituitary is responsible. Secondary gonadal insufficiency, that is, hypogonadotropic hypogonadism, requires the demonstration of end-organ failure, with low testosterone levels in men and low estrogen levels in women, as well as low or normal levels of the gonadotropins, LH and FSH.

Insufficiency of antidiuretic hormone requires the documentation of urine hyposmolality in the face of a stimulus to concentrate urine, usually water restriction. Subsequently, an increase in urine osmolality in response to ADH administration must be demonstrated. Prolactin deficiency is documented by low basal levels of the hormone and its failure to increase after an injection of TRH, chlorpromazine, or other stimulating agents.

Growth hormone excess is documented by the failure to suppress GH concentration after a glucose load. Prolactin excess is documented by measurement of elevated basal levels of prolactin. Inappropriate secretion of ADH is documented by hyponatremia with inappropriately elevated urine osmolality, in the presence of normal cardiac, renal, adrenal, and thyroid function.

10.2c Criteria for Rating Permanent Impairment Due to Hypothalamic-Pituitary Axis Disorders

The assessment of permanent impairment of the whole person from disorders of the hypothalamic-pituitary axis requires evaluation of (1) primary abnormalities related to GH, prolactin, or ADH; (2) secondary abnormalities in other endocrine glands, such as thyroid, adrenal, and gonads; and (3) structural and functional disorders of the central nervous system caused by anatomic abnormalities of the pituitary.

The examiner must evaluate each disorder separately, using the guidelines in this or other chapters, such as those on the visual system (Chapter 12), nervous system (Chapter 13), or mental and behavioral disorders (Chapter 14). The estimated impairments of the various organ systems then should be combined by means of the Combined Values Chart (p. 604). Criteria for evaluating permanent impairment resulting from hypothalamic-pituitary axis disorders are given in Table 10-1.

Table 10-1 Criteria for Rating Permanent Impairment Due to Hypothalamic-Pituitary Axis Disorders

Class 1 0%-15% Impairment of the Whole Person	Class 2 16%-25% Impairment of the Whole Person	Class 3 26%-50% Impairment of the Whole Person
Disease controlled effectively with continuous treatment, with minimal impact on ability to perform activities of daily living	Related symptoms and signs from disease inadequately controlled by treatment and impact ability to perform activities of daily living	Severe symptoms and signs of disease persist despite treatment and significantly impact ability to perform activities of daily living

Class 1 0%-15% Impairment of the Whole Person
Disease controlled effectively with continuous treatment, with minimal impact on ability to perform activities of daily living

An individual with hypothalamic-pituitary disease belongs in class 1 when the disease can be controlled effectively with continuous treatment, with minimal impact on the ability to perform activities of daily living. If a person does not take the medication, a different degree of impairment may result.

Example 10-1
0% to 15% Impairment Due to Traumatic Diabetes Insipidus

Subject: 19-year-old man.

History: Head trauma from a motor vehicle crash 15 months earlier. Fluid intake and output ranged from 4 to 7 L/d.

Current Symptoms: Severe thirst; increased frequency of urination. Nocturia occurred three to six times, and thirst during the night is marked. General health excellent except for fatigue related to interrupted sleep. Symptoms recur if a dose of desmopressin (DDAVP) is missed. No other endocrine disease found; able to carry out ordinary daily activities.

Physical Exam: Normal.

Clinical Studies: On initial assessment, serum osmolality: 292 mmol/kg H_2O (292 mOsm/kg H_2O); serum sodium concentration: 142 mmol/L (142 mEq/L); urine osmolality: 120 mmol/kg H_2O (120 mOsm/kg H_2O); specific gravity: 1.003. No glycosuria. Attempt at water deprivation led to severe thirst with a serum osmolality of 302 mmol/kg H_2O (302 mOsm/kg H_2O) and urine osmolality of 150 mmol/kg H_2O (150 mOsm/kg H_2O). After an initial antidiuretic hormone (ADH) injection, urine osmolality rose to 450 mmol/kg H_2O (450 mOsm/kg H_2O) and urine volume diminished. Individual was placed on regimen of DDAVP, 0.1 mL (10 µg) twice daily by nasal spray; on this regimen, feels well and urine output is well controlled.

Diagnosis: Traumatic diabetes insipidus controlled by treatment.

Impairment Rating: 5% impairment due to diabetes insipidus; combine with assessment for any additional behavioral effects from the head injury (see *Guides* Chapter 14, Mental and Behavioral Disorders, and the Combined Values Chart, p. 604) to determine whole person impairment.

Comment: Minimal effects on ability to perform activities of daily living when the diabetes insipidus is controlled by treatment.

Class 2 16%-25% Impairment of the Whole Person
Related symptoms and signs from disease inadequately controlled by treatment and impact ability to perform activities of daily living

An individual with hypothalamic-pituitary disease belongs in class 2 when the related symptoms and signs are inadequately controlled by treatment and impact ability to perform activities of daily living.

Example 10-2
16% to 25% Impairment Due to Acromegaly

Subject: 57-year-old man.

History: After treatment of a growth hormone–secreting tumor, headaches were relieved, but symptoms of fatigue, excess perspiration, and joint discomfort continued. Despite an attempt at surgical excision and ionizing radiation therapy, growth hormone (GH) level remained elevated at 4400 pmol/L (100 ng/mL) and individual unable to tolerate bromocriptine therapy. Testosterone level was low, but thyroid and adrenal function remained normal. Libido improved with bimonthly injections of testosterone; carpal tunnel syndrome required surgical therapy.

Current Symptoms: Pain in knees and back; decreased libido.

Physical Exam: Clinical hyperhidrosis; carpal tunnel syndrome; enlargement of hands, feet, and nose.

Clinical Studies: Enlarged sella turcica with suprasellar extension of a pituitary tumor. No visual field abnormalities. GH level: 25 300 pmol/L (575 ng/mL)—markedly elevated.

Diagnosis: Moderately severe acromegaly, inadequately controlled by therapy.

Impairment Rating: 16% impairment due to acromegaly and 5% impairment due to testosterone deficiency combine to 19% impairment of the whole person (see Combined Values Chart, p. 604).

Comment: Combine endocrine impairment with upper extremity impairment from carpal tunnel syndrome.

Example 10-3
16% to 25% Impairment Due to Hypothalamic-Pituitary Axis Disease

Subject: 26-year-old woman.

History: Following a delivery complicated by excessive blood loss and hypotension, failed to lactate; was not seen again until 6 months later.

Current Symptoms: Failure to resume menstrual cyclicity; progressively worsening fatigue, anorexia, and weight loss.

Physical Exam: Blood pressure (BP): 90/60 mm Hg; pulse rate (PR): 100 BPM. Sparse pubic and axillary hair; cool, dry skin; slow return of Achilles' deep tendon reflexes; visual fields: normal.

Clinical Studies: Prolactin and thyrotropin (TSH) levels: low and unresponsive to 500 µg intravenous protirelin (TRH). Follicle-stimulating hormone (FSH) and luteinizing hormone (LH): unresponsive to administration of luteinizing hormone-releasing hormone (LHRH). Attenuated response of cortisol to insulin-induced hypoglycemia and growth hormone unresponsive. Serum free thyroxine: low—7.7 pmol/L (0.6 ng/dL); TSH not elevated—0.2 µIU/L (0.2 µU/mL).

Diagnosis: Postpartum pituitary apoplexy (Sheehan's syndrome) with panhypopituitarism.

Impairment Rating: 20% impairment due to panhypopituitarism; 10% impairment due to replacement for multiple hormones; combine (see Combined Values Chart, p. 604) to obtain whole person impairment.

Comment: Panhypopituitarism will remain permanent, requiring lifelong hormone replacement. With levothyroxine, hydrocortisone, and dehydroepiandrosterone replacement, normal adrenal and thyroid balance are established, but additional hydrocortisone is required at physiologically stressful times. The individual remains infertile and unable to lactate. Growth hormone replacement requires daily injections of very expensive human growth hormone. Fertility may be induced by hormonal stimulation of the ovary, but this is not always successful.

Class 3
26%-50% Impairment of the Whole Person
Severe symptoms and signs of disease persist despite treatment and significantly impact ability to perform activities of daily living

An individual with hypothalamic-pituitary disease belongs in class 3 when severe symptoms and signs persist despite treatment and significantly impact ability to perform activities of daily living.

Example 10-4
26% to 50% Impairment Due to Hypothalamic-Pituitary Axis Disease

Subject: 55-year-old man.

History: Seen initially at age 45 because of an enlarged sella turcica. Evaluation revealed testosterone deficiency; no suprasellar extension of the tumor. Individual was not treated; was lost to follow-up. Several years later, hospitalized with complaints of excruciating headache, visual loss, and impotence. Underwent emergency transsphenoidal pituitary decompression under coverage with glucocorticoids. Vision was unchanged, and mild headaches persisted. Unable to tolerate bromocriptine. Despite testosterone administration, continued to have erectile dysfunction.

Physical Exam: Beard markedly diminished; had a female escutcheon. Testing of visual fields showed nearly complete loss of vision in left eye and temporal field defect in right eye with macular involvement. After decompression, visual acuity in left eye limited to finger counting; temporal field loss in right eye remained.

Clinical Studies: Skull roentgenogram: massively enlarged sella turcica. CT scan: extensive suprasellar growth of the tumor, with a suggestion of hemorrhage into the tumor. Preoperative prolactin concentration: 1000 µg/L (1000 ng/mL); postoperative prolactin level: remained elevated at 660 µg/L (660 ng/mL). In postoperative period, received course of ionizing radiation to the sella turcica. Subsequent evaluation revealed elevated prolactin concentration of 280 µg/L (280 ng/mL), low testosterone concentration, deficient cortisol response to hypoglycemia, and decreased thyroid function.

Diagnosis: Prolactin-secreting pituitary adenoma with pituitary apoplexy, secondary panhypopituitarism, and vision loss.

Impairment Rating: 26% impairment due to pituitary dysfunction, secondary adrenal dysfunction, and secondary testosterone deficiency; combine with impairments from loss of visual acuity and from persistent headaches (see Combined Values Chart, p. 604) to determine whole person impairment.

Comment: Regular monitoring and lifelong medication required.

10.3 Thyroid

10.3a Interpretation of Symptoms and Signs

The thyroid gland, through its secretion of hormones, influences the metabolic rate of many organ systems. Hypersecretion and hyposecretion of thyroid hormones cause impairments. Hypersecretion by the thyroid gland results in hyperthyroidism and may be manifested by nervousness, weight loss, heat intolerance, goiter, tachycardia, palpitation, atrial fibrillation, frequent bowel movements, tremor, and muscle weakness. Eye changes, such as exophthalmos and double vision, may also be present. Hyposecretion by the thyroid gland results in hypothyroidism and may be manifested by lethargy, slowing of mental processes, weakness, cold intolerance, dry skin, constipation, and myxedema. Late complications include myocardial insufficiency, effusions into body cavities, and coma. Hypothyroidism in infancy may be associated with failure of physical and mental development.

10.3b Description of Clinical Studies

These include, but are not limited to, determination of (1) circulating thyroid hormone levels, including total thyroxine, free thyroxine, triiodothyronine, and free triiodothyronine; (2) circulating pituitary thyrotropin level measured by a sensitive assay; (3) radioiodine uptake of the thyroid gland; (4) thyroid antibodies; and (5) radiotriiodothyronine resin or red blood cell uptake. The nature of thyroid nodules is often best evaluated by needle aspiration or biopsy.

10.3c Criteria for Rating Permanent Impairment Due to Thyroid Disease

In practically all individuals with hyperthyroidism, the condition can be corrected by treatment and there is no loss in the ability to perform activities of daily living. However, the ophthalmopathy seen in some cases of hyperthyroidism may persist after treatment of the thyrotoxic state and result in permanent cosmetic disfigurement or visual impairment. In severe cases, loss of vision may result. These conditions should be evaluated as described in the chapters on the ear, nose, throat, and related structures (Chapter 11) and the visual system (Chapter 12). When atrial fibrillation persists following adequate treatment of hyperthyroidism, this condition should be evaluated as described in the chapters on the cardiovascular system (Chapters 3 and 4).

In most instances, hypothyroidism can be controlled satisfactorily by the administration of thyroid medication. Occasionally, because of associated disease in other organ systems, full hormone replacement may not be possible. Table 10-2 gives the criteria for rating permanent impairment due to thyroid disease.

Table 10-2 Criteria for Rating Permanent Impairment Due to Thyroid Disease

Class 1 0%-15% Impairment of the Whole Person	Class 2 16%-25% Impairment of the Whole Person
Continuous thyroid therapy required for correction of thyroid insufficiency or for maintenance of normal thyroid anatomy *and* no objective physical or laboratory evidence of inadequate replacement therapy	Symptoms and signs of thyroid disease present *or* anatomic loss or alteration *and* continuous thyroid hormone replacement therapy required for correction of confirmed thyroid insufficiency *and* presence of a disease process in another body system permits only partial replacement of the thyroid hormone

Class 1 0%-15% Impairment of the Whole Person
Continuous thyroid therapy required for correction of thyroid insufficiency or for maintenance of normal thyroid anatomy *and* no objective physical or laboratory evidence of inadequate replacement therapy

An individual belongs in class 1 when (1) continuous thyroid therapy is required for correction of the thyroid insufficiency or for maintenance of normal thyroid anatomy and (2) there is no objective physical or laboratory evidence of inadequate replacement therapy.

Example 10-5
0% to 15% Impairment Due to Hashimoto's Thyroiditis

Subject: 45-year-old woman.

History: Symptoms of mild hypothyroidism of 2 years' duration. Required daily therapy with 0.20 mg of levothyroxine to maintain normal-sized thyroid, although symptoms of hormone deficiency were relieved by a lower dose.

Current Symptoms: Easily fatigued; feels cold often.

Physical Exam: Enlarged thyroid.

Clinical Studies: Needle biopsy: indicated lymphoepithelial goiter (Hashimoto's thyroiditis).

Diagnosis: Hashimoto's thyroiditis controlled by treatment.

Impairment Rating: 5% impairment of the whole person.

Comment: Regular monitoring of thyroid disease.

Class 2 16%-25% Impairment of the Whole Person
Symptoms and signs of thyroid disease present *or* anatomic loss or alteration *and* continuous thyroid hormone replacement therapy required for correction of confirmed thyroid insufficiency *and* presence of a disease process in another body system permits only partial replacement of the thyroid hormone

An individual belongs in class 2 when (1) symptoms and signs of thyroid disease are present or (2) there is anatomic loss or alteration, and (3) continuous thyroid hormone replacement therapy is required for correction of the confirmed thyroid insufficiency, and (4) the presence of a disease process in another body system permits only partial replacement of the thyroid hormone.

Example 10-6
16% to 25% Impairment Due to Hypothyroidism

Subject: 65-year-old man.

History: Severe hypothyroidism of 16 months' duration, with pronounced mental slowing, loss of memory, and apathy. Also had severe coronary artery disease with angina pectoris that could be precipitated by walking only 50 ft. Repeated trials and careful adjustment of doses of levothyroxine indicated that a dose larger than 0.05 mg/d caused aggravation of the angina. Significant debility due to hypothyroidism persisted.

Current Symptoms: Angina; persistent fatigue; inability to maintain concentration; constipation.

Physical Exam: BP: 105/70 mm Hg. Dry skin; slowed reflexes.

Clinical Studies: Total thyroxine level: 6.4 nmol/L (0.5 mcg/dL). Thyrotropin level: 100 µIU/L (100 mIU/mL).

Diagnosis: Partially treated hypothyroidism.

Impairment Rating: 20% impairment due to hypothyroidism; combine with an appropriate value for the cardiovascular impairment (see Combined Values Chart, p. 604) to determine whole person impairment.

Comment: If the cardiovascular disease were treated, for instance, by angioplasty or bypass surgery, it might be possible to fully replace the thyroid hormone level, in which case the impairment rating would need to be reevaluated.

10.4 Parathyroids

The secretion of parathyroid hormone from the four parathyroid glands regulates the levels of serum calcium and phosphorus, which are essential to the proper functioning of the skeletal, digestive, renal, and nervous systems. The major abnormalities of the glands include hyperfunction, hypofunction, and carcinoma.

10.4a Interpretation of Symptoms and Signs

Hypersecretion of parathyroid hormone, or hyperparathyroidism, may be due to the hyperfunctioning of one gland, as with an adenoma, or that of all four glands, as with hyperplasia, or may result from a parathyroid carcinoma. Manifestations of this condition include lethargy, constipation, nausea, vomiting, and polyuria, and, in extreme cases, bone pain, renal calculi, renal failure, and coma.

Hyposecretion of parathyroid hormone, or hypoparathyroidism, may be congenital in origin or due to inadvertent removal of the parathyroid glands during thyroidectomy, surgical excision for the treatment of hyperparathyroidism, or unknown causes. Manifestations include chronic fatigue, paresthesia, tetany, and seizures. Additionally, in idiopathic cases, there may be cataracts, chronic moniliasis of the skin, alopecia, and hypofunction of other endocrine organs, including hypothyroidism, diabetes mellitus, adrenal insufficiency, hypogonadism, and pernicious anemia.

10.4b Description of Clinical Studies

Techniques for evaluating parathyroid gland function include determinations of serum calcium, phosphorus, albumin, creatinine, magnesium, parathyroid hormone levels, $1,25(OH)_2$ vitamin D, calcium concentration in urine, and urinary cyclic adenosine monophosphate response to intravenously administered parathyroid hormone. Intravenous pyelography, skeletal roentgenography, and bone density studies may be useful. Ultrasonography, MRI, and CT and sestamibi scanning are useful tools in localizing parathyroid adenomas.

10.4c Criteria for Rating Permanent Impairment Due to Parathyroid Disease

Hyperparathyroidism

In most cases of hyperparathyroidism, surgical treatment results in correction of the primary abnormality, although secondary symptoms and signs may persist, such as fracture, renal calculi, or renal failure. The latter signs should be evaluated according to criteria in the chapters on the urinary and reproductive systems (Chapter 7) or musculoskeletal system (Chapters 15 through 17). If surgery fails, or if the individual cannot undergo surgery, long-term therapy may be necessary, in which case the permanent impairment may be classified according to the criteria in Table 10-3.

Table 10-3 Impairments Related to Hyperparathyroidism

Severity	% Impairment of the Whole Person
Symptoms and signs easily controlled with medical therapy	0%-14%
Persistent mild hypercalcemia with mild nausea and polyuria	15%-29%
Severe hypercalcemia with nausea and lethargy	30%-90%

Example 10-7
0% to 14% Impairment Due to Hyperparathyroidism

Subject: 45-year-old woman.

History: Hypercalcemia of 11.8 mg/dL was found on routine blood chemistry analysis.

Current Symptoms: No symptoms of hypercalcemia.

Physical Exam: Normal.

Clinical Studies: Repeat serum calcium: 2.90 mmol/L (11.6 mg/dL); serum phosphorus: 0.90 mmol/L (2.8 mg/dL); hypercalciuria: 376 mg/24 h. Serum parathyroid hormone (PTH) by immunoradiometric assay (IRMA): elevated—110 pg/mL. Complete blood count, electrolytes, and serum urea nitrogen (BUN): normal. Serum levels of calcium, phosphorus, and PTH returned to normal following surgical removal of a single parathyroid adenoma.

Diagnosis: Primary hyperparathyroidism.

Impairment Rating: 0% impairment of the whole person.

Comment: Surgical removal of the adenoma resulted in a cure, leaving no detrimental impact on the individual's ability to perform activities of daily living.

Example 10-8
0% to 14% Impairment Due to Hyperparathyroidism

Subject: 28-year-old man.

History: Subsequent to an episode of renal colic and passing a calcium oxalate stone, hypercalcemia of 12.3 mg/dL was found with mild hypophosphatemia and an elevated serum PTH level, which were corrected following surgical treatment of parathyroid hyperplasia.

Current Symptoms: 3 months postoperatively, asymptomatic other than periodic episodes of vague left flank pain.

Physical Exam: Normal.

Clinical Studies: Serum calcium, phosphorus, and PTH levels, as well as urinary calcium excretion: normal. Renal ultrasound: a large calculus in the left renal pelvis.

Diagnosis: Primary hyperparathyroidism with ureterolithiasis and a residual large renal calculus.

Impairment Rating: 10% impairment of the whole person due to hyperparathyroidism and continued risk of the renal calculus.

Comment: Impairment will decrease if the stone can be removed and the symptoms abate.

Example 10-9
15% to 29% Impairment Due to Hyperparathyroidism

Subject: 38-year-old man.

History: Consequent to diagnosis of primary hyperparathyroidism, neck exploration did not reveal presence of a parathyroid adenoma; treatment consisted of removal of 3½ parathyroid glands.

Current Symptoms: Persistent fatigue, mild nausea, polyuria, and nocturia.

Physical Exam: Normal.

Clinical Studies: Serum calcium: 3.50 mmol/L (14.0 mg/dL); phosphorus: 0.65 mmol/L (2.0 mg/dL); PTH by IRMA: 23.2 pmol/L (220 pg/mL); urinary calcium excretion: 190 mg/24 h. Complete blood count, BUN, and electrolytes: normal other than mild depression of bicarbonate to 19 mmol/L (19 mEq/L). Ultrasonography and sestamibi and CT scans failed to reveal presence of parathyroid tissue in either neck or chest.

Diagnosis: Primary hyperparathyroidism.

Impairment Rating: 20% impairment of the whole person.

Comment: Impairment remains until the source of hyperparathyroidism can be ascertained and corrected.

Example 10-10
15% to 29% Impairment Due to Hyperparathyroidism

Subject: 76-year-old woman.

History: Chronic obstructive pulmonary disease (COPD) treated with inhaled bronchodilators and sporadic use of systemic glucocorticoids; was noted to have a serum calcium level of 3.05 mmol/L (12.2 mg/dL).

Current Symptoms: Mild anorexia, nocturia three times, and lethargy, in addition to respiratory distress symptoms of COPD.

Physical Exam: Physical signs of poor respiratory air exchange with sporadic wheezes. No palpable neck mass.

Clinical Studies: Serum calcium: 3.10 mmol/L (12.4 mg/dL); phosphorus: 0.67 mmol/L (2.1 mg/dL); PTH by IRMA: elevated—165 pg/mL; urinary calcium excretion: 380 mg/24 h. Sestamibi scanning and MRI suggested presence of a retroesophageal parathyroid adenoma.

Diagnosis: Primary hyperparathyroidism due to an ectopic location of a parathyroid adenoma.

Impairment Rating: 25% impairment of the whole person.

Comment: Due to the comorbid state of COPD, intrathoracic surgery was felt to carry too great a risk. Therefore, medical treatment consisting of adequate hydration and exercise, as well as avoidance of prolonged immobilization, use of diuretics, and calcium ingestion in excess of 800 mg per day was advised.

Example 10-11
30% to 90% Impairment Due to Hyperparathyroidism

Subject: 72-year-old man.

History: Diagnosis of parathyroid carcinoma made at time of surgical resection 1 year ago.

Current Symptoms: Progressive fatigue, lethargy, mild confusion, polyuria, nocturia, and one episode of ureterolithiasis 3 months ago.

Physical Exam: Elderly appearing, thin, pale male who was lethargic but easily arousable, slow in mentation, and spoke with a hoarse voice. Presence of a 3×5-cm irregularly hard mass in lower right anterior portion of the neck; causes deviation of the trachea to the left.

Clinical Studies: Serum calcium: 4.25 mmol/L (17.0 mg/dL); phosphorus: 0.52 mmol/L (1.6 mg/dL); alkaline phosphatase: 350 U/L; urinary calcium excretion: 510 mg/24 h.

Diagnosis: Hyperparathyroidism due to recurrent parathyroid carcinoma.

Impairment Rating: 50% impairment of the whole person.

Comment: Treated with intravenous hydration and pamidronate and then referred for surgical "debulking" of the tumor. Prognosis of this disease is poor, and recurrent severe hypercalcemia can be expected.

Hypoparathyroidism

Hypoparathyroidism is a chronic condition of variable severity that requires long-term medical therapy in most cases. The degree of severity determines the estimated permanent impairment rating, as Table 10-4 indicates.

Table 10-4 Impairments Related to Hypoparathyroidism

Severity	% Impairment of the Whole Person
Symptoms and signs easily controlled by medical therapy	0%-9%
Intermittent hypercalcemia or hypocalcemia; symptoms more frequent than with above category, despite careful medical attention	10%-20%

Example 10-12
0% to 9% Impairment Due to Hypoparathyroidism

Subject: 42-year-old man.

History: 24 hours postoperatively for removal of a large parathyroid adenoma, develops hypocalcemia.

Current Symptoms: Perioral and peripheral paresthesias.

Physical Exam: Sutured surgical incision in lower anterior portion of the neck; Chvostek's sign present.

Clinical Studies: Serum calcium: 1.90 mmol/L (7.6 mg/dL); phosphorus: 1.45 mmol/L (4.5 mg/dL).

Diagnosis: Transient hypoparathyroidism.

Impairment Rating: 0% impairment of the whole person.

Comment: Hypoparathyroidism, which often occurs in this situation, is transient and due to the suppressive effect of the overactive parathyroid adenoma on the remaining parathyroid tissue. Full recovery occurs within several weeks.

Example 10-13
0% to 9% Impairment Due to Hypoparathyroidism

Subject: 62-year-old woman.

History: Surgical treatment for parathyroid hyperplasia 5 years ago. Due to persistent mild hypocalcemia since surgery, has required daily replacement with 1000 mg of elemental calcium, which has kept her asymptomatic and with normal calcium levels.

Current Symptoms: Over the past week, ran out of calcium supplement and has developed mild perioral and peripheral paresthesias.

Physical Exam: Unremarkable with the exception of bilateral Chvostek's sign.

Clinical Studies: Serum calcium: 2.05 mmol/L (8.2 mg/dL); phosphorus: 1.55 mmol/L (4.8 mg/dL); both returned to normal with resumption of calcium replacement.

Diagnosis: Surgically induced hypoparathyroidism; mild.

Impairment Rating: 3% impairment of the whole person.

Comment: With continual daily use of safe and inexpensive calcium replacement, remains asymptomatic and with no increased likelihood of morbidity.

Example 10-14
10% to 20% Impairment Due to Hypoparathyroidism

Patient: 58-year-old man.

History: Surgical removal of 3½ parathyroid glands, as treatment for hyperparathyroidism due to parathyroid hyperplasia; 3 months later, remains hypocalcemic despite daily ingestion of 1000 mg of elemental calcium and 0.25 µg of calcitriol.

Current Symptoms: Frequent episodes of peripheral paresthesias and muscular irritability, worsened with physical exercise.

Physical Exam: Well-healed surgical scar present in mid-lower anterior neck. Chvostek's and Trousseau's signs easily elicited.

Clinical Studies: Serum calcium: 1.80 mmol/L (7.2 mg/dL); phosphorus: 1.48 mmol/L (4.6 mg/dL); serum levels of creatinine, albumin, and electrolytes: normal. Serum calcium and phosphorus levels corrected to normal upon raising the daily doses of elemental calcium and calcitriol to 1500 mg and 0.5 µg, respectively.

Diagnosis: Surgically induced hypoparathyroidism.

Impairment Rating: 20% impairment of the whole person.

Comment: Due to persistence of hypocalcemia 3 months postoperatively, despite use of calcitriol and calcium supplementation, hypoparathyroidism will most probably be permanent. The individual requires lifelong treatment and can perform many activities of daily living.

10.5 Adrenal Cortex

The adrenal cortex synthesizes and secretes adrenocortical hormones. These hormones participate in the regulation of electrolyte and water metabolism and in the intermediate metabolism of carbohydrate, fat, and protein. They also affect inflammatory response, cell membrane permeability, and immunologic responses, and they play a role in the development and maintenance of secondary sexual characteristics.

Impairment may result from either hypersecretion or hyposecretion of the cortical hormones. Such abnormalities may be associated with dysfunction of another endocrine gland, for example, the pituitary. If this occurs, the adrenal impairment and the impairment related to the other gland are both evaluated, and the impairments are combined by means of the Combined Values Chart (p. 604) to determine the whole person impairment.

10.5a Interpretation of Symptoms and Signs

Hypersecretion of adrenocortical hormones results from hyperplasia or from benign or malignant tumors of the adrenal cortex. The symptoms and signs of adrenocortical disease may arise from hypersecretion of one or more of the following hormones: (1) glucocorticoids, (2) mineralocorticoids, (3) androgens, and (4) estrogens. In some instances, there may be hypersecretion of hormones in one category and hyposecretion of those in another. Iatrogenic Cushing's syndrome secondary to supraphysiologic doses of glucocorticoids administered for systemic diseases such as bronchial asthma, systemic lupus erythematosus, or rheumatoid arthritis is the most common condition related to adrenal hormonal excess.

Among the diseases caused by hypersecretion of the adrenocortical hormones are Cushing's syndrome, the adrenogenital syndrome, and primary aldosteronism. Hypersecretion of the adrenal cortex caused by hyperplasia may be associated either with a tumor of the anterior pituitary gland or with a malignant tumor that arises outside the endocrine system and causes ectopic corticotropin secretion.

Hyposecretion of adrenocortical hormones may be primary, resulting from surgical removal or destruction of the adrenals, as with Addison's disease or by metastatic cancer; secondary, resulting from decreased production of corticotropin; or tertiary, resulting from decreased production of corticotropin-releasing hormone by the hypothalamus. Therapy is guided by the number of hormonal deficiencies, which may be single, as in hypoaldosteronism, or multiple, as in adrenocortical destruction. One normal adrenal gland can compensate for the loss of the other.

10.5b Description of Clinical Studies

These techniques include (1) measurement of adrenocortical hormones in the urine, such as free cortisol and aldosterone, and of hormones in the plasma, such as cortisol and aldosterone; (2) measurement of corticotropin, serum electrolytes, plasma glucose, and creatinine; (3) measurement of the effects of suppression and stimulation of adrenocortical function; and (4) roentgenography of the adrenal glands, CT scanning, MRI, arteriography, and venography of the pituitary drainage.

10.5c Criteria for Rating Permanent Impairment Due to Adrenal Cortex Disease

Hypoadrenalism is a lifelong condition that requires long-term **replacement therapy** with glucocorticoids and/or mineralocorticoids for proven hormonal deficiencies. Evaluation of improvement may be difficult because a person may be fully functional on an everyday basis while taking **replacement medication** but not be able to respond properly to the stress of fever, trauma, infection, or very warm weather. This impaired ability to respond to stress needs careful consideration. Impairments should be classified according to Table 10-5.

Table 10-5 Impairments Related to Hypoadrenalism

Severity	% Impairment of the Whole Person
Symptoms and signs controlled with medical therapy	0%-14%
Symptoms and signs controlled inadequately, especially during acute illnesses	15%-29%
Severe symptoms of adrenal crisis during major illnesses*	30%-90%

*This would be considered a permanent impairment only if the episodes recurred and could not be controlled with therapy.

Example 10-15
0% to 14% Impairment Due to Hypoadrenalism

Subject: 28-year-old woman.

History: Severe poison ivy; treated with 40 mg of prednisone daily for 7 days; subsequent tapering of the dose and discontinuation after 16 days of treatment.

Current Symptoms: Marked fatigue and weakness, especially in the erect position.

Physical Exam: BP: 120/80 mm Hg with PR 72 BPM when supine; 100/65 mm Hg and 92 BPM when erect.

Clinical Studies: Serum sodium: 128 mmol/L (128 mEq/L); potassium: 5.6 mmol/L (5.6 mEq/L); plasma cortisol at 8 AM: 221 mmol/L (8 μg/dL) and poorly responsive to the administration of cosyntropin (Cortrosyn). Replacement dose of prednisone was started, more gradually tapered, and discontinued over the next 6 months, resulting in complete restoration of adrenal function.

Diagnosis: Adrenal insufficiency due to the administration of exogenous glucocorticoid.

Impairment Rating: 0% impairment of the whole person.

Comment: Individual was relatively adrenal insufficient during treatment, but following tapering and discontinuation of prednisone treatment, had normal adrenal function.

Example 10-16
0% to 14% Impairment Due to Hypoadrenalism

Subject: 32-year-old woman.

History: 10-year history of autoimmune thyroiditis; mother has pernicious anemia.

Current Symptoms: Over the past year has developed progressive fatigue, weakness, and periodic nausea; weight loss of 6.75 kg (15 lb). Also has periodic postural dizziness and has developed a craving for salt.

Physical Exam: Thin female weighing 49.5 kg (110 lb), with sporadic areas of vitiligo and hyperpigmentation, most notable in creases of the hands, elbows, knees, neck, and face. BP: 120/80 mm Hg in the supine position; decreased to 100/65 mm Hg in the erect position, with a compensatory tachycardia. Both axillary and pubic hair sparse.

Clinical Studies: Serum sodium: 122 mmol/L (122 mEq/L); potassium: 6.0 mmol/L (6.0 mEq/L); BUN: 10.71 mmol/L (30 mg/dL). Plasma corticotropin at 8 AM: elevated—44 pmol/L (200 pg/mL); plasma cortisol: low for 8 AM: 221 nmol/L (8 μg/dL), rising only to 276 nmol/L (10 μg/dL) following intramuscular injection of 250 μg of cosyntropin (Cortrosyn). Serum levels of dehydroepiandrosterone sulfate (DHEA-S) and free testosterone: low; thyroid hormone levels: normal.

Diagnosis: Addison's disease.

Impairment Rating: 10% impairment of the whole person.

Comment: Hypoadrenalism will be permanent, with the individual requiring lifelong treatment with an adrenal glucocorticoid and mineralocorticoid in order to perform usual activities of daily living. Dermatologic changes may remain and, if significant, can be evaluated in the skin chapter (Chapter 8) and combined with the endocrine impairment.

Example 10-17
15% to 29% Impairment Due to Hypoadrenalsim

Subject: 55-year-old man.

History: 8-year history of Addison's disease and 3-year history of depression exacerbated by the death of his mother. As a result of his depression, he often skipped his glucocorticoid and mineralocorticoid replacement medication, sometimes for as long as 3 or 4 days at a time.

Current Symptoms: Weakness, malaise, nausea, and vomiting for the past 3 days.

Physical Exam: BP: 105/60 mm Hg with PR 92 BPM when supine; 80/40 mm Hg and 112 BPM when erect. Moderately dehydrated with hyperpigmentation, most notable in creases of the hands, elbows, knees, neck, and face.

Clinical Studies: Serum sodium: 120 mmol/L (120 mEq/L); potassium: 5.6 mmol/L (5.6 mEq/L); BUN: 11.4 mmol/L (32 mg/dL). With resumption of usual steroid regimen, metabolic abnormalities of adrenal insufficiency abated.

Diagnosis: Addison's disease; depression.

Impairment Rating: 20% due to Addison's disease; combine with appropriate rating for depression (see Combined Values Chart, p. 604) to determine whole person impairment.

Comment: Due to depression and its impairment of the individual's ability to take medications regularly, he suffers a greater impairment from Addison's disease.

Example 10-18
15% to 29% Impairment Due to Hypoadrenalism

Subject: 68-year-old woman.

History: 20-year history of Addison's disease and 5-year history of diverticulosis. During treatment of frequent episodes of diverticulitis, her glucocorticoid dose requires adjustment due to the accompanying state of relative adrenal insufficiency.

Current Symptoms: 3 days of progressively worsening left lower quadrant abdominal pain, with fever to 38.4°C (101°F); accompanied by weakness, malaise, nausea, and vomiting.

Physical Exam: Marked tenderness in left lower quadrant of the abdomen, without rebound. BP: 110/70 mm Hg with PR 86 BPM when supine; 95/55 mm Hg and 108 BPM when erect. Mucous membranes dry.

Clinical Studies: Serum sodium: 126 mmol/L (126 mEq/L); potassium: 5.2 mmol/L (5.2 mEq/L); BUN: 10.7 mmol/L (30 mg/dL); Westergren erythrocyte sedimentation rate (WSR): 64 mm/h; white blood cell count: 15 000 10³/μL), with predominance of neutrophilic leukocytes. All symptoms, physical signs, and metabolic abnormalities of adrenal insufficiency abated with her maintaining fludrocortisone dosage at 0.1 mg per day and increasing hydrocortisone dosage to 90 mg per day, which was later decreased to her usual dosage as the diverticulitis responded to treatment.

Diagnosis: Addison's disease with intercurrent febrile illness.

Impairment Rating: 25% impairment of the whole person.

Comment: Continuing to take her daily adrenal hormone replacement. There were minimal effects on this individual's ability to perform activities of daily living. However, these frequent episodes of an intercurrent illness illustrate the degree of adrenal insufficiency with its increase in morbidity and possibly mortality.

Example 10-19
30% to 90% Impairment Due to Hypoadrenalism

Subject: 72-year-old man.

History: 20-year history of Addison's disease. Myocardial infarction 2 years ago, followed by congestive heart failure requiring treatment with digoxin, ACE inhibitor, and diuretics. With worsening periods of congestive heart failure, glucocorticoid and mineralocorticoid replacement requirement increased, often contributing to the fluid-retentive state.

Current Symptoms: Dyspnea on exertion, orthopnea, dependent edema, weakness, fatigue, and nausea.

Physical Exam: BP: 105/70 mm Hg with PR 104 BPM when supine; 90/55 mm Hg and 120 BPM when erect. Bibasilar rales, 3+ bipedal edema, vitiligo on back and chest, hyperpigmentation of appendectomy scar and in the creases of elbows, knees, and hands.

Clinical Studies: Serum sodium: 122 mmol/L (122 mEq/L); potassium: 3.6 mmol/L (3.6 mEq/L); BUN: 14.9 mmol/L (42 mg/dL).

Diagnosis: Addison's disease; congestive heart failure.

Impairment Rating: 60% impairment due to Addison's disease; combine with appropriate rating for congestive heart failure (see Combined Values Chart, p. 604) to determine whole person impairment.

Comment: Difficult to adequately control adrenal insufficiency due to its detrimental effect on the status of congestive heart failure.

Example 10-20
30% to 90% Impairment Due to Hypoadrenalism

Subject: 46-year-old man.

History: 40-year history of type 1 diabetes mellitus with poor glycemic control during most of this period; accompanied by proliferative retinopathy, nephropathy, neuropathy, and a hypnotic bladder. 10-year history of Addison's disease, well controlled with physiologic amounts of hydrocortisone and fludrocortisone acetate. Periodic infections, including pyelonephritis, have required adjustments of both insulin and hydrocortisone doses. Admitted to hospital because of pyelonephritis due to *Candida albicans* with sepsis.

Current Symptoms: Fever with shaking chills, fatigue, weakness, and nausea.

Physical Exam: Temperature: 38.9°C (102°F); BP: 110/80 mm Hg, PR: 76 BPM when supine; BP: 80/85 mm Hg, PR: 76 BPM when erect. Hyperpigmentation of lower extremity scars and in the creases of the elbows, hands, and knees.

Clinical Studies: Serum sodium: 123 mmol/L (123 mEq/L); potassium: 5.8 mmol/L (5.8 mEq/L); three blood cultures grew out *Candida albicans*.

Diagnosis: Addison's disease; type 1 diabetes mellitus; *Candida* sepsis and pyelonephritis.

Impairment Rating: 70% impairment due to Addison's disease; combine with rating due to *Candida* sepsis to determine whole person impairment.

Comment: Hydrocortisone dose increased to 50 mg/d; has not been replaced to the full physiologic requirement due to its interference with host defense mechanisms and the effect of masking signs of infection. Difficult to adequately control adrenal insufficiency due to its detrimental effect on the status of *Candida* sepsis.

Hyperadrenocorticism caused by the chronic side effects of supraphysiologic doses of glucocorticoids, that is, iatrogenic Cushing's syndrome, is related to dosage and duration of treatment and may cause osteoporosis, hypertension, diabetes mellitus, and the catabolic effects that result in cataracts, aseptic necrosis, myopathy, striae, and easy bruising. Permanent impairments may range from 0% to 100%, depending on the severity and chronicity of the disease process for which the steroids are given. Impairments from diseases of the pituitary-adrenal axis should be estimated according to Table 10-6.

Table 10-6 Impairments Related to Hyperadrenocorticism*

Severity	% Impairment of the Whole Person
Minimal, as with hyperadreno-corticism that is surgically corrected by removal of a pituitary or adrenal adenoma or due to moderate pharmacologic doses of glucocorticoids	0%-14%
Moderate, as with bilateral hyperplasia that is treated with medical therapy or adrenalectomy or due to large pharmacologic doses of glucocorticoids	15%-39%
Severe, as with aggressively metastasizing adrenal carcinoma	Variable†

* This table should be used to evaluate impairments due to the general effects of adrenal steroids, such as myopathy, easy bruising, and obesity. The estimated percentages should be combined with those related to specific impairments, such as diabetes or fractures due to osteoporosis, by means of the Combined Values Chart (p. 604).

† The degree of estimated impairment will depend on the effects of the tumor on other organ systems; appropriate *Guides* chapters should be consulted

Example 10-21
0% to 14% Impairment Due to Hyperadrenocorticism

Subject: 30-year-old woman.

History: Unremarkable other than the delivery of two children, who are now 6 and 4 years old.

Current Symptoms: 2 years of progressive weakness, easy bruisability, hirsutism, facial acne, weight gain, and depression.

Physical Exam: BP: 160/95 mm Hg; PR: 68 BPM. Marked central obesity with moderate peripheral muscle wasting and notable proximal muscle weakness. Rounded and acne-covered face. Red striae present over buttocks, flanks, and lower abdomen, bilaterally. Mildly increased vellus hair growth on face and lower arms; dark terminal hair on upper chest and upper abdomen.

Clinical Studies: Diurnal variation of cortisol secretion was lost as suggested by plasma cortisol concentrations: 690 nmol/L (25 µg/dL) and 607 nmol/L (22 µg/dL) at 8 AM and 4 PM, respectively. Urinary free cortisol excretion: elevated—966 nmol/d (350 µg/24 h); plasma corticotropin (ACTH): unmeasurable. Plasma cortisol and urinary free cortisol excretion failed to suppress during standard 2-day suppression tests, utilizing 2- and 8-mg dexamethasone doses. CT scan of the abdomen: a 3-cm tumor in left adrenal gland. With proper preoperative preparation, left adrenal gland was removed by open flank incision. Glucocorticoid replacement, followed by tapering doses over 6 months, resulted in complete resolution of the hyperadrenal state.

Diagnosis: Cushing's syndrome due to adrenocortical tumor.

Impairment Rating: 0% impairment of the whole person after resolution of clinical symptoms and signs.

Comment: Since the surgical cure rate for adrenal adenoma is virtually 100%, this individual should be considered cured.

Example 10-22
0% to 14% Impairment Due to Hyperadrenocorticism

Subject: 21-year-old woman.

History: Unremarkable past medical history.

Current Symptoms: Since puberty, at age 13, persistent acne and progressive hirsutism, with irregular menstrual cyclicity. Feels self-conscious and depressed regarding her physical appearance and has difficulty socializing.

Physical Exam: BP: 120/80 mm Hg; PR: 80 BPM. Height: 167.6 cm (5 ft 6 in); weight: 72 kg (160 lb), which is diffusely distributed. Markedly increased dark terminal hairs on lower back, upper chest including periareolar, upper and lower abdomen, and upper thighs; dark vellus hairs on face and lower arms. No striae or purpura. No evidence of muscular weakness.

Clinical Studies: Plasma DHEA-S: elevated—108.0 µmol/L (4000 µg/mL); free testosterone: 12.2 pg/mL; normal levels of estradiol, luteinizing hormone (LH), and cortisol, which suppresses following administration of 1 mg of dexamethasone. Plasma: slightly elevated level (120 µg/dL) of 17α-hydroxyprogesterone had an exaggerated response (12.0 nmol/L [400 ng/dL]) to administration of cosyntropin. Administration of 12 mg of prednisone every other day has resulted in normalization of the biochemical parameters, resolution of the acne, and marked diminution of the hirsutism, but not complete remission. Menstrual cyclicity returned to normal.

Diagnosis: Adult-onset 21-hydroxylase deficiency.

Impairment Rating: 14% impairment of the whole person.

Comment: The hirsutism may never completely resolve, leaving individual's self-image and ability to socialize in a compromised state. Assess severity in chapter on mental and behavioral disorders (Chapter 14).

Example 10-23
15% to 39% Impairment Due to Hyperadrenocorticism

Subject: 56-year-old woman.

History: 10-year history of worsening bronchial asthma with diminishing responsiveness to bronchodilators and requiring 15 to 20 mg of prednisone daily for the past year.

Current Symptoms: 6.75-kg (15-lb) weight gain and dependent edema over the past year. Facial acne, easy bruising, recurrent vaginal candidiasis, and acute low back pain, which has been persistent for the past month.

Physical Exam: Cushingoid body habitus, several ecchymotic areas over distal upper extremities, tinea versicolor on chest, tenderness over the L4 vertebra with bilateral paralumbar muscle spasm. "Cheesy" vaginal discharge, suggestive of monilial infection.

Clinical Studies: Vaginal discharge containing heavy growth of *Candida albicans*. Lumbar x-ray reveals marked osteoporosis and compression fracture of the L2 vertebra.

Diagnosis: Iatrogenic Cushing's syndrome.

Impairment Rating: 20% impairment due to Cushing's syndrome; combine with appropriate ratings for vertebral collapse, pulmonary impairment, and any permanent gynocologic impairment (see Combined Values Chart, p. 604) to determine whole person impairment.

Comment: Individual is subject to further impairment from hypercortisolism if glucocorticoid cannot be discontinued or, at least, diminished.

Example 10-24
15% to 39% Impairment Due to Hyperadrenocorticism

Subject: 54-year-old man.

History: Transsphenoidal microadenomectomy 2 years ago as treatment for Cushing's disease.

Current Symptoms: Past 6 months, 9.0-kg (20-lb) weight gain, acne, ankle edema, proximal muscle weakness, and generalized fatigue.

Physical Exam: BP: 150/100 mm Hg; PR: 84 BPM. Central obesity with rounded plethoric facies; red striae on abdomen and flanks; prominent proximal muscle weakness.

Clinical Studies: Serum sodium: 148 mmol/L (148 mEq/L); potassium: 2.8 mmol/L (2.8 mEq/L; BUN: 5.0 mmol/L (14 mg/dL). Plasma corticotropin (ACTH): elevated—33 pmol/L (150 pg/mL); urinary free cortisol: elevated—828 nmol/d (300 µg/24 h). Plasma cortisol at 8 AM: 552 nmol/L (20 µg/dL); at 4 PM: 607 nmol/L (22 µg/dL). Whereas there was no suppression of plasma cortisol and urinary free cortisol excretion with low-dose dexamethasone, there was adequate suppression with high-dose dexamethasone. MRI of the pituitary failed to reveal the presence of an adenoma, but CT scanning of the abdomen demonstrated bilateral adrenal hyperplasia. The individual was treated with 4500 rad of conventional megavoltage radiation to the pituitary gland, in addition to 4 g of mitotane daily and prednisone as replacement therapy.

Diagnosis: Recurrent Cushing's disease.

Impairment Rating: 25% impairment of the whole person.

Comment: Radiation therapy was used to spare the individual a surgical procedure and the possibility of developing Nelson's syndrome. Mitotane, as an adrenolytic agent, was used to achieve immediate control of the hypercortisolism since it may take up to 18 months to achieve maximum benefit from the radiation. Common complaints with the use of mitotane are nausea, vomiting, and anorexia. If signs and symptoms resolve, impairment rating may decrease.

Example 10-25
90% Impairment Due to Hyperadrenocorticism

Subject: 62-year-old man.

History: 15 months postoperative for adrenal carcinoma.

Current Symptoms: Marked fatigue and weakness, with recurrence of weight gain and edema.

Physical Exam: BP: 170/110 mm Hg; PR: 84 BPM. Facial plethora and acne; central obesity, 2+ bilateral lower extremity edema; palpable mass in left lateral portion of the abdomen.

Clinical Studies: Urinary free cortisol: elevated—635 nmol/d (230 µg/24 h); 17-ketosteroid (17-KS): markedly elevated—62 mg/24 h. Serum sodium: 146 mmol/L (146 mEq/L); potassium: 2.6 mmol/L (2.6 mEq/L). MRI: a large adrenal mass extending into the surrounding tissue, consistent with adrenal carcinoma.

Diagnosis: Recurrent infiltrative adrenal carcinoma.

Impairment Rating: 90% impairment of the whole person.

Comment: Although the individual was treated with mitotane to control the symptoms of hyperadrenalism, the disease is progressive with a survival expectancy of no more than 6 months.

Example 10-26
90% Impairment Due to Hyperadrenocorticism

Subject: 74-year-old man.

History: 18 months postoperative for adrenal carcinoma.

Current Symptoms: Marked fatigue and weakness, weight gain, edema, chest pain, and shortness of breath; uncomfortable with minimal exertion or self-care activities.

Physical Exam: BP: 160/100 mm Hg; PR: 80 BPM. Facial plethora and acne; central obesity, 3+ bilateral lower extremity edema; palpable mass in left lateral portion of the abdomen; left pleural effusion.

Clinical Studies: Urinary free cortisol: elevated—828 nmol/d (300 µg/24 h); 17-KS: markedly elevated—70 mg/24 h. Serum sodium: 148 mmol/L (148 mEq/L); potassium: 2.6 mmol/L (2.6 mEq/L). Chest x-ray: a large mass in left lower lung field and a large pleural effusion. MRI of the abdomen: a large adrenal mass extending into the surrounding tissue, consistent with adrenal carcinoma.

Diagnosis: Adrenal carcinoma, recurrent and metastatic to lung.

Impairment Rating: 95% impairment of the whole person.

Comment: Although mitotane may control the symptoms of hyperadrenalism, the disease is progressive with a survival expectancy of no more than 6 months. Combine this impairment with that of lung impairment due to metastatic cancer.

10.6 Adrenal Medulla

10.6a Interpretation of Symptoms and Signs

The adrenal medulla synthesizes and secretes primarily epinephrine, which functions in the regulation of blood pressure and cardiac output and, to some extent, affects the intermediary metabolism of the body. The adrenal medulla is usually not essential to the maintenance of life or well-being. Its absence may constitute a permanent impairment rating if an abnormality is detected in the individual's ability to perform activities of daily living, especially in the response to stress. Hyperfunction of the adrenal medulla may be caused by pheochromocytomas or, rarely, by hyperplasia of the chromaffin cells. Pheochromocytomas may arise at any site in the body that has sympathetic nervous tissue. The presence of a pheochromocytoma is usually associated with paroxysmal or sustained hypertension and may produce manifestations of coronary artery disease. Pheochromocytomas may be multiple in an individual and may occur in families in association with medullary carcinoma of the thyroid and hyperplasia of the parathyroids; this constitutes the syndrome of multiple endocrine neoplasia. Approximately 10% of pheochromocytomas are malignant.

10.6b Description of Clinical Studies

These techniques include (1) measurement of unmetabolized urinary catecholamines, including total catecholamines, epinephrine, and norepinephrine, and of their degradation products in urine, vanillylmandelic acid, and metanephrines; (2) measurement of the plasma catecholamines, epinephrine, norepinephrine, and dopamine; (3) suppressive response of catecholamines to oral clonidine; (4) radiography of the adrenals by CT scanning and MRI; and (5) nucleotide scanning with ^{123}I/^{131}I-metaiodobenzylguanidine (MIBG).

10.6c Criteria for Evaluating Permanent Impairment Due to Adrenal Medulla Disease

Permanent impairment related to a pheochromocytoma may be classified by means of Table 10-7.

Table 10-7 Permanent Impairment Related to Pheochromocytoma

Severity	% Impairment of the Whole Person
Minimal, as when the duration of hypertension has not led to cardiovascular disease and a benign tumor can be removed surgically	0%-14%
Moderate, as with an inoperable malignant pheochromocytoma; signs and symptoms of catecholamine excess can be controlled with blocking agents	15%-29%
Severe, as with a widely metastatic malignant pheochromocytoma, in which symptoms of catecholamine excess cannot be controlled	30%-90%

Example 10-27
0% to 14% Impairment Due to Pheochromocytoma

Subject: 42-year-old man.

History: 1-year history of high blood pressure, inadequately controlled by various antihypertensive medications.

Current Symptoms: Episodes consisting of headache, palpitations, diaphoresis, and a feeling of apprehension, lasting for up to several hours and occurring from zero to three times per day.

Physical Exam: BP: 130/85 mm Hg (170/110 mm Hg during an episode); PR: 76 BPM (112 PBM during an episode).

Clinical Studies: 24-hour urine specimen: contained large amounts of vanillylmandelic acid (VMA) and free catecholamines, 101 μmol/d (20 mg/24 h) and 350 μg/24 h, respectively. Plasma concentration of catecholamines: elevated—5 pg/mL, did not suppress following oral ingestion of 0.3 mg of clonidine. CT scan: a 3-cm tumor in left adrenal gland, which, after proper preoperative preparation, was successfully removed.

Diagnosis: Intra-adrenal pheochromocytoma.

Impairment Rating: 0% impairment of the whole person.

Comment: Subsequent to surgery, all blood pressure readings were normal. With the complete removal of the tumor and with no further symptoms or blood pressure elevation, the individual is considered cured.

Example 10-28
15% to 29% Impairment Due to Pheochromocytoma

Subject: 64-year-old man.

History: Progressively worsening hypertension, poorly responsive to various antihypertensive medications.

Current Symptoms: At least three episodes per day consisting of throbbing headache, palpitations, nausea, diaphoresis, tremulousness, and weakness; occasionally associated with chest pain.

Physical Exam: BP: 170/120 mm Hg, PR: 108 BPM (supine position); BP: 150/105 mm Hg, PR: 120 BPM (erect position).

Clinical Studies: 24-hour urine specimen: contained large amounts of VMA and free catecholamines, 151 μmol/d (30 mg/24 h) and 450 μg, respectively. Plasma concentration of catecholamines: elevated—8 pg/mL, did not suppress following oral ingestion of 0.3 mg of clonidine. CT scan: a large tumor in left adrenal gland and extending into the retroperitoneum. Hypertension and symptoms were well controlled with use of 20 mg of phenoxybenzamine twice a day and 50 mg of metoprolol twice a day.

Diagnosis: Malignant pheochromocytoma.

Impairment Rating: 20% impairment of the whole person.

Comment: As the disease progresses, symptoms and elevated blood pressure may recur, with the individual requiring larger doses of medication and experiencing a greater percentage of impairment.

Example 10-29
30% to 90% Impairment Due to Pheochromocytoma

Subject: Same as in Example 10-28, 2 years later.

History: Despite continued use of medication, during the past 3 months individual has had rising blood pressure and progressively worsening episodes.

Current Symptoms: Episodes consist of throbbing headaches, palpitations, nausea, diaphoresis, tremulousness, weakness, and chest pain. Unable to perform most activities of daily living.

Physical Exam: BP: 195/130 mm Hg; PR: 100 BPM.

Clinical Studies: 24-hour urine specimen: contained 202 μmol/d (40 mg/24 h) of VMA and 620 μg/24 h of free catecholamines. CT scan: further peritoneal extension of left adrenal gland tumor. ^{131}I-MIBG scan: skeletal metastases. With 100 mg of phenoxybenzamine twice a day and 100 mg of metoprolol twice a day, blood pressure was controlled only to 160/95 mm Hg, with continuation of symptomatic episodes, although milder in severity.

Diagnosis: Metastatic pheochromocytoma, inadequately controlled by medical therapy.

Impairment Rating: 90% impairment of the whole person.

Comment: Very poor prognosis.

10.7 Pancreas (Islets of Langerhans)

Insulin and glucagon are among the hormones secreted by the islets of Langerhans. Both hormones are required for the maintenance of normal metabolism of carbohydrates, lipids, and proteins. Permanent impairment may result from a deficiency or an excess of either hormone. Removal of normal pancreatic tissue during the resection of an islet cell neoplasm does not constitute an endocrine impairment if, after the operation, the individual's carbohydrate tolerance is normal.

10.7a Interpretation of Symptoms and Signs

Abnormalities of islet cell function may be manifested by high plasma glucose levels, as in diabetes mellitus, or by low plasma glucose levels, as in hypoglycemia. Diabetes mellitus is classified into two main groups: type 1 diabetes and type 2 diabetes. The complications of diabetes mellitus fall into two general categories: (1) those that are directly related to the degree of hyperglycemia and (2) the chronic complications resulting from inadequate control of hyperglycemia and lipid metabolism over many years.

People with type 1, if untreated, will develop severe hyperglycemia and ketonemia, resulting in dehydration, weight loss, and severe weakness, ultimately progressing into stupor, coma, and then death. This type of diabetes mellitus usually begins in young persons, but it may occur at any age.

People with type 2 generally are over 40 years old and overweight. In the early years of this disease, these people do not develop severe hyperglycemia and its associated symptoms and, indeed, may not experience any symptoms of the disease. In later years, when insulin production falls significantly, the hyperglycemic symptoms become more evident.

The main chronic complications of diabetes mellitus and associated impairments are (1) retinopathy, causing visual impairment; (2) nephropathy, causing renal impairment; (3) neuropathy, causing various neuropathic impairments; and (4) atherosclerosis, causing atherosclerotic heart disease, as well as cerebrovascular and peripheral vascular disease.

Hypoglycemia occasionally causes impairment. It may result from excessive insulin that either is produced endogenously or administered by injection. Hypoglycemia may be manifested by weakness, sweating, tachycardia, headache, confusion, muscular incoordination, blurred vision, loss of consciousness, and convulsions. Prolonged hypoglycemia or repeated severe attacks of hypoglycemia may lead to mental deterioration and brain damage.

10.7b Diabetes Mellitus

Description of Clinical Studies

These techniques include, but are not limited to (1) determination of fasting and postprandial plasma glucose levels; (2) determination of hemoglobin A_{1c} level; (3) measurements of levels of triglycerides, low-density lipoprotein (LDL) cholesterol, and other lipids; (4) electrocardiogram or cardiac stress testing; (5) ophthalmologic examination; (6) tests of renal function, including measurement of serum creatinine and urinary protein excretion; (7) Doppler testing of the peripheral circulation; (8) roentgenograms of the chest, gastrointestinal tract, pelvis, or extremities, including arteriograms; and (9) neurologic testing.

Although it may be useful to examine the results from blood glucose testing done by the individual at home in order to obtain an additional measure of the degree of glucose control, one must recognize that these measurements may be less objective than laboratory methods such as self-hemoglobin A_{1c} measurement.

Much of the impairment that results from diabetes is related to the chronic complications. Therefore, the examiner must not only determine the presence or absence of retinopathy, nephropathy, and neuropathy, but also evaluate the other systems that may be involved. Impairments of other systems would be expressed as whole person impairments and then combined with an impairment percent resulting from instability of glucose control by means of the Combined Values Chart (p. 604).

Criteria for Rating Permanent Impairment Due to Diabetes Mellitus

Permanent impairment from diabetes mellitus can be rated using the criteria given in Table 10-8.

Table 10-8 Criteria for Rating Permanent Impairment Due to Diabetes Mellitus

Class 1 0%-5% Impairment of the Whole Person	Class 2 6%-10% Impairment of the Whole Person	Class 3 11%-20% Impairment of the Whole Person	Class 4 21%-40% Impairment of the Whole Person
Type 2 diabetes mellitus that can be controlled by diet *and* may or may not have evidence of diabetic microangiopathy, as indicated by presence of retinopathy or albuminuria greater than 30 mg/dL	Type 2 diabetes mellitus *and* satisfactory control of plasma glucose level requires both a restricted diet and hypoglycemic medication (either an oral agent or insulin) *and* evidence of microangiopathy, as indicated by retinopathy or by albuminuria of greater than 30 mg/dL, may or may not be present; if retinopathy has led to visual impairment, evaluate as described in Chapter 12, The Visual System	Type 1 diabetes mellitus, with or without evidence of microangiopathy	Type 1 diabetes mellitus *and* hyperglycemia or hypoglycemia occurs frequently despite conscientious efforts of both individual and physician

| Class 1 |
| 0%-5% Impairment of the Whole Person |
| Type 2 diabetes mellitus that can be controlled by diet |
| *and* |
| may or may not have evidence of diabetic microangiopathy, as indicated by presence of retinopathy or albuminuria greater than 30 mg/dL |

Example 10-30
0% to 5% Impairment Due to Type 2 Diabetes Mellitus

Subject: 40-year-old man.

History: Diabetes discovered on a routine medical examination.

Current Symptoms: Feels well; lost 2.25 kg (5 lb) within the last year. Able to perform all desired activities.

Physical Exam: Moderately obese. Retinal examination showed no diabetic retinopathy. Remainder of exam: normal.

Clinical Studies: Medical examinations during a 2-year period disclosed 1+ glucosuria. Fasting plasma glucose level: 8.9 mmol/L (160 mg/dL) on two occasions; no albumin in the urine. After 3 months on a special diet, weight: normal; fasting plasma glucose level: 6.1 mmol/L (110 mg/dL).

Diagnosis: Type 2 diabetes mellitus controlled by diet, without evidence of microangiopathy.

Impairment Rating: 0% impairment of the whole person.

Comment: Impairment would increase if manifestations of diabetes develop over time.

Example 10-31
0% to 5% Impairment Due to Type 2 Diabetes Mellitus

Subject: 45-year-old woman.

History: Repeated *Candida* infections during the past year.

Current Symptoms: Easily fatigued; polyuria; polydipsia. No impairment of vision.

Physical Exam: Obese; retinal microaneurysms and "dot and blot" hemorrhages.

Clinical Studies: Fasting plasma glucose level: elevated on initial evaluation. No impairment of vision.

Diagnosis: Type 2 diabetes mellitus with early diabetic retinopathy.

Impairment Rating: 5% impairment of the whole person.

Comment: Evaluate control of diabetes after diet; regular ophthalmologic evaluations.

Example 10-32
0% to 5% Impairment Due to Type 2 Diabetes Mellitus

Subject: 55-year-old man.

History: Several-year history of signs and symptoms of type 2 diabetes mellitus.

Current Symptoms: Feels less fatigued when glucose level is lower and when following diet.

Physical Exam: No retinopathy or proteinuria. Although he lost weight on a prescribed diet, plasma glucose level could not be maintained within normal limits on that diet. When on a restricted diet and taking an oral agent, fasting serum glucose level was 6.7 mmol/L (120 mg/dL) and hemoglobin A_{1c} was 0.07 proportion of total hemoglobin (7.5% of total hemoglobin); normal = 0.06 proportion of total hemoglobin (6.3% of total hemoglobin).

Diagnosis: Type 2 diabetes mellitus, reasonably well controlled by diet and oral agent.

Impairment Rating: 5% impairment of the whole person.

Class 2
6%-10% Impairment of the Whole Person

Type 2 diabetes mellitus

and

satisfactory control of plasma glucose level requires both a restricted diet and hypoglycemic medication (either an oral agent or insulin)

and

evidence of microangiopathy, as indicated by retinopathy or by albuminuria of greater than 30 mg/dL, may or may not be present; if retinopathy has led to visual impairment, evaluate as described in Chapter 12, The Visual System

Class 3
11%-20% Impairment of the Whole Person

Type 1 diabetes mellitus, with or without evidence of microangiopathy

Example 10-33
6% to 10% Impairment Due to Type 2 Diabetes Mellitus

Subject: 50-year-old man.

History: Type 2 diabetes mellitus for 5 years. At onset, had a fasting plasma glucose level of 10.5 mmol/L (190 mg/dL) when on a restricted diet and taking an oral hypoglycemic agent. Right leg was amputated above the knee because of gangrene of the foot due to severe peripheral vascular disease 4 years ago.

Current Symptoms: Adheres to prescribed diet and takes 16 U of isophane (NPH) insulin daily. No symptoms; no glucosuria or acetonuria.

Physical Exam: Right knee amputee; decreased sensation in stocking-glove distribution over left lower extremity.

Clinical Studies: On this regimen, fasting plasma glucose level: 6.9 to 7.8 mmol/L (125 to 140 mg/dL); hemoglobin A_{1c}: 0.09 proportion of total hemoglobin (8.9% of total hemoglobin).

Diagnosis: Type 2 diabetes with complications, requiring insulin to control hyperglycemia. Plasma glucose level is fairly well controlled by diet and one daily injection of insulin.

Impairment Rating: 10% impairment due to type 2 diabetes mellitus; combine with impairment due to midthigh amputation above the knee joint to give impairment of the whole person (see Combined Values Chart, p. 604).

Comment: Subsequent complications likely; impairment will need to be reassessed.

Example 10-34
11% to 20% Impairment Due to Type 1 Diabetes Mellitus

Subject: 33-year-old woman.

History: Type 1 diabetes mellitus for 5 years. Originally presented with polyuria, polydipsia, and weight loss, in addition to a plasma glucose level of 22.2 mmol/L (400 mg/dL) and marked ketonuria. Condition was satisfactorily controlled with a prescribed diet and an injection of insulin before both breakfast and dinner. Meals and insulin had to be taken at prescribed times to maintain adequate glycemic control.

Current Symptoms: Cheesy vaginal discharge; pruritus; occurs every few months.

Physical Exam: No evidence of microangiopathy; vaginal candidiasis.

Clinical Studies: Fasting glucose: 8.9 mmol/L (160 mg/dL).

Diagnosis: Type 1 diabetes mellitus, vaginal candidiasis satisfactorily controlled by insulin and diet.

Impairment Rating: 15% impairment of the whole person.

Comment: Aim for improved control.

Example 10-35
11% to 20% Impairment Due to Type 1 Diabetes Mellitus

Subject: 40-year-old woman.

History: Onset of type 1 diabetes mellitus 20 years earlier. Originally presented with polydipsia, polyuria, weight loss, and a plasma glucose level of 19.4 mmol/L (350 mg/dL).

Current Symptoms: Occasional visual changes with floaters, flashes, and decreased visual acuity.

Physical Exam: Ophthalmologic examination discloses background retinopathy.

Clinical Studies: Hemoglobin A_{1c}: 0.10 proportion of total hemoglobin (10.5% of total hemoglobin).

Diagnosis: Type 1 diabetes mellitus with diabetic microangiopathy.

Impairment Rating: 20% impairment of the whole person.

Comment: Referral to ophthalmologist for regular assessments; combine any visual impairment (see Chapter 12 and Combined Values Chart, p. 604) with endocrine impairment.

Example 10-36
11% to 20% Impairment Due to Type 1 Diabetes Mellitus

Subject: 45-year-old man.

History: Type 1 diabetes mellitus for 25 years. Plasma glucose level was controlled by a mixture of isophane (NPH) and regular insulin, given twice daily: 12 U before breakfast and 6 U before dinner.

Current Symptoms: Blurred vision; decreased acuity.

Physical Exam: Proliferative retinopathy.

Clinical Studies: Creatinine level: elevated; diminished creatinine clearance (see Chapter 7, The Urinary and Reproductive Systems).

Diagnosis: Type 1 diabetes mellitus with complications; plasma glucose level is satisfactorily controlled by diet and insulin.

Impairment Rating: 20% impairment due to diabetes mellitus; combine with ratings for the visual and urinary system impairments (see Combined Values Chart, p. 604) to determine whole person impairment.

Comment: Monitor for progressive renal and visual impairment.

Class 4
21%-40% Impairment of the Whole Person
Type 1 diabetes mellitus
and
hyperglycemia or hypoglycemia occurs frequently despite conscientious efforts of both individual and physician

Example 10-37
21% to 40% Impairment Due to Type 1 Diabetes Mellitus

Subject: 24-year-old man.

History: Labile type 1 (insulin-dependent) diabetes mellitus for 10 years. Ability to perform physical activities varied greatly from day to day. Despite adherence to a prescribed diet that included between-meal and bedtime snacks and a carefully planned insulin program with both premeal and bedtime injections, results of home plasma glucose tests varied greatly. Severe hypoglycemic reactions occurred without warning.

Current Symptoms: Intermittent fatigue; episodes of hypoglycemia and severe hypoglycemic reactions.

Physical Exam: 10% underweight. Hemoglobin A_{1c}: elevated.

Clinical Studies: No clinical or laboratory evidence of complications.

Diagnosis: Type 1 diabetes mellitus, not adequately controlled by diet and insulin.

Impairment Rating: 35% impairment of the whole person.

Comment: Monitor for complications.

Example 10-38
21% to 40% Impairment Due to Type 1 Diabetes Mellitus

Subject: 35-year-old woman.

History: Poorly controlled type 1 diabetes mellitus for 15 years. Took injections of 30 U of isophane (NPH) insulin before breakfast and 10 U of isophane (NPH) insulin before dinner.

Current Symptoms: Severe hypoglycemic reactions occur unpredictably several times each week. Fatigues easily and complains of burning foot pain and difficulty walking.

Physical Exam: Malnourished on a 12 552-kJ (3000-kcal) diet. Vibratory sensation and deep tendon reflexes absent below the knees. Examination of the fundi disclosed numerous microaneurysms, but there was no visual impairment.

Clinical Studies: Fasting plasma glucose level: >11.1 mmol/L (>200 mg/dL).

Diagnosis: Type 1 (insulin-dependent) diabetes mellitus with complications, not adequately controlled by diet and insulin.

Impairment Rating: 40% impairment due to diabetes mellitus; combine with impairment due to peripheral neuropathy to determine impairment of the whole person (see Combined Values Chart, p. 604).

10.7c Hypoglycemia

Description of Clinical Studies
Distinction must be made between the presence of postprandial and postabsorptive hypoglycemia, since postabsorptive hypoglycemia suggests the possibility of a severe or even fatal disorder, whereas postprandial hypoglycemia is usually self-limited and rarely produces physical impairment.

The techniques used include, but are not limited to (1) measurement of plasma glucose and insulin or C-peptide after overnight or longer periods of fasting, on several occasions; (2) roentgenograms of the skull and chest and CT scan or MRI of the upper abdomen; (3) tests of liver function; and (4) tests of adrenocortical and pituitary gland function. Documented hypoglycemia requires a detailed medical evaluation to determine the specific cause.

Criteria for Rating Permanent Impairment Due to Hypoglycemia
The criteria for rating permanent impairment due to hypoglycemia are given in Table 10-9.

Table 10-9 Criteria for Rating Permanent Impairment Due to Hypoglycemia

Class 1 0%-5% Impairment of the Whole Person	Class 2 6%-50% Impairment of the Whole Person
Surgical removal of an islet cell adenoma results in complete remission of symptoms and signs of hypoglycemia *and* no postoperative sequelae	Symptoms and signs of hypoglycemia; severity depends on degree of control obtained with diet and medications, other coexisting conditions, and how the condition affects ability to perform activities of daily living

Class 1 0%-5% Impairment of the Whole Person
Surgical removal of an islet cell adenoma results in complete remission of symptoms and signs of hypoglycemia *and* no postoperative sequelae

Example 10-39
0% to 5% Impairment Due to Postprandial Hypoglycemia

Subject: 23-year-old woman.

History: Unremarkable medical history with no family history of diabetes mellitus; no excessive use of ethanol.

Current Symptoms: For past 2 to 3 months, several episodes per week consisting of lightheadedness, tachycardia, anxiety, hunger, and diaphoresis, which resolve 10 to 20 minutes after eating; typically occur 3 to 4 hours following a meal.

Physical Exam: Unremarkable.

Clinical Studies: 5-hour oral glucose tolerance test with 100 g of glucose: glucose concentration nadir of 2.5 mmol/L (46 mg/dL) at the 4th hour; was associated with the above-described symptoms. Thyrotropin (TSH), sodium, potassium, alanine aminotransferase (ALT), and alkaline phosphatase: normal.

Diagnosis: Postprandial (reactive) hypoglycemia. Diet consisting of limited quantities of refined carbohydrate and ingestion of snacks between meals and at bedtime resulted in abatement of symptomatic episodes.

Impairment Rating: 0% impairment of the whole person.

Comment: With proper diet, there should be minimal impact on the ability to perform activities of daily living.

Example10-40

0% to 5% Impairment Due to Hypoglycemia

Subject: 45-year-old man.

History: Bad temper upon arising; outlook improved after breakfast. Did not use alcohol or tobacco. Late one morning while at work, suddenly became agitated and lost consciousness. On emergency admission to a hospital, plasma glucose level was 1.1 mmol/L (20 mg/dL). Remained weak and irritable before breakfast, despite a high carbohydrate intake that included a large feeding at bedtime.

Current Symptoms: Asymptomatic.

Physical Exam: Abdominal examination: normal.

Clinical Studies: Fasting plasma glucose level: never exceeded 1.9 mmol/L (35 mg/dL). Plasma insulin, C-peptide, and proinsulin levels: elevated during hypoglycemic episodes. Chest roentgenogram: no abnormalities. Pituitary, adrenal, and liver functions: normal. A small, benign insulinoma was excised from the head of the pancreas.

Diagnosis: Benign functioning islet cell adenoma (insulinoma), with remission after excision.

Impairment Rating: 0% impairment of the whole person.

Comment: After a 3-month recovery period, individual remained without symptoms.

Class 2
6%-50% Impairment of the Whole Person
Symptoms and signs of hypoglycemia; severity depends on degree of control obtained with diet and medications, other coexisting conditions, and how the condition affects ability to perform activities of daily living

Example 10-41

6% to 50% Impairment Due to Hypoglycemia

Subject: 55-year-old man.

History: Alarming personality changes during a period of a few weeks; had a seizure. A diagnosis of insulinoma was made. Experienced no impairment of hepatic function, and recovery from surgery was uneventful except for persistence of mild fasting hypoglycemia. Hypoglycemia responded well to frequent feedings of a high-protein, high-carbohydrate diet and 40 mg of prednisone, taken daily. Still had occasional transient mental lapses 10 months after returning to work, during one of which the plasma glucose level was 1.5 mmol/L (28 mg/dL). When daily dosage of prednisone was increased to 60 mg, symptomatic hypoglycemia improved, but manifestations of Cushing's syndrome became more prominent.

Curent Symptoms: Episodes of irritability; light-headedness; anxiety; diaphoresis.

Physical Exam: Physical central obesity; mild facial acne; 1+ bipedal edema; firm, palpable right upper quadrant mass.

Clinical Studies: Laparotomy: a large islet cell adenocarcinoma in the tail of the pancreas, with metastases in the liver. The spleen and the main tumor mass were resected.

Diagnosis: Metastatic islet cell adenocarcinoma with incomplete control of symptoms.

Impairment Rating: 50% impairment due to pancreatic malignant neoplasm and hypoglycemia and 10% impairment due to steroid-induced Cushing's syndrome; because they involve different parts of the endocrine system, combine to give 55% impairment of the whole person (see Combined Values Chart, p. 604).

Comment: Poor prognosis; impairment will likely increase.

Example 10-42
6% to 50% Impairment Due to Hypoglycemia

Subject: 52-year-old man.

History: 38-year history of type 1 diabetes mellitus with nonproliferative retinopathy, albuminuria, distal symmetric polyneuropathy, and autonomic neuropathy, including gastroparesis and hypoglycemic unawareness. Without prior warning symptoms, has had many severe hypoglycemic episodes, one leading to an auto accident.

Current Symptoms: Easily fatigued; numbness of both lower extremities from toes to knees; periodic postprandial abdominal bloating and vomiting.

Physical Exam: BP: 150/95 mm Hg; PR: 84 BPM. Decreased sensory and vibratory perception below the knees, bilaterally.

Clinical Studies: Hemoglobin A_{1c}: 0.98 proportion of total hemoglobin (9.8% of total hemoglobin); fasting blood glucose: 18.2 mmol/L (328 mg/dL). Upper gastrointestinal radiographic study: prolonged gastric emptying.

Diagnosis: Type 1 diabetes mellitus with gastroparesis diabeticorum and hypoglycemic unawareness.

Impairment Rating: 30% impairment due to hypoglycemia; combine with rating from gastroparesis and peripheral neuropathy to determine whole person impairment.

Comment: Treatment with metoclopramide resulted in limited success with the symptoms of gastroparesis with continued hypoglycemic events.

10.8 Gonads

In addition to producing sex hormones that affect male and female physical and sexual development and behavior, the gonads produce either spermatozoa or ova. The major hormone of the testes is testosterone, whereas those of the ovaries are estrogen and progesterone. Dysfunction of the gonads can be caused by tumors, trauma, infection, chemotherapy, irradiation, autoimmune disease, abnormal XY chromatin, and surgical removal. Gonadal function may also vary with disorders of the pituitary-hypothalamic axis.

10.8a Interpretation of Symptoms and Signs

Precocious puberty in boys is accompanied by early and rapid somatic development and an increased rate of skeletal maturation and height velocity, but, paradoxically, it results in short adult height. It may result from various central nervous system disorders, adrenal enzyme defects, virilizing tumors, or—occasionally—as a familial condition.

Precocious puberty in girls may also be caused by various central nervous system disorders, as well as by ovarian and adrenal tumors. Often, a cause is not identified. As in boys, precocious puberty in girls results in early and rapid somatic development and an increased rate of skeletal maturation and height velocity, with ultimately short adult height. Some ovarian tumors may cause masculinization.

Some adrenal enzyme defects and neoplasms, as well as some gonadal neoplasms, may produce contrasexual precocity. Certain ovarian conditions produce irregular menstrual periods with heavy bleeding and anemia. Polycystic ovarian syndrome and several types of ovarian neoplasms may produce severe hirsutism and virilization, in addition to anovulation.

Testicular hypofunction that occurs before adolescence results in eunuchoidism, which is accompanied by diminished sexual function, infertility, and failure to develop or maintain secondary sexual characteristics. Growth of the body extends beyond the usual age because of delayed epiphyseal closure. Individuals with this condition usually lack endurance and strength. Testicular hypofunction that occurs in adulthood results in varying degrees of regression of secondary sexual characteristics, sexual function, strength, and endurance, and it may also be accompanied by infertility.

Ovarian hypofunction, with onset before adolescence, may be characterized by primary amenorrhea, anovulation, poor development of secondary sexual characteristics, and growth beyond the usual age because of delayed maturation of the skeleton. Menopause is a natural occurrence in older women, but it also may follow surgical removal of the ovaries. It may be accompanied by such symptoms as hot flashes, irritability, fatigue, and headaches. If not treated, osteoporosis and an enhancement of atherosclerosis may occur during later years.

10.8b Description of Clinical Studies

These techniques include, but are not limited to (1) measurements of plasma gonadotropins, prolactin, testosterone, estrogen, progesterone, DHEA-S, androstenedione, and occasionally 17-ketosteroids in the urine; (2) radiographic determinations of skeletal age in children and adolescents; (3) CT scans or MRI to evaluate the pituitary, adrenals, and ovaries; (4) sex chromatin and chromosome studies; (5) testicular biopsy; (6) semen analysis; (7) vaginal cytologic examination; (8) culdoscopy or laparoscopy; (9) endometrial biopsy; (10) ovarian biopsy; and (11) pelvic ultrasound in women.

10.8c Criteria for Rating Permanent Impairment Due to Disorders of the Gonads

An individual with anatomic loss or alteration of the gonads that results in an absence, or an abnormally high level, of gonadal hormones would have 0% to 35% impairment of the whole person, as detailed in Chapter 7, The Urinary and Reproductive Systems. Impairment resulting from inability to reproduce, and other impairments associated with gonadal dysfunction, should be evaluated in accordance with the criteria set forth in Chapter 7.

Example 10-43
10% Impairment Due to Hypogonadism

Subject: 31-year-old man.

History: Lack of sexual development and function, high-pitched voice, and no growth of beard. Tall, with relatively long arms and legs. Responded well to continuous treatment with testosterone. Penis became larger, and there was adequate sexual functioning; increase in body and facial hair; voice became deeper.

Current Symptoms: Embarrassed about limited sexual development; socially isolated.

Physical Exam: Penis was tiny; scrotum and testes were small.

Clinical Studies: Bone age: 18 years. Plasma testosterone level: 2.4 nmol/L (70 ng/mL); plasma gonadotropin level: low.

Diagnosis: Hypogonadotropic hypogonadism.

Impairment Rating: 10% impairment of the whole person.

Comment: If social isolation doesn't improve, psychiatric evaluation appropriate.

Example 10-44
30% Impairment Due to Turner Syndrome

Subject: 19-year-old woman.

History: Has been one the shortest in height among her peers since childhood. Primary amenorrhea without breast development.

Current Symptoms: Failure to grow to anticipated height and absence of menstrual periods.

Physical Exam: Height: 1680 cm (4 ft 8 in); sparse pubic and axillary hair; Tanner 1 breast development; bilateral short fourth metacarpals; short, webbed neck.

Clinical Studies: Follicle-stimulating hormone (FSH): 84 IU/L (84 mIU/mL); 45,XO karyotype; renal ultrasound echocardiogram and TSH: normal. Treated with replacement doses of estrogen and progesterone, inducing development of secondary sexual characteristics and menses.

Diagnosis: Gonadal dysgenesis (Turner syndrome).

Impairment Rating: 30% impairment due to gonadal loss and inability to reproduce as set forth in Chapter 7, The Urinary and Reproductive Systems; combine with any mental and behavioral impairment (see Chapter 14 and the Combined Values chart, p. 604) to determine whole person impairment.

Comment: Monitor for continued sexual development.

10.9 Mammary Glands

The mammary glands make, store, and secrete milk. Absence of the mammary glands does not cause impairment of the whole person in males, but in females it will prevent nursing. In some endocrine disorders, there may be galactorrhea in females and gynecomastia in males. Gynecomastia in males may be accompanied by galactorrhea.

10.9a Criteria for Rating Permanent Impairment Due to Mammary Gland Disorders

A female of childbearing age with absence of the breasts, an individual with galactorrhea sufficient to require the use of absorbent pads, and a male with painful gynecomastia that interferes with performance of activities of daily living each would have 0% to 5% impairment of the whole person. If there were a coexisting psychiatric impairment, the whole person impairment would be greater (see Chapter 14, Mental and Behavioral Disorders).

Example 10-45
5% Impairment Due to Microadenoma of the Pituitary

Subject: 32-year-old woman.

History: 1-year history of prolactin-producing microadenoma of the pituitary; using no medications.

Current Symptoms: Irregular menstrual cyclicity and profuse galactorrhea, sufficient to require the use of absorbent pads. Both bromocriptine and cabergoline cause nausea, precluding use of either drug.

Physical Exam: Easily expressible milky breast discharge; thyroid normal to palpation.

Clinical Studies: Serum prolactin: 120 μg/L (120 ng/mL); TSH: 1.2 μIU/L (1.2 μU/mL); BUN: 5.7 mmol/L (16 mg/dL); alkaline phosphatase: 35 IU/L.

Diagnosis: Prolactin-producing microadenoma of the pituitary.

Impairment Rating: 5% impairment of the whole person.

Comment: Impairment results from the persistent embarrassment of galactorrhea and alteration of some activities of daily living.

10.10 Metabolic Bone Disease

Metabolic bone disease usually does not result in impairment unless there is fracture, pain, deformity, or peripheral nerve entrapment. Hyperparathyroidism, hypogonadism, glucocorticoid excess, hyperthyroidism, nutritional deficiencies, and certain drugs may cause osteoporosis, which is reversible with treatment, and are discussed elsewhere, as are multiple myeloma and other malignancies. The treatment of renal osteodystrophy may be highly successful, but even after renal transplantation, bone disease may persist. In order to prevent progressive skeletal deterioration, continuous treatment may be required for primary osteoporosis, hypogonadism, Paget's disease, and vitamin D-resistant osteomalacia. Permanent deformity may result from rickets, osteoporotic fractures, and osteogenesis imperfecta.

10.10a Interpretation of Symptoms and Signs

Metabolic bone disease is usually asymptomatic unless complications occur, such as fractures, accompanied by pain.

10.10b Description of Clinical Studies

These include, but are not limited to (1) dual-energy x-ray absorptiometry (DEXA); (2) biochemical markers such as alkaline phosphatase, osteocalcin, and collagen cross-links; (3) urinary calcium excretion; (4) radiographs and bone scans; and (5) bone biopsy.

10.10c Criteria for Rating Permanent Impairment Due to Metabolic Bone Disease

Unless accompanied by pain, skeletal deformity, or peripheral nerve involvement, 0% impairment exists since activities of daily living are not affected. When continuous hormone and mineral therapy gives complete relief of symptoms, impairment of the whole person may be considered to be 0% to 3%. When continuous therapy is required to relieve pain and the activities of daily living are restricted, the estimate should be 5% to 15% impairment of the whole person.

Impairment from fracture, spinal collapse, or other complications of metabolic bone disease is discussed in the chapters on the musculoskeletal system (Chapters 15-17) and pain (Chapter 18). In general, the impairment percents shown in the *Guides* chapters make allowance for the pain that may accompany the impairing conditions. Any associated loss of motion should be evaluated in accordance with the criteria set forth in the chapters on the musculoskeletal system.

Example 10-46
0% to 3% Impairment Due to Metabolic Bone Disease

Subject: 62-year-old woman.

History: 20 years postmenopausal; never used hormone replacement therapy due to strong family history of breast malignancy.

Current Symptoms: Asymptomatic.

Physical Exam: Unremarkable.

Clinical Studies: Bone density by DEXA: lumbar T score of -2.32 SD; hip -2.64 SD. TSH, parathyroid hormone (PTH), complete blood count, BUN, AM and PM cortisol, and urinary excretion of calcium: normal. Treatment was initiated with 10 mg of alendronate daily.

Diagnosis: Osteoporosis secondary to hypogonadism.

Impairment Rating: 0% impairment of the whole person.

Comment: Bone density should improve and risk of fracture decrease with continued use of alendronate.

Example 10-47
5% to 15% Impairment Due to Metabolic Bone Disease

Subject: 68-year-old woman.

History: Considerable local pain with motion of the back and spine, along with some generalized backache and spasm related to partial collapse of T4 and T12. Pain persisted despite prolonged therapy with anabolic agents, estrogens, vitamin D, and calcium.

Current Symptoms: Pain that limits the ability to do activities of daily living.

Physical Exam: Scoliosis; stooped posture; arthritic and slow gait.

Clinical Studies: Severe osteoporosis of the axial skeleton and, to a lesser extent, of the extremities.

Impairment Rating: 15% impairment due to metabolic bone disease; combine with the estimated rating for musculoskeletal system impairment (see Combined Values Chart, p. 604) to determine whole person impairment.

10.11 Endocrine System Impairment Evaluation Summary

See Table 10-10 for an evaluation summary for the assessment of endocrine system impairment.

Table 10-10 Endocrine System Impairment Evaluation Summary

Disorder	History, Including Selected Relevant Symptoms	Examination Record	Assessment of Endocrine Function
General	Change in growth; fatigue; weakness; nausea; irritability; etc	Height; weight; blood pressure; pulse rate; skin temperature, texture, and moisture; general muscle strength and mass	As indicated below
Hypothalamic-Pituitary Axis	Discuss symptoms such as menstrual cyclicity, galactorrhea, polyuria, fatigue, weakness, and headache	Note breast discharge Visual field examination and assessment of target organs as described below	Measure prolactin, growth hormone, IGF-1, urine specific gravity, serum osmolality, CT or MRI of pituitary, and function of target organs
Thyroid	Fatigue; weakness; slowing of mental process; cold or heat intolerance; nervousness; weight loss; palpitations; eye changes, such as exophthalmos and diplopia; goiter; change in bowel habits	Achilles' deep tendon reflexes; thyroid size and nodularity; presence of tremor; anxiety or generalized slowness; proptosis of eyes and their movement	Serum free thyroxine, total triiodothyronine, and TSH Radioiodine uptake and scan of thyroid; ultrasound of thyroid; fine needle aspiration of thyroid nodule
Parathyroids	Fatigue; weakness; nausea, polyuria; renal calculi; muscular irritability; paresthesias; tetany; seizures	Chvostek's and Trousseau's signs	Serum calcium; phosphorus; parathyroid hormone Urinary calcium excretion; renal ultrasound; bone densitometry; ultrasound; MRI; sestamibi scan of parathyroid gland
Adrenal Cortex	Weakness; easy bruisability; hirsutism; acne; weight gain; depression; menstrual irregularities; fungal infections	Blood pressure; weight and its body distribution; skin; muscle strength; edema	Plasma cortisol and aldosterone; urinary cortisol excretion; suppression and stimulation tests of cortisol; plasma ACTH; measurement of other steroid metabolites; serum electrolytes; urinary 17-KS excretion; bone densitometry; CT or MRI examination of abdomen
Adrenal Medulla	Episodes of headache, palpitations, diaphoresis, apprehension, and weakness	Blood pressure; pulse rate	Urinary measurement of catecholamines and their metabolites; plasma catecholamines and suppressive response to clonidine; CT or MRI exam of the adrenals
Pancreas (Islets of Langerhans)	Polyuria; polydipsia; weight loss; weakness; diaphoresis; tachycardia; blurred vision; confusion; loss of consciousness; convulsions; symptoms relevant to dysfunction of end organs of diabetes mellitus (eg, eyes, kidneys, nervous system, heart, and vascular system)	Blood pressure; pulse rate; weight; skin; eyes; neurologic; heart; presence of pulses	Plasma glucose; insulin or C-peptide; HbA_{1c}; lipids; urinalysis; CT or MRI exam of pancreas
Gonads	Lack of secondary sexual development; irregular menstrual cycles or amenorrhea; infertility; precocious development of secondary sexual characteristics; hirsutism and virilization; lack of endurance and strength	Gonads; secondary sexual characteristics; height	Plasma gonadotropins; testosterone; estradiol; progesterone; semen analysis; pelvic ultrasound; x-ray for determination of skeletal age
Mammary Glands	Inappropriate milk production; growth in the male; lack of development in the female; medication history	Breast	Estradiol; testosterone; free thyroxine; liver function tests
Metabolic Bone Disease	Fractures; medications; malignancies; renal disease	Skeletal abnormalities	Bone densitometry, such as DEXA; urinary calcium excretion; skeletal metabolic markers

End-Organ Damage	Diagnosis(es)	Degree of Impairment
Include assessment of sequelae, including end-organ damage and impairment	Record all pertinent diagnosis(es); note if they are at maximal medical improvement; if not, discuss under what conditions and when stability is expected	Criteria outlined in this chapter
Dysfunction of relevant organs, such as ovaries, testes, thyroid, adrenal, skeleton, and heart Is often reversible to varying degrees with treatment	Diabetes insipidus, prolactinoma, acromegaly, Cushing's disease, panhypopituitarism, or deficiency of any one or more pituitary hormones	See Table 10-1
Eye muscles and other retro-orbital tissue Other end-organ dysfunction usually reversible with treatment	Hyperthyroidism; hypothyroidism; thyroid nodule; goiter; carcinoma	See Table 10-2
Renal; skeletal	Hypoparathyroidism; hyperparathyroidism	See Tables 10-3 and 10-4
Skeletal; possible fracture Other end-organ dysfunction usually reversible with treatment	Addison's disease; Cushing's syndrome; adult-onset adrenal hyperplasia	See Tables 10-5 and 10-6
Possible cerebrovascular accident from severely elevated blood pressure	Pheochromocytoma	See Table 10-7
Eyes; kidneys; nervous system; cardiovascular; skin	Diabetes mellitus; insulinoma; reactive hypoglycemia	See Tables 10-8 and 10-9
Gonads; skin; skeletal	Gonadal dysgenesis; premature ovarian failure; precocious puberty; polycystic ovarian syndrome; seminiferous tubule dysgenesis; orchitis	See Section 10.8 and Chapter 7, The Urinary and Reproductive Systems
Breast	Galactorrhea; hypoplasia; gynecomastia	See Section 10.9
Skeleton	Osteoporosis; osteomalacia	See Section 10.10

Bibliography

1. Wilson JD, Foster DW, eds. *Williams Textbook of Endocrinology.* 9th ed. Philadelphia, Pa: WB Saunders Co; 1985.

2. Felig P, Baxter J, Broadus A, Frohman L. *Endocrinology and Metabolism.* 2nd ed. New York, NY: McGraw-Hill Book Co; 1987.

3. Marble A, Krall LP, Bradley RF, Christlieb AR, Soeldner JS, eds. *Joslin's Diabetes Mellitus.* 12th ed. Philadelphia, Pa: Lea & Febiger; 1985.

4. Levin ME, O'Neal LW, eds. *The Diabetic Foot.* 3rd ed. St Louis, Mo: CV Mosby Co; 1983.

5. Davidson JK, ed. *Clinical Diabetes Mellitus: A Problem-Oriented Approach.* 2nd ed. New York, NY: Thieme Medical Publishers; 1991.

6. Braverman LE, Utiger RD, eds. *Werner and Ingbar's The Thyroid.* 6th ed. Philadelphia, Pa: JB Lippincott Co; 1991.

7. Burger HG, McLachlan RI, eds. Gonadal Disorders. *Endocrinol Metab Clin North Am.* Philadelphia, Pa: WB Saunders Co; December 1998.

8. Service JF, McMahon MM, O'Brien PC, Ballard DJ. Functioning insulinoma—incidence, recurrence and long-term survival of patients: a 60-year study. *Mayo Clin Proc.* 1991;66:711-719.

9. Orth DN. Cushing's syndrome: review article. *N Engl J Med.* 1995;332:791-803.

10. Bravo EL. Evolving concepts in the pathophysiology, diagnosis, and treatment of pheochromocytoma. *Endocrinol Rev.* 1994;15:356-367.

11. Silverberg SJ, Bilezikian JP. Evaluation and management of primary hyperparathyroidism. *J Clin Endocr Metab.* 1996;81:2036-2040.

12. Watts NB, ed. Osteoporosis. *Endocrinol Metab Clin North Am.* Philadelphia, Pa: WB Saunders Co; June 1998;419-439.

Chapter 11

Ear, Nose, Throat, and Related Structures

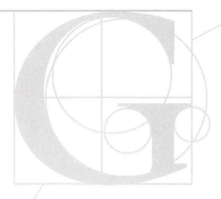

Introduction

This chapter provides criteria for evaluating permanent impairments resulting from principal dysfunction of the ear, nose, throat, and related structures. Assess permanent impairment ratings of these structures by evaluating losses in structure or the following functions: hearing; equilibrium; respiration; mastication, olfaction, and taste; speech and voice; and the effect of these losses on the ability to perform activities of daily living. Impairment criteria, listed in earlier editions of the *Guides,* were adapted from the American Academy of Otolaryngology–Head and Neck Surgery.[1] Abbreviations and their definitions are listed in the Glossary.

The following sections have been revised for the fifth edition: a new section has been added on the evaluation of voice impairment, facial disorders and disfigurements have been combined, and case examples have been added to the impairment classes.

11.1 Principles of Assessment

Before using the information in this chapter, the *Guides* user should become familiar with Chapters 1 and 2 and the Glossary. Chapters 1 and 2 discuss the *Guides'* purpose, applications, and methods for performing and reporting impairment evaluations. The Glossary provides definitions of common terms used by many specialties in impairment evaluations.

Assistive devices *must not* be used during the determination of a hearing impairment rating. The use of such devices might give a false impression of a subject's sensitivity and distort the need to take hearing conservation or other indicated measures. As stated in Chapter 1, report measured hearing with and without an assistive device. However, only the measurement without the assistive device should be used to determine the impairment rating.

11.1a Interpretation of Symptoms and Signs

Begin the evaluation with an inquiry into specific symptoms and their severity, duration, and manner of onset. The history, physical examination, and diagnostic studies may enable identification of the diagnosis, a management plan, and prognosis. Since the ear, nose, throat, and related structures have distinct functions, disorders of each system will be covered separately in this chapter. Permanent impairments of each system with nonoverlapping functional losses are evaluated separately and then combined.

Some impairment classes refer to limitations in the ability to perform daily activities. When this information is subjective and possibly misinterpreted, it should not serve as the sole criterion upon which decisions about impairment are made. Rather, obtain objective data about the severity of the findings and the limitations and integrate the findings with the subjective data to estimate the degree of permanent impairment.

11.1b Description of Clinical Studies

Multiple and diverse tests are used to investigate the ear, nose, throat, and related structures. Some of these tests are discussed in the relevant organ system section and summarized in Table 11-10.

11.2 The Ear

The ear consists of the auricle, the external canal, the tympanic membrane, the ossicles, the middle ear, the eustachian tube, the mastoid, and the internal ear. The auditory and vestibular systems include the ear and central nervous system pathways.

The ear provides sensorineural input critical to the senses of hearing and balance. Hearing enables contact with environmental cues (eg, those that alert) and enables us to communicate socially. Balance contributes to maintenance of equilibrium in relation to the environment. Balance function is mediated by dynamically monitoring information about the position of the head, eyes, trunk, and joints at rest and with activity. Although hearing and balance disturbances can be objectively measured, other conditions, such as chronic otorrhea, otalgia, and tinnitus,[2] are subjective, should be noted, but cannot be measured independently of the individual's self-reports.

Permanent hearing impairment is a permanently reduced hearing sensitivity, outside the range of normal for the individual or based on population normal values.[3] Hearing should be evaluated after maximum rehabilitation has been achieved and when the impairment is no longer accelerating beyond an age-appropriate rate.[4] Evaluate hearing impairment based upon the individual's binaural hearing, determined from the pure-tone audiogram.

11.2a Criteria for Rating Impairment Due to Hearing Loss

Criteria for evaluating hearing impairment are established through hearing threshold testing, which serves as the most reproducible of the measures of hearing. Therefore, estimate an impairment percentage based on the severity of the hearing loss, which accounts for changes in the ability to perform activities of daily living. **Tinnitus** in the presence of unilateral or bilateral hearing impairment may impair speech discrimination. Therefore, add up to 5% for tinnitus in the presence of measurable hearing loss if the tinnitus impacts the ability to perform activities of daily living.

In the calculation of a hearing impairment rating, no correction for presbycusis should be made because: (1) the method below calculates the degree of hearing and assigns a rating, regardless of cause (eg, age, injury, or noise exposure); (2) age correction would result in a reduced binaural impairment score that would thus underestimate the true magnitude of the hearing impairment; and (3) estimation of the relative contributions of various causes of binaural hearing impairment is a clinical process (apportionment or allocation) that is separate from the calculation of binaural hearing impairment.

Hearing impairment is measured by evaluating hearing in each ear separately and both ears together, based on audiometric measurements. Hearing impairment is reported in each ear separately and both ears together.

Audiometric Measurements to Determine Hearing Impairment

In determining impairments, the following steps should be taken.

1. Test each ear separately with a pure-tone audiometer and record the hearing levels at 500, 1000, 2000, and 3000 Hz. It is necessary that the hearing level for each frequency be determined in every subject. The following rules apply for extreme values:
   a. If the hearing level at a given frequency is greater than 100 dB or is beyond the range of the audiometer, the level should be taken as 100 dB.
   b. If the hearing level for a given frequency has a negative value (eg, –5 dB), the level should be taken as 0 dB.
2. Add the four hearing levels (dB) for each ear separately. Hearing levels are determined according to ANSI Standard S3.6-1996.[4]
3. Consult Table 11-1 to determine the percentages of monaural hearing impairment for each ear.
4. Consult Table 11-2 to convert the monaural hearing impairment percentages to a binaural hearing impairment rating.
5. Consult Table 11-3 to determine the impairment of the whole person.

Table 11-1 Monaural Hearing Loss and Impairment*

DSHL†	%	DSHL†	%	DSHL†	%
100	0	190	33.8	285	69.3
		195	35.6	290	71.2
105	1.9	200	37.5	295	73.1
110	3.8			300	75.0
115	5.6	205	39.4		
120	7.5	210	41.2	305	76.9
		215	43.1	310	78.8
125	9.4	220	45.0	315	80.6
130	11.2			320	82.5
135	13.1	225	46.9		
140	15.0	230	48.8	325	84.4
		235	50.6	330	86.2
145	16.9	240	52.5	335	88.1
150	18.8			340	90.0
155	20.6	245	54.4		
160	22.5	250	56.2	345	91.9
		255	58.1	350	93.8
165	24.4	260	60.0	355	95.6
170	26.2			360	97.5
175	28.1	265	61.9	365	99.4
180	30.0	270	63.8	≥370	100.0
		275	65.6		
185	31.9	280	67.5		

*Audiometers are calibrated to ANSI Standard S3.6-1996 reference levels.[4]
†Decibel sum of the hearing threshold levels at 500, 1000, 2000, and 3000 Hz.

Chapter 11

Table 11-2 Computation of Binaural Hearing Impairment*

	≥100	105	110	115	120	125	130	135	140	145	150	155	160	165	170	175	180	185	190	195	200	205	210	215	220	225	230
≤100	0.0																										
105	0.3	1.9																									
110	0.6	2.2	3.8																								
115	0.9	2.5	4.1	5.6																							
120	1.3	2.8	4.4	5.9	7.5																						
125	1.6	3.1	4.7	6.3	7.8	9.4																					
130	1.9	3.4	5.0	6.6	8.1	9.7	11.3																				
135	2.2	3.8	5.3	6.9	8.4	10.0	11.6	13.1																			
140	2.5	4.1	5.6	7.2	8.8	10.3	11.9	13.4	15.0																		
145	2.8	4.4	5.9	7.5	9.1	10.6	12.2	13.8	15.3	16.9																	
150	3.1	4.7	6.3	7.8	9.4	10.9	12.5	14.1	15.6	17.2	18.8																
155	3.4	5.0	6.6	8.1	9.7	11.3	12.8	14.4	15.9	17.5	19.1	20.6															
160	3.8	5.3	6.9	8.4	10.0	11.6	13.1	14.7	16.3	17.8	19.4	20.9	22.5														
165	4.1	5.6	7.2	8.8	10.3	11.9	13.4	15.0	16.6	18.1	19.7	21.3	22.8	24.4													
170	4.4	5.9	7.5	9.1	10.6	12.2	13.8	15.3	16.9	18.4	20.0	21.6	23.1	24.7	26.3												
175	4.7	6.3	7.8	9.4	10.9	12.5	14.1	15.6	17.2	18.8	20.3	21.9	23.4	25.0	26.6	28.1											
180	5.0	6.6	8.1	9.7	11.3	12.8	14.4	15.9	17.5	19.1	20.6	22.2	23.8	25.3	26.9	28.4	30.0										
185	5.3	6.9	8.4	10.0	11.6	13.1	14.7	16.3	17.8	19.4	20.9	22.5	24.1	25.6	27.2	28.8	30.3	31.9									
190	5.6	7.2	8.8	10.3	11.9	13.4	15.0	16.6	18.1	19.7	21.3	22.8	24.4	25.9	27.5	29.1	30.6	32.2	33.8								
195	5.9	7.5	9.1	10.6	12.2	13.8	15.3	16.9	18.4	20.0	21.6	23.1	24.7	26.3	27.8	29.4	30.9	32.5	34.1	35.6							
200	6.3	7.8	9.4	10.9	12.5	14.1	15.6	17.2	18.8	20.3	21.9	23.4	25.0	26.6	28.1	29.7	31.3	32.8	34.4	35.9	37.5						
205	6.6	8.1	9.7	11.3	12.8	14.4	15.9	17.5	19.1	20.6	22.2	23.8	25.3	26.9	28.4	30	31.6	33.1	34.7	36.3	37.8	39.4					
210	6.9	8.4	10.0	11.6	13.1	14.7	16.3	17.8	19.4	20.9	22.5	24.1	25.6	27.2	28.8	30.3	31.9	33.4	35	36.6	38.1	39.7	41.3				
215	7.2	8.8	10.3	11.9	13.4	15	16.6	18.1	19.7	21.3	22.8	24.4	25.9	27.5	29.1	30.6	32.2	33.8	35.3	36.9	38.4	40	41.6	43.1			
220	7.5	9.1	10.6	12.2	13.8	15.3	16.9	18.4	20.0	21.6	23.1	24.7	26.3	27.8	29.4	30.9	32.5	34.1	35.6	37.2	38.8	40.3	41.9	43.4	45		
225	7.8	9.4	10.9	12.5	14.1	15.6	17.2	18.8	20.3	21.9	23.4	25.0	26.6	28.1	29.7	31.3	32.8	34.4	35.9	37.5	39.1	40.6	42.2	43.8	45.3	46.9	
230	8.1	9.7	11.3	12.8	14.4	15.9	17.5	19.1	20.6	22.2	23.8	25.3	26.9	28.4	30.0	31.6	33.1	34.7	36.3	37.8	39.4	40.9	42.5	44.1	45.6	47.2	48.8
235	8.4	10.0	11.6	13.1	14.7	16.3	17.8	19.4	20.9	22.5	24.1	25.6	27.2	28.8	30.3	31.9	33.4	35.0	36.6	38.1	39.7	41.3	42.8	44.4	45.9	47.5	49.1
240	8.8	10.3	11.9	13.4	15.0	16.6	18.1	19.7	21.3	22.8	24.4	25.9	27.5	29.1	30.6	32.2	33.8	35.3	36.9	38.4	40.0	41.6	43.1	44.7	46.3	47.8	49.4
245	9.1	10.6	12.2	13.8	15.3	16.9	18.4	20.0	21.6	23.1	24.7	26.3	27.8	29.4	30.9	32.5	34.1	35.6	37.2	38.8	40.3	41.9	43.4	45.0	46.6	48.1	49.7
250	9.4	10.9	12.5	14.1	15.6	17.2	18.8	20.3	21.9	23.4	25.0	26.6	28.1	29.7	31.3	32.8	34.4	35.9	37.5	39.1	40.6	42.2	43.8	45.3	46.9	48.4	50.0
255	9.7	11.3	12.8	14.4	15.9	17.5	19.1	20.6	22.2	23.8	25.3	26.9	28.4	30.0	31.6	33.1	34.7	36.3	37.8	39.4	40.9	42.5	44.1	45.6	47.2	48.8	50.3
260	10.0	11.6	13.1	14.7	16.3	17.8	19.4	20.9	22.5	24.1	25.6	27.2	28.8	30.3	31.9	33.4	35.0	36.6	38.1	39.7	41.3	42.8	44.4	45.9	47.5	49.1	50.6
265	10.3	11.9	13.4	15.0	16.6	18.1	19.7	21.3	22.8	24.4	25.9	27.5	29.1	30.6	32.2	33.8	35.3	36.9	38.4	40.0	41.6	43.1	44.7	46.3	47.8	49.4	50.9
270	10.6	12.2	13.8	15.3	16.9	18.4	20.0	21.6	23.1	24.7	26.3	27.8	29.4	30.9	32.5	34.1	35.6	37.2	38.8	40.3	41.9	43.4	45.0	46.6	48.1	49.7	51.3
275	10.9	12.5	14.1	15.6	17.2	18.8	20.3	21.9	23.4	25.0	26.6	28.1	29.7	31.3	32.8	34.4	35.9	37.5	39.1	40.6	42.2	43.8	45.3	46.9	48.4	50.0	51.6
280	11.3	12.8	14.4	15.9	17.5	19.1	20.6	22.2	23.8	25.3	26.9	28.4	30.0	31.6	33.1	34.7	36.3	37.8	39.4	40.9	42.5	44.1	45.6	47.2	48.8	50.3	51.9
285	11.6	13.1	14.7	16.3	17.8	19.4	20.9	22.5	24.1	25.6	27.2	28.8	30.3	31.9	33.4	35.0	36.6	38.1	39.7	41.3	42.8	44.4	45.9	47.5	49.1	50.6	52.2
290	11.9	13.4	15.0	16.6	18.1	19.7	21.3	22.8	24.4	25.9	27.5	29.1	30.6	32.2	33.8	35.3	36.9	38.4	40.0	41.6	43.1	44.7	46.3	47.8	49.4	50.9	52.5
295	12.2	13.8	15.3	16.9	18.4	20.0	21.6	23.1	24.7	26.3	27.8	29.4	30.9	32.5	34.1	35.6	37.2	38.8	40.3	41.9	43.4	45.0	46.6	48.1	49.7	51.3	52.8
300	12.5	14.1	15.6	17.2	18.8	20.3	21.9	23.4	25.0	26.6	28.1	29.7	31.3	32.8	34.4	35.9	37.5	39.1	40.6	42.2	43.8	45.3	46.9	48.4	50.0	51.6	53.1
305	12.8	14.4	15.9	17.5	19.1	20.6	22.2	23.8	25.3	26.9	28.4	30.0	31.6	33.1	34.7	36.3	37.8	39.4	40.9	42.5	44.1	45.6	47.2	48.8	50.3	51.9	53.4
310	13.1	14.7	16.3	17.8	19.4	20.9	22.5	24.1	25.6	27.2	28.8	30.3	31.9	33.4	35.0	36.6	38.1	39.7	41.3	42.8	44.4	45.9	47.5	49.1	50.6	52.2	53.8
315	13.4	15.0	16.6	18.1	19.7	21.3	22.8	24.4	25.9	27.5	29.1	30.6	32.2	33.8	35.3	36.9	38.4	40.0	41.6	43.1	44.7	46.3	47.8	49.4	50.9	52.5	54.1
320	13.8	15.3	16.9	18.4	20.0	21.6	23.1	24.7	26.3	27.8	29.4	30.9	32.5	34.1	35.6	37.2	38.8	40.3	41.9	43.4	45.0	46.6	48.1	49.7	51.3	52.8	54.4
325	14.1	15.6	17.2	18.8	20.3	21.9	23.4	25.0	26.6	28.1	29.7	31.3	32.8	34.4	35.9	37.5	39.1	40.6	42.2	43.8	45.3	46.9	48.4	50.0	51.6	53.1	54.7
330	14.4	15.9	17.5	19.1	20.6	22.2	23.8	25.3	26.9	28.4	30.0	31.6	33.1	34.7	36.3	37.8	39.4	40.9	42.5	44.1	45.6	47.2	48.8	50.3	51.9	53.4	55.0
335	14.7	16.3	17.8	19.4	20.9	22.5	24.1	25.6	27.2	28.8	30.3	31.9	33.4	35.0	36.6	38.1	39.7	41.3	42.8	44.4	45.9	47.5	49.1	50.6	52.2	53.8	55.3
340	15.0	16.6	18.1	19.7	21.3	22.8	24.4	25.9	27.5	29.1	30.6	32.2	33.8	35.3	36.9	38.4	40.0	41.6	43.1	44.7	46.3	47.8	49.4	50.9	52.5	54.1	55.6
345	15.3	16.9	18.4	20.0	21.6	23.1	24.7	26.3	27.8	29.4	30.9	32.5	34.1	35.6	37.2	38.8	40.3	41.9	43.4	45.0	46.6	48.1	49.7	51.3	52.8	54.4	55.9
350	15.6	17.2	18.8	20.3	21.9	23.4	25.0	26.6	28.1	29.7	31.3	32.8	34.4	35.9	37.5	39.1	40.6	42.2	43.8	45.3	46.9	48.4	50.0	51.6	53.1	54.7	56.3
355	15.9	17.5	19.1	20.6	22.2	23.8	25.3	26.9	28.4	30.0	31.6	33.1	34.7	36.3	37.8	39.4	40.9	42.5	44.1	45.6	47.2	48.8	50.3	51.9	53.4	55.0	56.6
360	16.3	17.8	19.4	20.9	22.5	24.1	25.6	27.2	28.8	30.3	31.9	33.4	35.0	36.6	38.1	39.7	41.3	42.8	44.4	45.9	47.5	49.1	50.6	52.2	53.8	55.3	56.9
365	16.6	18.1	19.7	21.3	22.8	24.4	25.9	27.5	29.1	30.6	32.2	33.8	35.3	36.9	38.4	40.0	41.6	43.1	44.7	46.3	47.8	49.4	50.9	52.5	54.1	55.6	57.2
≥370	16.7	18.2	19.8	21.4	22.9	24.5	26.0	27.6	29.2	30.7	32.3	33.9	35.4	37.0	38.5	40.1	41.7	43.2	44.8	46.4	47.9	49.5	51.0	52.6	54.2	55.7	57.3
ANSI 1969	≥100	105	110	115	120	125	130	135	140	145	150	155	160	165	170	175	180	185	190	195	200	205	210	215	220	225	230

*The axes are the sum of hearing levels at 500, 1000, 2000, and 3000 Hz. The sum for the worse ear is read at the side; the sum for the better ear is read at the bottom. At the intersection of the row for the worse ear and the column for the better ear is the hearing impairment (%).

Chapter 11

235	240	245	250	255	260	265	270	275	280	285	290	295	300	305	310	315	320	325	330	335	340	345	350	355	360	365	≥368
50.6																											
50.9	52.5																										
51.3	52.8	54.4																									
51.6	53.1	54.7	56.3																								
51.9	53.4	55.0	56.6	58.1																							
52.2	53.8	55.3	56.9	58.4	60.0																						
52.5	54.1	55.6	57.2	58.8	60.3	61.9																					
52.8	54.4	55.9	57.5	59.1	60.6	62.2	63.8																				
53.1	54.7	56.3	57.8	59.4	60.9	62.5	64.1	65.6																			
53.4	55.0	56.6	58.1	59.7	61.3	62.8	64.4	65.9	67.5																		
53.8	55.3	56.9	58.4	60.0	61.6	63.1	64.7	66.3	67.8	69.4																	
54.1	55.6	57.2	58.8	60.3	61.9	63.4	65.0	66.6	68.1	69.7	71.3																
54.4	55.9	57.5	59.1	60.6	62.2	63.8	65.3	66.9	68.4	70.0	71.6	73.1															
54.7	56.3	57.8	59.4	60.9	62.5	64.1	65.6	67.2	68.8	70.3	71.9	73.4	75.0														
55.0	56.6	58.1	59.7	61.3	62.8	64.4	65.9	67.5	69.1	70.6	72.2	73.8	75.3	76.9													
55.3	56.9	58.4	60.0	61.6	63.1	64.7	66.3	67.8	69.4	70.9	72.5	74.1	75.6	77.2	78.8												
55.6	57.2	58.8	60.3	61.9	63.4	65.0	66.6	68.1	69.7	71.3	72.8	74.4	75.9	77.5	79.1	80.6											
55.9	57.5	59.1	60.6	62.2	63.8	65.3	66.9	68.4	70.0	71.6	73.1	74.7	76.3	77.8	79.4	80.9	82.5										
56.3	57.8	59.4	60.9	62.5	64.1	65.6	67.2	68.8	70.3	71.9	73.4	75.0	76.6	78.1	79.7	81.3	82.8	84.4									
56.6	58.1	59.7	61.3	62.8	64.4	65.9	67.5	69.1	70.6	72.2	73.8	75.3	76.9	78.4	80.0	81.6	83.1	84.7	86.3								
56.9	58.4	60.0	61.6	63.1	64.7	66.3	67.8	69.4	70.9	72.5	74.1	75.6	77.2	78.8	80.3	81.9	83.4	85.0	86.6	88.1							
57.2	58.8	60.3	61.9	63.4	65.0	66.6	68.1	69.7	71.3	72.8	74.4	75.9	77.5	79.1	80.6	82.2	83.8	85.3	86.9	88.4	90.0						
57.5	59.1	60.6	62.2	63.8	65.3	66.9	68.4	70.0	71.6	73.1	74.7	76.3	77.8	79.4	80.9	82.5	84.1	85.6	87.2	88.8	90.3	91.9					
57.8	59.4	60.9	62.5	64.1	65.6	67.2	68.8	70.3	71.9	73.4	75.0	76.6	78.1	79.7	81.3	82.8	84.4	85.9	87.5	89.1	90.6	92.2	93.8				
58.1	59.7	61.3	62.8	64.4	65.9	67.5	69.1	70.6	72.2	73.8	75.3	76.9	78.4	80.0	81.6	83.1	84.7	86.3	87.8	89.4	90.9	92.5	94.1	95.6			
58.4	60.0	61.6	63.1	64.7	66.3	67.8	69.4	70.9	72.5	74.1	75.6	77.2	78.8	80.3	81.9	83.4	85.0	86.6	88.1	89.7	91.3	92.8	94.4	95.9	97.5		
58.8	60.3	61.9	63.4	65.0	66.6	68.1	69.7	71.3	72.8	74.4	75.9	77.5	79.1	80.6	82.2	83.8	85.3	86.9	88.4	90.0	91.6	93.1	94.7	96.3	97.6	99.4	
58.9	60.4	62.0	63.5	65.1	66.7	68.2	69.8	71.4	73.0	74.5	76.0	77.6	79.2	80.7	82.3	83.9	85.4	87.0	88.5	90.1	91.7	93.2	94.8	96.4	97.9	99.5	100

Evaluation of Monaural Hearing Impairment

If the average of the hearing levels at 500, 1000, 2000, and 3000 Hz is 25 dB or less, according to 1996 American National Standards Institute (ANSI) audiometric standards,[4] no impairment rating is assigned since there is no change in the ability to hear everyday sounds under everyday listening conditions (Table 11-1). At the other extreme, if the average of the hearing levels at 500, 1000, 2000, and 3000 Hz is more than 91.7 dB, the binaural hearing impairment rating is 100% since the individual has lost the ability to perform an activity of daily living—the ability to hear everyday speech.[1]

The data from which this formula[1] was developed indicate that the ability to hear everyday sounds under everyday listening conditions is not impaired when the average of the hearing levels at 500, 1000, 2000, and 3000 Hz is 25 dB or less. The 25-dB "fence" represents this finding; it is not a compensatory adjustment for presbycusis, the hearing loss that occurs with age.

This method of evaluating hearing impairment should be applied only to adults who have acquired language skills. Evidence suggests that language acquisition by children who do not have language skills may be delayed when the average hearing level is in the range of 15 to 25 dB.

According to the above standards for monaural hearing impairment, for every decibel that the average hearing level or loss for speech exceeds 25 dB, 1.5% of monaural impairment is assigned. Thus, with an average hearing level loss of 67 dB above 25 dB, monaural impairment is 100% (Table 11-1).

Evaluation of Binaural Hearing Impairment

Hearing impairment of both ears, referred to as binaural impairment, indicates a loss of hearing of greater than 25 dB in both ears at frequencies of 500, 1000, 2000, and/or 3000 Hz.

Binaural impairment is determined by the following formula:

$$\text{binaural hearing impairment (\%)} = \frac{[5 \times (\% \text{ hearing impairment better ear}) + (\% \text{ hearing impairment poorer ear})]}{6}$$

To calculate binaural impairment when only one ear exhibits hearing impairment, use the above formula, allowing 0% impairment for the unimpaired ear (the ear with the better hearing).

Table 11-3 Relationship of Binaural Hearing Impairment to Impairment of the Whole Person

% Binaural Hearing Impairment	% Impairment of the Whole Person	% Binaural Hearing Impairment	% Impairment of the Whole Person
0.0- 1.7	0	50.0-53.1	18
1.8- 4.2	1	53.2-55.7	19
4.3- 7.4	2	55.8-58.8	20
7.5- 9.9	3	58.9-61.4	21
10.0-13.1	4	61.5-64.5	22
13.2-15.9	5	64.6-67.1	23
16.0-18.8	6	67.2-70.0	24
18.9-21.4	7	70.1-72.8	25
21.5-24.5	8	72.9-75.9	26
24.6-27.1	9	76.0-78.5	27
27.2-30.0	10	78.6-81.7	28
30.1-32.8	11	81.8-84.2	29
32.9-35.9	12	84.3-87.4	30
36.0-38.5	13	87.5-89.9	31
38.6-41.7	14	90.0-93.1	32
41.8-44.2	15	93.2-95.7	33
44.3-47.4	16	95.8-98.8	34
47.5-49.9	17	98.9-100.0	35

Alternatively, use Table 11-2, which is derived from the formula given above, to calculate the value for binaural hearing impairment. Then apply the value for binaural hearing impairment to Table 11-3, which converts binaural hearing impairment to impairment of the whole person.

Example 11-1
5% Impairment Due to Hearing Loss

Subject: 70-year-old woman.

History: Chronic recurrent ear infections since teens. Occasional drainage from right ear. Right ear now dry but feels "like stuffed with cotton." Has occasional tinnitus in right ear; not bothersome. No dizziness.

Current Symptoms: Difficulty hearing, especially in right ear, with no impact on activities of daily living. No recent drainage.

Physical Exam: Scarred, retracted right tympanic membrane. Left tympanic membrane is thickened and retracted. Pneumo-otoscopy shows motion of left tympanic membrane, but no motion on right.

Clinical Studies: Tympanograms: B pattern for right ear and C pattern for left ear. Speech discrimination score: 95% for right ear; 80% for left ear. Acoustic immitance: reveals normal external auditory canal volumes for both ears. Pure tone audiometry reveals the following threshold levels in decibels (dB):

	Right Ear (thousands)						Left Ear (thousands)					
Frequency, Hz	0.5	1	2	3	4	6	8	0.5	1	2	3	4	6	8
Air Conduction	40	55	60	70	80	95	NR	25	30	30	40	40	60	70
Bone Conduction	20	30	15	—	35	—	—	Not tested in left ear

Diagnosis: Mixed (sensorineural + conductive) hearing impairment, right ear. Mild sensorineural hearing impairment, left ear.

Impairment Rating: 5% impairment of the whole person.

Comment: The decimal sum of hearing threshold levels (DSHL) for the right ear is 225 (40 + 55 + 60 + 70), and the DSHL for the left ear is 125 (25 + 30 + 30 + 40). Combine 225 (worse ear) and 125 (better ear) using Table 11-2 for a binaural hearing impairment rating (BI) of 15.6%. Use Table 11-3 to obtain the 5% whole person impairment rating.

Example 11-2
8% Impairment Due to Hearing Loss

Subject: 65-year-old woman.

History: Repeated ear infections for many years. Hearing loss in both ears and roaring, pulsing, rushing-water tinnitus in both ears. No history of dizziness. Tympanoplasty, left ear, 4 months ago.

Current Symptoms: Difficulty hearing in both ears, but hearing much improved in left ear since tympanoplasty. Still has tinnitus in both ears, which impacts some activities of daily living.

Physical Exam: Retracted right tympanic membrane.

Clinical Studies: Left tympanic membrane shows well-healed graft. Tympanograms: B pattern for right ear. Tympanometry was not performed for left ear due to recent otologic surgery. Speech discrimination scores: 80% for right ear; 85% for left ear. Pure tone audiometry reveals the following threshold levels in decibels (dB):

	Right Ear (thousands)						Left Ear (thousands)					
Frequency, Hz	0.5	1	2	3	4	6	8	0.5	1	2	3	4	6	8
Air Conduction	50	50	55	55	60	85	NR	25	30	40	40	40	60	85
Bone Conduction	15	35	35	—	20	—	—	0	5	25	—	15	—	—

Diagnosis: Mixed (sensorineural + conductive) hearing impairment, bilaterally.

Impairment Rating: 8% impairment of the whole person.

Comment: The DSHL for the right ear is 210 (50 + 50 + 55 + 55), and the DSHL for the left ear is 135 (25 + 30 + 40 + 40). Combine 210 (worse ear) and 135 (better ear) using Table 11-2 for a BI of 17.8%. Add 5% for the presence of tinnitus, giving a BI of 22.8%. Use Table 11-3 to obtain the 8% whole person impairment.

Example 11-3
8% Impairment Due to Hearing Loss

Subject: 64-year-old man.

History: Progressive hearing loss for 13 years. Worked in several noisy environments; used hearing protectors fairly regularly. Exposure to gunfire during 4 years of service in the Marines. General health good. No history of tinnitus or vertigo.

Current Symptoms: Difficulty with communication at home, in restaurants, driving a car, and in noisy environments.

Physical Exam: No abnormalities.

Clinical Studies: Audiologic tests: speech reception threshold of 20 dB. Pure tone audiometry reveals the following threshold levels in decibels (dB):

	Right Ear (thousands)						Left Ear (thousands)					
Frequency, Hz	0.5	1	2	3	4	6	8	0.5	1	2	3	4	6	8
	20	15	60	80	85	85	70	25	15	60	60	65	65	60

Diagnosis: Sensorineural hearing impairment, bilateral.

Impairment Rating: 8% impairment of the whole person.

Comment: The impairment calculated from this audiogram is based on the DSHL. The DSHL for the right ear is 175 (20 + 15 + 60 + 80), and the DSHL for the left ear is 160 (25 + 15 + 60 + 60). Combine 175 (worse ear) and 160 (better ear) using Table 11-2 for a binaural hearing impairment of 23.4%. Use Table 11-3 to obtain the 8% whole person impairment.

Chapter 11

11.2b Equilibrium

Equilibrium, or orientation in space, is maintained by the visual, kinesthetic, and vestibular mechanisms. When impairments of equilibrium are predominantly due to or have effects on other organ systems, the impairment should be evaluated in the relevant organ system, eg, disorders of the nervous system (Chapter 13), cardiovascular system (Chapters 3 and 4), and visual system (Chapter 12).

Disturbances of equilibrium may be classified as follows: (1) **vertigo,** a sensation of rotation of the subject or of objects about the subject in any plane; (2) giddiness or lightheadedness, distinguished from vertigo by the absence of feelings of movement[2]; and (3) abnormalities of postural stability and/or standing balance with or without vertigo. Vertigo may be produced by disorders of the vestibular mechanism and its central nervous system components, including the cerebral cortex, cerebellum, and brain stem, and by eye movements.

Permanent impairment may result from any disorder causing vertigo or disorientation in space. Three regulatory systems—vestibular, ocular (visual), and kinesthetic (proprioceptive)—are related to the vestibulo-ocular reflex. The evaluation of impairments of equilibrium may include consideration of one or more of these mechanisms.[5,6] This chapter addresses only disturbances in equilibrium due to vestibular disorders.

Clinical evaluations may include electronystagmography,[2] caloric irrigation, positional and rotatory tests, dynamic posturography, Romberg and tandem Romberg tests, and radiological brain imaging studies. The results of these laboratory tests should be correlated with validated clinical measures of balance and ambulation to determine the true state of equilibratory dysfunction. For other causes of disequilibrium, see the relevant chapter, such as the neurologic system (Chapter 13), for central nervous system disorders.

Vestibular System

Permanent impairment can result from defects of the vestibular (labyrinthine) mechanism and its central connections. The defects are evidenced by loss of equilibrium produced by disturbance or loss of vestibular function.

Complete loss of vestibular function may be unilateral or bilateral. When the loss is unilateral, adequate central nervous system compensation may or may not occur. With total bilateral loss of vestibular function, equilibrium is totally dependent on the kinesthetic and visual systems, which usually are unable to compensate fully for movement or ambulation. Depending on the ability to perform activities of daily living, the percentage of permanent impairment of the whole person may range from 0% to 95%.

Disturbances of vestibular function are evidenced by vertigo (vestibular dysequilibrium) as defined above. Lightheadedness and abnormalities of gait not associated with vertigo are not defined here as being disturbances of vestibular function.

Vertigo may be accompanied by varying degrees of nausea, vomiting, headache, immobility, ataxia, and nystagmus. Movement may increase the vertigo and the accompanying signs and symptoms. Peripheral vestibular (labyrinthine) disorders are often associated with hearing loss and tinnitus. Vestibular disorders may result in temporary or permanent impairments. Evaluation of vestibular impairment should be performed when the condition is stable and maximum adjustment has been achieved, which generally is considered to occur months after resolution of the disease or injury.[5,6]

The classification in Table 11-4 has been developed for evaluation of those individuals with permanent disturbances of the vestibular mechanism. The impairment ratings reflect the severity of the permanent impairment and the ability of the individual to perform activities of daily living. Since vestibular disorders are dynamic, assessment of permanent impairment should be based on determination of the person's condition after it is stable. Although symptoms may be intermittent, the examiner needs to gauge functioning during episodes with exacerbations. Vestibular impairment as defined here is rated similarly in Chapter 13.

Table 11-4 Criteria for Rating Impairment Due to Vestibular Disorders

Class 1 0% Impairment of the Whole Person	Class 2 1%-10% Impairment of the Whole Person	Class 3 11%-30% Impairment of the Whole Person	Class 4 31%-60% Impairment of the Whole Person	Class 5 61%-95% Impairment of the Whole Person
Symptoms or signs of vestibular dysequilibrium present without supporting objective findings *and* activities of daily living can be performed without assistance	Symptoms or signs of vestibular dysequilibrium present with supporting objective findings *and* activities of daily living can be performed without assistance, except for complex activities (eg, riding a bicycle) or certain types of demanding activities related to the individual's work (eg, walking on girders or scaffolds)	Symptoms or signs of vestibular dysequilibrium present with supporting objective findings *and* activities of daily living cannot be performed without assistance, except for simple activities (eg, self-care, some household duties, walking, and riding in a motor vehicle operated by another person)	Symptoms or signs of vestibular dysequilibrium present with supporting objective findings *and* activities of daily living cannot be performed without assistance, except for self-care	Symptoms or signs of vestibular dysequilibrium present with supporting objective findings *and* activities of daily living cannot be performed without assistance, except for self-care not requiring ambulation *and* home confinement is necessary

Class 1 0% Impairment of the Whole Person
Symptoms or signs of vestibular dysequilibrium present without supporting objective findings *and* activities of daily living can be performed without assistance

Class 2 1%-10% Impairment of the Whole Person
Symptoms or signs of vestibular dysequilibrium present with supporting objective findings *and* activities of daily living can be performed without assistance, except for complex activities (eg, riding a bicycle) or certain types of demanding activities related to the subject's work (eg, walking on girders or scaffolds)

Example 11-4
0% Impairment Due to Floating Vestibular Otoconia

Subject: 70-year-old man.

History: Retired physician; onset of **dizziness** last week when leaning head to right or to left side. Sensation of giddiness with positional change of body but not with turning of head when upright. No nausea or vomiting. Uses the Epley maneuver to reposition otoconia.

Current Symptoms: Asymptomatic; the dizziness has not recurred; no disruption of activities of daily living.

Clinical Studies: ENG study: normal. Dix-Hallpike test: positive, with head rotation to the left and to the right.

Diagnosis: Floating vestibular otoconia.

Impairment Rating: 0% impairment of the whole person.

Comment: Treatment to be repeated as necessary.

Example 11-5
1% to 10% Impairment Due to Labyrinthitis

Subject: 50-year-old-woman.

History: Sudden onset of severe vertigo, nausea, and vomiting. No history of upper respiratory infection, fever, cough, or chills. Confined to bed. Spontaneous nystagmus to left noted. Hearing normal; no tinnitus. Treated with vestibular suppressors. Gradual, slow recovery of ability to ambulate, but unable to walk in the dark for about 1 year.

Current Symptoms: Can perform activities of daily living without assistance. Slightly unsteady when fatigued. Does not tolerate rocking motion (sailboat) without visual fixation of horizon. Unable to ride bicycle, but can drive automobile at night.

Physical Exam: Normal.

Clinical Studies: ENG and caloric studies: no vestibular function of right ear. Other neuro-otologic findings: within normal limits. Audiogram: normal hearing bilaterally. Mastoid X-rays: normal. CT scans of temporal bones: normal.

Diagnosis: Labyrinthitis, probably viral, with total loss of vestibular function, right ear.

Impairment Rating: 10% impairment of the whole person.

Comment: Class 2 impairment, with moderate loss of function.

Class 3
11%-30% Impairment of the Whole Person

Symptoms or signs of vestibular dysequilibrium present with supporting objective findings

and

activities of daily living cannot be performed without assistance, except for simple activities (eg, self-care, some household duties, walking, and riding in a motor vehicle operated by another person)

Example 11-6
11% to 30% Impairment Due to Vestibular Disorders

Subject: 40-year-old woman.

History: Nurse; progressive hearing loss in left ear, increased difficulty with gait, some loss of balance with falling to the left, and slurred speech when fatigued for 3 months. History of hypertension, controlled with beta-blockers. Audiogram showed normal hearing in right ear, 80-dB sensorineural hearing loss in left ear. Tympanograms were type A bilaterally. Acoustic reflex was absent in left ear. Vestibular tests suggested marked left peripheral end-organ lesion. Changes in oculomotor testing suggested brainstem involvement on the left side. Other neuro-otologic tests showed minimal left facial nerve weakness. MRI studies showed large left cerebellopontine angle (CPA) mass involving the left internal auditory canal. At surgery, via the translabyrinthine route, a 4-cm tumor of the left CPA, with secondary brain stem compression, was removed.

Current Symptoms: Walks with broad-based gait with slight limp. Has fallen twice since surgery.

Physical Exam: Slight weakness in lower extremities and control motions of left upper and lower extremities. Left facial paralysis. Total hearing loss in left ear. Left cerebellar tremor, in the upper extremity more than in the lower. Ophthalmologic exam reveals exposure keratopathy without microbial keratitis, left eye.

Clinical Studies: Neuro-otologic and neurologic: total loss of hearing and of vestibular function, left ear. No evident tumor, but changes in brain stem area noted on MRI. Electroencephalogram: no evidence of epileptiform activity. Gait and

balance scores: abnormal for age. Left lateral canthoplasty with insertion of gold weights in left upper eyelid was performed, plus a cross-face sural nerve graft to the left face.

Diagnosis: Large left acoustic neuroma with postoperative total left auditory and vestibular impairments and left facial nerve paralysis.

Impairment Rating: 30% impairment due to vestibular disorders; combine with appropriate ratings for other impairments to determine whole person impairment (see Combined Values Chart, p. 604).

Comment: Preoperatively active. Exercises; walks with some difficulty; can perform self-care and limited household activities; unable to drive a car or to continue to work.

Class 4
31%-60% Impairment of the Whole Person

Symptoms or signs of vestibular dysequilibrium present with supporting objective findings

and

activities of daily living cannot be performed without assistance, except for self-care

---

Example 11-7
31% to 60% Impairment Due to Chronic Vestibular Disorder

Subject: 43-year-old woman.

History: Dizziness for the past 6 years. Has consulted many physicians. In the past has had gall bladder problems and recurrent renal infections. No history of trauma or surgery. No history of chronic drug ingestion, but currently taking an antidepressant. Nonsmoker.

Current Symptoms: Occasional double vision during past year. Cannot drive. Does self-care slowly because of dizziness. Denies hearing loss. Self-rated as moderately impaired. Requires assistance with daily tasks.

Physical Exam: Hearing within normal limits. Blood pressure is normal.

Clinical Studies: Posturography: abnormal. Exhibits 50% caloric weakness in right ear. No directional preponderance. Rotatory tests: normal. Dix-Hallpike test: normal. Oculomotor tests: normal. Responded poorly to habituation exercises.

Diagnosis: Chronic vestibular disorder.

Impairment Rating: 31% to 60% impairment of the whole person.

Comment: Ophthalmologic evaluation required to evaluate visual complaints.

11.3 The Face

The face, its parts, and its structural components serve multiple functions: protection of underlying structures and organs (such as the eyes), portals of entry for deglutition and respiration, and communication through expression and speech.

The skin covers the body, acts as a physical barrier to underlying structures, provides sensory perception, regulates temperature and body fluids, and resists trauma. See Chapter 8 for primary skin impairments.

The portal for deglutition is the mouth and lips. Disturbances in function can result in drooling or inability to keep food or liquid in the mouth while eating. The lips and mouth also serve in vocal articulation, adding intelligibility to speech. The nose and mouth are the portals of entry for respiration. Impairment may be a result of neurologic disorders, such as partial or complete paralysis of the lips; scar formation and contracture of the lips; or loss of tissue.

The face plays a unique role in communication. No other part of the body serves as specific a function for personal identity and for the expression of thought and emotion. Facial expressions are an integral part of normal living postures. A degree of normalcy is needed for effective verbal and nonverbal communication. Facial anatomy contributes to identity, expression, and normal functioning, and to the appearance of the forehead and cheeks; eyes, eyelids, and eyebrows; lips and mouth; nose; and chin and neck. The face is such a prominent feature that it plays a critical role in the individual's physical, psychological, and emotional makeup. Facial disfigurement can affect all of these components and can result in social and vocational handicaps and even psychiatric impairment.

11.3a Criteria for Rating Impairment Due to Facial Disorders and/or Disfigurement

To evaluate permanent impairment due to a disorder or disfigurement of the face, consider changes in anatomy and function and the effect of the impairment on the ability to perform activities of daily living. This section deals with permanent impairment as it relates mainly to the face's structural integrity. For loss of function involving other aspects of the functioning of the face, refer to the specific organ system involved and combine the structural integrity loss with the relevant loss of function. Loss of structural integrity can result from cutaneous disfigurement, such as that due to abnormal pigmentation or scars, or from loss of supporting structures, such as soft tissue, bone, or cartilage of the facial skeleton. Other information on cutaneous disfigurement appears in Chapter 8 (The Skin).

Disfigurement of the face can result from many causes, particularly burns, traumatic injury, surgery, infections, or dysplasia. Effects on individuals can vary tremendously, as can remaining function. Total disfigurement of the face after treatment should be deemed a 16% to 50% impairment of the whole person, dependent also upon the degree of functional loss. For the assessment of psychosocial impairment due to disfigurement, refer to Chapter 14 on mental and behavioral disorders.

Facial disfigurement may be considered total if it is severe and grossly deforming of the face and features. Such disfigurement must involve at least the entire area between the brow line and the upper lip on both sides. Severe disfigurement above the brow line should be deemed to be, at a maximum, 1% impairment of the whole person. If disfigurement is severe below the upper lip, it may be deemed to be 8% impairment of the whole person. Specific, prominent facial disfigurements are estimated as shown in Table 11-5.

Table 11-5 Criteria for Rating Impairment Due to Facial Disorders and/or Disfigurement

Class 1 0%-5% Impairment of the Whole Person	Class 2 6%-10% Impairment of the Whole Person	Class 3 11%-15% Impairment of the Whole Person	Class 4 16%-50% Impairment of the Whole Person
Facial abnormality limited to disorder of cutaneous structures, such as visible scars or abnormal pigmentation (refer to Chapter 8 for skin disorders) *or* mild, unilateral, total facial paralysis *or* nasal distortion that affects physical appearance	Facial abnormality involves loss of supporting structure of part of face, with or without cutaneous disorder (eg, depressed cheek, nasal, or frontal bones)	Facial abnormality involves absence of normal anatomic part or area of face, such as loss of eye or loss of part of nose, with resulting cosmetic deformity; combine with any functional loss, eg, vision (Chapter 12) *or* severe, unilateral, total facial paralysis *or* mild, bilateral, total facial paralysis	Massive or total distortion of normal facial anatomy with disfigurement so severe that it precludes social acceptance; combine with any mental and behavioral impairment (Chapter 14) *or* severe, bilateral, total facial paralysis *or* loss of a major portion of or entire nose

---

Class 1 0%-5% Impairment of the Whole Person
Facial abnormality limited to disorder of cutaneous structures, such as visible scars or abnormal pigmentation (refer to Chapter 8 for skin disorders) *or* mild, unilateral, total facial paralysis *or* nasal distortion that affects physical appearance

Example 11-8
0% to 5% Impairment Due to Facial Disorders and/or Disfigurement

Subject: 25-year-old woman.

History: Struck in nose with baseball bat 1 year previously; sustained 2-cm laceration across dorsum of nose with minimally displaced nasal bone fractures. Underwent closed reduction of fractures of nasal bones and repair of laceration. Returned to normal activities after normal recovery.

Current Symptoms: Small scar on top of nose.

Physical Exam: Normal nasal region except for well-healed, stable 1.5-cm scar across glabellar region. Scar falls in skinfold lines.

Clinical Studies: None.

Diagnosis: Residual scar on dorsum of nose from compound nasal bone fracture.

Impairment Rating: 1% impairment of the whole person.

Comment: No loss of nasal function or nasal bone structural integrity. Appearance of nose did not change. Scar falls in skinfold line and is barely visible.

Example 11-9
0% to 5% Impairment Due to Facial Disorders and/or Disfigurement

Subject: 36-year-old man.

History: Fell off tractor at work 18 months previously and sustained deep abrasion over right cheek and fracture of right zygomatic arch. Surgery was performed with closed reduction of zygomatic arch fracture and debridement of right cheek wound. Fracture healed well and maintained its normal anatomical position. Deep abrasion healed well with additional topical wound care. Returned to normal activities shortly after injury.

Current Symptoms: Injured skin area on right cheek is lighter than normal surrounding skin, especially after sun exposure, but does not require medical care, even with prolonged sun exposure.

Physical Exam: 3- to 4-cm area of skin on right cheek is lighter than uninjured skin. Injured skin has irregular, rough "cobblestone" appearance in some areas. Right zygomatic arch has normal appearance and projection compared to left side.

Clinical Studies: None.

Diagnosis: Stable scar on right cheek with loss of normal skin color and residual skin texture changes. Healed fracture.

Impairment Rating: 3% impairment of the whole person.

Comment: No permanent loss of structural integrity of arch. Injured skin area has lost some structural integrity, but healed without surgery. Area has abnormal pigmentation and appearance compared to surrounding skin.

Class 2
6%-10% Impairment of the Whole Person

Facial abnormality involves loss of supporting structure of part of face, with or without cutaneous disorder (eg, depressed cheek, nasal, or frontal bones)

Example 11-10
6% to 10% Impairment Due to Facial Disorders and/or Disfigurement

Subject: 35-year-old woman.

History: Struck across nasal region 19 months previously by a box that had fallen off a shelf in a store. Sustained crush injury to face with compound fracture of nasal bones and compound fracture of frontal bone that goes into frontal sinus. Fractures and wounds were surgically repaired. Wounds and bones healed well. Frontal sinus and nasal respiratory function returned to normal. No additional surgery. Returned to normal activities.

Current Symptoms: Affected area is darker than surrounding skin; hollow area over nasofrontal region.

Physical Exam: Slightly brown discoloration of skin over superior dorsal nasal and glabellar regions. 3-cm depression 3 to 4 mm deep over frontal sinus region.

Clinical Studies: None.

Diagnosis: Healed compound nasal and frontal bone fractures. Residual skin pigmentation changes. Loss of structural integrity of frontal bone.

Impairment Rating: 6% impairment of the whole person.

Comment: Although initial injury required extensive surgery, permanent loss of structural integrity of skin and frontal bone involves relatively small area, with no anticipated problems with function of nose or nasal passages.

Example 11-11
6% to 10% Impairment Due to Facial Disorders and/or Disfigurement

Subject: 35-year-old man.

History: Struck on right side of face with a heavy pipe 14 months previously. Sustained crush injury to right facial region; deep laceration along inferior orbital rim; and fractures of malar ("tripod"), orbital floor, and nasal bones. Refused additional surgery. Quickly recovered and returned to normal activities after surgical repair of injuries.

Current Symptoms: Scars on right lower eyelid and lateral orbital regions. Sunken appearance of right eye and right cheekbone. Nose is wider and flatter than it was before injury. Individual is embarrassed by his appearance but has no complaints of loss of vision or nasal function.

Physical Exam: Well-healed, stable, 1- to 2-cm scars over right inferior and lateral orbital rim regions, with palpable metal plates beneath scars. 1-cm depression of right malar eminence (compared to left side). Mild to moderate enophthalmos of right orbit. Nasal bones have smooth, flat depression in nasofrontal region.

Clinical Studies: None.

Diagnosis: Depression of right malar bone and nasal bones; enophthalmos of right orbit; scars on right lower eyelid and lateral orbital skin.

Impairment Rating: 10% impairment of the whole person.

Comment: Structural integrity of right orbital and nasal regions was lost, leaving permanent, measurable depressions and enophthalmos.

Class 3
11%-15% Impairment of the Whole Person

Facial abnormality involves absence of normal anatomic part or area of face, such as loss of eye or loss of part of nose, with resulting cosmetic deformity; combine with any functional loss, eg, vision (Chapter 12)

or

severe, unilateral, total facial paralysis

or

mild, bilateral, total facial paralysis

Example 11-12
11% to 15% Impairment Due to Facial Disorders and/or Disfigurement

Subject: 35-year-old woman.

History: Sustained gunshot wound to face 9 months previously. Bullet blew off portion of left side of nose and created open, deep wound on left cheek. Returned to most normal activities after undergoing several operations.

Current Symptoms: Scar on left cheek. Missing tip of nose on left side. She is uncomfortable with her appearance.

Physical Exam: Significant depression on left tip of nose due to loss of left lateral cartilage and nasal tissue. Alar region on left has significant shortening compared to right side and partially consists of grafted tissue, which has whiter, thicker appearance than skin on right side. Left cheek has a stable, soft scar approximately 4 cm long by 2 mm wide running from left nasolabial fold to left lateral orbital region.

Clinical Studies: None.

Diagnosis: Loss of skin and cartilage on left tip of nose and scar on left cheek.

Impairment Rating: 15% impairment of the whole person.

Comment: Reconstructive surgery was able to somewhat correct cosmetic defect. But loss of an anatomical part and a significant scar on left cheek have affected self-image.

Example 11-13
11% to 15% Impairment Due to Facial Disorders and/or Disfigurement

Subject: 55-year-old man.

History: Struck with large hook in left eye while working on fishing boat 18 months previously. Eye was destroyed due to injury and replaced with prosthetic eye. Returned to most normal activities.

Current Symptoms: Loss of function of left eye.

Physical Exam: Loss of left eye.

Clinical Studies: None.

Diagnosis: Loss of left eye.

Impairment Rating: 15% impairment of the whole person.

Comment: Combine impairment with impairment resulting from total loss of vision in left eye, as determined according to criteria in Chapter 12.

Class 4
16%-50% Impairment of the Whole Person

Massive or total distortion of normal facial anatomy with disfigurement so severe that it precludes social acceptance; combine with any mental and behavioral impairment (Chapter 14)

or

severe, bilateral, total facial paralysis

or

loss of entire nose

Example 11-14
16% to 50% Impairment Due to Facial Disorders and/or Disfigurement

Subject: 34-year-old man.

History: Thrown and kicked in face by a bull 26 months previously. Sustained crush injury to right side of face and compound fractures of mandible, nasal bones, and orbital bones. Subsequently developed severe infection in face, which required multiple surgical procedures. Operations resulted in loss of most of the normal skin and muscle on right side of nose, right cheek, and right side of upper lip. Nasal septum cartilage and tip were lost. Bones of right side of nose, right half of mandible, and right anterior maxillary region were lost. Underwent no further reconstructive procedures but has been fitted with facial prostheses. Condition is stable. Required speech therapy due to loss of articulatory function. Required help in management of diet because of permanent dietary restriction to semisolid or soft foods.

Current Symptoms: Altered speech with loss of ability to speak well. Loss of skin and bones on right side of face. Loss of ability to eat normal food.

Physical Exam: Loss of normal skin, muscles, and bone structures on right side of nose and in right mandibular and right anterior maxillary regions. Speech is poorly articulated and has low intensity due to loss of skin and muscle on right side of mouth.

Clinical Studies: None.

Diagnosis: Massive loss of normal structural integrity of right side of face and loss of normal speech function and mastication.

Impairment Rating: 25% impairment of the whole person.

Comment: Combine with other impairments for loss of speech (Section 11.4d) and mastication (Section 11.4b).

Example 11-15
16% to 50% Impairment Due to Facial Disorders and/or Disfigurement

Subject: 45-year-old woman.

History: Sustained severe electrical injury to face 26 months previously with loss of left orbital structures, skin on left cheek, and anterior maxillary sinus bones.

Current Symptoms: Lost vision in left eye and is missing left side of face. Individual says she looks like a freak.

Physical Exam: Loss of left orbital structures with open orbital region. No bones remain on orbital floor or inferior orbital rim. Left anterior maxillary sinus regions and overlying skin and muscles are gone, leaving large, residual, open orbital and maxillary cavity.

Clinical Studies: None.

Diagnosis: Massive loss of normal facial structural integrity.

Impairment Rating: 40% impairment of the whole person.

Comment: Combine with other impairments from the vision chapter (Chapter 12) and mental and behavioral chapter (Chapter 14).

11.4 The Nose, Throat, and Related Structures

The nasal region includes the external part of the nose, the nasal cavity, and the nasopharynx. The oral region includes the mouth and lips, teeth, temporomandibular joint, tongue, hard and soft palate, region of the palatine tonsil, and oropharynx. The neck and chest region includes the hypopharynx, larynx, trachea, esophagus, and bronchi.

The functions of these structures, and the order in which they will be discussed, are as follows: (1) respiration, (2) mastication and deglutition, (3) olfaction and taste, and (4) speech. Permanent impairment may result from a deviation from normal in any of the above functions, and, because of their close relationship, more than one structure may be involved.

11.4a Respiration

Respiration may be defined as the act or function of breathing, that is, the act by which air is inspired and expired from the lungs. The respiratory mechanism includes the lungs and the air passages; the latter includes the nares, nasal cavities, mouth, pharynx, larynx, trachea, and bronchi.

In this chapter, discussion of permanent impairments related to respiration is limited to defects of the air passages. Refer to Chapter 5 on the respiratory system for a discussion of impairments of the lower airways and lung parenchyma.

The most commonly encountered defect of the air passages is obstruction, which may be partial, as with stenosis, or complete, as with occlusion. Obstructions and other air passage defects are evidenced primarily by dyspnea or so-called unusual breathlessness. Sleep apnea, which is covered in Chapter 5, may be related to functional upper-airway obstruction.

Dyspnea is a cardinal factor that contributes to an individual's diminished capacity to carry out activities of daily living and to permanent impairment. This subjective complaint or symptom, which indicates an awareness of respiratory distress, usually is noted first and is most severe during exercise. When dyspnea occurs at rest, respiratory dysfunction probably is severe. Dyspnea may or may not be accompanied by related signs or symptoms.

Individuals with air passage defects may be evaluated in accordance with the classification in Table 11-6. Permanent impairments involving obstructive sleep apnea should be evaluated with the respiratory system criteria described in Chapter 5.

Table 11-6 Criteria for Rating Impairment Due to Air Passage Defects

Class 1 0%-10% Impairment of the Whole Person	Class 2 11%-29% Impairment of the Whole Person	Class 3 30%-49% Impairment of the Whole Person	Class 4 50%-89% Impairment of the Whole Person	Class 5 90%+ Impairment of the Whole Person
Dyspnea *does not occur* at rest *and* dyspnea is not produced by walking freely, climbing stairs freely, or performance of other usual activities of daily living *and* dyspnea is not produced by stress, prolonged exertion, hurrying, hill-climbing, or recreational or similar activities requiring intensive effort* *and* examination reveals partial obstruction of the oropharynx, laryngopharynx, larynx, upper trachea (to the fourth cartilaginous ring), lower trachea, bronchi, or complete (bilateral) obstruction of the nose or nasopharynx	Dyspnea *does not occur* at rest *and* dyspnea is not produced by walking freely on a level surface, climbing one flight of stairs, or performance of other usual activities of daily living *but* dyspnea is produced by stress, prolonged exertion, hurrying, hill-climbing, or recreational or similar activities (except sedentary forms) *and* examination reveals partial obstruction of the oropharynx, laryngopharynx, larynx, upper trachea (to the fourth cartilaginous ring), lower trachea, bronchi, or complete (bilateral) obstruction of the nose or nasopharynx	Dyspnea *does not occur* at rest *and* dyspnea is produced by walking more than one or two level blocks, climbing one flight of stairs even with periods of rest, or performance of other usual activities of daily living *and* dyspnea is produced by stress, prolonged exertion, hurrying, hill-climbing, or recreational or similar activities *and* examination reveals partial obstruction of the oropharynx, laryngopharynx, larynx, upper trachea (to the fourth cartilaginous ring), lower trachea, or bronchi	Dyspnea *occurs* at rest, although individual is not necessarily bedridden *and* dyspnea is aggravated by the performance of any of the usual activities of daily living (beyond personal cleansing, dressing, or grooming) *and* examination reveals partial obstruction of the oropharynx, laryngopharynx, larynx, upper trachea (to the fourth cartilaginous ring), lower trachea, and/or bronchi	Severe dyspnea *occurs* at rest and spontaneous respiration is inadequate *and* respiratory ventilation is required *and* examination reveals partial obstruction of the oropharynx, laryngopharynx, larynx, upper trachea (to the fourth cartilaginous ring), lower trachea, and/or bronchi

*Prophylactic restriction of activity, such as strenuous competitive sport, does not exclude subject from class 1.

Note: Individuals with successful permanent tracheostomy or stoma should be rated at 25% impairment of the whole person.

Class 1 0%-10% Impairment of the Whole Person
Dyspnea *does not occur* at rest
and
dyspnea is not produced by walking freely, climbing stairs freely, or performance of other usual activities of daily living
and
dyspnea is not produced by stress, prolonged exertion, hurrying, hill-climbing, or recreational or similar activities requiring intensive effort
and
examination reveals partial obstruction of the oropharynx, laryngopharynx, larynx, upper trachea (to the fourth cartilaginous ring), lower trachea, bronchi, or complete (bilateral) obstruction of the nose or nasopharynx

Class 2 11%-29% Impairment of the Whole Person
Dyspnea *does not occur* at rest
and
dyspnea is not produced by walking freely on a level surface, climbing one flight of stairs, or performance of other usual activities of daily living
but
dyspnea is produced by stress, prolonged exertion, hurrying, hill-climbing, or recreational or similar activities (except sedentary forms)
and
examination reveals partial obstruction of the oropharynx, laryngopharynx, larynx, upper trachea (to the fourth cartilaginous ring), lower trachea, bronchi, or complete (bilateral) obstruction of the nose or nasopharynx

Example 11-16
0% to 10% Impairment Due to Right Vocal Fold Paralysis

Subject: 26-year-old man.

History: Spinal cord tumor removed 4 years ago, with right anterior cervical fusion. Persistent hoarseness since surgery. Had to give up coaching.

Current Symptoms: Voice stable, but weak, with poor volume and projection. Coughing and clearing of throat develop after drinking cold liquids. No shortness of breath or difficulty swallowing.

Physical Exam: Ear, nose, and throat examination: within normal limits.

Clinical Studies: Fiberoptic laryngoscopy: right vocal cord in paramedian position, with a 2-3-mm gap on attempted phonation.

Diagnosis: Right vocal fold paralysis.

Impairment Rating: 5% to 10% impairment due to vocal fold paralysis; combine with appropriate rating for musculoskeletal impairment to determine whole person impairment (see Combined Values Chart, p. 604).

Comment: Partial obstruction of the laryngeal airway.

Example 11-17
11% to 29% Impairment Due to Bilateral Vocal Fold Paralysis and Permanent Tracheostomy

Subject: 29-year-old man.

History: Tracheostomy performed 10 years ago after traumatic tracheal intubation. Diagnosed with Arnold-Chiari syndrome and underwent successful neurosurgical decompression. Developed meningitis of unknown etiology, hemiparesis, and other neurologic sequellae. Past history reveals hearing loss, hypertension, and diabetes. 20-year cigarette use.

Current Symptoms: Wheelchair dependent. Metal tracheotomy tube in place. With tube occluded, has good voice but poor airway.

Physical Exam: Right-side hemiparesis and right-side hearing loss.

Clinical Studies: Fiberoptic laryngoscopy: both vocal folds in midline position with very poor abduction.

Diagnosis: Bilateral vocal fold paralysis with poor airway. Permanent tracheostomy.

Impairment Rating: 29% impairment due to vocal fold paralysis; combine with appropriate ratings for musculoskeletal and hearing impairments to determine whole person impairment (see Combined Values Chart, p. 604).

Comment: Monitor for tracheostomy patency.

11.4b Mastication and Deglutition

The act of eating includes mastication and deglutition. Numerous conditions of nongastrointestinal origin, singly or in combination, may interfere with these functions.

Dysfunction of the temporomandibular joint may impede mastication, affect speech, cause lower facial deformity, and produce pain.[7,8] In this section, the effect of temporomandibular joint dysfunction on eating is considered; other effects may be considered in conjunction with parts of the *Guides* that deal with the nervous system or pain.

In accordance with the philosophy of the *Guides*, when mastication and deglutition are evaluated, the ability to eat should be stable and maximal rehabilitation should have been achieved. When mastication or deglutition is impaired, the imposition of dietary restrictions usually results. Such restrictions are the most objective criteria by which to evaluate permanent impairment of these functions.[9-14] The relationship of the restrictions to impairments of mastication and deglutition are shown in Table 11-7.

Table 11-7 Relationship of Dietary Restrictions to Permanent Impairment

Type of Restriction	% Impairment of the Whole Person
Diet is limited to semisolid or soft foods	5%-19%
Diet is limited to liquid foods	20%-39%
Ingestion of food requires tube feeding or gastrostomy	40%-60%

Example 11-18
5% to 19% Impairment Due to Inflammation and Scarring of the Left Temporomandibular Joint

Subject: 58-year-old woman.

History: Following removal of an impacted upper left third molar, individual developed a left oro-antral fistula and acute left maxillary sinusitis, confirmed by x-ray. Dental films confirmed a tooth remnant in the maxillary area. Despite use of antibiotics, she developed persistent drainage from the fistula and pain in the left maxillary area of the face. Severe pain was noted in the left temporomandibular joint (TMJ), and she experienced progressive loss of mobility of the mandible, with the ability to open the jaws limited to a 1-cm excursion. The left oro-antral fistula was explored surgically 6 weeks later, and the residual tooth fragment was removed. A left naso-antral window was placed in the inferior meatus for drainage of the maxillary sinus. Extensive scarring in and about the left TMJ was found. The scars were released, but full mobility of the mandible was not obtained until the left coronoid process was released from the surrounding tissues. She received postoperative steroid therapy; physical therapy exercises maintained mandibular mobility. A stent to keep the jaws apart was created and used for several months while individual was sleeping.

Current Symptoms: On a soft diet because of discomfort in the left TMJ.

Physical Exam: Maxillary mobility limited to about 60% of mobility noted at surgery, with a well-healed oral fistula area.

Clinical Studies: Paranasal sinus x-rays: normal.

Diagnosis: Inflammation and scarring of the left TMJ; reduced mandibular mobility.

Impairment Rating: 10% impairment of the whole person.

Comment: Individual is able to talk satisfactorily, but dietary choices are limited. Speech is not affected. No facial deformity, but she may need to continue exercises to maintain maxillary mobility. No problem in maintaining body weight.

11.4c Olfaction and Taste

Only rarely does complete loss of the closely related senses of olfaction and taste seriously affect an individual's performance of the usual activities of daily living. For this reason, a value of 1% to 5% impairment of the whole person is suggested for use in cases involving partial or complete bilateral loss of either sense due to peripheral lesions. This value is to be combined with any other impairment of the individual (see the Combined Values Chart, p. 604).

11.4d Speech

In this chapter, speech is defined as the capacity to produce vocal signals that can be heard, understood, and sustained over a useful period of time. Speech ought to allow effective communication in the activities of daily living.

This chapter does not consider the causes and characteristics of abnormal speech. Rather, it considers how an impairment relates to the individual's ability or efficiency in using speech to make himself or herself understood in activities of daily living. It is assumed that speech evaluation pertains to the production of voice and articulate speech and not to the language content or structure of the individual's communication. On the basis of these assumptions, the primary problem is estimating proficiency in the use of oral language or measuring the utility of speech as defined above. This section also considers esophageal speech.

At this time there is no single, acceptable, proven test that will measure objectively the degrees of impairment due to the many varieties of speech disorders. Therefore, it is recommended that speech impairment be evaluated by examining the audibility, intelligibility, and functional efficiency of speech.

- Audibility is based on the ability to speak at a level sufficient to be heard.
- Intelligibility is based on the ability to articulate and to link phonetic units of speech with sufficient accuracy to be understood.
- Functional efficiency is based on the ability to produce a satisfactorily rapid rate of speaking and to sustain this rate over a useful period of time.

Other definable attributes of speech–such as voice quality, pitch, and melodic variation–are evaluated only when they affect one of the three primary characteristics noted above.

The classification chart, oral reading paragraph, and examining procedure used in estimating speech impairment are described below.

Classification Chart

Judgments as to the amount of impairment should be made with reference to the classes, percentages, and examples provided in the classification chart (Table 11-8). The 15 categories in the chart suggest activities or situations with different levels of impairment. Data gathered from direct observation of the individual or from interviews should be compared with these categories, and values should be assigned on the basis of the specific impairments that are present.

Oral Reading Paragraph

The following paragraph, entitled "The Smith House," is composed of 100 words and 10 sentences. It provides a uniform means of comparing a speech sample of the person being evaluated with the speech of normal speakers. The phonetic elements of the paragraph are selected particularly for their relevance to the intelligibility of the person's speech.

The Smith House

Larry and Ruth Smith have been married nearly 14 years. They have a small place near Long Lake. Both of them think there's nothing like the country for health. Their two boys would rather live here than any other place. Larry likes to keep some saddle horses close to the house. These make it easy to keep his sons amused. If they wish, the boys can go fishing along the shore. When it rains, they usually want to watch television. Ruth has a cherry tree on each side of the kitchen door. In June they enjoy the juice and jelly.

Examining Procedure

General Orientation

The examiner should have normal hearing as defined in the earlier section in this chapter on hearing. The setting of the examination should be a reasonably quiet room that approximates the noise levels of everyday living.

The examiner should base judgments of impairment on two kinds of evidence: (1) attention to and observation of the individual's speech in the office—for example, during conversation, during the interview, and while reading and counting aloud—and (2) reports pertaining to the individual's performance in everyday living situations. The reports or the evidence should be supplied by reliable observers who know the person well. The standard of evaluation is an average speaker's performance in average situations of everyday living. It is assumed in this context that an average speaker can usually perform according to the following criteria:

- Talk in a loud voice when the occasion demands it.
- Sustain phonation for at least 10 seconds after one breath.
- Complete at least a 10-word sentence in one breath.
- Form all of the phonetic units of American speech and join them intelligibly.
- Maintain a speech rate of at least 75 to 100 words per minute and sustain a flow of speech for a reasonable length of time. A speech rate of 125 words per minute enables a speaker to read approximately one $8\frac{1}{2}$ x 11-inch page of double-spaced text in 2 minutes.

Specific Instructions

1. Place the individual approximately 8 ft from the examiner.

2. Interview the individual. This will permit observation of his or her speech in ordinary conversation while pertinent historical information is obtained.

3. Have the individual's back toward the examiner and keep a separation of 8 ft between the examiner and the examinee. Instruct the person as follows: "You are to read this passage so I can hear you plainly. Be sure to speak so I can understand you." Then ask him or her to read aloud the short paragraph, "The Smith House."

4. If additional reading procedures are required, simple prose paragraphs from a magazine may be used. A person who cannot read may be requested to give his or her name and address and name all the days of the week and months of the year. Additional evidence regarding the person's rate of speech and ability to sustain it may be obtained by noting the time required to count to 100 by ones. Completion of this task in 60 to 75 seconds is accepted as normal.

5. Record judgment of the individual's speech capacity with regard to each of the three rows of the classification chart (Table 11-8). The degree of impairment of speech is equivalent to the greatest percentage of impairment recorded in any one of the three rows of the classification chart.

For example, a person's speech capacity is judged to be the following: audibility, 10% (class 1); intelligibility, 50% (class 3); and functional efficiency, 30% (class 2). The individual's speech impairment is judged to be equivalent to the greatest impairment (50%). A speech impairment of 50% is judged to be an 18% impairment of the whole person, according to Table 11-9.

11.4e Voice

Voice, as the term is used in this section, refers to the production of audible sounds by the vibration of the true vocal folds of the larynx. Voice, or phonation, is therefore the generator of speech—the shaping of sounds into intelligible words. Alternative physiological sound generators, such as the false vocal folds or the esophagus, are not considered here.

This section does not consider the causes of voice disorders. Rather, it recognizes that voice disorders may present such definable symptoms as abnormal volume (voice fatigue, weakness, or low sound intensity), abnormal control (pitch and/or melodic variation), and/or abnormal quality (hoarseness, harshness, or breathiness). These symptoms indicate abnormal physiological functioning of the phonatory mechanism and may contribute to impairment of speech.

At this time, there is no single, acceptable, proven test that will measure objectively the degrees of impairment associated with the many varieties of voice disorders. Tests such as laryngoscopy, acoustical analysis of voice, strobovideolaryngoscopy, analysis of phonatory function, and laryngeal electromyography are recognized as appropriate and useful.[15-17] The significance of current normative data is unclear when confined to consideration of impairment.

Table 11-8 Classification of Voice/Speech Impairment

	Class 1 0%-14% Voice/ Speech Impairment	Class 2 15%-34% Voice/ Speech Impairment	Class 3 35%-59% Voice/ Speech Impairment	Class 4 60%-84% Voice/ Speech Impairment	Class 5 85%-100% Voice/ Speech Impairment
Audibility	Can produce speech of an intensity sufficient for *most* needs of everyday speech, although this sometimes may require effort and occasionally may be beyond individual's capacity	Can produce speech of an intensity sufficient for *many* needs of everyday speech and is usually heard under average conditions; however, may have difficulty being heard in noisy places—such as cars, buses, trains, train stations, or restaurants	Can produce speech of an intensity sufficient for *some* needs of everyday speech such as close conversation; however, has considerable difficulty at a distance or in noisy places—such as cars, buses, trains, train stations, or restaurants—because the voice tires easily and tends to become inaudible after a few seconds	Can produce speech of an intensity sufficient for a *few* needs of everyday speech, but can barely be heard by a close listener or over the telephone and may be able to whisper audibly but with no louder voice	Can produce speech of an intensity sufficient for *no* needs of everyday speech
Intelligibility	Can perform *most* articulatory acts necessary for everyday speech, but may occasionally be asked to repeat and find it difficult or impossible to produce some phonetic units	Can perform *many* articulatory acts necessary for everyday speech and be understood by a stranger, but may have numerous inaccuracies and sometimes appears to have difficulty articulating	Can perform *some* articulatory acts necessary for everyday speech and can usually converse with family and friends, but may be understood by strangers only with difficulty and often may be asked to repeat	Can perform a *few* articulatory acts necessary for everyday speech, can produce some phonetic units, and may have approximations for a few words such as names of own family members, but is unintelligible out of context	Can perform *no* articulatory acts necessary for everyday speech
Functional Efficiency	Can meet *most* demands of articulation and phonation for everyday speech with adequate speed and ease, but occasionally may hesitate or speak slowly	Can meet *many* demands of articulation and phonation for everyday speech with adequate speed and ease, but sometimes speaks with difficulty and speech may be discontinuous, interrupted, hesitant, or slow	Can meet *some* demands of articulation and phonation for everyday speech with adequate speed and ease, but can sustain consecutive speech only for brief periods and may give the impression of being easily fatigued	Can meet a *few* demands of articulation and phonation for everyday speech with adequate speed and ease (such as single words or short phrases), but cannot maintain uninterrupted speech flow; speech is labored and rate is impractically slow	Can meet *no* demands of articulation and phonation for everyday speech with adequate speed and ease

For voice and/or speech impairments, the classifications in Table 11-8 and Table 11-9 should be used. Note that the impairment ratings for speech and/or voice impairments are not evaluated separately. The degree of impairment of speech and/or voice is equivalent to the greatest percentage of impairment recorded in any one of the three sections (audibility, intelligibility, or functional efficiency) of the classification chart (Table 11-8).

Table 11-9 Voice/Speech Impairment Related to Impairment of the Whole Person

% Voice/ Speech Impairment	% Impairment of the Whole Person	% Voice/ Speech Impairment	% Impairment of the Whole Person
0	0	50	18
5	2	55	19
10	4	60	21
15	5	65	23
20	7	70	24
25	9	75	26
30	10	80	28
35	12	85	30
40	14	90	32
45	16	95	33
		100	35

Class 1:
0%-14% Voice/Speech Impairment

Audibility: Can produce speech of an intensity sufficient for most needs of everyday speech, although this sometimes may require effort and occasionally may be beyond individual's capacity

Intelligibility: Can perform most articulatory acts necessary for everyday speech, but may occasionally be asked to repeat and find it difficult or impossible to produce some phonetic units

Functional efficiency: Can meet most demands of articulation and phonation for everyday speech with adequate speed and ease, but occasionally may hesitate or speak slowly

Example 11-19
0% to 14% Voice/Speech Impairment

Subject: 47-year-old woman.

History: Professional operatic soprano and voice teacher; had sudden onset of dysphonia 1 year previously; diagnosis was vocal fold hemorrhage. Developed vocal fold mass secondary to hemorrhage. Gastroesophageal reflux. Five vocal fold surgeries for repeated vocal fold masses. Had operations to attempt to reduce vocal fold scar. Advised to undergo another surgical procedure that would implant fat into vocal fold.

Current Symptoms: Husky speaking voice; lowered pitch; oral dryness; postnasal drip. Unable to sing or perform professionally since vocal fold hemorrhage.

Physical Exam: Voice is mildly hoarse, mildly soft, and slightly breathy. Left vocal fold posthemorrhagic cyst, right vocal fold mass, left vocal fold scar, possible mild superior laryngeal nerve paresis, muscular tension dysphonia, and gastro-esophageal reflux disease on laryngeal examination by strobovideolaryngoscopy. Singing technique was very good and was able to correct minor technical deficiencies.

Clinical Studies: Mild decrease in maximum phonation time and air-conduction flow.

Diagnosis: Recurrent vocal fold hemorrhage and vocal fold scar. Intermittently uncontrolled gastroesophageal reflux disease. Obesity. Inability to regain singing voice she had prior to the vocal fold injury. Altered and diminished self-image.

Impairment Rating: 0% to 14% voice/speech impairment; 0% to 5% impairment of the whole person.

Comment: Afraid her career is over. Traumatic change in self-image. Unable to resume her living as an internationally known opera star. Resigned her teaching position in Europe and moved to the

United States to receive necessary voice care. Voice is now of a sufficient intensity for most everyday speech needs. However, because of her emotional distress, loss of her previous occupation as an international opera star, and change in activities of daily living, an impairment rating is warranted.

Example 11-20
0% to 14% Voice/Speech Impairment

Subject: 58-year-old man.

History: Attorney; underwent thoracoscopic excision of mediastinal schwannoma 2 months previously. Postoperatively immediately developed hoarseness, breathiness, and dysphagia. Was diagnosed with bilateral vocal fold weakness. Underwent speech therapy but voice did not improve. Computed tomography (CT) scan of larynx 1 month later revealed dislocated arytenoid cartilage.

Current Symptoms: Hoarseness; breathiness; decreased volume; lower pitch; voice fatigue. Cannot effectively communicate with clients in courtroom.

Physical Exam: All symptoms were noted, but examination of head and neck was otherwise normal. Left arytenoid dislocation and left vocal fold paresis on strobovideolaryngoscopy. Sulcus vocalis.

Clinical Studies: Laryngeal electromyogram: left superior laryngeal nerve paresis with 50% decreased recruitment of left posterior cricoarytenoid and vocalis muscle and 70% decreased recruitment response of left cricothyroid muscle. Normal right superior laryngeal nerve function. Evidence of right recurrent laryngeal nerve paresis. CT scan of larynx: widening of left cricoarytenoid joint with anteromedial rotation of left arytenoid cartilage.

Diagnosis: Markedly decreased intensity, frequency range, and phonation time. All acoustic measurements were severely abnormal.

Impairment Rating: 0% to 14% voice/speech impairment; 0% to 5% impairment of the whole person.

Comment: Had surgical correction of arytenoid dislocation. After surgery his voice was nearly normal, with only slight voice breaks and slightly decreased volume.

> **Class 2**
> **15%-34% Voice/Speech Impairment**
>
> **Audibility:** Can produce speech of an intensity sufficient for many needs of everyday speech and is usually heard under average conditions; however, may have difficulty being heard in noisy places—such as cars, buses, trains, train stations, or restaurants
>
> **Intelligibility:** Can perform many articulatory acts necessary for everyday speech and be understood by a stranger, but may have numerous inaccuracies and sometimes appears to have difficulty articulating
>
> **Functional efficiency:** Can meet many demands of articulation and phonation for everyday speech with adequate speed and ease, but sometimes speaks with difficulty and speech may be discontinuous, interrupted, hesitant, or slow

Example 11-21
15% to 34% Voice/Speech Impairment

Subject: 28-year-old man.

History: Rock-and-roll singer/songwriter; developed new onset of vocal difficulties while recording album 1 year previously. Had been singing and performing for 10 years with no prior vocal difficulties. Loss of midrange, decreased volume, breathiness, and hoarseness while singing. Diagnosed with left vocal fold polyp 3 months later. Underwent surgical excision of lesion 1 month after that. Treated for laryngopharyngeal reflux with usual medical therapy.

Current Symptoms: Breathiness; hoarseness; loss of vocal stamina; loss of volume; loss of lower range. Voice is worse in morning, with frequent throat-clearing and sensation of lump in throat.

Physical Exam: Right vocal fold mass, left vocal fold scar, reflux laryngitis, and neurolaryngologic asymmetries on strobovideolaryngoscopy. Excess tension in jaw and tongue, hoarseness, and decreased range while singing.

Clinical Studies: Laryngeal electromyogram: 20% decreased function of left superior laryngeal nerve. Abnormalities in electroglottogram (EGG), quasi-open quotient, air-conduction flow, minimal flow, maximum flow rate, S/Z ratio, maximum phonation time, and acoustic measurements.

Diagnosis: Persistent vocal fold mass and vocal fold scar after recent vocal fold surgery; superior laryngeal nerve paresis; laryngopharyngeal reflux disease.

Impairment Rating: 15% to 34% voice/speech impairment; 5% to 12% impairment of the whole person.

Comment: Class 2 on the basis of audibility and activities of daily living, not including work. Unhappy with his vocal progress. Totally disabled as a professional singer because of this work-related injury.

Example 11-22
15% to 34% Voice/Speech Impairment

Subject: 46-year-old man.

History: Voice teacher/singer; involved in motor vehicle collision 4 months ago in which he screamed loudly and seat belt tightened across anterior part of neck. Experienced immediate hoarseness and throat pain. Seen for treatment of sore throat 3 days later. Negative cultures. Attempted to give two 30-minute performances 3 days after collision. Voice became hoarse, strained, and fatigued quickly. Experienced problems with pitch control. Has not performed or sung since. Does not smoke or drink. Had direct laryngoscopy and biopsy, flexible bronchoscopy, and rigid esophagoscopy.

Current Symptoms: Hoarseness; voice fatigue; pain. Unable to sing or speak extensively. Weak, strained voice. Unable to project voice.

Physical Exam: Gastroesophageal reflux disease, height disparity of vocal folds, and white, irregular, firm, vocal fold mass on laryngeal exam by strobovideolaryngoscopy.

Clinical Studies: Laryngeal electromyogram: left superior laryngeal nerve paresis with 50% decreased recruitment response and left recurrent laryngeal nerve paresis with 30% decreased recruitment, both from vocalis and posterior cricoarytenoid muscles. Objective voice measures: mild acoustic abnormalities including increased mean flow rate and decreased maximum phonation time. Laryngeal CT scan: normal cricoarytenoid joint and no focal lesions. Normal magnetic resonance imaging (MRI) scan with gadolinium of larynx.

Diagnosis: Infiltrating keratinizing squamous cell carcinoma of left vocal fold with evidence of focal chronic inflammatory infiltrate. Lesion was classified T2 N0 M0. Has undergone radiation therapy, reflux treatment, and voice therapy.

Impairment Rating: 15% to 34% voice/speech impairment; 5% to 12% impairment of the whole person.

Comment: May not be able to continue as a voice teacher and singer, with subsequent loss of income and life alteration. Will have to make frequent visits to physician for cancer surveillance, probably for life. Motor vehicle collision probably caused hemorrhage into previously asymptomatic cancerous tumor. Reflux was the only known risk factor in this nonsmoker. Voice became worse after surgery and radiation therapy.

Class 3
35%-59% Voice/Speech Impairment

Audibility: Can produce speech of an intensity sufficient for some needs of everyday speech such as close conversation; however, has considerable difficulty at a distance or in noisy places—such as cars, buses, trains, train stations, or restaurants—because the voice tires easily and tends to become inaudible after a few seconds

Intelligibility: Can perform some articulatory acts necessary for everyday speech and can usually converse with family and friends, but may be understood by strangers only with difficulty and often may be asked to repeat

Functional efficiency: Can meet some demands of articulation and phonation for everyday speech with adequate speed and ease, but can sustain consecutive speech only for brief periods and may give the impression of being easily fatigued

---

Example 11-23
35% to 59% Voice/Speech Impairment

Subject: 52-year-old woman.

History: Chronic hoarseness and dysphonia for 10 years. Gastroesophageal reflux disease for at least 10 years. Multiple laryngeal surgeries, including vocal fold polypectomy, microlaryngoscopy, excision of left vocal fold mass, and vaporization of laryngeal vocal fold varices. Initial improvement with voice therapy; deteriorated after heavy voice use in classroom. Developed recurrent vocal fold mass. Had vocal fold hemorrhage after yelling. Multiple bouts of acute laryngitis secondary to voice overuse. Recurrent vocal fold nodules that were initially treated with voice therapy. Experienced voice fatigue by Wednesday of each week. Developed severe upper respiratory infection that resulted in vocal fold hemorrhage. Vocal fold stiffness and scar secondary to recurrent vocal fold hemorrhages. Relatively asymptomatic for about a year.

Thereafter had ongoing treatment for reflux disease and underwent voice therapy. Reflux disease became more problematic. Referred to gastroenterologist for problem with gastroesophageal reflux. Considered surgical treatment of reflux disease.

Current Symptoms: Recurrent hoarseness, despite strictly adhering to antireflux treatment and voice therapy modifications.

Physical Exam: Left vocal fold scar, new right vocal fold mass (probably a cyst), evidence of reflux laryngitis, and muscle-tension dysphonia on strobovideolaryngoscopy. Voice hoarse, soft, and strained.

Clinical Studies: Abnormal acoustic measures, including harmonic measures and harmonic to noise ratio.

Diagnosis: Vocal fold mass and scar; muscle-tension dysphonia; reflux laryngitis.

Impairment Rating: 35% to 59% voice/speech impairment; 12% to 21% impairment of the whole person.

Comment: Direct microlaryngoscopy and excision of right vocal fold mass; left vocal fold autologous fat injection and, possibly, fat implantation for treatment of scar recommended. Rated class 3 on basis of audibility.

Example 11-24
35% to 59% Voice/Speech Impairment

Subject: 40-year-old man.

History: Recurrent sinusitis and progressive hoarseness for 2 years. Voice worse after vocal fold "polypectomy" for leukoplakia. Had septoplasty and functional endoscopic sinus surgery. No complaint of nasal/sinus disease. Speaks about 14 hours a day over loud noise. Must talk loudly or yell frequently. Is regularly exposed to car fumes, asbestos, and aerosols. Does not smoke. Rarely drinks alcohol.

Current Symptoms: Constant hoarseness. Difficulty speaking, but without pain, by afternoon. Frequently clears throat. Complains of lump in throat.

Physical Exam: Leukoplakia on left vocal fold and stiffness of vibratory margin secondary to scar on strobovideolaryngoscopy. Erythema and edema of glottis consistent with gastroesophageal reflux disease. Improper speaking technique and significant muscle-tension dysphonia.

Clinical Studies: Laryngeal electromyogram: left superior laryngeal nerve paresis and muscle-tension dysphonia. No evidence of neuromuscular junction abnormalities. Severely abnormal harmonic to noise ratios, decreased intensity, decreased frequency range, and decreased phonation time.

Diagnosis: Vocal fold scar, leukoplakia (hyperkeratosis), muscle-tension dysphonia, and gastroesophageal reflux disease.

Impairment Rating: 35% to 59% voice/speech impairment; 12% to 21% impairment of the whole person.

Comment: Leukoplakia requires biopsy. Hoarseness caused by scarring from previous injury and from surgery is permanent.

Class 4
60%-84% Voice/Speech Impairment

Audibility: Can produce speech of an intensity sufficient for a few needs of everyday speech, but can barely be heard by a close listener or over the telephone and may be able to whisper audibly but with no louder voice

Intelligibility: Can perform a few articulatory acts necessary for everyday speech, can produce some phonetic units, and may have approximations for a few words such as names of own family members, but is unintelligible out of context

Functional efficiency: Can meet a few demands of articulation and phonation for everyday speech with adequate speed and ease (such as single words or short phrases), but cannot maintain uninterrupted speech flow; speech is labored and rate is impractically slow

---

Example 11-25
60% to 84% Voice/Speech Impairment

Subject: 40-year-old man.

History: Involved in motor vehicle collision 20 years previously. Sustained massive brain stem trauma and multiple injuries including fractured clavicle, shoulder, and hands. Was comatose for 8 weeks. Underwent tracheotomy and gastrostomy 3 days after collision. Left hemiparesis, cognitive deficits, memory loss, and "personality change." Completed occupational therapy, physical therapy, and speech and cognitive rehabilitation.

Current Symptoms: Unable to be heard on telephone; cannot carry on sustained conversation; cannot raise voice above soft whisper.

Physical Exam: Extremely breathy, soft voice. Halting speech pattern. Short phrasing. Can only count up to "eight" on one breath. Has left facial weakness, dysphagia, and chronic cough. Bilateral vocal fold immobility with patent but narrow airway on strobovideolaryngoscopy.

Clinical Studies: Laryngeal electromyogram: bilateral vocal fold paralysis. Severely short phonation times. All acoustic measures: highly abnormal.

Diagnosis: Bilateral vocal fold paralysis.

Impairment Rating: 60% to 84% impairment due to bilateral vocal fold paralysis; 21% to 30% whole person impairment. Combine with appropriate ratings due to other impairments to determine whole person impairment (see Combined Values Chart, p. 604).

Comment: Underwent voice therapy. Conservative, anterior vocal fold medializations. Cannot be heard in office setting or anywhere with background noise. Is dysfluent and has halting speech (often interpreted by others as intellectual deficits). Unable to use the telephone. Unable to carry on sustained conversation. Unlikely to ever regain voice he had prior to motor vehicle collision. Requires ongoing medical care (not only for voice) and will require multiple laryngeal surgical procedures for voice improvement. Is prone to aspiration pneumonia secondary to vocal fold paralysis. Requires ongoing voice therapy and voice-assistive devices.

Example 11-26
60% to 84% Voice/Speech Impairment

Subject: 42-year-old woman.

History: Taught elementary school 7 years previously. Experienced sudden onset of hoarseness 1 month after starting teaching. Continued to teach for several months with hoarseness before seeking medical attention. Otolaryngologist diagnosed vocal fold nodules and recommended resting voice for 4 days. She complied, but with no improvement in voice. Saw speech therapist weekly for 2 years with minimal voice improvement. Underwent excision of bilateral vocal fold masses. Voice improved until 6 months later, when recurrent hoarseness developed. Had recurrent vocal fold masses. Diagnosed with gastroesophageal reflux disease. Had surgery after aggressive medical treatment for reflux disease and after voice therapy. No improvement in appearance of vocal fold lesions. Had excisional biopsy for definitive pathology.

Current Symptoms: Constant hoarseness and voice fatigue. Unable to project voice well and unable to sing. Year-round allergy symptoms.

Physical Exam: Moderately hoarse and breathy voice. Broad-based, solid, white mass of right vocal fold and fibrotic mass of left vocal fold on strobovideolaryngoscopy. Arytenoid erythema and edema consistent with gastroesophageal reflux disease, bilateral superior surface varicosities, and scars on stroboscopy. No neuromuscular junction abnormalities were noted.

Clinical Studies: Laryngeal electromyogram: mild bilateral superior laryngeal nerve paresis. Decreased intensity, phonation time, harmonic to noise ratio, acoustic measures, and S/Z ratio.

Diagnosis: Adult-onset laryngeal papillomatosis.

Impairment Rating: 60% to 84% voice/speech impairment; 21% to 30% impairment of the whole person.

Comment: Required two subsequent laryngeal surgeries in attempt to eradicate disease and improve phonatory function. Requires ongoing surveillance by laryngologist for recurrence of papillomas and surveillance for development of laryngeal carcinoma. Requires ongoing voice therapy and treatment for reflux disease. Will require personal amplification system to help with vocal projection for job. Vocal prognosis is guarded.

Class 5
85%-100% Voice/Speech Impairment

Audibility: Can produce speech of an intensity sufficient for no needs of everyday speech

Intelligibility: Can perform no articulatory acts necessary for everyday speech

Functional efficiency: Can meet no demands of articulation and phonation for everyday speech with adequate speed and ease

---

Example 11-27
85% to 100% Voice/Speech Impairment

Subject: 38-year-old man.

History: Worked with rubber, plastics, and chemicals for 20 years (described as responsible for "everything that blows up"). Suffered inhalation injury from heavy exposure to vinyl chloride fumes due to reactor malfunction. Had microlaryngoscopy and excision of bilateral vocal fold polyps 1 year after inhalation injury. Voice improved after surgery; remained off work for 6 weeks after operation. Exposed to ammonia fumes 1 month after returning to work. Experienced immediate dyspnea and sudden and severe hoarseness. Required a second microlaryngoscopy and vocal fold polypectomy. Became aphonic after 3 days back at work. Required two vocal fold surgeries since initial injury. Undergoing psychological counseling for stress-related problems secondary to voice problems. Quit smoking.

Current Symptoms: Voice deterioration after using voice and after any exposure to fumes, perfume, smoke, or gasoline; hoarseness associated with shortness of breath; chronic sensation of lump in throat.

Physical Exam: Voice is harsh, hoarse, slightly breathy, and strained. Bilateral vocal fold scarring, decreased mucosal wave, hypervascularity, and mucosal irregularities on strobovideolaryngoscopy.

Clinical Studies: Marked abnormalities in harmonic to noise ratio, shimmer, and maximum flow rate.

Diagnosis: Mucosal vocal fold injury secondary to inhalation of noxious fumes, initially vinyl chloride. Airway hyperactivity that causes dysphonia and dyspnea.

Impairment Rating: 85% to 100% voice/speech impairment; 30% to 35% impairment of the whole person.

Comment: Third surgery is recommended. Vocal fold mucosa and voice quality have never returned to normal. Had progressive dysplastic vocal fold changes (leukoplakia) 5 years later. Would be rated class 3 on basis of audibility if in an environment (such as home) protected from fumes or pollution. However, in activities of daily living, has a class 5 impairment.

Example 11-28
85% to 100% Voice/Speech Impairment

Subject: 50-year-old man.

History: Had large endolaryngeal tumor without airway obstruction. Hoarseness for 1 year. Enlarging anterior neck mass for 2 weeks. Dysphagia and 4.5-kg (10-lb) weight loss over 2 months. Forty to 50 pack-year history of smoking. Moderately heavy alcohol user. Underwent total laryngectomy with radical neck dissection and excision of malignant laryngeal cutaneous fistula. Surgery was followed by radiation therapy. Underwent four esophageal dilatations and stomal revisions in preparation for Singer-Blom prosthesis after laryngectomy and radiation therapy. Had submental swelling that required full mouth dental extraction and alveoloplasty. Smokes through tracheostoma. Eats well; weight is stable. Has virtually no family to assist him in his care.

Current Symptoms: Unable to speak. Unable to develop esophageal speech or use electrolarynx. Remains totally aphonic.

Physical Exam: No evidence of cancer. Has very dense and deep scarring of neck musculature. Stoma appears epithelialized and open.

Clinical Studies: Four esophageal dilatations. Stoma remains open, but he has not been able to accommodate Singer-Blom prosthesis.

Diagnosis: Laryngeal cancer; laryngectomy.

Impairment Rating: 85% to 100% voice/speech impairment; 30% to 35% impairment of the whole person.

Comment: Altered self-image secondary to disfigurement from cancer, radical neck surgery, and tracheostomy. Unable to achieve speech with Singer-Blom assistive device or by alternative means. Lacks motivation and dexterity for use of assistive voicing devices due to chronic alcohol abuse.

11.5 Ear, Nose, Throat, and Related Structures Impairment Evaluation Summary

See Table 11-10 for an evaluation summary for the assessment of impairmnent of the ear, nose, throat, and related structures.

Table 11-10 Ear, Nose, Throat, and Related Structures Impairment Evaluation Summary

Disorder	History, Including Selected Relevant Symptoms	Examination Record	Assessment of Physical Function
General	Ear, nose, and throat symptoms (eg, hearing loss, dizziness, or vertigo) and general symptoms; impact of symptoms on function and ability to do daily activities; prognosis if change anticipated; review medical history and any resulting limitation of physical function	Comprehensive physical examination; detailed relevant system assessment	Data derived from relevant studies (eg, audiometry)
Hearing Impairment	Comprehensive history including family history, developmental history of trauma, noise, and drug exposure; surgical procedures; symptoms of imbalance (eg, unsteadiness or vertigo); ear-popping; history of tinnitus; age; associated metabolic and/or endocrine disorders	General physical examination; ear, nose, and throat examination; findings from pneumonotoscopy, tuning-fork tests, hearing tests, balance function tests, and radiographic tests; metabolic evaluation	Otologic examination on tuning-fork tests; tympanometry; behavioral, audiometry, and auditory brain (evoked) response tests; electrocochleography tests; electronystagmography; metabolic and endocrine studies as necessary
Vestibular Impairment	Discuss symptoms and antecedent events; determine associated symptoms (eg, nausea, vomiting, or tinnitus); review medications; trauma; disorders associated with dizziness	Complete physical examination findings; audiologic evaluation; balance tests; electronystagmogram; blood pressure; radiologic studies	Blood pressure tests; provocative maneuvers; audiometry; electronystagmogram tests; x-rays as appropriate
Structural Facial Impairment	Case history (including symptoms) relative to facial structure and integrity; relate to other organ systems (eg, skin, eye, alimentary tract, and upper airway); social acceptability	Description of comprehensive examination of head and neck, especially the face; cutaneous abnormalities; description of supporting structures of the face such as lips; record of eye examination; photographic records; radiologic records; records of psychosocial behavior	Consider data from relevant physical findings; assess cutaneous findings, structural abnormalities, and neurologic impairments
Facial Disfigurement	History of burns, trauma, or infection; dysplasia; social factors	Records of physical findings of face, head, and neck; neurologic studies; photographic records	Consider data from clinical examination of face and facial nerve studies; photographic studies
Impairment of Respiration (Air Passage Defects)	Medical history (especially respiratory function) related to upper airway, lower airway, and lungs; consider signs and symptoms of breathiness and dyspnea; limitations of exercise; sleep disorders; consider related systems (eg, pulmonary, cardiac, allergy, metabolic, neurologic, or psychological systems)	Data from examination of head and neck, especially nasal, oropharyngeal, and tracheobronchial airways; rhinometric studies; endoscopic findings; pulmonary function tests; radiologic findings; ultrasound studies	Examination of airway; rhinometry; endoscopy; pulmonary function tests; radiologic studies; ultrasound studies of airway

Physical Findings	Diagnosis	Degree of Impairment
Assessment of sequelae including end-organ damage and impairment	Record all pertinent diagnoses; note if they are at maximal medical improvement; if not, discuss under what conditions and when stability is expected	Criteria outlined in this chapter
Assess relevant organs; external ear and middle ear functions; eustachian tube function; status of hearing by audiometry; status of electrophysiologic tests as applicable	Conductive, sensorineural, mixed, and functional hearing loss; tinnitus; Meniere's disease	See Table 11-5
Signs of otitis media and head trauma; audiogram; auditory brain (evoked) response findings; electronystagmogram findings; evidence of cardiovascular, endocrine, metabolic, and/or ocular disorders	Otitis media; head trauma; drug side effects; vestibular neuronitis; seizure disorder; syncope; hyperventilation; benign positional vertigo; endolymphatic hydrops; CPA tumor Cardiovascular, endocrine, metabolic, functional, and/or ocular disorders	See Table 11-4
Examine cutaneous aspects of face; examine supporting (structural) aspects of face, head, and neck; consider integrity and appearance of lips, nose, eyebrows, and eyelids; radiologic studies of head and neck; CT scans; MRI scans; assess related systems (eg, visual, cutaneous, respiratory, neurologic, and psychosocial)	Visible scars; abnormal pigmentation; depressed fracture of facial bones and/or nasal cartilage; mutilation of nose or ear; distortion of anatomic facial structure; notable facial distortion; loss of social acceptance	See Table 11-5
Examine face; assess physical findings; perform facial nerve function tests; make photographic records	Facial nerve paresis or paralysis; deformity or loss of external ear or nose	See Table 11-5
Partial obstruction of nose and/or oropharynx, larynx, trachea, or bronchi; complete obstruction of nose and/or nasopharynx; tracheotomy or tracheostomy	Air passage defect with no, mild, moderate, severe, or profound dyspnea; permanent tracheotomy or tracheostomy	See Table 11-6

Table 11-10 continued

Disorder	History, Including Selected Relevant Symptoms	Examination Record	Assessment of Physical Function
Impairment of Mastication and Deglutition	History and symptoms of mastication and/or deglutition difficulty; history of dietary habits and restrictions; history of burns or trauma; records of related systems (eg, gastrointestinal, neurologic, endocrine, or dental systems)	Comprehensive examination of nose and throat; records of temporomandibular joint function; results of speech articulation tests; esophageal function tests; endocrine studies; neurologic reports; assessment of pain if present; dental reports	Examination of nose, throat, and oropharynx; examination of temporomandibular joint function; x-rays of head and neck; swallowing studies; esophageal examination; esophageal studies; dental findings
Impairment of Olfaction and/or Taste	Ear, nose, and throat infections; head trauma; structural or foreign body nasal obstruction; nasal allergy; infections of nose and sinuses; history of head and neck tumors; drug use	Tests for odor identification; tests for taste identification; results of x-rays of head and neck; results of MRI and CT studies of head and neck; allergy tests	Subjective tests for odor identification; subjective tests for taste identification; electrical taste tests; x-rays of head and neck; MRI and CT studies of head; cranial nerve function tests; test for nasal allergens
Voice and Speech Impairment	History of general health and development; history of speech development and dysfluency; history of onset of speech and/or voice symptoms; history of surgery, trauma, infections, tumors, and treatment	Records of general medical examination; ear, nose, and throat examination; reports of hearing tests, neurologic evaluations, and pulmonary function studies; reports of laryngeal surgery and endocrine and metabolic evaluations	Records of general medical examination; examination of ears, nose, throat, and larynx; laryngoscopy; voice analysis; strobovideolaryngoscopy; speech analysis; pulmonary function tests; laryngeal electromyography

References

1. American Academy of Otolaryngology Committee on Hearing and Equilibrium and American Council of Otolaryngology Committee on the Medical Aspects of Noise. Guide for the evaluation of hearing handicap. *JAMA.* 1979;241:2055-2059.

2. Sataloff RT, Sataloff J. *Occupational Hearing Loss.* 2nd ed. New York, NY: Marcel Dekker; 1993:443-472.

   A clinical overview of the subjects listed in this reference.

3. Glorig A, Roberts J. *Hearing Levels of Adults by Age and Sex: United States, 1960-1962.* Washington, DC: National Center for Health Services Research and Development, US Dept of Health, Education, and Welfare; 1965. DHEW-PUB-1000-SER-11-11.

4. American National Standards Institute. *American National Standards Specification for Audiometers.* ANSI Standard S3.6-1996. New York, NY: American National Standards Institute; 1996.

5. Herdman SJ. *Vestibular Rehabilitation.* Philadelphia, Pa: FA Davis; 1994:47-180, 206-242.

   A presentation of vestibular function, adaptation, assessment, and medical management of vestibular disorders. A chapter on the assessment and treatment of vestibular deficits in children with developmental disorders is included.

6. Shepard NT, Telian SA. *Practical Management of the Balance Disorder Patient.* San Diego, Calif: Singular Publishing Group; 1996:33-168.

   Presents the basics of vestibular system function, clinical diagnosis, treatment planning, and rehabilitation of vestibular disorders. The discussion of normative data is helpful.

7. Dworkin SF, Kimberly KH, LeResche L, et al. Epidemiology of signs and symptoms in temporomandibular disorders: clinical signs in cases and controls. *J Am Dent Assoc.* 1990;120:273-281.

   An epidemiologic study of signs and symptoms of temporomandibular disorders (TMD) in a probability sample of adults enrolled in a major health maintenance organization.

8. McNeil C. Epidemiology. In: McNeil C, ed. *Temporomandibular Disorders: Guidelines for Classification, Assessment, and Management.* 2nd ed. Chicago, Ill: Quintessence Books; 1993.

   Discusses prevalence of TMJ disorders in nonpatient populations and the need to assess chronic pain and headache related to TMJ dysfunction.

9. Burakoff R. Epidemiology. In: Kaplan AS, Assael LA, eds. *Temporomandibular Disorders: Diagnosis and Treatment.* Philadelphia, Pa: WB Saunders Co; 1991.

   Presents the need for long-term studies of TMJ disorders.

Physical Findings	Diagnosis	Degree of Impairment
Abnormal temporomandibular joint function; pain (see Chapter 18); contributory dental conditions; gastroenterologic findings (see Chapter 6)	Temporomandibular joint disorder; pain (see Chapter 18); neurologic diagnoses (see Chapter 13); gastroenterologic diagnoses (see Chapter 6)	See Table 11-7
Nasal obstruction due to mucosal edema, nasal polyps, septal or turbinate occlusion of airway, or nasal tumor; physical findings may be normal except for presenting symptom; surgery sequela	Nasal septal deviation; nasal airway occlusion by turbinate bone; allergic rhinitis; nasal polyps; sinusitis; foreign body in nose; traumatic anosmia; drug toxicity; dermoid encephalocele; meningocele; intracranial or other tumor	See Olfaction and Taste (Section 11.4c)
Assess laryngeal structures; assess vocal cord function and articulators of oropharynx; assess palatal function; assess phonation, articulation, and speech intelligibility; consider esophageal speech; include assessment of respiratory, neurologic, and psychiatric findings when applicable	Pulmonary function disorder; phonatory disorder (eg, voice fatigue, weak voice, abnormal pitch, melodic variation, hoarseness, harshness, or breathiness); articulatory disorder; larynx or airway tumor; myasthenia gravis; esophageal speech	See Table 11-8

10. Carlsson GE, deBoever JA. Epidemiology. In: Zarb GA, ed. *Temporomandibular Joint Function and Dysfunction.* Copenhagen, Denmark: Munksgaard; 1994.

    Presents the need for better definition of principles of diagnosis and treatment of TMJ disorders.

11. Okeson JP. Current terminology and diagnostic classification schema. deBont LGM. Epidemiology and natural progression of temporomandibular joint intracapsular and arthritic conditions. Stohler CS. Epidemiology and natural progression of muscular temporomandibular disorder conditions. In: National Institutes of Dental Research and the NIH Office of Medical Applications of Research. *NIH Technology Assessment Conference on Management of Temporomandibular Disorders.* Bethesda, Md: National Institutes of Health; 1996:21-26, 33-39.

    Stresses the need for reliable diagnostic instrumentation compatible with both diagnostic and therapeutic purposes.

12. Norman JE, Bramley P, Painter DM. Medico-legal implications: post-traumatic disorders. In: Norman JE, Bramley P, eds. *Textbook and Color Atlas of the Temporomandibular Joint.* Chicago, Ill: Year Book Medical Publishers, Inc; 1990:134-135.

    A brief commentary on some medicolegal aspects of posttraumatic TMJ disorders.

13. Widmer CG. Evaluation of diagnostic tests for TMD. In: *Clinics in Physical Therapy: Temporomandibular Disorders.* London, England: Churchill Livingstone; 1994.

    An overview of the reliability and validity of diagnostic tests for temporomandibular disorders (TMD).

14. Kaplan AS, Assael LA. *Temporomandibular Disorders: Diagnosis and Treatment.* Philadelphia, Pa: WB Saunders Co; 1991:106-117.

15. Hirano M. *Clinical Examination of the Voice.* New York, NY: Springer-Verlag; 1981:1-98.

    Overview of standard methods for clinical examination of the voice.

16. Sataloff RT. *Professional Voice: The Science and Art of Clinical Care.* 2nd ed. San Diego, Calif: Singular Publishing Group, Inc; 1997.

    An extensive review of the current information on diagnosis and treatment of voice disorders. Data on normative values is limited.

17. Baken RJ. *Clinical Measurement of Speech and Voice.* Boston, Mass: College-Hill Press; 1987:518.

    Clinical measurements of speech and voice with emphasis on methods of measurement.

Chapter 12

The Visual System

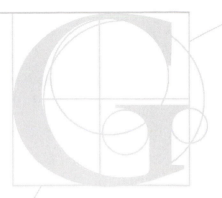

Chapter 12

Introduction

This chapter provides criteria for evaluating permanent impairment of the visual system as it affects an individual's ability to perform activities of daily living. The visual system consists of the eyes and supporting structures, the neural pathways, and the visual cortex of the brain. The visual system is unique in that it combines the input from two separate eyes into a single visual perception.

This chapter focuses on functional impairment of the visual system as a whole. The impairment ratings in this chapter estimate the severity of the effects of certain types of vision loss on the ability to perform activities of daily living. Changes due to abnormalities in the optic nerve or visual cortex are also discussed in Chapter 13, The Central and Peripheral Nervous System.

This chapter has been significantly revised from the fourth edition of the *Guides*. The revision was based on a consensus within the international community of experts in low vision. Individuals interested in further discussion, including an emphasis on ability, can refer to the *Guide for the Evaluation of Visual Impairment*, published for the International Society for Low Vision Research and Rehabilitation.[12] A summary of revisions follows.

1. The Visual Efficiency Scale that was used up to the fourth edition of the *Guides to the Evaluation of Permanent Impairment*[22, 23] was developed by Snell in 1925.[19-21] This scale was replaced with the **Functional Vision Score (FVS).**[17] The FVS provides an estimate of the effect of certain types of vision loss on the ability to perform activities of daily living. On this scale, 20/200 is rated as a 50% impairment.

2. The FVS is based on an assessment of visual acuity and visual field. The FVS allows for individual adjustments for other functional deficits, such as contrast and glare sensitivity, color vision, binocularity, stereopsis, suppression, and diplopia, if these deficits cause a significant ability loss that is not reflected in a visual acuity or visual field loss.

3. The extra scale and losses for diplopia and aphakia have been removed. Recommendations to make adjustments on an individual basis, if needed, have been added.

4. Near vision measurements are optional; the last section of this chapter contains a discussion on how to make the assessment of reading acuity more accurate.

5. Visual field is recalculated using a new Visual Field Score (VFS). To better account for the functional significance of losses in the two lower quadrants, the lower visual field carries 50% more weight than the upper field. Hemianopia is also scored more appropriately.

6. Visual impairment ratings are calculated using the formula $(3 \times OU + OD + OS)/5$ instead of the prior formula $(3 \times better\ eye + 1 \times lesser\ eye)/4$. The new formula better accounts for situations where the binocular function is not identical to the function of the better eye. This can be particularly important for dissimilar field losses.

7. This edition also calculates a binocular impairment value for visual acuity and for field loss before combining these into an estimate of total visual loss and functional vision.

8. The impairment rating for the visual system = 100 – the FVS.

12.1 Principles of Assessment

Before using the information in this chapter, the *Guides* user should become familiar with Chapters 1 and 2 and the Glossary. Chapters 1 and 2 discuss the *Guides'* purpose, applications, and methods for performing and reporting impairment evaluations. The Glossary provides definitions of common terms used by many specialties in impairment evaluation.

A permanent visual impairment is defined as a permanent loss of vision that remains after maximal medical improvement of the underlying medical condition has been reached. Ophthalmology has the capability to measure organ functions such as visual acuity and visual field rather precisely. Accordingly, this chapter uses a numerical assessment of visual functions to derive an estimate of their effect on functional vision (ie, on the ability to perform generic activities of daily living). The process is summarized in Table 12-1.

Table12-1 Calculation of the Impairment Rating for the Visual System

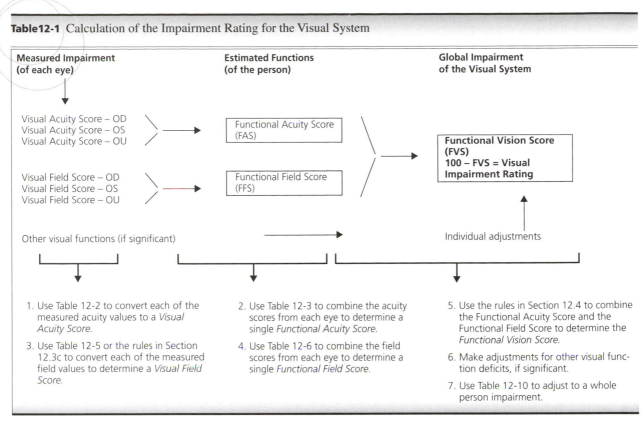

Note that the prefix *visual* is used when the score refers to each eye. The prefix *functional* refers to the estimated performance of the individual.
The term *vision score* combines visual acuity and visual field estimates (and individual adjustments, if significant).

12.1a Steps to Calculate the Visual Impairment Rating

1. Measure visual acuity. Use Table 12-2 to convert each of the measured acuity values to a Visual Acuity Score (VAS).

2. Use Table 12-3 to combine the acuity scores from each eye to determine a single **Functional Acuity Score (FAS).** *Note:* If the visual fields are normal and no individual corrections are made, the impairment rating for the visual system is equal to the acuity-related impairment rating (100 – FAS).

3. Measure the visual fields. Use Table 12-5 or the detailed instructions in Section 12.3c to convert each of the measured field values to a Visual Field Score (VFS).

4. Use Table 12-6 to combine the field scores from each eye to determine a single **Functional Field Score (FFS).**

5. Use the rules in Section 12.4 to combine the Functional Acuity Score and the Functional Field Score to determine a Functional Vision Score (FVS).

6. Subtract the Functional Vision Score from 100 to obtain the impairment rating for the visual system.

7. If additional visual impairments are not reflected in the reduction of visual acuity or visual field, the examiner may make an adjustment as explained in Section 12.4. The need for such adjustment must be well documented.

The procedure as outlined in Table 12-1 reduces a complex reality to a single number. This number ignores individual differences in adjustment to vision loss. This approach can be helpful for administrative and legal purposes because it does not penalize the individual who has made a good adjustment with a reduction of the impairment rating. By the same token, this approach cannot be used for individualized rehabilitation plans. Such plans must be based on an ability profile detailing each of the various skills and abilities of the specific individual. As the rehabilitation proceeds, successful adaptations will reduce further rehabilitation needs. Thus, the ability profile may change while the generic impairment rating will remain the same.

12.1b Interpretation of Symptoms and Signs

Subjective symptoms of vision loss usually are the result of objective changes in visual acuity and/or visual field.

Visual acuity describes the ability of the eye to perceive details. Visual acuity loss will manifest itself in an inability to perform detail-oriented tasks, such as reading and face recognition. A lay term for visual acuity loss is *blurred vision*. Visual acuity loss affects many activities of daily living. Although visual acuity is governed by only a small area of the retina (the fovea, the central-most area), it occupies a major part of the visual cortex.

Visual field refers to the ability to detect objects in the periphery of the visual environment. A lay term for peripheral field loss is *tunnel vision*. Visual field loss will manifest itself in an inability to detect peripheral objects and, often, in a reduced ability to avoid obstacles. The peripheral visual field occupies the largest part of the retina, but it occupies a smaller part of the visual cortex.

Good visual acuity and good visual field are both needed for the performance of daily living skills. A person with tunnel vision may not notice when someone enters the room. A person with visual acuity loss, on the other hand, may notice the newcomer but may have difficulty recognizing the person's face. Once an object has been detected in peripheral vision, central vision will be used to recognize it. A person with a visual field defect (ie, tunnel vision) may not notice a sign on the road or on a wall but could read the sign once found, assuming the individual had good visual acuity. A person with normal visual fields but a visual acuity loss will detect the sign but will not be able to read it.

Another important function is contrast sensitivity. Whereas visual acuity is generally measured with small objects of high contrast, **contrast sensitivity** refers to the ability to detect larger objects of poor contrast. This ability is often needed for daily living skills. Facial characteristics are an example of typical low-contrast objects. Contrast sensitivity loss often accompanies visual acuity loss, but it can occur separately. Because measurement methods for contrast sensitivity are not standardized, this function is not included in the impairment ratings. Where indicated, contrast sensitivity loss that exceeds the effects of the visual acuity loss may be handled as an individual adjustment.

Other symptoms may result from deficits in glare sensitivity, color vision, night vision, binocularity, stereopsis, suppression, and diplopia. If these deficits cause a significant ability loss that is not reflected in a visual acuity or a visual field loss, they may also be handled as adjustments to the impairment rating.

12.1c Description of Clinical Studies

To obtain the required information, the physician needs to perform a detailed visual assessment, including the cause, severity, and prognosis of the underlying disorder and the expected or documented effects of the vision loss on the ability to perform activities of daily living. Such a visual assessment includes the following.

- Medical history, with particular emphasis on preexisting conditions and treatments and on the major cause of the current vision loss.
- Current condition of the eyes and visual system, with documentation of relevant anatomic findings.
- Visual acuity measurement with best correction, binocularly and for each eye separately. Accurate measurement of distance visual acuity (letter chart acuity) is mandatory; measurement of near acuity (reading acuity) is optional.
- Visual field measurement for each eye.
- Other visual functions, such as contrast sensitivity or color vision, if considered relevant.
- Calculation of an initial impairment rating (visual ability estimate), as detailed in this chapter.
- Other factors that may affect the individual's ability to perform activities of daily living.
- Discussion (with documentation) of factors that might justify an adjustment of the initial ability estimate and discussion of apportionment considerations, if relevant.

In addition to the equipment needed for a standard ophthalmologic evaluation, the following tools are required for the functional evaluation.
- *Standardized letter chart.* A lighted chart in a lighted room is preferred because it is more representative of normal viewing conditions than is a projector chart in a semidark room. Charts with five letters per line, proportional spacing, and a geometric progression of letter sizes are preferred.[5-10] For vision in the normal and near-normal ranges, testing at 6 m (20 ft) is recommended. For testing in the low-vision range, testing at 1 m is recommended (see Table 12-2). Test charts for this distance are commercially available.[24]

- *Standardized reading tests.* Such tests are optional. If performed, they should be standardized tests with continuous text segments as specified in the last section of this chapter. A geometric progression of letter sizes is preferred. Letter size designations should be in M-units[24] because the implementation of point size and Jaeger numbers has been shown to be inconsistent from chart to chart.
- *Visual field equipment.* If a restriction of the visual field is claimed or suspected, formal visual field testing on standardized equipment is required. If no visual field restriction is claimed, a confrontation visual field is acceptable to confirm the absence of field restrictions.
- Other functional tests, such as a contrast sensitivity test or glare test, if problems in these areas are reported.
- Samples of actual job-related tasks, if these tasks are different from average reading tasks.

12.2 Impairment of Visual Acuity

12.2a Visual Acuity Notations

Visual acuity is usually recorded as a fraction comparing the individual's performance to a performance standard. If the individual needs letters that are twice as large or twice as close as those needed by a standard eye (ie, 2x angular magnification), the visual acuity is 1/2. If letters are needed that are five times larger or five times closer than those needed by a standard eye, the visual acuity is 1/5, etc. In the United States, it is customary to standardize the numerator at 20. Thus, a visual acuity of 1/2 is recorded as 20/40 and one of 1/5 is recorded as 20/100.

12.2b Test Procedures

Visual acuity is usually measured with symbols (letters, numbers, pictures, or other symbols) presented in a letter chart format. Because visual acuity values can vary widely, the optimum testing distance is not the same for all groups.

12.2b.1 Testing in the Normal Range

Individuals in the normal and near-normal range of vision (20/60 or better, *ICD-9-CM*[2], Table 12-2) represent the majority of all patients. The traditional letter charts and projector charts were designed for this group. The most common testing distance is 6 m (20 ft) because at this distance the optical difference with infinity may be ignored. When a printed chart is used, the indicated visual acuity values are valid only if the individual is located at the distance for which the chart was designed. If a projector chart is used, the individual must be located at the distance for which the projector was adjusted. Charts with a geometric progression of letter sizes, five letters on each row, and letter spacing that is equal to the letter size (often referred to as *ETDRS-type charts*) are the preferred standard.[9, 10]

The individual is placed at the distance for which the chart was designed and encouraged to read as far down as possible. The line is considered read when more than half of the characters (eg, three of five) are read correctly. Most charts will indicate the visual acuity level that corresponds to the ability to read each line. When visual acuity is measured in this way, the result should be recorded using the standard US notation (ie, 20/…). The individual should be tested with the best available refractive correction.

When testing for visual acuities around the 20/200 level (**legal blindness**), the choice of letter chart is particularly important because it affects the assignment of benefits. On traditional charts that have no lines between 20/100 and 20/200, the descriptor 20/200 or less becomes, effectively, less than 20/100, so individuals with 20/125 would be recorded as 20/200. On newer charts, 20/200 or less is more appropriately interpreted as less than 20/160. If only an older printed chart is available, the individual can be brought to 10 ft so that less than 20/160 can be interpreted as less than 10/80. The individual with 20/125 (10/63) is then reported appropriately as better than 20/200. Note that the term *legal blindness* is a misnomer because 90% of individuals who have 20/200 or less visual acuity are not blind. The term *severe vision loss* as used in *ICD-9-CM* should replace the term *legal blindness*.

12.2b.2 Testing in the Low-Vision Range

Use of the *Guides* will often involve individuals whose visual acuity has dropped to less than 20/60 (ie, to the low-vision range in *ICD-9-CM*,[2] Table 12-2). Individuals in the low-vision range form a minority of the general population but may represent the majority of those for whom visual impairment evaluations are requested.

Traditional letter charts often have only a few letters for visual acuities worse than 20/100. Such charts are inadequate for the low-vision range and have promoted the use of vague statements such as "count fingers" and "hand motions." More accurate results can be obtained by bringing the chart closer. Testing at 1 m is recommended because it can cover the entire low-vision range, down to 1/50 (20/1000).

When visual acuity is measured at 1 m, it should be recorded as a metric Snellen fraction in which the numerator records the test distance in meters (in this case 1 m, thus 1/…) and the denominator indicates the smallest letter size read in "M-units" (1 M = 1.45 mm = about 1/16 in). The standard US notation may be added in parentheses. Thus, the ability to read 8 M characters at 1 m should be recorded as 1/8 (20/160). Charts with a cord attached and labeled for 1-m testing are available commercially.[24]

12.2b.3 Correction for Refractive Error

The visual acuity without correction may be reported as part of the general eye examination. The impairment ratings should be based on the *best-corrected* visual acuity. It is important, therefore, to ensure that the refractive correction is appropriate for the testing distance. This is especially true for the short viewing distances used for low-vision individuals. If uncorrected and best-corrected visual acuity are the same, this should be stated explicitly.

12.2b.4 Monocular vs Binocular Acuity

Because binocular viewing represents the most common viewing condition in daily life, the impairment rating should consider the best-corrected binocular visual acuity as well as the best-corrected acuity for each eye separately.

Under most circumstances, best-corrected visual acuity measured binocularly will be determined by the acuity of the better eye. There are exceptions, however. People with latent nystagmus may have better eye stability, and hence better acuity, when viewing binocularly than when one eye is occluded. Some people with diplopia or with distortions in one eye may see better when the poorer eye is occluded.

12.2b.5 Incomplete Data

Whenever possible, determination of an impairment rating should be based on direct examination of the individual. Occasionally, it may be necessary to determine a tentative impairment rating based on chart review, where complete data may not be available. If no better information is obtainable, use the following:

Interpret CF	… ft	as	… /200.
Interpret CF	… m	as	… /60.
Interpret HM	… ft	as	… /1000.
Interpret HM	… m	as	… /300.

Therefore, CF 3 ft is interpreted as 3/200, and HM 5 ft is interpreted as 5/1000.

12.2b.6 Use of Realistic Conditions

The evaluation of visual functions should be based on performance under optimal conditions. An exception can be made, however, when the best possible conditions are not feasible in daily life. Examples include individuals who would see better with contact lenses but who cannot tolerate them; those with a large interocular difference in refractive error who cannot tolerate full correction of both eyes; and those who can achieve better acuity with an extremely high or extremely low illumination level that cannot be achieved under daily living conditions or in the workplace.

Under these and similar conditions, the evaluation should be based on measurements obtained under realistic daily living conditions. Document why testing under suboptimal conditions is most appropriate. When testing multihandicapped individuals, a distinction must be made between failure to see and failure to respond.

12.2c Steps for Assigning a Visual Acuity–Based Impairment Rating

1. Assign a Visual Acuity Score for each eye.
Measure visual acuity as outlined above. Use Table 12-2 to replace the visual acuity value with a score value.

The left part of Table 12-2 lists the **ranges of visual acuity loss** used in *ICD-9-CM*.[2] At the top of the scale are those with normal vision (20/20 or better), and at the bottom are those who are **blind** (no light perception). In between are those who have lost part of their vision. This group is said to have **low vision** (the word *vision* indicates that they are not blind; the word *low* indicates that they have less than normal vision). The visual acuity values follow a geometric progression—each line differs from the adjacent lines by a fixed ratio (25%, 10 steps = 10x).

The central part of Table 12-2 lists impairment ratings. This conversion is based on Weber-Fechner's law, which states that a proportional increase in the stimulus corresponds to a linear increase in sensation. The Visual Acuity Score (VAS) has fixed increments (5 points) based on counting 1 point for each letter read on a standard acuity chart with 5 letters per line. The VAS is an *ability* scale on which higher values indicate better function. The impairment rating, which is a scale of *ability loss*, is obtained by subtracting the VAS from 100. Note that the VAS extends beyond 100 (as does normal visual acuity), but that ability loss is counted only when visual acuity is less than 20/20.

The right part of Table 12-2 lists the estimated impact of visual acuity loss on reading ability. These ranges are based on a general ability scale with the following gradations.[17]

100 ± 10	Range of normal	Normal function, with reserve capacity
80 ± 10	Mild loss (near-normal)	Normal function, but loss of reserve capacity
60 ± 10	Moderate loss	Normal function, but need for some aids
40 ± 10	Severe loss	Restricted function, slower than normal, even with aids
20 ± 10	Profound loss	Restricted function, marginal performance, even with aids
0 ± 10	(Near-) total loss	Cannot perform; needs substitution skills

The three parts of Table 12-2 fit well with each other. This confirms that the VAS is a reasonable estimate of acuity-related visual abilities and that the impairment rating is a reasonable estimate of acuity-related performance loss. If no visual acuity data were obtainable, the right side of Table 12-2 might be used to obtain a very rough impairment estimate.

2. Combine the acuity values.
After the best-corrected visual acuity values for binocular vision (OU), for the right eye (OD), and for the left eye (OS) have been obtained and converted to Visual Acuity Scores, these values need to be combined to a single Functional Acuity Score (FAS). The FAS provides an estimate of the ability of the person to perform acuity-dependent daily living tasks. This is done using Table 12-3.

Note that VAS and FAS may differ. For example, an individual with one blind eye will have a 0 VAS for that eye. However, if the other eye is normal, the FAS will be near-normal, indicating normal performance but loss of reserves (see Examples 12-2 and 12-14).

The acuity-related impairment rating (IR) is calculated by subtracting the FAS from 100. Note that the FAS can be larger than 100 but that the impairment rating is truncated at 0.

3. Consider reading acuity (optional).
Determination of reading acuity (near vision) is optional and is explained in more detail in the last section of this chapter. Reading acuity is typically determined binocularly, but it may be determined monocularly if this gives better results.

If reading acuity is significantly worse than letter acuity, the functional acuity score may be adjusted to the average of the letter chart (or distance) acuity score and the reading (or near) acuity score. The probable reason for the discrepancy should be explored and explained.

Chapter 12

Table 12-2 Impairment of Visual Acuity*

Impairment Classes (Based on *ICD-9-CM*)		Visual Acuity		Visual Acuity Score (ability)	Visual Acuity Impairment Rating (%) (ability loss)	Estimated Reading Ability
		US Notation	1 m Notation			
(Near-) Normal Vision	Range of Normal Vision	20/12.5 20/16 20/20 20/25	1/0.63 1/0.8 1/1 1/1.25	110 105 100 95	... ... 0 5	Normal reading speed Normal reading distance Reserve capacity for small print
	Near-Normal Vision	20/32 20/40 20/50 20/63	1/1.6 1/2 1/2.5 1/3.2	90 85 80 75	10 15 20 25	Normal reading speed Reduced reading distance No reserve for small print
Low Vision	Moderate Low Vision	20/80 20/100 20/125 20/160	1/4 1/5 1/6.3 1/8	70 65 60 55	30 35 40 45	Near-normal with reading aids Uses low-power magnifier or large-print books
	Severe Low Vision	20/200 20/250 20/320 20/400	1/10 1/12.5 1/16 1/20	50 45 40 35	50 55 60 65	Slower than normal with reading aids Uses high-power magnifiers
	Profound Low Vision	20/500 20/630 20/800 20/1000	1/25 1/32 1/40 1/50	30 25 20 15	70 75 80 85	Marginal with reading aids Uses magnifiers for spot reading but may prefer talking books
(Near-) Blindness	Near-Blindness	20/1250 20/1600 20/2000 or less	1/63 1/80 1/100 or less	10 5	90 95	No visual reading Must rely on talking books, Braille, or other nonvisual sources
	Total Blindness	No light perception		0	100	

*Use this table to determine a Visual Acuity Score for each eye. Proceed to Table 12-3 to combine the scores from each eye to a single Functional Acuity Score.
Note: The visual acuity values used in this table follow a strict geometric progression. For clinical use, values such as 20/32 and 20/63 may be rounded to 20/30 and 20/60.

Table 12-3 Calculation of the Acuity-Related Impairment Rating *

Measured Snellen Values   **Calculated Visual Acuity Scores**

OU: letter chart acuity: 20/____ → VAS_{OU}: _____ × 3 = ____

OD: letter chart acuity: 20/____ → VAS_{OD}: _____ × 1 = ____

OS: letter chart acuity: 20/____ → VAS_{OS}: _____ × 1 = ____

Add OU, OD, and OS   = ____

Divide by 5 to calculate the weighted average   = ____ = Functional Acuity Score (FAS)

Acuity-Related Impairment Rating = 100 – FAS   = ____

Optionally, calculate a Visual Acuity Score for reading (near) acuity. If the outcome is significantly different from the letter chart acuity score, document the differences and calculate the average:

$FAS_{global} = (FAS_{letter\ chart} + FAS_{reading})/2$

*If visual fields are normal and no individual adjustments are made, the acuity-related impairment rating equals the whole person impairment rating.

Table 12-4 Classification of Visual Acuity Impairment*

Class 1 0%-9% Impairment of Visual Acuity	Class 2 10%-29% Impairment of Visual Acuity	Class 3 30%-49% Impairment of Visual Acuity	Class 4 50%-69% Impairment of Visual Acuity	Class 5 70%-89% Impairment of Visual Acuity	Class 6 90%-100% Impairment of Visual Acuity
FAS: ≥ 91	FAS: 90-71	FAS: 70-51	FAS: 50-31	FAS: 30–11	FAS: ≤ 10
Range of normal vision	Near-normal vision (mild vision loss)	Moderate vision loss	Severe vision loss	Profound vision loss	(Near-) Total vision loss
Both eyes have visual acuity of 20/25 or better	Both eyes have visual acuity of 20/60 or better	Both eyes have visual acuity of 20/160 or better	Both eyes have visual acuity of 20/400 or better	Both eyes have visual acuity of 20/1000 or better	Both eyes have visual acuity worse than 20/1000
	One eye has 20/200 or less; the other eye is normal	One eye has 20/200 or less; the other eye has 20/80	One eye has 20/200 or less; the other eye has 20/200		

*This table assumes that the visual fields are normal and provides general impairment ranges for the listed conditions. Use Tables 12-2 and 12-3 to calculate a more exact impairment rating and to handle cases of visual acuity loss that are not listed. Proceed to Tables 12-5 and 12-6 if visual field loss is present.

12.2d Calculation Examples for Visual Acuity Loss

Note: In the following examples it is assumed that the visual acuity loss is the only deficit. Visual fields and other visual functions are presumed to be normal.

Example 12-1
15% Impairment Due to Visual Acuity Loss

Subject: 18-year-old man.

History: Driving instructor questioned student's visual acuity. Student always liked to sit in front of the class to see the blackboard.

Current Symptoms: Has difficulty with distant road signs.

Physical Exam: No ocular abnormalities.

Clinical Studies: Best-corrected acuities: VOU: 20/40, VOD: 20/40, VOS: 20/40.

Visual fields are normal in both eyes; no other deficits in visual functions.

Functional Acuity Score (use Table 12-2 to determine the Visual Acuity Score for each eye; use Table 12-3 to combine the values to a Functional Acuity Score):

VOU	20/40	85 × 3	=	255
VOD	20/40	85 × 1	=	85
VOS	20/40	85 × 1	=	85
Functional Acuity Score		=	425/5 = 85	

Diagnosis: Unexplained amblyopia, possibly congenital.

Impairment Rating: 100 – 85 = 15% visual impairment.

Comment: This rating places the person in the range of near-normal vision or mild vision loss. Persons in this range can generally function normally, but they need to bring reading material close.

Example 12-2
16% Impairment Due to Visual Acuity Loss

Subject: 45-year-old woman.

History: Office worker; left eye was enucleated in childhood.

Current Symptoms: Can perform all office functions.

Physical Exam: Left eye replaced by good-fitting prosthesis.

Clinical Studies: Best-corrected acuities: VOU: 20/15, VOD: 20/15, VOS: NLP.

Functional Acuity Score (use Tables 12-2 and 12-3, as above):

VOU	20/15	105 × 3	=	315
VOD	20/15	105 × 1	=	105
VOS	NLP	0 × 1	=	0
Functional Acuity Score			=	420/5 = 84

Diagnosis: History of retinoblastoma.

Impairment Rating: 100 – 84 = 16% visual impairment.

Comment: Based on visual acuity, this person's condition is in the near-normal range. The visual field in the left eye is also lost (see Section 12.3). However, because this loss is not independent of the visual acuity loss (see the previous section) and does not exceed the visual acuity–based loss, the Functional Vision Score will still be equal to the Functional Acuity Score (see Example 12-12).

Chapter 12

Example 12-3
25% Impairment Due to Visual Acuity Loss

Subject: 35-year-old man.

History: Farm worker; scratched the left eye on a branch several years ago.

Current Symptoms: Farm work is OK; no interest in reading or fine crafts.

Physical Exam: Dense corneal scar in OS.

Clinical Studies: Best-corrected acuities: VOU: 20/40, VOD: 20/40, VOS: 20/400.

Functional Acuity Score (use Tables 12-2 and 12-3, as above):

VOU	20/40	85×3	=	255
VOD	20/40	85×1	=	85
VOS	20/400	35×1	=	35
Functional Acuity Score			=	375/5 = 75

Diagnosis: Vision loss due to corneal opacity.

Impairment Rating: $100 - 75 = 25\%$ visual impairment.

Comment: Even though the left eye has much poorer vision than in Example 12-1, this person is still in the range of near-normal vision or mild vision loss. Note that the impairment rating is influenced much more by binocular function than by the function of the lesser eye.

Example 12-4
36% Impairment Due to Visual Acuity Loss

Subject: 70-year-old woman.

History: Noticed gradual vision loss over several years. Afraid of surgery.

Current Symptoms: Increasing difficulties with reading.

Physical Exam: Early lens opacity OD; dense cataract OS.

Clinical Studies: Best-corrected acuities: VOU: 20/60, VOD: 20/60, VOS: 20/800.

Functional Acuity Score (use Tables 12-2 and 12-3, as above):

VOU	20/60	75×3	=	225
VOD	20/60	75×1	=	75
VOS	20/800	20×1	=	20
Functional Acuity Score			=	320/5 = 64

Diagnosis: Vision loss due to cataract.

Impairment Rating: $100 - 64 = 36\%$ visual impairment.

Comment: Although 20/60 is still in the near-normal range, the very poor condition of the other eye drops the person to the range of moderate vision loss. Persons in this range can perform activities of daily living but may require some aids, such as a hand-held magnifier, to perform detail-oriented tasks, such as reading. If the VOU were not available, assume the VOU = VOD and proceed as above.

Example 12-5
52% Impairment Due to Visual Acuity Loss

Subject: 25-year-old woman.

History: College student; vision loss since teens.

Current Symptoms: Relies on talking books and videomagnifier for her studies.

Physical Exam: Irregular foveal reflex OU.

Clinical Studies: Best-corrected acuities: VOU: 20/200, VOD: 20/300, VOS: 20/200.

Functional Acuity Score (use Tables 12-2 and 12-3, as above):

VOU	20/200	50×3	=	150
VOD	20/300	40×1	=	40
VOS	20/200	50×1	=	50
Functional Acuity Score			=	240/5 = 48

Diagnosis: Stargardt juvenile maculopathy.

Impairment Rating: $100 - 48 = 52\%$ visual impairment.

Comment: This person is in the range of severe vision loss (sometimes called legal blindness in the United States) and will have limitations in the ability to perform activities of daily living even with aids. Persons in this range need to rely more heavily on assistive devices.

12.3 Impairment of the Visual Field

12.3a Test Procedures

If no visual field impairment is claimed or suspected (impairment rating = 0), a confrontation visual field may be used to confirm a normal field. In all other circumstances (impairment rating > 0), formal visual field tests should be performed by qualified personnel according to the instructions provided with the equipment.

12.3a.1 Confrontation Visual Field

This method uses only the examiner's hands. Seated in front of the individual, the examiner moves his or her hands from the periphery inward to test for the peripheral field limits. This method is an acceptable way to confirm a normal visual field in individuals in whom no field loss is claimed, but it is too gross for detailed evaluation if a field loss is claimed or suspected.

12.3a.2 Tangent Screen Testing

This method uses a black screen on which variously sized objects may be moved. This method is difficult to standardize and loses accuracy beyond 45°. It is not acceptable for the accurate assessment of permanent impairment.

12.3a.3 Goldmann-Type Testing

The Goldmann visual field equipment provided the first standardized measurement technique. Testing is done in a bowl so that all testing distances are equal while the background and stimulus luminances can be controlled tightly. The usual mode of testing is known as *kinetic perimetry* because a test stimulus of constant size and intensity is moved by an operator.

The test results are plotted as *isopters*, contour lines that outline the areas where stimuli of various intensity can be perceived. The functional implications of certain isopter patterns are relatively easy to interpret. Agencies, such as the Social Security Administration, often require testing of the Goldmann III4e isopter for eligibility determinations.

12.3a.4 Automated Perimetry

In recent decades, there has been a move from manual to automated perimetry. (Commonly used equipment includes Humphrey, Octopus, Dicon, and other brands.) This has been accompanied by a move to static perimetry. In static perimetry, the presentations are limited to various fixed locations where stimulus size and intensity are varied.

Automated perimetry results are commonly plotted as a gray scale. Such reports are better suited for automated statistical analysis. They are less intuitive for human interpretation with regard to functional vision. Most clinical tests are limited to the central 30° because this is the most important area for medical diagnostic purposes. For the functional assessment of visual field loss, however, testing to 60° or beyond is mandatory.

12.3a.5 Binocular Fields

Considering both monocular and binocular function is even more important for a functional assessment of the field of vision than it is for visual acuity because intact field areas in one eye may compensate for field loss in the other eye. In cases of asymmetric field loss, the binocular field of view may be substantially better than the field of view of either eye alone.

Direct testing of the binocular visual field presents problems, however, because the amount of convergence in a bowl perimeter cannot be monitored and fixation monitoring devices will not work when the head, rather than the eye, is centered. Therefore, the fields of each eye should be measured separately, and a binocular field plot should be derived from the superimposition of the two monocular field plots.

12.3a.6 Tests Used

When Goldmann equipment is used, the III4e isopter should be plotted. If only a larger isopter is available, this isopter may be used (this may result in an underestimation of the field loss). If only smaller isopters are available, the test cannot be used for impairment evaluation.

If automated equipment is used, a pseudoisopter equivalent to the Goldmann III4e isopter should be constructed (see Example 12-9). On the Humphrey equipment, this would be the isopter for a 10-dB stimulus. Plots of the central 30° may only be used when the remaining field radius is smaller than 20° and confrontation testing indicates no further peripheral vision.

12.3b The Visual Field Score (VFS)

The **Visual Field Score (VFS),** which is the basis for the calculation of visual field–based impairment ratings, parallels the **Visual Acuity Score (VAS).** The VAS can be determined by counting the letters read correctly on a standardized visual acuity chart. Similarly, the VFS can be determined by counting the points seen on a standardized visual field grid. The combination rules are also similar.

12.3b.1 Testing Grid

The testing grid is constructed by drawing 10 meridians: 2 in each of the upper quadrants and 3 in each of the lower quadrants. The optimal positions for the 10 meridians are as follows: 25°, 65° (upper right), 115°, 155° (upper left), 195°, 225°, 255° (lower left), 285°, 315°, and 345° (lower right). Along these meridians, 5 points (spaced 2° apart) are assigned to the central 10° and 5 points (spaced 10° apart) are assigned to the periphery beyond 10°; thus, a 60° radius will represent 10 points. The nasal and superior meridians may not reach 60°, but the lateral field will extend further. Thus, the average normal field will score about 100 points.

Figure 12-1 summarizes the point assignments. The circle represents a 10° radius.

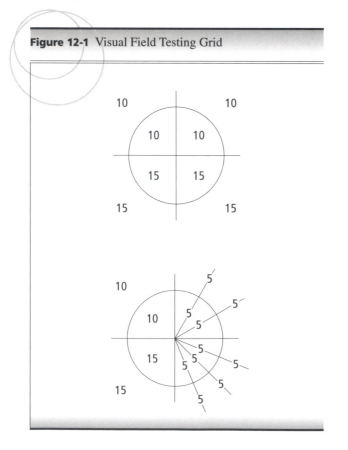

Figure 12-1 Visual Field Testing Grid

This arrangement has the following effects:

- The visual field score for the central 10° is 50 points. This reflects that the central 10° of the visual field correspond to 50% of the primary visual cortex. This also maintains the traditional assumption that a visual field loss to a 10° radius is equally disabling as a visual acuity loss to 20/200.
- Choosing the measured meridians within the quadrants rather than along the horizontal and vertical meridians avoids the need for special rules for hemianopias.
- A complete homonymous hemianopia receives a 50-point score. This implies that it is considered equally disabling as a field restriction to a 10° radius or as a visual acuity loss to 20/200.
- Choosing 3 meridians in the lower quadrants and 2 in the upper ones acknowledges the functional importance of the lower field by giving it 50% extra weight.
- *ICD-9-CM* defines severe, profound, and near-total visual field loss as concentric restriction to a 10°, 5°, and 2.5° field radius.[2] These categories fit the VFS scale.

The VFS is summarized in Table 12-5, which is similar to Table 12-2 in organization.

Use Table 12-5 or the detailed rules in Section 12.3c to determine a Visual Field Score for each eye. Proceed to Table 12-6 to combine the scores from each eye to determine a single Functional Field Score.

Table 12-5 Impairment of the Visual Field*

Impairment Classes (Based on *ICD-9-CM*)		Special Conditions	Average Radius If Loss Is Concentric	Visual Field Score (ability)	Visual Field Impairment Rating (%) (ability loss)	Estimated Ability for Visual Orientation and Mobility (O + M) Tasks
(Near-) Normal Vision	Range of Normal Vision			110	...	Normal visual orientation
				105	...	Normal mobility skills
			60°	100	0	
				95	5	
	Near-Normal Vision		50°	90	10	Normal O + M performance
				85	15	Needs more scanning
		Loss of 1 eye	40°	80	20	Occasionally surprised by events
				75	25	on the side
Low Vision	Moderate Low Vision		30°	70	30	Near-normal performance
				65	35	Requires scanning for obstacles
		Lost upper field	20°	60	40	
				55	45	
	Severe Low Vision	Hemianopia	10°	50	50	Visual mobility is slower than normal
				45	55	
		Lost lower field	8°	40	60	Requires continous scanning
				35	65	May use cane as adjunct
	Profound Low Vision		6°	30	70	Must use long cane for detection of obstacles
				25	75	
			4°	20	80	May use vision as adjunct for identification
				15	85	
(Near-) Blindness	Near-Blindness		2° or less	10	90	Visual orientation unreliable
				5	95	Must rely on long cane, sound, guide dog, and other blind mobility skills
			0°			
	Total Blindness	No visual fields		0	100	

*This table follows the clinical usage of describing field losses on the basis of the remaining radius. In the rehabilitation and disability literature, field losses are often described on the basis of the remaining diameter (eg, a concentric field loss to a radius of 10° leaves a field with a diameter of 20°).

Table 12-6 Calculation of the Field-Related Impairment Rating

Measured Field Plots		Calculated Visual Field Scores
Binocular field plot (OU)	→	VFS$_{OU}$: _____ × 3 = _____
Field plot right eye (OD)	→	VFS$_{OD}$: _____ × 1 = _____
Field plot left eye (OS)	→	VFS$_{OD}$: _____ × 1 = _____
Add OU, OD, and OS		= _____
Divide by 5 to calculate the weighted average		= _____ = Functional Field Score (FFS)
Field-related Impairment Rating = 100 − FFS		= _____

Table 12-7 Classification of Visual Field Impairment*

Class 1 0%-9% **Impairment of Visual Field**	Class 2 10%-29% **Impairment of Visual Field**	Class 3 30%-49% **Impairment of Visual Field**	Class 4 50%-69% **Impairment of Visual Field**	Class 5 70%-89% **Impairment of Visual Field**	Class 6 90%-100% **Impairment of Visual Field**
FFS: ≥ 91	FFS: 90-71	FFS: 70-51	FFS: 50-31	FFS: 30–11	FFS: ≤ 10
Range of normal vision	Near-normal vision (mild vision loss)	Moderate vision loss	Severe vision loss	Profound vision loss	(Near-) Total vision loss
Both eyes have visual fields > 50°	Both eyes have visual fields ≤ 50° and > 30°	Both eyes have visual fields ≤ 30° and > 10°	Both eyes have visual fields ≤ 10° and > 6°	Both eyes have visual fields ≤ 6° and > 2°	Both eyes have visual fields of 2° or less
	One eye is lost (the other eye is normal)	Both eyes have lost the upper half-field	Both eyes have lost the lower half-field Homonymous hemianopia		

*This table assumes that the visual acuity is still normal. It can be used to determine the general impairment range for the listed conditions. Use Tables 12-5 and 12-6 or the detailed rules in Section 12.3c to calculate a more exact figure and to handle other visual field loss. Use Tables 12-2 and 12-3 if visual acuity loss is present.

12.3c Assigning a Field-Based Impairment Rating

Calculation of a visual field–based impairment rating requires the following steps.

1. Determine the extent of the visual field for each eye.
If Goldmann visual field plots are available, determine the III4e isopter for each eye. If only automated visual field plots are available, determine a pseudoisopter by drawing a line surrounding all points with a sensitivity of 10 dB or better, excluding points with < 10-dB sensitivity. If automated field plots are used, these should be full-field plots (Humphrey 60-2 or the equivalent). The 30° plot may be used only if confrontation testing has determined that there are no peripheral islands of vision and if a 30° central field plot (Humphrey 30-2 or the equivalent) shows that there is no vision beyond 20°.

2. Determine the Visual Field Score for each eye.
Use the pattern explained in Figure 12-1. This pattern can be implemented in several ways, explained below.

2.a. Paper and pencil
Starting with a visual field plot of the III4e isopter (or the equivalent), draw 10 meridians, 2 in each upper quadrant and 3 in each lower quadrant. To space the meridians evenly, use the following approximate positions: 25°, 65° (upper right), 115°, 155° (upper left), 195°, 225°, 255° (lower left), 285°, 315°, and 345° (lower right).

Determine the extent of each meridian. Within 10° from fixation, round to the nearest 2° value; outside 10° round to the nearest 10° value. Convert the rounded extent to a subscore using Table 12-8.

Table 12-8 Conversion of Field Radius to Field Score

Rounded Peripheral Field limits:

Extent:	0°	2°	4°	6°	8°	10°	20°	30°	40°	50°	60°	70° or more
Score:	0	1	2	3	4	5	6	7	8	9	10	11

Subtract for scotomata within 10°:

Radial Extent:	1°	2°	3°	4°	5°	6°	7°	8°	9°
Subtract:	0	1	1	2	2	3	3	4	4

Subtract for scotomata outside 10°:

Radial Extent:	1°-4°	5°-14°	15°-24°	25°-34°	35°-44°	45°-54°
Subtract:	0	1	2	3	4	5

If a scotoma interrupts the meridian, round the extent of the scotoma to the nearest 2° or 10° value and subtract the corresponding point value. In the presence of scotomata, use of the overlay grid is the preferred method.

Add the 10 subscores to obtain the VFS for that eye. The average normal field will score about 100 points.

2.b. Overlay grid

Create an overlay grid with 10 meridians (see step 2.a) and grid points on each meridian at 1°, 3°, 5°, 7°, 9°, 15°, 25°, 35°, 45°, 55°, and 65°. Place the overlay grid over the field plot. Count the grid points enclosed by the III4e isopter (or the equivalent). Grid points within scotomata should not be counted. The total number of points seen is the Visual Field Score (VFS).

2.c. Automated calculation

A pilot study in 1992 conducted with a Humphrey Field Analyzer and controlled by an IBM-PC has shown the feasibility of a fully automated test sequence using the points of the overlay grid as stimulus positions.[16] Such a program is not yet available commercially.

3. Determine the Functional Field Score (FFS).

Determine the binocular field by superimposing the monocular fields. For the binocular field, points are counted as seen if seen by both eyes or by one of the eyes. This determines the binocular VFS.

Combine the Visual Field Scores for OU, OD, and OS (see Table 12-6):

$$FFS = (3 \times VFS_{OU} + VFS_{OD} + VFS_{OS})/5.$$

4. The visual field–based impairment rating is 100 – FFS.

12.3d Calculation Examples for Visual Field Loss

The following examples calculate the Visual Field Score for a single eye. This calculation needs to be followed by the same calculation for the other eye and for the binocular field (see Examples12-10 and 12-11). Finally, use Table 12-6 to combine these values to determine a Functional Field Score.

Example 12-6
0% Impairment Due to Visual Field Loss

Request: Determine the Visual Field Score for an eye with the following Goldmann III4e isopter.

Method 1: Draw 10 meridians (see instruction 2.a in section 12.3c).

Measure the extent in degrees of each meridian.

Use Table 12-8 to convert the extents to subscores.

Add the subscores: $(10 + 9) + (9 + 11) + (11 + 11 + 11) + (10 + 9 + 9) = 100$.

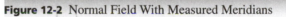

Figure 12-2 Normal Field With Measured Meridians

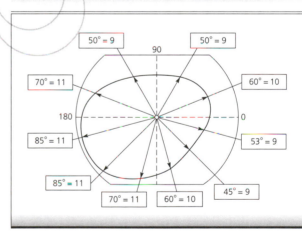

Method 2: Create an overlay grid (see instructions in Section 12.3c).

Count the points within the III4e isopter. The diagram has 100 solid dots within the 60° circle and 8 open dots outside. The score is easily counted as: 100 – solid dots missed (symbol ×) + open dots seen (symbol heavy o). For this field plot: FFS = 100 – 4 + 4 = 100.

Comment: The Visual Field Score is 100; therefore, the impairment rating is 0%. Note that the extra points seen laterally compensate for the points missed nasally and superiorly.

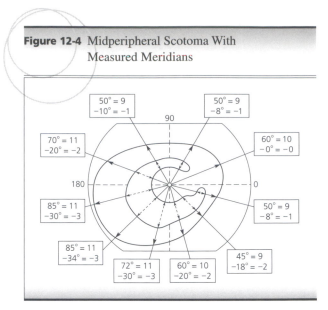

Figure 12-4 Midperipheral Scotoma With Measured Meridians

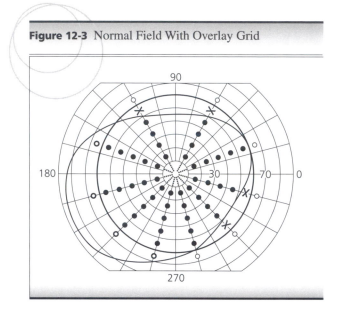

Figure 12-3 Normal Field With Overlay Grid

Method 2: Using the overlay grid as in Example 12-6, do not count the 18 points within the scotoma.

Comment: The Visual Field Score is reduced by 18 points from 100 to 82 (18% impairment). This places the individual in the near-normal range. Because the scotoma is in the midperiphery, central vision is not affected and far peripheral vision still warns of obstacles. Thus, the effect on daily living skills is relatively minor. The effect on the whole person depends on the exact condition of the other eye.

Example 12-7
18% Impairment Due to Visual Field Loss

Request: Determine the Visual Field Score for an individual with a midperipheral ring scotoma due to early RP. The central field is not affected. The Goldmann III4e isopter is as indicated.

Method 1: Determine the peripheral field limits and the peripheral subscore as in Example 12-6.

(For simplicity, the peripheral score is kept the same.)

Determine the extent of the scotoma in each of the sample meridians.

Subtract the amounts indicated in Table 12-8.

The Visual Field Score is 90.

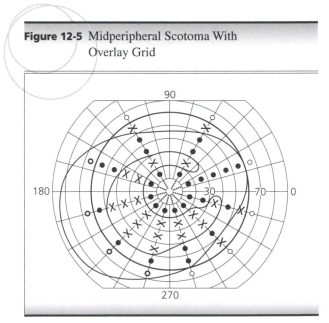

Figure 12-5 Midperipheral Scotoma With Overlay Grid

Example 12-8
20% Impairment Due to Visual Field Loss

This individual has a juxtafoveal scotoma due to early macular degeneration. Letter chart acuity is still unaffected.

Request: Determine the Visual Field Score.

Method 1: Subtract points from each meridian as indicated in Figure 12-6.

100 − 20 = 80 (20% impairment).

Figure 12-6 Juxtafoveal Scotoma With Measured Meridians

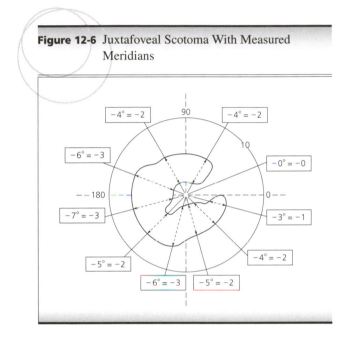

Method 2: Subtract the solid dots that are not seen (see Figure 12-7).

100 − 20 = 80 (20% impairment).

Comment: Although this scotoma is far smaller than the one in the previous example, it will significantly interfere with reading and similar tasks. This justifies a significant decrease of the Functional Field Score and a corresponding increase in the impairment rating. (See also Examples 12-13 and 12-14.)

Figure 12-7 Juxtafoveal Scotoma With Overlay Grid

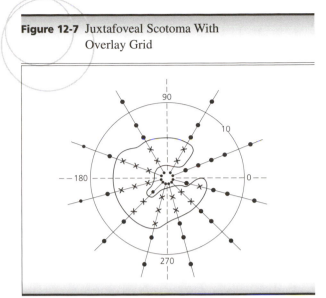

Example 12-9
72% Impairment Due to Visual Field Loss

A Goldmann visual field test is not available for this individual. Automated static perimetry has been performed with the result indicated in Figure 12-8.

Figure 12-8 Tunnel Vision: Automated Perimetry Plot

			4	0	0	0			
		0	16	18	0	5	0		
	0	6	14	22	18	18	16	11	
0	0	12	21	18	24	25	20	0	0
0	0	12	14	18	28	22	22	18	16
0	0	0	0	0	23	0	0	16	18
0	0	0	0	0	0	0	0	0	0
	0	0	0	0	0	0	0	0	
		0	0	0	0	0	0		
			0	0	0	0			

Follow these steps:
1. Construct a pseudoisopter around the points with better than 10-dB sensitivity.
2. Measure the extent in the 10 meridians. If this is a Humphrey 30-2 plot, the test points are 6° apart. The subscores are shown in Figure 12-9.

Figure 12-9 Extent of the Pseudoisopters for the Automated Perimetry Plot in Figure 12-8

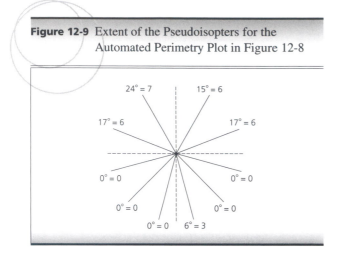

The Visual Field Score is 28. The field-related impairment rating is 100 − 28 = 72.

Comment: This may be a case of advanced retinitis pigmentosa. The automated field test did not test points beyond 30° from fixation. The calculated Visual Field Score is acceptable only if there is additional evidence that there is no further peripheral vision. A full-field automated test is preferred. In the absence of such a test and in advanced cases like this one, evidence from a confrontation visual field may be acceptable.

12.3e Calculating the Binocular Field

Existing perimeters are not equipped to provide reliable measurements of the binocular visual field. Therefore, the binocular visual field is constructed by superimposing the two monocular plots. On the superimposed plot, areas seen by either eye are counted as seen; only areas not seen by either eye are counted as defects. The resulting binocular score can vary dramatically, depending on the location of the defects.

Figure 12-10 Effect of Nasal Field Loss on the Binocular Field

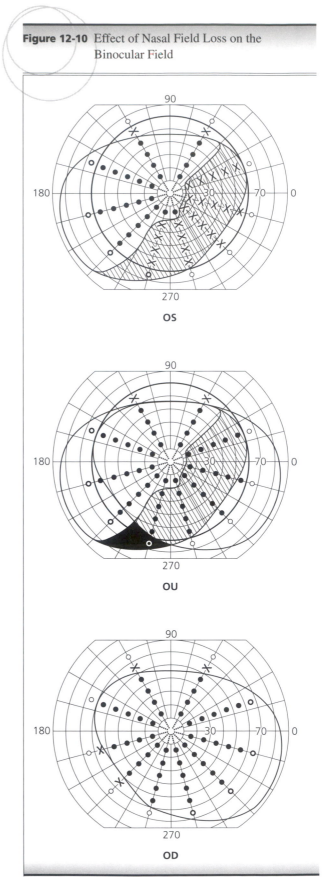

Example 12-10
2% Impairment With Consideration of Binocular Visual Field Loss

An individual has a nasal defect in the left eye. The right eye is normal (see Figure 12-10).

Visual Field Score: Visual Field Score, using the overlay grid (100 – solid dots missed + open dots seen).

OS: $100 - 24 + 3 =$ 79
OU: $100 -\ \ 2 + 7 = 105 \times 3 = 315$
OD: $\underline{100}$
                            $494 / 5 = 99$

(1% impairment rating)

Comment: Because the defect in the left eye corresponds to a seeing area of the right eye, the scotoma is not counted in the binocular plot. Because the binocular field carries 60% of the weight of the Functional Field Score, the Functional Field Score is affected little.

Example 12-11
4% Impairment With Consideration of Binocular Visual Field Loss

An individual has a temporal defect in the left eye (see Figure 12-11).

Visual Field Score: Visual Field Score, using the overlay grid (100 – solid dots missed + open dots seen).

OS: $100 - 20 =$ 80
OU: $100 - 4 + 4 = 100 \times 3 = 300$
OD: $\underline{100}$
                            $380 / 5 = 96$

(4% impairment rating)

Comment: Because the temporal defect in the left eye extends beyond the area seen by the right eye, both the left eye score and the binocular score are affected. Thus, the Functional Field Score is affected more than in Example 12-10.

Figure 12-11 Effect of Temporal Field Loss on the Binocular Field

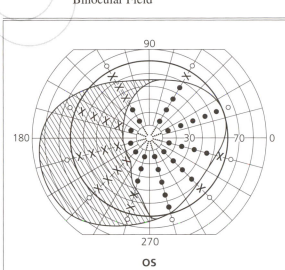

OS

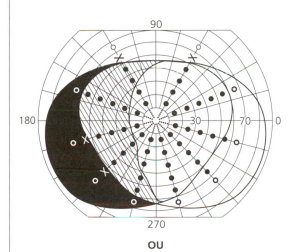

OU

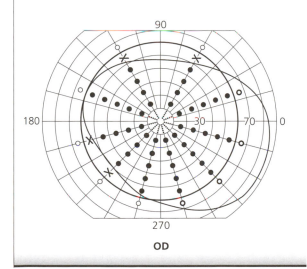

OD

12.4 Impairment of the Visual System

The preceding calculations have provided us with two separate impairment estimates. The FAS provides an estimate for visual acuity–related abilities, such as reading, while the FFS provides an estimate for visual field–related abilities, such as orientation and mobility. To obtain an overall estimate of visual impairment, the two impairment estimates must be combined to a single Functional Vision Score (FVS). Subtracting the FVS from 100 then provides the **visual impairment rating** for the visual system. See below (Section 12.4c, Table 12-10) for the whole person impairment rating.

Because the calculations outlined so far consider only the visual acuity and visual field aspects of vision, there must be room for individual adjustments in cases where functional vision is limited by factors other than visual acuity and visual field. The procedure was summarized in Table 12-1.

12.4a Calculating an Impairment Rating for the Visual System

The FAS and the FFS were calculated as weighted averages. This is appropriate because a good visual acuity or good visual field in one eye can compensate for loss of the same function in the other eye. Visual acuity–related functions and visual field–related functions, however, are largely independent. Good visual acuity cannot compensate for a loss of visual field, and vice versa. Therefore, the FAS and the FFS are combined using a multiplication formula.

12.4a.1 Basic Rule

To calculate the FVS, the FAS and the FFS are multiplied as if they represented percentage scores:

$$FVS = (FAS \times FFS)/100$$

For example, if the FAS is 80 (a 20% impairment) and the FFS is 75 (a 25% impairment), the FVS is calculated as: $80\% \times 75\% = 60\%$ (a 40% impairment).

Note that this calculation can be performed only on the basis of *residual ability* scores. Adding or multiplying the impairment ratings (which indicate *ability loss*) gives erroneous answers.

12.4a.2 Additional Rules

Some additional rules are needed to avoid unrealistic calculations.

1. For the purpose of this calculation, Functional Acuity and Functional Field Scores that are > 100 are treated as if they were 100. Thus, losses are counted only if the performance drops below the performance standard. The average performance of healthy eyes often is better than the performance standard. This better performance is taken into account in calculating the Functional Scores (see Example 12-2), but it is not counted as a reduction of the impairment rating.

2. If visual field data are not available and if there is no clinical reason to suspect visual field loss, the FFS may be assumed to be 100. In this case, the FVS is the same as the FAS, and the impairment rating for the visual system is the same as the impairment rating for the visual acuity loss.

12.4a.3 Rule for Central Scotomata (Field Loss and Acuity Loss Are Not Independent)

The dense array of points in the central 10° area of the visual field grid means that paracentral scotomata (blind spots adjacent to the point of fixation) will be counted even if they do not affect the central acuity. This is appropriate because it has been shown that such scotomata can interfere significantly with reading ability and with other activities of daily living.

However, if the scotoma is central (ie, it covers the point of fixation), it affects both visual acuity and visual field and the two impairment ratings can no longer be treated as independent. Using the basic formula, central scotomata would be counted twice: once through their effect on visual acuity and once through their effect on the central field. Therefore, an additional rule is needed.

3. If visual acuity is reduced, some central visual field losses will not be counted, as specified in Table 12-9.

Thus, for every 10 points of VAS loss, field losses in one ring of 10 grid points are ignored. This means that these points are *counted as if they were seen*. This adjustment is made for each eye separately. The effect of this rule is that individuals with a small island of good acuity within a pericentral scotoma will get credit for this scotoma, but that those with a central scotoma that affects visual acuity will not get double benefits. The adjustment does not affect peripheral field losses. Thus, a person with peripheral field loss due to glaucoma who also develops a

Table 12-9 Correction for Central Scotomata

If the Visual Acuity Score is	100-90	89-80	79-70	69-60	59-50	49 or less
(that is, if the VAS loss is	0-10	11-20	21-30	31-40	41-50	51 or more
and visual acuity is	> 20/30	> 20/50	> 20/80	> 20/125	> 20/200	≤ 20/200)
ignore central field loss up to	—	2°	4°	6°	8°	10°

central loss due to macular degeneration will get credit for the central loss as well as for the peripheral field loss (see Examples 12-13, 12-14, and 12-15).

12.4b Individual Adjustments

Although visual acuity loss and visual field loss represent significant aspects of visual impairment, they are not the only factors that can lead to a loss of functional vision. This edition of the *Guides* does not provide detailed scales for other functions, such as:

- *Contrast sensitivity.* This is the ability to perceive larger objects of poor contrast. Loss of this ability can interfere significantly with many activities of daily living. It is often, but not always, associated with a loss of visual acuity.
- *Glare sensitivity (veiling glare), delayed glare recovery, photophobia (light sensitivity), and reduced or delayed light and dark adaptation.* These are other functions that may interfere with proper contrast perception.
- *Color vision defects.* These defects are not uncommon but usually do not interfere significantly with generic activities of daily living. Severe color vision defects (achromatopsia) are usually accompanied by visual acuity loss. In some vocational settings the impact of minor color vision deficiencies can be significant. This could be a case where the generic impairment rating does not reflect the job-specific employability rating.
- *Binocularity, stereopsis, suppression, and diplopia.* These functions vary in their effect on activities of daily living. Their significance often depends on the environment and on vocational demands.

Standardized measurement techniques on which standardized ability estimates can be based have not yet been developed for most of these functions. Furthermore, their effect may be partially accounted for by a loss of visual acuity and may vary significantly according to environmental demands.

If significant factors remain that affect functional vision and that are not accounted for through visual acuity or visual field loss, a further adjustment of the impairment rating of the visual system may be in order. The need for the adjustment, however, must be well documented. The adjustment should be limited to an increase in the impairment rating of the visual system (reduction of the FVS) by, at most, 15 points.

The same rule should be observed as in the case of central scotomata: Deficits should only be counted to the extent that their effect exceeds the effect of the related visual acuity or visual field deficit. Note the following examples.

1. An individual with a congenital dark adaptation deficit with normal acuity and normal fields may be given a limited impairment rating based on this deficit. In someone with rod dystrophy (RP) manifested by field loss as well as dark adaptation problems, the impairment rating will be determined by the field loss and no additional rating is given for the dark adaptation deficit.

2. Most people with visual acuity loss due to macular degeneration also have a loss of contrast sensitivity. Because the impairment rating is dominated by the visual acuity loss, no additional rating is given for the contrast sensitivity loss. Occasionally, individuals will have a bothersome contrast sensitivity loss while the visual acuity is still normal. In these cases, a limited impairment rating may be given based on the contrast sensitivity loss.

3. Minor color vision deficits exist in about 5% of males. These deficits do not interfere with generic activities of daily living and do not receive an impairment rating. A printer with such a deficit would have no problems with black-and-white printing, but he or she may have difficulty judging the accuracy of color prints. This is a deficit that affects employability in a specific job, but it does not enter into the generic impairment considerations in this chapter (see Chapters 1 and 2). Total color blindness (achromatopsia) is extremely rare. It is accompanied by visual acuity loss, in which case the visual acuity loss will determine the impairment rating.

12.4c Impairment of the Whole Person

In classes 1, 2, and 3, individuals may benefit from vision enhancement techniques such as large print, better illumination, and better contrast. In classes 4, 5, and 6, a shift to vision substitution techniques occurs; this may include talking books, Braille, long cane, etc. Because of these techniques, a totally blind person is not totally incapacitated. In the previous section, a downward adjustment of the Functional Vision Score of up to 15 points was allowed for additional impairments whose effect exceeds that of the visual acuity and/or visual field loss. A similar, but opposite, adjustment may be made in classes 4, 5, and 6 to account for the effects of vision substitution skills that alleviate the effects of the permanent vision loss.

This adjustment affects the translation of the impairment rating of the visual system to an impairment rating of the whole person as shown in Table 12-10. Since the effectiveness of vision substitution skills will vary from person to person and cannot be predicted from the visual acuity and visual field measurements, the adjustments in Table 12-10 are generalized estimates.

That the whole person impairment rating is not reduced further, even for blind persons who have made very effective adjustments, reflects the fact that vision substitution skills alleviate the effects of vision loss but do not eliminate the vision loss itself.

12.4d Calculation Examples Combining Visual Acuity Loss and Visual Field Loss

Example 12-12 (See also Example 12-2)
16% Impairment Due to Visual Acuity Loss Combined With Visual Field Loss

Subject: 45-year-old woman.

History: As stated in Example 12-2, the individual lost the left eye (enucleated in childhood); the right eye is normal.

Current Symptoms: Can perform all office functions.

Physical Exam: Left eye replaced by good-fitting prosthesis.

Table 12-10 Classification of Impairment of the Visual System and of the Whole Person*

Class 1 0%-9% Impairment of the Whole Person	Class 2 10%-29% Impairment of the Whole Person	Class 3 30%-49% Impairment of the Whole Person	Class 4 50%-61% Impairment of the Whole Person	Class 5 62%-73% Impairment of the Whole Person	Class 6 74%-85% Impairment of the Whole Person
Visual System Impairment Rating (estimate of visual ability loss)					
0%-9%	10%-29%	30%-49%	50%-69%	70%-89%	90%-100%
Functional Vision Score (estimate of visual abilities)					
FFS: ≥ 91 points	FFS: 90-71 points	FFS: 70-51 points	FFS: 50-31 points	FFS: 30–11 points	FFS: ≤ 10 points
Range of normal vision	Near-normal vision (mild vision loss)	Moderate vision loss	Severe vision loss	Profound vision loss	(Near-) Total vision loss
Both eyes have normal visual fields and					
visual acuity of 20/25 or better	visual acuity of 20/60 or better	visual acuity of 20/160 or better	visual acuity of 20/400 or better	visual acuity of 20/1000 or better	visual acuity worse than 20/1000
Both eyes have normal visual acuity and					
visual fields better than 50°	visual fields better than 30°	visual fields better than 10°	visual fields of 10° or less	visual fields of 6° or less	visual fields of 2° or less
	One eye has 20/200 or less; the other eye is normal	One eye has 20/200 or less; the other eye has 20/80	One eye has 20/200 or less; the other eye has 20/200		
	One eye lost (other eye normal)	Both eyes lost the upper half-field	Both eyes lost the lower half-field		
			Homonymous hemianopia		
Estimated ability to perform activities of daily living					
Normal (or near-normal) performance			Restricted (or failing) performance		
Has reserve capacity	Lost reserve capacity	Need for vision enhancement aids	Slower than normal, even with enhancement aids	Marginal visual performance, even with aids	Cannot perform visually; needs substitution aids

* The examples in this table refer to visual acuity loss alone or to visual field loss alone. Use Tables 12-2, 12-3, 12-5, and 12-6 and the rules in this section to calculate an impairment value when there is both visual acuity loss and visual field loss. If VSI ≤50%, WPI = VSI. If VSI >50%, WPI is adjusted based on the formula WPI = 50 + 0.7 × (VSI − 50).

Clinical Studies: Best-corrected acuities:
VOU: 20/15, VOD: 20/15, VOS: NLP.

Functional Acuity Score: 84 (as calculated in Example 12-2).

Functional Field Score:

Field OD	full field	100 × 1	=100
Field OS	no field	0 × 1	= 0
Field OU	full field	100 × 3	=300
Functional Field Score		400/5	= 80

Functional Vision Score: In this case, the visual acuity loss and the visual field loss are not independent. Multiplying the two ratings, FAS × FFS/100 → (84 × 80)/100 = 67, would count the same deficit twice. Because the field loss includes the point of fixation, the rule for central scotomata applies. Because the 100% field loss in the left eye does not exceed the 100% visual acuity loss in that eye, the field loss is ignored for the FVS calculation (counted as FFS = 100, ie, 0% impairment). The Functional Vision Score thus equals the Functional Acuity Score. The Functional Vision Score = (84 × 100)/100 = 84.

Diagnosis: History of retinoblastoma.

Impairment Rating: 100 – 84 = 16% impairment of the visual system, which is also the impairment of the whole person (see Table 12-10).

Comment: The loss of one eye reduces the Functional Vision Score to the near-normal range, indicating a significant loss of reserves but not a significant restriction of the ability to perform activities of daily living.

Note: To simplify the presentation of the following cases, the assumption is made that both eyes have identical conditions so that the Functional Acuity and Field Scores equal the Visual Acuity and Field Scores of the eye that is discussed. In real cases there usually will be differences in the scores.

Example 12-13
16% Impairment Due to Perifoveal Visual Field Loss

Subject: 65-year-old man.

History: No prior history of eye disease.

Current Symptoms: Reading is no longer enjoyable.

Physical Exam: Atrophic macular degeneration (geographic atrophy).

Clinical Studies: Best-corrected acuities:
VOU: 20/20, VOD: 20/20, and VOS: 20/20.
Visual field studies reveal a central island of good foveal vision surrounded by a scotoma; beyond this scotoma the peripheral field is normal.

Functional Acuity Score: Normal visual acuity means Functional Acuity Score = 100.

Functional Field Score: The grid points at 3° and 5° are missed in all 10 meridians (20 points lost). The Visual Field Score is 100 – 10 × 2 = 80.

Functional Vision Score: Because the field loss does not include the center of fixation, the rule for central scotomata does not apply. The Functional Vision Score is
FAS × FFS/100 → 100 × 80/100 = 80.

Diagnosis: Age-related maculopathy.

Impairment Rating: 100 – 80 = 20% impairment of the visual system, which is also the impairment of the whole person (see Table 12-10).

Comment: The impairment rating reflects the significant effect of a perifoveal scotoma on reading ability and other daily living skills. Without the perifoveal scotoma, the impairment would have been 0%.

Example 12-14
45% Impairment Due to Visual Acuity Loss Combined With Visual Field Loss

Subject: 68-year-old man described in Example 12-13.

History: Prior history of macular degeneration.

Current Symptoms: Has lost the central island of his vision. Reading is possible only with a strong magnifier.

Physical Exam: Progressive macular degeneration, now including the foveal area.

Clinical Studies:

Functional Acuity Score: Visual acuity dropped to 20/160. The Visual Acuity Score, considered alone, is 20/160 = 55 (45% impairment rating).

Functional Field Score: All grid points at 1°, 3°, and 5° are lost. The Visual Field Score, considered alone, is 100 – 10 × 3 = 70 (30% impairment rating).

Functional Vision Score: Because the field loss now includes the center of fixation, the rule for central scotomata applies. For the calculation of the Functional Vision Score, the central field loss of 30% is ignored because it does not exceed the 45% visual acuity loss. Therefore, the Functional Field Score is entered into the calculation as if it were 100. The calculation is: FAS × FFS/100 → 55 × 100/100 = 55.

Diagnosis: Progressive age-related maculopathy.

Impairment Rating: 100 – 55 = 45% impairment of the visual system, which is also the impairment of the whole person (see Table 12-10).

Comment: In Example 12-13, the impairment rating was determined by the visual field loss. In this case, the visual acuity loss dominates.

Example12-15
59% Impairment Due to Visual Acuity Loss Combined With Visual Field Loss

Subject: 75-year-old man described in Examples 12-13 and 12-14.

History: Prior history of macular degeneration. In recent years the individual has also been followed for glaucoma.

Current Symptoms: Reading remains possible with a strong magnifier, but the individual complains of being startled by objects in his peripheral vision.

Physical Exam: The macular degeneration appears stationary. The optic disc shows cupping.

Clinical Studies:

Functional Acuity Score: The Visual Acuity Score is still 20/160 = 55 (45% impairment rating).

Functional Field Score: In addition to the 30 central points, 25 peripheral points are now lost. The Visual Field Score, considered alone, is 100 – 30 (central loss) – 25 = 45 (55% impairment rating).

Functional Vision Score: Although the visual field loss alone (55%) is worse than the visual acuity loss alone (45%), for the calculation of the Functional Vision Score the central field loss is ignored since this part of the vision loss is already accounted for in the visual acuity impairment rating (see Table 12-9 and the example above). The peripheral field loss, which is independent of the visual acuity loss, is not ignored. Therefore, the Functional Field Score is now entered into the calculation as if it were 100 – 25 = 75. Therefore: FVS = FAS × FFS/100 → 55 × 75/100 = 41 (59% impairment rating).

Diagnosis: Age-related maculopathy. Chronic open-angle glaucoma.

Impairment Rating: 100 – 41 = 59% impairment of the visual system, which might be rated as 56% impairment of the whole person (see Table 12-10).

Comment: The impairment rating is now affected by the visual acuity loss as well as by the peripheral field loss.

12.5 Visual Acuity Measurement at Near (Reading Acuity)

Consideration of reading acuity in the calculation of the FAS is optional. It is warranted only if the reading acuity is significantly different from the distance acuity. In that case, it is appropriate to use the average of the FAS for letter chart acuity and the FAS for reading as indicated in Table 12-11. This section contains instructions for accurate reading acuity measurement.

12.5a Near Acuity vs Distance Acuity (Reading Acuity vs Letter Chart Acuity)

Near acuity may be measured with a reduced-size letter chart or with continuous text. When the objective is the assessment of functional vision—as is the purpose of the *Guides*—continuous textual reading material should be used.

Under most circumstances, letter chart acuity and reading acuity—if measured appropriately and with the proper refractive correction—will be similar. If significant differences between reading acuity and letter chart acuity exist, measurement errors, inappropriate refractive correction, and/or other complicating factors should first be suspected. The nature of these factors needs to be explored, documented, and corrected where possible. Accurate calculation of the reading acuity requires accurate measurement of the letter size as well as the viewing distance. Many practitioners record only the letter size read and not the reading distance. Table 12-11 shows that this is inappropriate because small changes in the reading distance can result in significant changes in visual acuity, especially if the reading distance is short.

One cause of a true discrepancy between reading acuity and letter chart acuity might be that the individual uses a small central island within a ring scotoma for letter acuity while using a larger, more eccentric area for reading. Another cause might be that when measuring letter chart acuity, people are usually pushed for threshold or marginal performance, whereas reading tests more often aim at a level of comfortable performance. For this reason, the magnification requirement for reading acuity may be somewhat greater than that for letter acuity. The difference is known as the magnification reserve needed for reading fluency.

12.5b Letter Size Notations
Another reason for discrepancies can be found in the use of inaccurate letter size notations. The commonly used Jaeger numbers refer to the labels on the boxes in the printing house in Vienna where Jaeger selected his print samples. They have no numerical value, and their implementation on various reading cards is notoriously variable. The J-numbers listed in Table 12-11 present the range of J-designations found for each letter size when a number of reading cards were surveyed.

Some charts use a notation in printer's points. Point sizes have a numerical value but may vary depending on the type style used. Many reading cards list distance equivalents. This notation is valid only if the card is used at the distance for which the card was designed. At any other distance, the use of distance equivalents is utterly confusing.

The only letter size unit that allows a comparison between letter chart acuity and reading acuity is the M-unit. M-units refer directly to the actual letter size (X-height for uppercase letters on a letter chart, x-height for lowercase letters in a reading segment). One M-unit subtends 5 minutes of arc at 1 m and equals 1.454 mm (10% less than 1/16 in).

12.5c Measurement Guidelines for Reading Acuity (Near-Vision Acuity)
Visual acuity measurement at near is more complex than visual acuity measurement at distance because both letter size and viewing distance can vary. When reading acuity is measured, follow these guidelines.

If binocular reading is possible, the binocular reading acuity should be recorded. If binocular reading is not possible or not preferred, the reading acuity of the eye that is preferred for actual reading should be used.

The measurement of reading acuity requires a reading card with calibrated reading segments. Cards with proportionally spaced segments of equal length are preferred. The preferred step size is the same as for letter charts. The viewing distance should be measured and recorded carefully. Measurement with a diopter ruler simplifies calculations (see Section 12.5d) and provides a direct comparison to the required accommodation or reading add. Letter size specification in M-units is mandatory if any calculations or comparisons are involved. One M-unit equals 1.454 mm, which is slightly smaller than

1/16 in. Measuring the letter size in units of 1/16 in overestimates the visual acuity by slightly less than half a standard step size.

To test reading acuity for the normal and near-normal range, many cards are available. Most will indicate distance equivalents. Note that these distance equivalents are valid only if the designated distance is used.

Many individuals undergoing impairment evaluation will fall in the low-vision range. They may require shorter reading distances and/or larger print sizes. Table 12-11 shows the proper visual acuity values and impairment ratings for many combinations of letter size and viewing distance.

12.5d Modified Snellen Formula
The visual acuity values found in Table 12-11 could be calculated using the standard Snellen fraction V = m/M, in which the viewing distance is specified in meters (1 m = 100 cm = 40 in, 1 in = 2.5 cm) and the letter size is in M-units. Use of the standard Snellen fraction becomes awkward when the viewing distance (in meters) is itself a fraction. In this case, it is more convenient to use the reciprocal of the viewing distance, which is known as the diopter (2 diopters = 1/2 m, 5 D = 1/5 m, etc). The use of reciprocal values turns the Snellen fraction into a multiplication, which is more easily calculated in one's head because it uses whole numbers instead of fractions within fractions.

The traditional formula

$$V = \frac{m}{M}$$

thus becomes

$$1/V = \frac{M}{m} = M \times \frac{1}{m} = M \times D,$$

where M = letter size in M-units, m = viewing distance in meters, and D = viewing distance in diopters.

12.5e Instructions
To find the optimal combination of reading distance and letter size, start at the reading distance that corresponds to the individual's current reading add and/or accommodative power. Increase the reading add (reduce the reading distance) to reach smaller print. Using Table 12-11, find the visual acuity at the intersection of the letter size row and the reading distance column. Alternatively, using the M × D formula and a diopter ruler, calculate the 1/V value.

For each combination of viewing distance and letter size read, compare the reading add to the viewing distance in diopters to verify the appropriate refractive correction. Also, compare the M × D value to verify that the visual acuity values are consistent.

12.5f Correction of Refractive Error

To verify that the refractive correction is appropriate for the viewing distance, it is often useful to ask the individual to move the card back and forth to find the best possible focus. If the refractive correction (reading add) is not optimal, the measured acuity will not be the best-corrected visual acuity. Measuring the reading distance in diopters has the advantage of easy comparison to the reading addition.

Table 12-11 Determination of Reading Acuity and Impairment Rating Using Letter Size and Viewing Distance*

Letter Size		5 cm 2" 20 D	6.3 cm 2.5" 16 D	8 cm 3.2" 12.5 D	10 cm 4" 10 D	12.5 cm 5" 8 D	16 cm 6.3" 6.3 D	20 cm 8" 5 D	25 cm 10" 4 D	32 cm 12.5" 3.2 D	40 cm 16" 2.5 D	50 cm 20" 2 D		100 cm 40" 1 D	ICD-9-CM
3.2p J1	0.4 M	45 20/160	40 20/125	35 20/100	30 20/80	25 20/63	20 20/50	15 20/40	10 20/32	5 20/25	0 20/20	20/16		20/8	Above
4p J1	0.5 M	50 20/200	45 20/160	40 20/125	35 20/100	30 20/80	25 20/63	20 20/50	15 20/40	10 20/32	5 20/25	0 20/20		20/10	
5p J1,2	0.63 M	55 20/250	50 20/200	45 20/160	40 20/125	35 20/100	30 20/80	25 20/63	20 20/50	15 20/40	10 20/32	5 20/25		20/12	
6.3p J2-5	0.8 M	60 20/320	55 20/250	50 20/200	45 20/160	40 20/125	35 20/100	30 20/80	25 20/63	20 20/50	15 20/40	10 20/32		20/160	Normal Range
8p J3-6	1 M	65 20/400	60 20/320	55 20/250	50 20/200	45 20/160	40 20/125	35 20/100	30 20/80	25 20/63	20 20/50	15 20/40		0 20/20	
10p J4-7	1.25 M	70 20/500	65 20/400	60 20/320	55 20/250	50 20/200	45 20/160	40 20/125	35 20/100	30 20/80	25 20/63	20 20/50		5 20/25	
12p J7,10	1.6 M	75 20/630	70 20/500	65 20/400	60 20/320	55 20/250	50 20/200	45 20/160	40 20/125	35 20/100	30 20/80	25 20/63		10 20/30	
16p J7,10	2 M	80 20/800	75 20/630	70 20/500	65 20/400	60 20/320	55 20/250	50 20/200	45 20/160	40 20/125	35 20/100	30 20/80		15 20/40	Near-Normal
20p J10,12	2.5 M	85 20/1000	80 20/800	75 20/630	70 20/500	65 20/400	60 20/320	55 20/250	50 20/200	45 20/160	40 20/125	35 20/100		20 20/50	
25p J14	3.2 M	90 20/1250	85 20/1000	80 20/800	75 20/630	70 20/500	65 20/400	60 20/320	55 20/250	50 20/200	45 20/160	40 20/125		25 20/63	
32p J16	4 M	95 20/1600	90 20/1250	85 20/1000	80 20/800	75 20/630	70 20/500	65 20/400	60 20/320	55 20/250	50 20/200	45 20/160		30 20/80	
40p J-	5 M	100 20/2000	95 20/1600	90 20/1250	85 20/1000	80 20/800	75 20/630	70 20/500	65 20/400	60 20/320	55 20/250	50 20/200		35 20/100	Moderate Low Vision
50p J-	6.3 M		100 20/2500	95 20/2000	90 20/1600	85 20/1250	80 20/1000	75 20/800	70 20/630	65 20/500	60 20/400	55 20/320		40 20/125	
63p J-	8 M			100 20/3200	95 20/2500	90 20/2000	85 20/1600	80 20/1250	75 20/1000	70 20/800	65 20/630	60 20/500		45 20/160	
80p J-	10 M				100 20/4000	95 20/3200	90 20/2500	85 20/2000	80 20/1600	75 20/1250	70 20/1000	65 20/800		50 20/200	
100p J-	12.5 M					100 20/5000	95 20/4000	90 20/3200	85 20/2500	80 20/2000	75 20/1600	70 20/1250		55 20/250	
		Near-Total Visual Acuity Loss							**Profound Low Vision**					**Severe Low Vision**	

*Columns indicate reading distances. Rows indicate letter sizes. The resulting reading acuity ratings are found at the intersections. The large number in each box represents the impairment rating (100 – Visual Acuity Score, truncated at 0 and at 100). The small number represents the Snellen distance equivalent. Note that the visual acuity values and impairment ratings are arranged in diagonal bands. The same visual acuity value can be represented by many different combinations of viewing distance and letter size. The outer edge of the table indicates the ranges of vision loss for each diagonal band in *ICD-9-CM*.

References

Classifications

1. World Health Organization. *International Classification of Diseases, 9th Revision (ICD-9)*. Geneva, Switzerland: World Health Organizations; 1977.

2. *International Classification of Diseases, 9th Revision: Clinical Modification (ICD-9-CM)*. First edition: Commission on Professional and Hospital Activities, Ann Arbor, 1978. Later editions: US Public Health Service, 1980 and others.

   ICD-9-CM is the official US health care classification required for all diagnostic reporting. *ICD-9-CM* follows the international edition *(ICD-9)* but contains additional detail. The impairment ranges used in this chapter are based on *ICD-9-CM*.

3. World Health Organization. *International Classification of Impairments, Disabilities, and Handicaps*. Geneva, Switzerland: World Health Organizations; 1980. (Also referred to as *ICIDH-80*, to distinguish it from *ICIDH-2*.)

4. World Health Organization. *ICIDH-2: International Classification of Impairments, Activities, and Participation, Beta-2*. Geneva, Switzerland: World Health Organizations; under development. Available at: www. who.ch/icidh.

   ICIDH is a companion classification to the *ICD*. The *ICD* classifies diseases and disorders; *ICIDH* classifies their functional consequences.

Standards and Related Documents

These documents provide additional detail regarding the scales used in this chapter.

5. International Council of Ophthalmology. Visual acuity measurement standard (approved 1984). *Ital J Ophthalmol*. 1988; II/I:1-15.

6. Sloan LL. New test charts for the measurement of visual acuity at far and near distances. *Am J Ophthalmol*. 1959; 48:807-813.

   Louise Sloan introduced the name *M-unit* to identify letter size based on Snellen's formula.

7. Bailey IL, Lovie JE. New design principles for visual acuity letter charts. *Am J Optom Physiol Ophthalmol*. 1976;53:740-745.

   Bailey and Lovie introduced the proportionally spaced layout with five letters per line that is now the standard.

8. National Academy of Sciences, National Research Council, Committee on Vision, Report of Working Group 39. Recommended standard procedures for the clinical measurement and specification of visual acuity. *Adv Ophthalmol*. 1980;41:103-148.

9. Ferris FL, Kassov A, Bresnick GH, Bailey I. New visual acuity charts for clinical research. *Am J Ophthalmol*. 1982;94:91-96.

10. National Eye Institute. *Measurement Guidelines for Collaborative Studies*. Bethesda, Md: National Eye Institute; 1982.

    The NEI (ETDRS) guidelines popularized the standardized layout. The NEI rules specify a rating system similar to the Visual Acuity Score.

11. Colenbrander A. Visual acuity measurement for low vision. In: Kooiman, et al, eds. *Low Vision: Research and New Developments in Rehabilitation*. Studies in Health Technology and Informatics. Amsterdam: IOS Press; 1994:542-551.

12. Workgroup for the International Society for Low Vision Research and Rehabilitation. *Guide for the Evaluation of Visual Impairment*. Available from Pacific Vision Foundation, San Francisco, 1999. ($5, fax: 415-346-6562).

Disability Ratings

These documents provide more detail about disability ratings that can be used for rehabilitation.

13. Colenbrander A. Dimensions of visual performance. *Trans AAOO*. Low Vision Symposium, American Academy of Ophthalmology. 1977;83:332-337.

14. Hyvärinen L. Classification of visual impairment and disability. *Bull Soc Belge Ophthalmol*. 1985;215:1-16.

15. Department of Health and Human Services. *Disability Evaluation Under Social Security*. Washington, DC: Department of Health and Human Services; 1986.

16. Colenbrander A, Lieberman MF, Schainholz DC. Preliminary implementation of the functional vision score on the Humphrey field analyzer. Proceedings of the International Perimetric Society. Kyoto, 1992. In: *Perimetry Update 1992/1993*. Kugler Publcations; 1993:487-496.

17. Colenbrander A. The Functional Vision Score: A coordinated scoring system for visual impairments, disabilities, and handicaps. In: Kooiman, et al, eds. *Low Vision: Research and New Developments in Rehabilitation*. Studies in Health Technology and Informatics. Amsterdam: IOS Press; 1994:552-561.

18. Mangioni CM, et al. Psychometric properties of the National Eye Institute visual function questionnaire (NEI-VFQ). *Arch Ophthalmol*. 1998;116:1496-1504.

Guides to the Evaluation of Permanent Impairment **and Its Precursors**

19. Snell AC. Visual efficiency of various degrees of subnormal visual acuity, its effect on earning ability. *JAMA*. 1925;85:1367-1373.

20. Snell AC, Sterling S. The percentage evaluation of macular vision. *Arch Ophthalmol*. 1925;54:443-461.

21. Report of the Committee on Compensation for Eye Injuries. *JAMA*. 1925;85:113-115.

22. Guides to the Evaluation of Permanent Impairment: committee report. *JAMA*. 1958;168:475-485.

23. American Medical Association. *Guides to the Evaluation of Permanent Impairment.* Chicago, Ill: American Medical Association; 1st ed, 1971; 2nd ed, 1984; 3rd ed, 1988; 3rd ed rev, 1990; 4th ed, 1993.

Test Chart

24. *Low Vision Test Chart.* One side: letter chart from 50 M to 1 M (acuity: 1/50, 20/1000 to 1/1, 20/20), 1 m cord attached. Other side: reading segments from 10 M to 0.6 M, diopter ruler included, standardized segments for reading rate measurements. Available in English, Spanish, Portuguese, German, Dutch, Finnish, Swedish. Precision Vision, 944 First St, LaSalle, IL 61301. Fax: 815-223-2224.

Chapter 13

The Central and Peripheral Nervous System

Introduction

This chapter provides criteria for evaluating permanent impairments due to documented dysfunction of the brain, cranial nerves, spinal cord, nerve roots, and/or peripheral nerves and muscles.

The following revisions have been made for the fifth edition: (1) an impairment evaluation summary is provided at the end of the chapter to allow easy access to the neurologic impairment in question; (2) a description of ancillary tests with some of their indications provides an understanding of abnormalities found on the neurologic examination; (3) there is more guidance in the assessment of cognition, gait and movement disorders, and cranial nerve disorders; and (4) additional cases are included to illustrate each area of impairment.

13.1 Principles of Assessment

This chapter emphasizes the deficits or impairments that may be identified during a neurologic evaluation.

For some nervous system impairments listed, hand dominance is critical to determine the degree of impairment. To evaluate distal nerve traumatic injury, refer to Chapter 16, The Upper Extremities. Because neurologic impairments are intimately related to mental and emotional processes and their functioning, the examiner should also understand Chapters 14, Mental and Behavioral Disorders, and 18, Pain (pain has been accounted for in neurologic-based impairment ratings). Additional impairments based on those chapters may need to be considered.

Before using the information in this chapter, the *Guides* user should become familiar with Chapters 1 and 2 and the Glossary. Chapters 1 and 2 discuss the *Guides'* purpose, applications, and methods for performing and reporting impairment evaluations. The Glossary provides definitions of common terms used by many specialties in impairment evaluations.

A permanent neurologic impairment is any anatomic, physiological, or functional abnormality or loss that remains after maximum medical improvement (MMI). Impairment rating criteria for neurologic impairments include an assessment of the ability to perform activities of daily living, as listed in Table 1-2. These limitations may involve physical performance (eg, walking, climbing, lifting, finger dexterity) or mental performance (eg, cognition or communication).

If impairments involve several nervous system areas (eg, the brain, spinal cord, and/or peripheral nerves), calculate separate whole person impairment ratings for each area and combine them using the Combined Values Chart (p. 604). As discussed in the following text, impairment of the brain is assessed differently. Because brain dysfunction will likely affect many overlapping functions, identify the most severe cerebral impairment. The impairment rating is based on the neurologic condition that causes the most severe impairment. Examples are provided later in the chapter.

13.1a Interpretation of Symptoms and Signs

Nervous system disorders can present with generalized or focal symptoms. Symptoms may include alterations in level of consciousness, confusion, memory loss, difficulties with language, headache, visual blurring, double vision, fatigue, facial pain and weakness, ringing in the ears, dizziness, vertigo, difficulty swallowing or speaking, weakness of one or multiple limbs, difficulty walking or climbing

stairs, shooting pain, numbness and tingling in the extremities, tremor, loss of coordination, loss of bladder or rectal control, and sexual dysfunction. Note that many of these symptoms describe the functional impairment experienced by the individual. The neurologic evaluation and ancillary clinical testing determine the origin of these symptoms. Difficulty walking, for example, may result from problems in different areas of the central and/or peripheral nervous system. The neurologic examination may find a spastic paraparesis associated with a spinal cord lesion. Magnetic resonance imaging (MRI) of the spine may show the etiology to be demyelinating plaques that also may show abnormal somatosensory evoked response since the pathway travels through the areas of demyelination in the spinal cord.

Some impairment classes refer directly to limitations in the ability to perform activities of daily living because of symptoms. When this information is subjective and open to misinterpretation, it should not serve as the sole criterion upon which decisions about impairment are made. Rather, obtain objective data about the severity of the findings and the limitations and integrate those findings with the subjective data to estimate the degree of permanent impairment.

13.1b Description of Clinical Studies:

A detailed neurologic examination enables the physician to identify the location of nervous system impairment. The purpose of ancillary testing is to assess the severity and location of the lesion and confirm the underlying pathology. It is important to remember that an abnormality found on ancillary testing (anatomic or physiologic) is an impairment but is not necessarily assigned an impairment rating if functions needed for activities of daily living are not affected. The nervous system is able to compensate for a variety of lesions due to its plasticity and redundancy, sometimes resulting in limited representation on the neurologic examination.

Common clinical studies for the central nervous system (brain and spinal cord) include those described below.

Neuropsychologic assessment can characterize cognitive and behavioral alterations and therefore is useful in the clinical assessment and planning of patient management. The results of this assessment must be interpreted in the context of clinical and other test information. Many factors affect neuropsychological performance—age, education, socioeconomic status, and cultural background—and they must therefore be considered for their influence on test results. Neuropsychological tests may be able to distinguish between abnormal and normal performance but cannot determine the cause of the problem. In other words, neuropsychological testing cannot demonstrate consistent diagnostic validity. Traumatic brain injury, for example, may have a profile similar to that of other forms of dementia.

Lumbar puncture (spinal tap) is a procedure by which cerebrospinal fluid is removed through a medium-sized needle, usually at the L3-4 interspace, in order to examine the presence of cells, proteins, glucose, or infection. This test may be performed when evaluating peripheral nerve disease. Other indications are infections of the nervous system and, sometimes, multiple sclerosis.

An *electroencephalogram (EEG)* records the spontaneous electrical activity generated by the cerebral cortex and is useful for recording the site and type of electrical discharge associated with seizure activity. Remember that a large percentage of cortical spikes are not recorded because they arise from deeper structures and there is significant attenuation by the cerebrospinal fluid and dura. Therefore, a seizure disorder is not necessarily accompanied by an abnormal EEG. Also, many diseases and metabolic abnormalities produce nonspecific EEG abnormalities. The EEG may be normal when the neurologic examination is clearly abnormal since many areas of the brain are inaccessible to the recording electrodes and the EEG is time specific, ie, normal between discharges.

Evoked potentials are able to record components of response in the nervous system following multiple somatosensory, visual, and auditory stimuli. The integrity of these afferent pathways is evaluated. These studies may be used in the clinical evaluation of multiple sclerosis, optic neuritis, and acoustic neuroma. Also, a variety of neurotoxins (eg, solvents, heavy metals) may produce alterations in the evoked potentials.

Carotid duplex examination includes Doppler flow velocity of different areas in the carotid artery and, thus, estimates the severity of stenosis in the carotid artery. It is performed in the evaluation of cerebrovascular disease.

Computed tomographic (CT) scan shows the anatomy of the brain, spinal cord, skull, and vertebral column. X-ray beams are used to differentiate densities of bone-calcified tissue, gray matter, white matter, cerebrospinal fluid, and air. Intravenous contrast demonstrates areas where the blood-brain barrier is disrupted. CT scans are not ideal for examination of soft tissue but are better used to detect fresh hemorrhage or bone lesions.

CT myelogram uses a CT scan, after contrast material is injected into the dural sac, to show alterations in the anatomy between the dural sac and the structures that surround it. Since this is an invasive technique, it may be used for diagnostic aid or preoperative planning.

Magnetic resonance imaging (MRI) uses a powerful magnetic field to align the protons of the tissue that are excited by a radio frequency, subsequently forming an image from the different intensities of radio waves emitted from the different tissues. T1-weighted images show soft tissue anatomy, while T2-weighted images demonstrate edema and cerebrospinal fluid. Contrast agents enhance lesions when there is disruption in the blood-brain barrier. A variety of MRI techniques enhance the ability to see different types of pathology.

Magnetic resonance angiography (MRA) allows vessel visualization with images of different intensities that reflect velocity and flow patterns. Basically, visualization of vessels reflects physical differences between moving and stationary protons.

Positron emission tomography (PET) allows examination of cerebral function by tomographic images. Because of the complexity, cost, and limitation of isotopes with short half-lives, most studies at present are limited to research protocols, although clinical studies are available to document, in some individuals, the presence of Parkinson's disease in its early stages.

Single-photon emission computed tomography (SPECT) assesses brain perfusion by use of tracers. Since there is a strong relationship between local metabolism and blood flow, SPECT provides indirect information about metabolism. Therefore, it may show abnormalities in dementia and neurodegenerative diseases.

The peripheral nervous system can be evaluated by means of the following tests.

Nerve conduction and *needle electromyography (EMG) studies* help to determine which nerves are involved and their anatomic location. Also evident will be whether sensory, motor, or both fibers are predominantly involved and whether axonal degeneration, deymelination, or a combination of both is present. Skillful differentiation of peripheral neuropathy and neuromuscular disorders may also be possible. Expert neuromuscular knowledge and understanding of pathologic manifestations of disease processes are necessary for the appropriate application and performance of these tests, particularly the EMG. These tests are objective and require minimal cooperation from the individual being tested. They reflect pathology in the largest, fastest-conducting nerve fibers. The interpretation of these tests must be correlated with a detailed neurologic evaluation.

Quantitative sensory tests are portable tests, easily conducted in the clinician's office, that provide a quantitative assessment of sensation. The integrity of large myelinated fibers is monitored with vibration threshold. Warm and cold temperature thresholds assess medium myelinated and unmyelinated fibers not reflected in nerve conduction studies. Since these are psychophysical tests, the cooperation of the individual being tested is required to process information from cutaneous receptors and provide the appropriate response. These tests can provide information about nerve fibers not examined by nerve conduction studies.

Autonomic function assessment is performed when cardiovascular, thermoregulatory, sphincter, and/or sexual dysfunction is believed to be caused by dysautonomia. For example, postural hypotension tests would include measuring heart rate and blood pressure response to the Valsalva maneuver and heart rate response to deep breathing, postural change, and stress. The integrity of both the central and efferent autonomic pathways is examined with these studies. Sweating abnormalities can be documented by warming the individual and then applying a powder that changes color when wet.

13.2 Criteria for Rating Impairment Due to Central Nervous System Disorders

The central nervous system (CNS) consists of the brain and spinal cord. When injury or illness affects the CNS, several areas of function may be impaired. Therefore, the most severe category of impairment is based on the neurologic evaluation and relevant clinical investigations in four categories: (1) state of consciousness and level of awareness, whether

permanent or episodic; (2) mental status evaluation and integrative functioning; (3) use and understanding of language; and (4) influence of behavior and mood. The motor and sensory systems, gait, and coordination are evaluated once the four categories of cerebral impairment have been determined.

The most severe of these four categories should be used to determine a cerebral impairment rating.

Step 1. The initial step in assessing cerebral function is to determine whether disturbance is present in the level of consciousness or awareness. This may be a permanent alteration or an intermittent alteration in consciousness, awareness, or arousal. See Table 13-2 (Criteria for Rating Impairment of Consciousness and Awareness); Table 13-3 (Criteria for Rating Impairment Due to Episodic Loss of Consciousness or Awareness); and Table 13-4 (Criteria for Rating Impairment Due to Sleep and Arousal Disorders).

Step 2. Evaluate mental status and highest integrative functioning (see Table 13-6, Criteria for Rating Impairment Related to Mental Status).

Step 3. Identify any difficulty with understanding and use of language (see Table 13-7, Criteria for Rating Impairment Due to Aphasia or Dysphasia).

Step 4. Evaluate any emotional or behavioral disturbances, such as depression, that can modify cerebral function (see Table 13-8, Criteria for Rating Impairment Due to Emotional or Behavioral Disorders).

Step 5. Identify the most severe cerebral impairment listed above. Combine the most severe impairment from catagories 1 through 4 with any or multiple distinct neurologic impairments listed in Table 13-1 using the Combined Values Chart (p. 604).

Table 13-1 Neurologic Impairments That Are Combined With the Most Severe Cerebral Impairment
Cranial nerve impairments
Station, gait, and movement disorders
Extremity disorders related to central impairment
Spinal cord impairments
Chronic pain
Peripheral nerve, motor, and sensory impairments
These are central nervous system or peripheral nervous system impairments, and all are combined when appropriate with the most severe cerebral impairment (see Tables 13-2 through 13-4, Tables 13-6 through 13-8, and the Combined Values Chart, p. 604).

13.3 Criteria for Rating Cerebral Impairments

13.3a Disturbances in Level of Consciousness and/or Awareness

Individuals experiencing disturbances in consciousness may be suffering from a range of symptoms from episodes of altered awareness to being in a persistent vegetative state or an unresponsive coma. These conditions are evaluated based on clinical findings on the neurologic examination and ancillary testing such as CT scan, MRI, SPECT, EEG, evoked potentials, and vestibular testing. The examination and tests will provide the extent of the underlying pathology and help examiners form a prognosis for patient management.

These neurologic disturbances may result in global loss of consciousness, responsiveness, or focal or lateral neurologic impairments. Table 13-2 lists criteria for determining permanent impairment ratings in individuals with these conditions, considering the severity of their condition and their ability to perform activities of daily living. For a class 1 rating, the individual is expected to perform activities of daily living (ADL) independently but may need assistance with activities that require fine motor dexterity (eg, buttoning). Class 2 impairment, in which individuals are moderately limited in ability to perform ADL, indicates the preservation of some independence but a need for assistance with transfers, bathing, and activities that require fine motor skills. Impairment classes 3 and 4 are assigned to individuals who require assistance in performing all ADL; different levels of participation by the individual differentiate the level of care required in the two classes.

Table 13-2 Criteria for Rating Impairment of Consciousness and Awareness

Class 1 0%-14% Impairment of the Whole Person	Class 2 15%-39% Impairment of the Whole Person	Class 3 40%-69% Impairment of the Whole Person	Class 4 70%-90% Impairment of the Whole Person
Brief repetitive or persistent alteration of state of consciousness *and* minimal limitation in performance of ADL	Brief repetitive or persistent alteration of state of consciousness *and* moderate limitation in performance of ADL	Prolonged alteration of state of consciousness, which diminishes capabilities in personal care and ADL	State of semicoma with complete dependency and subsistence on nursing care and artificial medical means of support *or* irreversible coma requiring total medical support

Class 1 0%–14% Impairment of the Whole Person
Brief repetitive or persistent alteration of state of consciousness *and* minimal limitation in performance of ADL

Example 13-1
0% to 14% Impairment Due to Parkinsonian Syndrome With Symptomatic Orthostatic Hypotension

Subject: 70-year-old man.

History: Right-handed; periodic episodes of sudden-onset drop attacks for the past 3 years. Paralysis agitans (Parkinson's disease) for the past 10 years; under treatment with appropriate medications.

Current Symptoms: Postural hypotension, dizziness, light-headedness with a resting tremor.

Physical Exam: BP: 140/90 mm Hg seated, 100/74 mm Hg standing, with minimal increase in pulse rate. Classic features of Parkinson's syndrome: flat facies, resting tremor and hesitant speech, cogwheeling, festinating gait and propulsion, and mild orofacial dyskinesia.

Clinical Studies: MRI: nonspecific mild widening of cortical sulci.

Diagnosis: Parkinsonian syndrome with symptomatic orthostatic hypotension.

Impairment Rating: 14% impairment due to drop attacks; combine with appropriate rating from movement Section 13.5 to determine whole person impairment (see Combined Values Chart, p. 604).

Comment: Despite many attempts to adjust medications to control both sets of symptoms, the individual has some dependence on his caregivers to prevent serious falls, limiting his ability to perform independently all activities of daily living.

Class 2
15%-39% Impairment of the Whole Person
Brief repetitive or persistent alteration of state of consciousness
and
moderate limitation in performance of ADL

Class 3
40%-69% Impairment of the Whole Person
Prolonged alteration of state of consciousness, which diminishes capabilities in personal care and ADL

Example 13-2
15% to 39% Impairment Due to Uremic Encephalopathy and Uremic Neuropathy

Subject: 55-year-old man.

History: Right-handed; 10-year history of progressive kidney failure, leading to thrice-weekly renal dialysis. Repeated episodes of lapse of concentration and alteration of awareness, as well as uremic encephalopathy, for the past 3 years.

Current Symptoms: Periodic episodes of forgetfulness, disorientation, apathy, wandering between dialysis treatments. Burning numb sensations in his feet.

Physical Exam: BP: 140/90 mm Hg; disheveled appearance, disoriented to time, person, and place; poor performance for three-word retention, spelling of *world* backward, serial 7s, and understanding of proverbs. Diminished strength 4/5 distally in both lower legs, with poor deep-tendon reflexes and decreased response to pin, cold, and vibration distally, and painful dysesthesias upon squeezing the soles of his feet.

Clinical Studies: EEG: poorly developed 8- to 13-Hz alpha activity with a preponderance of 4- to 7-Hz theta activity diffusely. CT scan: normal. Blood studies: elevated blood urea nitrogen (BUN), creatinine, and calcium, and lowered phosphorus.

Diagnosis: Uremic encephalopathy with episodes of confusion and uremic neuropathy.

Impairment Rating: 30% impairment due to dialysis dementia, confusion, and uremic neuropathy; combine with appropriate ratings due to kidney disease and peripheral neuropathy to determine whole person impairment (see Combined Values Chart, p. 604).

Comment: The most limiting symptom of the renal failure is the individual's periodic state of altered mentation and awareness, with a baseline dementia. This moderately interferes with his ability to perform activities of daily living in addition to the moderate limitations due to his peripheral neuropathy, which is mild, and his renal failure and periodic dialysis treatments.

Example 13-3
40% to 69% Impairment Due to Dementia and Nondominant-Side Hemiplegia

Subject: 65-year-old man.

History: Right-handed; third episode of sudden-onset left hemiparesis, hemianopia, hemisensory defects with poor subsequent recovery, which had followed previous episodes, persisting for the past 2 months.

Current Symptoms: Total nursing care for most activities of daily living. Attempts to feed himself but has no ability to transfer bed to chair. Poor control over bowel and bladder functions. He is not on a respirator and cardiac function is stable on medications.

Physical Exam: Disoriented; cannot follow directions and has a poor fund of knowledge; has naming difficulties. Flaccid left hemiparesis and hemisensory loss with hemianopia.

Clinical Studies: CT scan of head: no evidence of hemorrhage, with a lucency in the right central-parietal area. EEG: slow waves in the same area without seizure activity.

Diagnosis: Dementia and hemiplegia of the nondominant side.

Impairment Rating: 49% impairment due to dementia; combine with appropriate ratings due to other neurologic impairments to determine whole person impairment (see Combined Values Chart, p. 604).

Comment: This is a persistent state requiring care, with almost constant attention, for all activities of daily living. He can watch TV and request help when he needs it.

Class 4
70%-90% Impairment of the Whole Person
State of semicoma with complete dependency and subsistence on nursing care and artificial medical means of support
or
irreversible coma requiring total medical support

Example 13-4
70% to 90% Impairment Due to Persistent Vegetative State

Subject: 39-year-old woman.

History: Right-handed; acute onset of coma 2 months ago following head trauma with subsequent cardiorespiratory arrest and cardioversion. Fluid/nutrition by artificial means.

Current Symptoms: Deep unresponsiveness to verbal and painful stimuli.

Physical Exam: No response to environment or purposeful response to stimuli. No comprehension of language, with intermittent wakefulness in sleep-wake cycles. Survival with medical nursing care. Bladder and bowel incontinence. Pupils react to bright light. Extraocular movements (EOM) conjugate but no doll's-eye movements (eyes did not move from primary position while head was rotated like a painted doll's eyes). Cold caloric response with nystagmus in either external ear canal. Regular cardiac rate; deep-tendon reflexes 1/5 and toes up-going.

Clinical Studies: CT scan: bilateral intracerebral hemorrhages with extension into ventricles. EEG: diffuse bilateral delta, slowing without paroxysmal events.

Diagnosis: Persistent vegetative state due to cerebral contusion and intracranial hemorrhage.

Impairment Rating: 90% impairment of the whole person.

Comment: Persistent vegetative state is defined as a "clinical condition of complete unawareness of the self and the environment accompanied by sleep-wake cycles with either complete or partial preservation of hypothalamic and brain stem autonomic functions."[1] The state is persistent 1 month after acute traumatic or nontraumatic brain injury.

13.3b Episodic Neurologic Impairments

The *Guides* rates episodic neurologic impairments that are persistent and permanent. Episodic conditions involve syncope or loss of awareness, convulsive disorders, and arousal and sleep disorders. Episodic indicates more than one occurrence. When these conditions originate from a problem in the nervous system, they should be evaluated according to the guidelines given in this chapter. For similar manifestations that originate in other body systems (eg, cardiovascular, respiratory) and secondarily affect the central nervous system, see the chapter(s) for the originating body system(s).

In assessing permanent impairment due to episodic conditions, first ensure that the individual's condition has reached MMI and is unlikely to change significantly. Document the pattern of occurrence, estimate the effect of the condition on the individual's ability to perform activities of daily living, and evaluate the effects of appropriate treatment. Record results from appropriate physiologic evaluations (eg, ECG, cardiologic evaluations, EEG) to document the disorder's severity and provide information about prognosis.

Describe episodic disorders according to their onset, frequency, duration, and effect on performance of daily activities. Document and describe the results of seizure control. Daytime loss of consciousness with tonic or clonic seizures, nocturnal episodes with daytime residua, or brief lapses of awareness/communication from minor seizures may interfere significantly with daily activities. Minor seizures with alterations of awareness or consciousness, transient manifestations of unconventional behavior, or interruptions of daytime activity can result in an inability to perform activities of daily living. Impairment ratings for major or minor seizures are calculated on the basis of how they affect the ability to perform activities of daily living.

The same criteria apply to impairments related to transient loss of awareness or consciousness (syncope, dizziness) after a period of cerebral ischemia that may be due to various mechanisms, including orthostasis, reflex actions, or cardiopulmonary disorders. Examiners may need to refer to other *Guides* chapters to estimate the magnitude of impairments related to cardiovascular disorders.

The criteria for evaluating episodic loss of consciousness or awareness are given in Table 13-3.

Table 13-3 Criteria for Rating Impairment Due to Episodic Loss of Consciousness or Awareness

Class 1 0%-14% Impairment of the Whole Person	Class 2 15%-29% Impairment of the Whole Person	Class 3 30%-49% Impairment of the Whole Person	Class 4 50%-70% Impairment of the Whole Person
Paroxysmal disorder with predictable characteristics and unpredictable occurrence that does not limit usual activities but is a *risk* to the individual or limits daily activities *or* blood pressure drop of 15/10 mm Hg without compensatory increase in pulse rate and lasting more than 2 minutes after precipitating event, with mild awareness loss that limits daily activities	Paroxysmal disorder that interferes with *some* daily activities *or* moderate blood pressure drop of 25/15 mm Hg, with loss of awareness or consciousness lasting 1 to 2 minutes and that interferes with *some* daily activities	Severe paroxysmal disorder of such frequency that it limits activities to those that are supervised, protected, or restricted *or* repeated severe blood pressure losses of 30/20 mm Hg, with loss of awareness or consciousness lasting 1 to 2 minutes *and* additional neurologic symptoms or signs of focal or generalized nature	Uncontrolled paroxysmal disorder of such severity and constancy that it severely limits the individual's daily activities *or* repeated severe blood pressure losses of 30/20 mm Hg, with uncontrolled loss of consciousness and muscle control without recognized cause and with risk of body injury

* This table is applicable to individuals receiving treatment.

Class 1 0%-14% Impairment of the Whole Person
Paroxysmal disorder with predictable characteristics and unpredictable occurrence that does not limit usual activities but is a *risk* to the individual or limits daily activities *or* blood pressure drop of 15/10 mm Hg without compensatory increase in pulse rate and lasting more than 2 minutes after precipitating event, with mild awareness loss that limits daily activities

Example 13-5
0% to 14% Impairment Due to Dizziness and Light-Headedness

Subject: 65-year-old man.

History: Right-handed; brief episodes of interruption of speech, pale appearance, and light sweatiness, with total recovery in minutes, for the past 2 years. These usually have occurred upon standing from a lying or seated position and are associated with a light-headed and/or dizzy sensation.

Current Symptoms: Continuation of the history without other sequelae or interruption of activities of daily living.

Physical Exam: BP: 130/80 mm Hg seated, 110/70 mm Hg upon standing, without increase in pulse rate.

Clinical Studies: No neurologic impairments.

Diagnosis: Dizziness and light-headedness.

Impairment Rating: 4% impairment of the whole person.

Comment: No additional impairments to combine.

Example 13-6
0% to 14% Impairment Due to Partial Epilepsy

Subject: 20-year-old woman.

History: Right-handed; onset of generalized tonic-clonic convulsions in middle school at age 13 years, with subsequent evaluations of these being of focal origin with sensations in the right hand, shaking progressing to generalized tonic-clonic convulsions and a brief postictal period of difficulty in expressing self, as well as slight weakness of the right hand and headache with confusional state for about 2 to 3 hours. Episodes initially occurred about two to three times a week.

Current Symptoms: Treatment with anticonvulsants, when taken regularly, has decreased the frequency to one to two minor, brief focal right-hand sensations and interruption in speech about every 2 to 3 months.

Physical Exam: Vital signs and physical/neurologic evaluations: normal.

Clinical Studies: EEG: rare spikes in the left temporal area; otherwise normal. MRI: normal.

Diagnosis: Partial epilepsy, with mention of impairment of consciousness.

Impairment Rating: 10% impairment of the whole person due to seizures.

Comment: Attempts to control episodes completely have not been successful; as a result, individual's license to operate a motor vehicle and work around moving machinery has been limited. Employment has been limited in view of the diagnosis and presumed risk of employment.

Example 13-7
0% to 14% Impairment Due to Partial Epilepsy

Subject: 29-year-old woman.

History: Individual was involved in a motor vehicle accident with resulting head impact injury. She had a seizure 1 week later. Seizures are characterized by onset in the left hand with a "funny" sensation, followed by rhythmic shaking that progresses to involve the entire arm. She has lip-smacking and talks inappropriately with postictal confusional state for about 5 to 10 minutes.

Current Symptoms: Treated with antiseizure mediction for 6 months with control of seizures, at which point medication was discontinued. Had a third seizure after 2 weeks off medication. Now back on an anticonvulsant with good control, but she periodically "feels funny."

Physical Exam: No neurologic impairment on examination.

Clinical Studies: EEG, brain CT scan, and MRI: normal.

Diagnosis: Partial epilepsy with impairment of consciousness.

Impairment Rating: 14% impairment of the whole person due to seizures.

Comment: Posttraumatic epilepsy, fairly well controlled. The seizures require control as demonstrated by the recurrence following withdrawal of medication.

Class 2
15%–29% Impairment of the Whole Person

Paroxysmal disorder that interferes with *some* daily activities

or

moderate blood pressure drop of 25/15 mm Hg, with loss of awareness or consciousness lasting 1 to 2 minutes and that interferes with *some* daily activities

---

Example 13-8
15% to 29% Impairment Due to Partial Epilepsy

Subject: 40-year-old man.

History: Left-handed mechanic; at age 30 was involved in a motor vehicle accident with significant head trauma. Unconscious and hospitalized for 3 weeks; recovered, with rehabilitation, with no neurologic impairment on examination over the course of a year. Subsequently took training and completed courses in motor mechanical repairs, but started having focal seizures with brief lapse of consciousness 5 years ago, occurring about twice a week until partially and intermittently controlled on medications.

Current Symptoms: Over the past year has taken his medication without fail with numerous attempts at modification by his neurologist. Continues to have brief episodes of left arm/hand weakness, lasting about 3 minutes, about once a month, resulting in limited activities at work and inability to drive.

Physical Exam: Normal vital signs and general physical examination. No cognitive or communication impairments; cranial nerve functions are normal. Mild weakness of dominant left hand, with poor dexterity in fine movements and strength 4/5. Deep-tendon reflexes are increased at the biceps area on the left; poor finger-nose fine dexterity.

Clinical Studies: EEG: periodic delta slowing in the right temporal-parietal area. MRI: old area of small infarction in the right posterior temporal-parietal region.

Diagnosis: Partial epilepsy without mention of impairment of consciousness.

Impairment Rating: 25% impairment of the whole person due to seizures; combine with appropriate rating due to neurologic impairments to determine whole person impairment (see Combined Values Chart, p. 604).

Comment: Seizures developed after apparent cerebral contusion as seen in the MRI and EEG, with persistent neurologic signs of impairment in his dominant hand. Seizures have not been controlled, and individual continues to have brief partial seizures in addition to hand impairment. The latter should be combined in the whole person evaluations using the guidelines given in Chapter 16, The Upper Extremities.

Chapter 13

Example 13-9
15% to 29% Impairment Due to Transient Alteration of Awareness and Orthostatic Hypotension

Subject: 75-year-old woman.

History: Right-handed African American; frequent episodes of loss of consciousness and falling or slumping with head dropping and pale appearance. These usually occur upon standing and never while lying down. Recovery in minutes without other problems. Previous history of cerebrovascular accident (CVA) with mild residual left hemiparesis. On antihypertensive medications.

Current Symptoms: Fairly frequent falls without injury and responsive immediately. Blood pressure very difficult to control with good compliance.

Physical Exam: BP: 160/90 mm Hg seated, 138/75 mm Hg on standing, with brief loss-of-awareness sensation. Mild left hemiplegia with sensory loss.

Clinical Studies: Tilt table testing: drop in BP 25/15 mm Hg without increased pulse.

Diagnosis: Transient alteration of awareness and orthostatic hypotension.

Impairment Rating: 25% impairment due to transient alteration of awareness and orthostatic hypotension; combine with an appropriate rating due to the hemiparesis with sensory loss to determine whole person impairment (see Combined Values Chart, p. 604).

Comment: Hypertension in African Americans may be difficult to control. With advancing age, the medications may need to be adjusted to allow adequate cerebral perfusion.

Example 13-10
15% to 29% Impairment Due to Partial Epilepsy

Subject: 22-year-old man.

History: Suffered blunt trauma to the right side of the head during a robbery attempt in the store at which he works. Admitted in status epilepticus, but control was rapidly established with intravenous phenytoin.

Current Symptoms: Maintained on phenytoin without further overt seizures, but he has frequent auras with derealization during which time he ceases activity. These episodes occur 0 to 8 times per day, last 5 to 10 minutes, and are followed by full recovery and resumption of activity.

Physical Exam: Normal neurologic evaluation.

Clinical Studies: MRI: left temporal lucency; EEG: left temporal rare spikes.

Diagnosis: Partial epilepsy without mention of impairment of consciousness.

Impairment Rating: 29% impairment of the whole person due to seizures.

Comment: Fairly frequent minor seizures that are not completely controlled and that interrupt individual's activities. Initial episode of status epilepticus.

| **Class 3** |
| **30%-49% Impairment of the Whole Person** |
| Severe paroxysmal disorder of such frequency that it limits activities to those that are supervised, protected, or restricted |
| *or* |
| repeated severe blood pressure losses of 30/20 mm Hg, with loss of awareness or consciousness lasting 1 to 2 minutes |
| *and* |
| additional neurologic symptoms or signs of focal or generalized nature |

Example 13-11
30% to 49% Impairment Due to Episodic Loss of Consciousness

Subject: 65-year-old man.

History: Right-handed; blunt head trauma with a skull fracture during a robbery 3 years ago. Decompressive surgery was followed by mild left hemiplegia, which improved with rehabilitation. Episodes of syncope for the past 5 years.

Current Symptoms: Episodes of syncope, at times followed by brief increase in left hemiplegia.

Physical Examination: BP: 170/96 mm Hg seated, 130/70 mm Hg upon standing, without compensatory tachycardia. Moderate left hemiplegia, which improves over the next 30 minutes to baseline mild left hemiplegia.

Clinical Studies: MRI of head: contusion of the right parietal area; EEG: slowing in the same region.

Diagnosis: Syncope and collapse, transient cerebral ischemia, late effect intracranial injury, and cerebral contusion.

Impairment Rating: 45% impairment due to above diagnosis; combine with an appropriate rating due to the hemiparesis to determine whole person impairment (see Combined Values Chart, p. 604).

Comment: With the drop in blood pressure, there was a decrease in cerebral perfusion with brief decompensation of the previous neurologic impairment and subsequent return to baseline. This is not really a transient ischemic attack (TIA), but rather transient cerebral ischemia (TCI) secondary to decreased cerebral perfusion into a previously damaged area.

Example 13-12
30% to 49% Impairment Due to Partial Epilepsy, Impairment of Consciousness, and Episodes of Intractable Epilepsy

Subject: 45-year-old man.

History: Right-handed; policeman was shot in the left frontal area while restraining a person with a gun. Hospitalized for surgery; recovered without neurologic paresis but continues to have seizures.

Current Symptoms: Frequent minor complex seizures of the right hand and leg, which progress periodically to almost continuous seizures with loss of consciousness.

Physical Exam: Mild right hand loss of dexterity and fine movement; slight dragging of right leg.

Clinical Studies: MRI: area of contusion left frontotemporal; EEG: slowing in the same area with frequent polyspike waves.

Diagnosis: Partial epilepsy, with mention of impairment of consciousness and with episodes of intractable epilepsy.

Impairment Rating: 45% impairment due to epilepsy and impairment of consciousness; combine with appropriate ratings for other neurologic impairments to determine whole person impairment (see Combined Values Chart, p. 604).

Comment: The bullet entered the individual's skull; there was good subsequent recovery following operation. The resultant seizures, unfortunately, are difficult to control with episodes of status epilepticus, in spite of good compliance.

Example 13-13
30% to 49% Impairment Due to Generalized Convulsive Epilepsy

Subject: 55-year-old man.

History: Man was rescued, in an unconscious state, from a burning building; had experienced significant smoke inhalation. Recovered consciousness; diagnosis of hypoxic encephalopathy. Hospitalized for a month with gradual recovery of mental function.

Current Symptoms: Has two to six generalized tonic-clonic seizures per week, usually with a 1- to 2-hour postictal state, in spite of good compliance with medications.

Physical Exam: No focal neurologic impairment; however, Mini-Mental State Examination (MMSE) was 23/30.

Clinical Studies: EEG: bitemporal sharp waves with hyperventilation.

Diagnosis: Generalized convulsive epilepsy without mention of intractable epilepsy.

Impairment Rating: 49% impairment due to generalized convulsive epilepsy; combine with any mental and behavioral impairments to determine whole person impairment (see Combined Values Chart, p. 604).

Comment: The event of being trapped in a burning building caused hypoxic encephalopathy with no other focal neurologic impairments except seizures and additional mental status changes that need to be combined.

Chapter 13

> **Class 4**
> **50%-70% Impairment of the Whole Person**
>
> Uncontrolled paroxysmal disorder of such severity and constancy that it severely limits the individual's daily activities
>
> *or*
>
> repeated severe blood pressure losses of 30/20 mm Hg, with uncontrolled loss of consciousness and muscle control without recognized cause and with risk of body injury

Example 13-14
50% to 70% Impairment Due to Uncontrolled Epilepsy

Subject: 50-year-old woman.

History: Right-handed; sudden onset of severe headache, right hemiparesis, and brief loss of consciousness 3 months ago. Subsequent improvement to stable state and rehabilitation.

Current Symptoms: Unable to use dominant hand for activities of daily living or to communicate needs or concerns. Frequent, uncontrolled, spontaneous right-sided clonic seizures with loss of consciousness and awareness and with postictal confusional state for about 5 to 10 minutes.

Physical Exam: Right hemiparesis, hemianopia, inability to express herself, and poor comprehension of spoken or written words.

Clinical Studies: CT scan of head: large intracerebral hematoma in the central area on the left side, with effacement on the ventricles; EEG: delta slowing in the same area.

Diagnosis: Late effect of cerebrovascular disease, secondary to traumatic intracerebral hematoma, with dysphasia, right hemiparesis, and partial epilepsy, and with mention of impairment of consciousness and episodes of status epilepticus.

Impairment Rating: 65% impairment due to seizures; combine with appropriate rating for other neurologic impairments to determine whole person impairment (see Combined Values Chart, p. 604).

Comment: Rating for uncontrolled seizures should be combined with rating for whole person based on other neurologic impairments.

Example 13-15
50% to 70% Impairment Due to Shy-Drager Syndrome With Orthostatic Hypotension

Subject: 45-year-old man.

History: Right-handed; 5-year history of very difficult to control parkinsonism with various medications and severe orthostatic hypotension, postprandial hypotension, constipation, and poor bladder control.

Current Symptoms: Frequent episodes of fainting and falling that require attendance, bed and wheelchair living, and assistance with all activities of daily living and feeding.

Physical Exam: BP: 110/80 mm Hg lying down, 70/40 mm Hg seated. Resting tremor with sweaty face, decrease in facial expression, rigidity of all four extremities, and unintelligible speech.

Clinical Studies: Tilt table test: positive for orthostatic hypotension.

Diagnosis: Multiple-system atrophy (Shy-Drager syndrome) with orthostatic hypotension.

Impairment Rating: 70% impairment due to Shy-Drager syndrome with orthostatic hypotension; combine with appropriate rating for parkinsonism to determine whole person impairment (see Combined Values Chart, p. 604).

Comment: A very serious condition, which is parkinsonlike but with more profound autonomic failure. It is very unresponsive to therapeutic attempts.

Example 13-16
50% to 70% Impairment Due to Partial Epilepsy With Impairment of Consciousness

Subject: 44-year-old man.

History: Drove a delivery truck; lost control of the vehicle on a wet road and struck a tree. Hit his head on the windshield and developed a left epidural hematoma requiring urgent evacuation.

Current Symptoms: More than 6 months following the accident, has frequent partial complex seizures characterized by decreased responsiveness, lip smacking, and rightward eye deviation. These occur up to five times per day despite the use of three anticonvulsant agents. May undergo secondary generalization with tonic-clonic seizures occurring once or twice per week.

Physical Exam: Mild right hemiparesis with a left craniotomy scar, well healed.

Clinical Studies: CT scan: left skull defect and underlying small lucency. EEG: rare spike/slow waves left temporal.

Diagnosis: Partial epilepsy with impairment of consciousness.

Impairment Rating: 70% impairment due to partial epilepsy with impairment of consciousness; combine with appropriate rating for hemiparesis to determine whole person impairment (see Combined Values Chart, p. 604).

Comment: The posttraumatic epidural hematoma was evacuated successfully; however, there was additional underlying brain contusion from the head trauma, which accounts for the mild hemiparesis.

13.3c Arousal and Sleep Disorders

Arousal and sleep disorders include disorders related to initiating and maintaining sleep or inability to sleep; excessive somnolence, including sleep-induced respiratory impairment; and sleep-wake schedules.

Impairment categories that may arise from sleep disorders relate to (1) the nervous system, with reduced daytime attention, concentration, and other cognitive abilities; (2) mental and behavioral factors, including depression, irritability, interpersonal difficulties, and social problems; (3) the cardiovascular system, with systemic and pulmonary hypertension, cardiac enlargement, congestive heart failure, or arrhythmias; and (4) the hematopoietic system. The Respiratory System (Chapter 5) also discusses impairment as it relates to obstructive sleep apnea.

Neurologic disorders associated with increased daytime sleepiness include central sleep apnea syndrome, narcolepsy, idiopathic hypersomnia, periodic limb movement disorder, restless leg syndrome, depression, brain tumors, posttraumatic hypersomnolence, multiple sclerosis, encephalitis and postencephalopathy, Alzheimer's disease, Parkinson's disease, multiple system atrophy, and neuromuscular disorders with sleep apnea. It is expected that the diagnosis of excessive daytime sleepiness has been supported by formal studies in a sleep laboratory.

The clinician can evaluate sleepiness with the Epworth Sleepiness Scale,[2] which assesses the likelihood of dozing (never = 0 to high chance = 3) in different situations: sitting and reading, watching television, sitting in a public place, riding as a passenger for an hour, taking an afternoon nap, sitting and talking to someone, sitting after a nonalcohol lunch, and stopped in traffic in a car. A score of 10/24 is equal to excessive sleepiness, or class 2 impairment. This scale correlates with the multiple sleep latency test (MSLT), which supports pathologic sleep in narcolepsy and idiopathic hypersomnia. See Table 13-4 for impairment due to sleep and arousal disorders.

Table 13-4 Criteria for Rating Impairment Due to Sleep and Arousal Disorders

Class 1 1%-9% Impairment of the Whole Person	Class 2 10%-29% Impairment of the Whole Person	Class 3 30%-69% Impairment of the Whole Person	Class 4 70%-90% Impairment of the Whole Person
Reduced daytime alertness; sleep pattern such that individual can perform most activities of daily living	Reduced daytime alertness; interferes with ability to perform some activities of daily living	Reduced daytime alertness; ability to perform activities of daily living significantly limited	Severe reduction of daytime alertness; individual unable to care for self in any situation or manner

Class 1
1%-9% Impairment of the Whole Person
Reduced daytime alertness; sleep pattern such that individual can perform most activities of daily living

Example 13-17
1% to 9% Impairment Due to Obstructive Sleep Apnea

Subject: 47-year-old man.

History: Right-handed; moderately obese; suffered a serious crush injury to the right foot. While the foot was healing, the man was unable to exercise and gained 20.25 kg (45 lb), whereupon he developed daytime somnolence. Despite his best efforts, he remains unable to lose the excess weight.

Current Symptoms: Able to complete most necessary work, but works less efficiently and cannot take on any new special projects.

Physical Exam: Normal.

Clinical Studies: Cranial CT scan: normal; polysomnogram: findings consistent with obstructive sleep apnea.

Diagnosis: Obstructive sleep apnea.

Impairment Rating: 9% impairment of the whole person.

Comment: Except for daytime somnolence, the individual has a normal neurologic exam.

Class 2
10%-29% Impairment of the Whole Person
Reduced daytime alertness; interferes with ability to perform some activities of daily living

Example 13-18
10% to 29% Impairment Due to Ideopathic Hypersomnolence

Subject: 31-year-old woman.

History: Right-handed; several lapses of awareness while driving; on one occasion she awakened with her car off the road, having no idea what had happened or how she had arrived there. No history of seizures.

Physical Exam: Normal.

Clinical Studies: EEG and brain MRI: normal; polysomnogram: marked hypersomnolence.

Diagnosis: Idiopathic hypersomnolence.

Impairment Rating: 19% impairment of the whole person.

Comment: The individual responds partially to stimulants but should not drive a vehicle, nor can she handle dangerous materials. Reduced daytime alertness interferes with ability to perform some daytime activities.

Class 3
30%-69% Impairment of the Whole Person
Reduced daytime alertness; ability to perform activities of daily living significantly limited

Example 13-19
30% to 69% Impairment Due to Narcolepsy

Subject: 37-year-old woman.

History: Left-handed; suffered two work demotions because of declining work performance and poor memory. Complains of morning headache and excessive daytime somnolence; experiences multiple daily episodes in which the urge to nap is irresistible. If this occurs while driving, she has to pull off the road. The naps last 10 or 15 minutes, after which she feels refreshed.

Physical Exam: Normal.

Clinical Studies: Brain MRI: normal; polysomnogram and MSLT: findings consistent with narcolepsy.

Diagnosis: Narcolepsy.

Impairment Rating: 39% impairment of the whole person

Comment: Reduced daytime alertness with sleep episodes uncontrolled.

Class 4
70%- 90% Impairment of the Whole Person
Severe reduction of daytime alertness; individual unable to care for self in any situation or manner

Example 13-20
70% to 90% Impairment Due to Brainstem Infarct

Subject: 62-year-old man.

History: Right-handed; could not be awakened in bed.

Current Symptoms: Severe somnolence with occasional brief periods of arousal.

Physical Exam: Flaccid bilateral paraparesis, loss of lateral gaze bilaterally, and loss of facial movement bilaterally.

Clinical Studies: MRI of the brain: occlusion of the basilar artery with extensive midbrain infarction.

Diagnosis: Brainstem infarct secondary to a basilar artery occlusion.

Impairment Rating: 90% impairment due to brainstem infarct and basilar artery occlusion; combine with appropriate ratings due to other neurologic impairments to determine whole person impairment (see Combined Values Chart, p. 604).

Comment: This individual could also have been rated using Table 13-2, Criteria for Rating Impairment of Consciousness and Awareness, assigning class 4 for 90% impairment due to semicoma. Using Table 13-4, the individual has severe reduction of daytime alertness and is unable to care for himself.

13.3d Mental Status, Cognition, and Highest Integrative Function

Mental status and integrative function deficits include the general effects of organic brain syndrome; dementia; and some specific, focal, and neurologic deficiencies. Mental status tests are used to screen and follow individuals, frequently with repeated testing. They usually cover measures of orientation, attention, immediate recall, calculations, abstraction, construction, information, and recall. Frequently used mental status tests that cover these domains include the 6-item, short Blessed Test,[3] the Neurobehavioral Cognitive Status Examination (NCSE),[4] and the Mini-Mental State Examination (MMSE).[5] These screening tests can identify severely impaired individuals and are used to determine whether further evaluation with neuropsychological testing is needed.

Neuropsychological test battery covers many functional domains—attention, language, memory, visuospatial skills, executive function, intelligence, motor speed, and educational achievement—using tests with established validity and reliability. Individuals with severe cognitive impairments that have been identified on mental status tests will usually not benefit from neuropsychological evaluation. It is the person with subtle cognitive changes who benefits from neuropsychological testing. Neurologic disorders that have different behavioral ramifications amenable to neuropsychological evaluation include traumatic brain injury, dementia, Parkinson's disease, human immunodeficiency virus, encephalopathy, multiple sclerosis, epilepsy, neurotoxic exposure, chronic pain, and personality assessment in individuals with neurologic disease.

The criteria for evaluating mental status and cognitive impairment are based on the amount of interference with the ability to perform activities of daily living. This information can be obtained from someone who has close and continual contact with the individual and can be documented using any one of numerous ADL indices that determine changes in activities of daily living (eg, Barthel ADL Index[6] and Blessed Dementia Scale[7]). A tool that combines both cognitive skills and function is the Clinical Dementia Rating (CDR),[8-10] which covers memory, orientation, judgment and problem solving, home and hobbies, community affairs, and personal care. This validated clinical assessment tool is reproduced in Table 13-5 to serve as an example of how to evaluate cognitive change in light of ADL impairment. One of the standardized mental status tests—the short Blessed, NCSE, or MMSE—can be used in conjunction with the CDR to rate the impairment. To use the CDR, score the individual's cognitive function for each category (M, O, JPS CA, HH, and PC) independently. The maximum CDR score is 3. Memory is considered the primary category; the other categories are secondary. If at least three secondary categories are given the same numeric score as memory, then CDR = M. If three or more secondary categories are given a score greater or less than the memory score, CDR = the score of the majority of secondary categories unless three secondary categories are scored on one side of M and two secondary categories are scored on the other side of M. In this case, CDR = M. [Adapted from 8]

Corresponding impairment ratings for CDR scores are listed in Table 13-6. A CDR score of 0.5 = class 1 impairment, CDR score of 1 = class 2, CDR score of 2 = class 3, and CDR score of 3 = class 4.

Table 13-5 Clinical Dementia Rating (CDR)

	Impairment Level and CDR Score		
	None 0	Questionable 0.5	Mild 1.0
Memory (M)	No memory loss or slight inconsistent forgetfulness	Consistent slight forgetfulness; partial recollection of events; "benign" forgetfulness	Moderate memory loss; more marked for recent events; defect interferes with everyday activities
Orientation (O)	Fully oriented	Fully oriented except for slight difficulty with time relationships	Moderate difficulty with time relationships; oriented for place at examination; may have geographic disorientation elsewhere
Judgment and Problem Solving (JPS)	Solves everyday problems and handles business and financial affairs well; judgment good in relation to past performance	Slight impairment in solving problems, similarities, and differences	Moderate difficulty in handling problems, similarities, and differences; social judgment usually maintained
Community Affairs (CA)	Independent function at usual level in job, shopping, volunteer and social groups	Slight impairment in these activities	Unable to function independently at these activities although may still be engaged in some; appears normal to casual inspection
Home and Hobbies (HH)	Life at home, hobbies, and intellectual interests well maintained	Life at home, hobbies, and intellectual interests slightly impaired	Mild but definite impairment of function at home; more difficult chores abandoned; more complicated hobbies and interests abandoned
Personal Care (PC)	Fully capable of self-care	Fully capable of self-care	Needs prompting

Source: Morris JC. The Clinical Dementia Rating (CDR): current version and scoring rules [see comment]. *Neurology*. 1993;43(11):2412-2414. Reprinted with permission.

Table 13-6 Criteria for Rating Impairment Related to Mental Status

Class 1 1%-14% Impairment of the Whole Person	Class 2 15%-29% Impairment of the Whole Person	Class 3 30%-49% Impairment of the Whole Person	Class 4 50%-70% Impairment of the Whole Person
Paroxysmal disorder with preimpairment exists, but is able to perform activities of daily living CDR = 0.5	Impairment requires direction of some activities of daily living CDR = 1.0	Impairment requires assistance and supervision for most activities of daily living CDR = 2.0	Unable to care for self and be safe in any situation without supervision CDR = 3.0

Class 2 15%-29% Impairment of the Whole Person
Impairment requires direction of some activities of daily living CDR = 1.0

Example 13-21
15% to 29% Impairment Due to Alzheimer's Disease

Subject: 75-year-old man.

History: Left-handed; 2 to 3 years' history of loss of interest in current events, inability to find his home or location, wandering out of the house, poor short-term memory, inability to balance checkbook, and inability to comprehend TV programs or newspapers.

Current Symptoms: No focal or lateral neurologic symptoms with loss of recent memory; failure to follow through on instructions; inability to calculate.

Physical Exam: Disoriented to time, person, and place; can't recall three unrelated words or spell *world* backward, but can identify objects, copy pentagons, and write a sentence. No focal or lateral neurologic impairments. Ambulatory; needs assistance feeding self and dressing. Speech is articulate. Cooperative and noncombative.

Clinical Studies: CT scan and MRI: normal except for mild widening of cortical sulci. EEG: poorly developed to absent rhythmic alpha activity without slowing or paroxysm.

	Moderate 2.0	Severe 3.0
	Severe memory loss; only highly learned material retained; new material rapidly lost	Severe memory loss: only fragments remain
	Severe difficulty with time relationships; usually disoriented to time, often to place	Oriented to person only
	Severely impaired in handling problems, similarities, and differences; social judgment usually impaired	Unable to make judgments or solve problems
	No pretense of independent function outside home	No pretense of independent function outside home
	Appears well enough to be taken to functions outside a family home	Appears too ill to be taken to functions outside a family home
	Only simple chores preserved; very restricted interests, poorly maintained	No significant function in home
	Requires assistance in dressing, hygiene, keeping of personal effects	Requires much help with personal care; frequent incontinence

Diagnosis: Alzheimer's disease.

Impairment Rating: 29% impairment of the whole person due to mental impairment.

Comment: Dementia is progressing and dependence is becoming more of a problem.

This case merits a CDR of 1.0.

Class 3
30%-49% Impairment of the Whole Person

Impairment requires assistance and supervision for most activities of daily living

CDR = 2.0

Example 13-22
30% to 49% Impairment Due to Traumatic Brain Injury

Subject: 25-year-old man.

History: Right-handed; 1 year ago was involved in a head-on collision of the car he was driving with another automobile, which had crossed the highway median. Did not have his seat belt on, and did not recall hitting his head on the steering wheel and windshield. Brought to the hospital unconscious; had sustained a fracture of the left arm. Over the next 4 weeks, gradually improved with rehabilitation; had no recall of the accident or immediate preceding events.

Current Symptoms: Moderate inability to follow commands and find his room. Disoriented to time, person, and place; wanders alone and gets lost in familiar surroundings. Loss of interest in home activities and current events. Sleep-wake cycle has been interrupted. Decreased ability to initiate responses, agitation, learning difficulties, impulsivity, and social disinhibition.

Physical Exam: No focal or lateral paralysis, but attention and gait are slow. The latter is not grossly ataxic, and Romberg sign is negative. Cranial nerve functions are intact. Mental status examination reveals 18/30 with poor orientation; difficulty with recall of three unrelated words and spelling *world* backward. No motor or sensory difficulties, and cerebellar testing is adequate.

Diagnosis: Traumatic brain injury.

Impairment Rating: 40% impairment due to mentation impairment; combine with ratings due to other neurologic impairments to determine whole person impairment (see Combined Values Chart, p. 604).

Comment: This case merits a CDR of 2.0. The concept of traumatic brain injury is being developed into mild, moderate, and severe categories resulting from "significant impairment of an individual's physical, cognitive, and psychosocial functions." The "more problematic consequences involve the individual's cognition, emotional functioning, and behavior."[11] If there are other impairments, the combined rating of those impairments should be added.

13.3e Communication Impairments: Dysphasia and Aphasia

Communication involves comprehension, understanding, language, and effective interaction between and among individuals. Aphasia is a condition in which language function is defective or absent. It includes a lack of comprehension with deficits in vision, hearing, and language (both spoken and written), and also the inability to implement discernible and appropriate language symbols by voice, action, writing, or pantomime. Dysphasia is a language impairment that is less severe than aphasia (which literally means "no speech") but still is associated with a lesion in the dominant parietal lobe. It presents as a communication problem due to receptive or expressive dysphasia or a combination of the two. Inability to have a meaningful conversation because no nouns are used is an example of dysphasia. Other common errors include errors of grammatical structure, word-finding difficulties, and word substitution. Dysphasia and aphasia are different from dysarthria, which is imperfect articulation of speech due to disordered muscle control. Dysphonia is an impairment of sound production that causes difficulty speaking and understanding. Speech and communication impairments due to nonneurologic primary problems are discussed in Chapter 11, Ear, Nose, Throat, and Related Structures.

Dysphasia is the most common diagnosis, since most individuals usually retain some ability to communicate. An inability to understand language has a poorer prognosis than an inability to express language. Speech therapy is of little value in the absence of comprehension; therefore, compensatory techniques may not be learned when a receptive aphasia or dysphasia exists. Tests for dysphasia should be conducted after it is established how confused or disoriented the individual is and which side of the brain is dominant for speech. Cognition should also be evaluated after dysphasia mechanisms have been excluded.

Aphasia and dysphasia test batteries are frequently devised by the clinician and cover the following simple tasks: (1) listening to spontaneous speech or responses to simple questions; (2) pointing commands and questions that can be answered "yes" or "no" to test comprehension; (3) repeating words and phrases; (4) naming objects that have high- and low-frequency use; (5) reading comprehension and reading aloud (reading is related to educational achievement, which must be known before interpreting reading comprehension and reading aloud results); and (6) writing and spelling.[12] If comprehension is relatively intact, the aphasia screening battery may be adequate to place an individual in class 1 or 2. However, individuals with dysphasia may score poorly on aphasia and dysphasia test batteries while they demonstrate communicative competency for activities of daily living. This communicative competency may be measured by means of the Communicative Abilities in Daily Living (CADL),[13] in which nonverbal communication is assessed. Table 13-7 describes the criteria for rating impairment due to aphasia or dysphasia.

Table 13-7 Criteria for Rating Impairment Due to Aphasia or Dysphasia

Class 1 0%-9% Impairment of the Whole Person	Class 2 10%-24% Impairment of the Whole Person	Class 3 25%-39% Impairment of the Whole Person	Class 4 40%-60% Impairment of the Whole Person
Minimal disturbance in comprehension and production of language symbols of daily living	Moderate impairment in comprehension and production of language symbols of daily living	Able to comprehend nonverbal communication; production of unintelligible or inappropriate language for daily activities	Complete inability to communicate or comprehend language symbols

Class 1 0%-9% Impairment of the Whole Person
Minimal disturbance in comprehension and production of language symbols of daily living

Example 13-23
0% to 9% Impairment Due to Dysphasia

Subject: 45-year-old woman.

History: Right-handed; head trauma while doing laundry in cellar; brief episode of loss of awareness.

Current Symptoms: Periodic difficulty expressing herself in conversations.

Physical Exam: Unable to name objects on sight, but can point to object when seen on a printed card. Able to read and comprehend language. Mild periodic dysnomia in trying to name objects.

Diagnosis: Dysphasia, mild intermittent Broca's dysphasia, and other speech disturbances as late effect of accident—striking against object accidentally.

Impairment Rating: 7% impairment of the whole person due to speech impairment.

Comment: Only neurologic impairment is a periodic inability to speak correctly. This case is rated for the speech impairment since this is the most severe cerebral criteria impairment.

Example 13-24
0% to 9% Impairment Due to Expressive Dysphasia

Subject: 47-year-old woman.

History: Right-handed; traveling by train when a sudden stop occurred. Individual was thrown forward, striking her head on a metal railing and suffering 10 minutes of loss of consciousness, with subsequent loss of ability to find the correct words to express herself.

Current Symptoms: Persistent difficulty finding correct words with loss of vocabulary.

Physical Exam: Inability to name objects on sight, but can point to the object when shown its name on a card. Understands verbal commands and can copy words. Orientation is difficult because of inability to express the date. No hemiparesis or sensory impairment.

Clinical Studies: Neuropsychological testing was limited due to individual's inability to correctly express herself.

Diagnosis: Expressive dysphasia.

Impairment Rating: 9% impairment of the whole person.

Comment: This is an example of traumatic brain injury with minimal residual impairment that involves production of language and is limiting daily activities. The rating was done at a time when this impairment was deemed to be stable (MMI), namely, 6 months following the injury.

Class 2 10%-24% Impairment of the Whole Person
Moderate impairment in comprehension and production of language symbols of daily living

Example 13-25
10% to 24% Impairment Due to Receptive Dysphasia

Subject: 45-year-old man.

History: Left-handed; individual's car was struck from the right frontal side while crossing an intersection. He wore no seat belt, and no air bag was present. His head hit the windshield and mirror; no loss of consciousness, but a bruise was noted over the left parietal area.

Current Symptoms: This individual apparently does not comprehend simple commands and therefore has difficulty both in his work area and at home.

Physical Exam: Able to name objects from sight but has difficulty understanding verbal and written commands.

Clinical Studies: MRI of the brain with enhancement: mild contusion of the left temporal parietal area; EEG: mild slowing in the same area.

Diagnosis: Receptive dysphasia as a late effect of a motor vehicle accident.

Impairment Rating: 20% impairment due to dysphasia; combine with appropriate ratings due to other neurologic impairments to determine whole person impairment (see Combined Values Chart, p. 604).

Comment: Trauma to the left temporal parietal area in a left-handed individual without clear dominance of side for development of speech has resulted in receptive dysphasia in speech and mild impairment in understanding.

Class 3
25%-39% Impairment of the Whole Person
Able to comprehend nonverbal communication; production of unintelligible or inappropriate language for daily activities

Example 13-26
25% to 39% Impairment Due to Hemiplegia, Homonymous Hemianopia, and Conduction Aphasia

Subject: 60-year-old woman.

History: Right-handed; progressive loss of function of the right arm, face, and leg over 2 days; fluent speech but poor understanding. Slow recovery to stable state 2 months later.

Current Symptoms: Walks with a stiff right leg and needs to use a cane. Right arm is flexed, and individual has difficulty expressing herself, substituting inappropriate words.

Physical Exam: Paraphrases words and reads poorly out loud. Also has difficulty writing from dictation, with substituted words and misspellings. Examination demonstrated a spastic right hemiplegia, hemianopia, and hemisensory impairment.

Clinical Studies: CT scan and MRI/MRA: large infarction in the area of the angular branch of the left middle cerebral artery.

Diagnosis: Late effect of CVA: hemiplegia affecting dominant side, aphasia, homonymous hemianopia, and conduction aphasia.

Impairment Rating: 30% impairment due to dysphasia; combine with appropriate ratings due to other neurologic impairments to determine whole person impairment (see Combined Values Chart, p. 604).

Comment: Major stroke in the dominant hemisphere due to occlusion of a branch of the middle cerebral artery by presumed thrombus. MMI has been achieved, and current state is stable.

Class 4
40%-60% Impairment of the Whole Person
Complete inability to communicate or comprehend language symbols

Example 13-27
40% to 60% Impairment Due to Hypoxic Encephalopathy With Focal Seizures

Subject: 35-year-old man.

History: Left-handed; fireman was trapped in a burning private home; he was brought out unconscious by another fireman and was revived onsite. He was taken to the hospital constant care unit, where he remained for 6 weeks with slow improvement to a stable state.

Current Symptoms: Needs complete ADL care, including bladder and bowel functions. In a chair and/or bed situation for all activities. Will occasionally respond but is completely unable to communicate or comprehend language symbols. Has periodic focal complex parietal seizures that are poorly controlled with medications.

Physical Exam: Complete inability to speak with comprehension; no paresis or seizures.

Clinical Studies: EEG: diffuse slow activity with discharges in the left temporal area. MRI and CT scan: normal.

Diagnosis: Hypoxic encephalopathy with focal seizures.

Impairment Rating: 60% impairment due to aphasia; combine with appropriate ratings due to other neurologic impairments to determine whole person impairment (see Combined Values Chart, p. 604).

Comment: This is a case of very serious hypoxic encephalopathy due to inhalation of fumes and gases in a burning building, resulting in severe generalized impairment of central nervous system control of many functions including swallowing, nutrition, and bladder and bowel function.

13.3f Emotional or Behavioral Impairments

Emotional, mood, and behavioral disturbances illustrate the relationship between neurology and psychiatry. Emotional disturbances originating in verifiable neurologic impairments (eg, stroke, head injury) are assessed using the criteria in this chapter. Psychiatric features may also exist with primary neurologic disorders. Psychiatric features can range from irritability to outbursts of rage or panic and from aggression to withdrawal. Neurologic impairments producing psychiatric conditions are assessed using the neurologic examination, with an expanded neuropsychiatric history and the necessary ancillary tests. Psychiatric impairments may include depression, manic states, emotional fluctuations, socially unacceptable behavior, involuntary laughing or crying, impulsivity, general disinhibition with obsessive and scatological behaviors, and other kinds of CNS responses.

Psychiatric manifestations and impairments that do not have documented neurologic impairments are evaluated using the criteria in the chapter on mental and behavioral impairments (See Table 13-8 and Chapter 14, Mental and Behavioral Disorders). Examples of neurologic conditions associated with changes in emotion and affect include (1) right hemisphere infarct and inappropriate jocularity; (2) left hemisphere infarct and deep dejection and dysphasia; (3) left-sided temporolimbic seizure foci and ideational disorders; and (4) right-sided temporolimbic seizure foci and mood disturbances. With the more diffuse pathology underlying the dementias, "no cognitive" behavioral symptoms (apathy, delusions, dysphoria, agitation/aggression, euphoria, hallucinations, irritability/lability, and aberrant motor behavior) may be assessed with the Neuropsychiatric Inventory (NPI).[14] This tool was evaluated for content and concurrent validity, has good test-retest reliability, and has good internal consistency among the items of the NPI. The NPI assesses behaviors' frequency and severity to assist in determining daily function.

Table 13-8 Criteria for Rating Impairment Due to Emotional or Behavioral Disorders

Class 1 0%-14% Impairment of the Whole Person	Class 2 15%-29% Impairment of the Whole Person	Class 3 30%-69% Impairment of the Whole Person	Class 4 70%-90% Impairment of the Whole Person
Mild limitation of activities of daily living and daily social and interpersonal functioning	Moderate limitation of some activities of daily living and some daily social and interpersonal functioning	Severe limitation in performing most activities of daily living, impeding useful action in most daily social and interpersonal functioning	Severe limitation of all daily activities, requiring total dependence on another person

> **Class 2**
> **15%-29% Impairment of the Whole Person**
>
> Moderate limitation of some activities of daily living and some daily social and interpersonal functioning

Example 13-28
15% to 29% Impairment Due to Traumatic Encephalopathy

Subject: 60-year-old man.

History: Right-handed; former competitive boxer; for the past 10 years has been a sparring partner for professional boxers. In the past, he frequently has been rendered unconscious in training sessions and boxing events.

Current Symptoms: Episodes of mild confusion and occasional unsteadiness of gait, with difficulty in speech and articulation; has a mild head tremor.

Physical Exam: No paresis or sensory defect, but has difficulty with neuropsychological testing, short-term memory, calculation, serial 7s or 3s subtraction. Difficulty with inappropriate jocularity and interpersonal relationships.

Clinical Studies: CT scan and MRI: very mild widening of the cerebral sulci. EEG: poor background alpha activity but no definite focal or generalized slowing.

Diagnosis: Traumatic encephalopathy.

Impairment Rating: 17% impairment of the whole person.

Comment: The problem in this case is the frequency of head trauma over the course of years, including occasional knockouts.

> **Class 3**
> **30%-69% Impairment of the Whole Person**
>
> Severe limitation in performing most activities of daily living, impeding useful action in most daily social and interpersonal functioning

Example 13-29
30% to 69% Impairment Due to Low-Grade Glioma

Subject: 35-year-old woman.

History: Right-handed; progressive irritability and periodic lethargy. Individual has had difficulty shopping for groceries, cooking, cleaning, and helping her children with their homework.

Current Symptoms: A new headache and very slight difficulty in handwriting. She has become labile, irritable, apathetic, and intermittently agitated.

Physical Exam: Diminished fine dexterity of the right hand with loss of 2-point discrimination in that hand and inability to properly identify coins. Unable to find right hand in space with the left hand. No definite paresis or other sensory defects.

Clinical Studies: MRI of the brain with contrast: mildly enhancing 2-cm area in the left parietal region with moderate ventricular compression. EEG: intermittent moderate-amplitude delta activity in the left parietal region.

Diagnosis: Probable low-grade glioma, left parietal region.

Impairment Rating: 45% impairment due to the glioma; combine with appropriate ratings due to other neurologic impairments to determine whole person impairment (see Combined Values Chart p. 604).

Comment: The major problem is the limitation of daily activities, social, interpersonal, and family functioning, with mild focalizing sensory neurologic impairments confirmed by clinical studies.

> **Class 4**
> **70%-90% Impairment of the Whole Person**
>
> Severe limitation of all daily activities, requiring total dependence on another person

Example 13-30
70% to 90% Impairment Due to Huntington's Chorea

Subject: 40-year-old man.

History: Right-handed; progressive difficulty with recent memory, keeping track of financial obligations, and maintaining checkbook over the past 2 years. Similar history in his father and, possibly, paternal grandfather.

Current Symptoms: Individual has recently developed a periodic, somewhat explosive, hand-arm movement with facial grimacing. He has begun to wander away from the house and recently was restricted in driving his automobile because he got lost in familiar areas.

Physical Exam: No cranial nerve signs or motor-sensory impairments except for chorea of both extremities and face and a dancing, arrhythmic gait. Mini-Mental State Exam was 15/30.

Clinical Studies: MRI: decrease of the area of the caudate. EEG: relatively poor background activity without focal or lateral abnormalities.

Diagnosis: Huntington's chorea.

Impairment Rating: 70% impairment due to Huntington's chorea; combine with appropriate ratings due to other neurologic impairments to determine whole person impairment (see Combined Values Chart, p. 604).

Comment: The major impairments here include all ADL, in addition to movement disorder and gait impairment.

The remainder of this chapter covers the impairments listed in Table 13-1. The following impairments are combined with the most severe category of cerebral impairment described previously. If no cerebral impairment exists, the following impairments can stand alone or be combined with each other using the Combined Values Chart (p. 604).

13.4 Criteria for Rating Impairments of the Cranial Nerves

13.4a Cranial Nerve I—the Olfactory Nerve

The olfactory nerve is responsible for the sense of smell and odor recognition. It is located on the floor of the skull's frontal fossa and is only occasionally impaired from trauma or other mechanism. Lack of sense of smell may reduce taste perception, which is mediated by cranial nerves VII and IX. Partial or complete right or left dysosmia or anosmia, or a perversion of the sense of smell, parosmia, may occur. Combine the estimate for anosmia or parosmia (given only if the anosmia interferes significantly with daily activities) with any other permanent impairment to determine the whole person impairment. The Smell Identification Test™[15] is a quantitative test for smell with an extensive normative database. The maximum impairment from anosmia is 3%.

Example 13-31
3% Impairment Due to Olfactory Tract Damage

Subject: 24-year-old man.

History: Right-handed; individual had a car accident without a seat belt 4 months ago and sustained a severe whiplash and subsequently struck his forehead on the windshield, with brief loss of consciousness.

Current Symptoms: Intermittent dizziness and headaches, but individual is more bothered by loss of smell and diminished appetite secondary to lack of taste.

Physical Exam: Normal except for 10/40 on the University of Pennsylvania Smell Identification Test, which is compatible with anosmia.

Clinical Studies: CT scan, MRI, and EEG: normal.

Diagnosis: Olfactory tract damage.

Impairment Rating: 3% impairment of the whole person.

Comment: It is important to remember not to use an irritant when testing smell, since this will stimulate trigeminal nerve endings and not reflect olfactory function. Appropriate bedside odorants include coffee, flowers, and some foods.

13.4b Cranial Nerve II—the Optic Nerve

The optic nerves carry visual information from the eyes to the visual cortex of the brain. Loss of visual input can have a profound influence on the ability to perform ADL. Impairment ratings for vision loss are discussed in general in this chapter and in more detail in Chapter 12 (The Visual System).

The optic nerve is one neural component of the visual system. The other components include the retina; the optic chiasm, which is unique in that only half of the nerve fibers cross to the contralateral side; the optic tracts; optic radiation; and visual cortex. This section discusses vision loss due to prechiasmal lesions, such as optic nerve dysfunction (eg, optic neuritis), as well as postchiasmal vision loss due to cortical lesions (eg, hemianopia).

General Principles of Vision Assessment (see Chapter 12 for more detail)

Tables 13-9 and 13-10 in this section and the tables in Chapter 12 have been significantly revised from previous editions to reflect the effect of vision changes on the ability to perform ADL as listed in

Table 1-2. When assessing vision, the ratings for visual acuity loss and visual field loss are combined to a global visual impairment rating as summarized in Table 12-1. Since vision in one eye still enables one to perform most ADL, binocular vision is weighted more heavily than monocular vision. Thus, vision loss in one eye will receive a much lower impairment rating than vision loss in both eyes.

As discussed in detail in Chapter 12, evaluation of near-vision is optional and visual acuity loss to 20/200 receives a 50% impairment rating (see Tables 12-2, 12-3, and 12-4). Visual field loss is sampled in 10 meridians, two in each superior quadrant, three in each inferior quadrant (Figure 12-1). Thus, a homonymous upper quadrantanopia will receive an impairment rating of about 20%; an inferior quadrantanopia will be rated at about 30%; a homonymous hemianopia, at about 50% (Tables 12-5, 12-6, and 12-7).

The whole person impairment rating results from the visual acuity impairment rating and the visual field impairment rating are detailed in Section 12-4. If acuity or visual fields are normal, the whole person impairment rating equals the abnormal visual impairment rating.

Vision Assessment Using Chapter 13

Due to the neurologic basis of vision, some conditions affecting vision may be evaluated using the guidelines in this chapter. Simple cases of visual acuity loss without peripheral field loss, such as those caused by optic neuritis, can be evaluated using Table 13-9. More complex conditions should be evaluated according to the methodology detailed in Chapter 12.

Simple cases of visual field loss, with normal acuity, may be evaluated using Table 13-10. Since postchiasmal lesions will result in vision loss in the contralateral hemifield of both eyes (eg, homonymous hemianopia or quadrantanopia), visual field tests can be an important diagnostic tool in localizing a lesion. For diagnostic purposes, a tangent screen test involving the central 30° is often sufficient. For complex vision loss patterns, especially those with some remaining peripheral vision and noncongruous patterns as may occur in chiasmal lesions, a full evaluation as detailed in Chapter 12 is required.

Table 13-9 Examples of Whole Person Impairment Due to Visual Acuity Loss (see also Table 12-4)

| Class 1
0%-9% Whole Person Impairment Due to Visual Acuity Loss | Class 2
10%-29% Whole Person Impairment Due to Visual Acuity Loss | Class 3
30%-49% Whole Person Impairment Due to Visual Acuity Loss | Class 4
50%-61% Whole Person Impairment Due to Visual Acuity Loss |
|---|---|---|---|
| Range of normal vision | Mild vision loss | Moderate vision loss | Severe vision loss |
| Both eyes have visual acuity of 20/25 or better | The affected eye has visual acuity of 20/200 or less; the other eye is normal (20/25 or better) | The affected eye is totally blind; the unaffected eye has reduced visual acuity of 20/40 or worse | Both eyes have visual acuity of 20/200 or worse |

Note: This table is based on the best corrected acuity and assumes that the visual fields are normal. See Chapter 12 for more complex cases of visual acuity loss. Note that the ability to perform ADL depends largely on the acuity of the better eye.

Table 13-10 Examples of Whole Person Impairment (WPI) Due to Visual Field Loss (see also Table 12-7)

| Class 1
0%-9% Whole Person Impairment Due to Visual Field Loss | Class 2
10%-29% Whole Person Impairment Due to Visual Field Loss | Class 3
30%-49% Whole Person Impairment Due to Visual Field Loss | Class 4
50%-61% Whole Person Impairment Due to Visual Field Loss |
|---|---|---|---|
| Range of normal vision | Mild vision loss | Moderate vision loss | Severe vision loss |
| Both eyes have full visual fields of > 50° radius

(no WPI) | Both eyes have lost an entire upper quadrant

(20% WPI) | Both eyes have lost an entire lower quadrant

(30% WPI) | Both eyes have tunnel vision of 20° diameter or less

(50% WPI)

Both eyes have lost an entire (L or R) hemifield

(50% WPI) |
| | One eye is lost; the other eye is normal

(20% WPI) | Both eyes have lost the upper hemifield

(40% WPI) | Both eyes have lost the lower hemifield

(60% WPI) |

Note: This table assumes that the visual acuity is still normal (as in hemianopia with macular sparing). See Chapter 12 for more complex cases, including noncongruous visual field loss and visual field loss combined with visual acuity loss. Note that the ability to perform ADL depends on the extent of the binocular field.

Lesions of the visual cortex may cause a homonymous visual field defect. Parietal lesions may cause visual neglect. Where possible, both these conditions should be evaluated for their effect on ADL skills. Because of brain plasticity, gradual improvement over a considerable period of time is possible. Ensure that the impairment is permanent, ie, unlikely to change significantly over the next year. If the vision loss is accompanied by other neurologic dysfunction, use the Combined Values Chart (p. 604) to combine the impairment rating from both conditions.

Example 13-32
10% Visual Acuity Impairment Due to Unilateral Optic Neuritis

Subject: 27-year-old woman.

History: Right-handed; enjoyed good health with accurate vision until 6 months ago, when she developed a painless progressive vision loss in the left eye. During the subsequent 6 months, visual clarity returned slightly.

Current Symptoms: Vision is blurred when she tries to read the newspaper with the affected eye; she has not been able to see television images clearly with this eye. She can perform all ADL functions with the unaffected eye.

Physical Exam: Near and far visual acuity of the left eye is 20/200; right eye, 20/20; binocular, 20/20. The eyes are externally normal; ophthalmoscopy reveals moderate pallor of the left optic disk. The pupil of the left eye is slightly dilated and poorly reactive to a direct light stimulus. No reaction in the right eye to left eye stimulation. When the right eye is stimulated with bright light, there is prompt constriction of the pupil of the left eye. No other cranial nerve signs.

Clinical Studies: Visual evoked potentials: prolongation of the P100 in the left eye.

Diagnosis: Optic neuritis, left eye.

Impairment Rating: 10% impairment of the whole person based on Table 13-9 and a left eye acuity of 20/200.

	Class 5 62%-73% Whole Person Impairment Due to Visual Acuity Loss	Class 6 74%-85% Whole Person Impairment Due to Visual Acuity Loss
	Profound vision loss	(Near-) Total vision loss
	Both eyes have visual acuity of 20/500 or worse	Both eyes have visual acuity worse than 20/1000

	Class 5 62%-73% Whole Person Impairment Due to Visual Field Loss	Class 6 74%-85% Whole Person Impairment Due to Visual Field Loss
	Profound vision loss	(Near-) Total vision loss
	Both eyes have tunnel vision of 10° diameter or less	Both eyes have tunnel vision of 5° diameter or less

Comment: Although this case represents a 50% visual acuity loss in the left eye, the impairment rating is much lower, since the ability to perform ADL depends largely on the better eye. If the right eye had the same loss, the impairment rating would be much worse.

13.4c Cranial Nerves III, IV, and VI— the Oculomotor, Trochlear, and Abducens Nerves

The oculomotor, trochlear, and abducens nerves innervate the muscles that move the eyeballs. The oculomotor nerve also controls pupil size and reaction to light. Malfunction of the oculomotor system results in strabismus, ie, misalignment of the visual axes. There are two main types of malfunction: ordinary or comitant strabismus, which occurs mainly in children, and paralytic or noncomitant strabismus, found mainly in adults.

Ordinary or comitant strabismus involves a malfunction of the oculomotor control centers. The angle of deviation is approximately the same in all directions of gaze. This type often results in visual acuity loss in one eye (amblyopia); diplopia is uncommon. The impairment rating is based on the visual acuity loss (see Chapter 12).

Paralytic or noncomitant strabismus is due to a paresis of one of the oculomotor nerves and muscles. The angle of deviation of the visual axes varies with the direction of gaze. Diplopia (double vision) is common. Occlusion of one eye eliminates the diplopia but may have undesirable side effects (such as reduction of the binocular field of vision).

If diplopia exists only in the extremes of gaze, it does not interfere with general ADL skills. If double vision exists at or near the primary direction of gaze, it (or the necessary occlusion) may interfere with ADL skills and would warrant an impairment rating. Assessment should be based on well-documented, individualized considerations as discussed in Chapter 12.

Example 13-33
25% Vision Impairment Due to Sixth Nerve Palsy, With Concurrent Peripheral Neuropathy

Subject: 55-year-old man.

History: Right-handed; 4-month history of seeing objects double, especially when looking to the right. He has also complained of burning, pins-and-needles sensation in his feet, mainly at night.

Current Symptoms: Persistent double vision on looking to the right interferes with performing some ADL. Burning sensation in his feet prevents him from obtaining a good night's sleep.

Physical Exam: Double vision is present on forward fixation and worsens upon looking to the right side. Poor abduction of the right eye on looking into the right lateral field. Decreased distal perception to pinprick and cold in both feet, with hyperesthesias of the soles of his feet to compression.

Clinical Studies: Showed type 2 diabetes mellitus, moderately controlled.

Diagnosis: Sixth nerve palsy and peripheral neuropathy associated with diabetes mellitus.

Impairment Rating: Chapter 12 has no specific scale for diplopia. This individual can still read normal print but has reduced reading endurance and no reserve for small print. He is in the range of *near-normal vision* (see Table 12-2), which warrants an impairment rating of up to 25%.

Comment: Combine the visual impairment from any impairment due to his peripheral neuropathy.

13.4d Cranial Nerve V—the Trigeminal Nerve

The trigeminal nerve is a mixed nerve with sensory fibers to the face, cornea, anterior scalp, nasal and oral cavities, tongue, and supratentorial dura mater. The nerve also transmits motor impulses to the mastication muscles.

Evaluate sensation in the parts served by the three major divisions of the trigeminal nerve with the usual techniques: pain, temperature, and touch. (See the description of loss of function due to sensory deficit, pain, or discomfort under section 13.9, Criteria for Rating Impairments of the Peripheral Nervous System, Neuromuscular Junction, and Muscular System.) Compare the two sides of the face or body. Bilateral facial sensation loss is uncommon. Combine the impairment percentage for sensation loss that involves the trigeminal nerve with the estimated impairment percentage for pain or motor loss. Pin, cold, and light touch are the best parameters for localization of sensory findings on the face. They can outline impairment of either side of the face, a branch of, or complete trigeminal nerve impairment.

Brief episodic trigeminal neuralgia or postherpetic neuralgia that involves a branch of the trigeminal nerve may be very severe and uncontrolled. Because there usually is no documented neurologic impairment except for a trigger point with trigeminal neuralgia or allodynia with postherpetic neuralgia, severe, uncontrolled, typical pain may be the impairment. Both atypical, episodic facial pain and typical, neuralgic pain may be evaluated (see Table 13-11) if they have occurred for months and interfere with daily activities. Motor impairment of the trigeminal nerve may affect chewing, swallowing, and speech articulation and may be accompanied by pain or a tic. Bilateral impairment is rare and may be severe. Daily activities may precipitate the pain. Speech, chewing, and swallowing impairments are considered in Chapter 9, Ear, Nose, Throat, and Related Structures.

Table 13-11 Criteria for Rating Impairment of Cranial Nerve V (Trigeminal Nerve)

Class 1 0%-14% Impairment of the Whole Person	Class 2 15%-24% Impairment of the Whole Person	Class 3 25%-35% Impairment of the Whole Person
Mild uncontrolled facial neuralgic pain that may interfere with activities of daily living	Moderately severe, uncontrolled facial neuralgic pain that interferes with activities of daily living	Severe, uncontrolled, unilateral or bilateral facial neuralgic pain that prevents performance of activities of daily living

Class 2 15%-24% Impairment of the Whole Person
Moderately severe, uncontrolled facial neuralgic pain that interferes with activities of daily living

Example 13-34
15% to 24% Impairment Due to Trigeminal Neuralgia

Subject: 60-year-old woman.

History: Right-handed; 3-month history of brief, sudden attacks of right-sided facial pain that radiates from the jaw to the mouth and up to the ear. These have occurred in the past with long remissions but now are more frequent.

Current Symptoms: Chewing, smiling, or hot or cold fluid touching the lower canine tooth triggers attacks of pain. Pain is described as a very severe, sudden, brief, electricity-like shock followed by severe pain. When the pain clears, she has no pain in her face until the next recurrence. No symptoms between these sudden brief episodes.

Physical Exam: Normal, without demonstrable sensory impairment. Light stimulation of upper lip reproduces lightning-like painful sensations similar to her history (trigger point).

Clinical Studies: None unless neurologic impairment is documented.

Diagnosis: Trigeminal neuralgia.

Impairment Rating: 15% impairment of the whole person.

Comment: Pain may respond to carbamazepine and/or Lioresal, but these medications may not be tolerated in the elderly. Surgical intervention, such as stereotactic thermocoagulation of the gasserian ganglion, may be required, but this may leave the face unpleasantly numb. In this case, the uncontrolled facial neuralgic pain interferes with daily, social, and interpersonal activities.

> **Class 3**
> **25%–35% Impairment of the Whole Person**
>
> Severe, uncontrolled, unilateral or bilateral facial neuralgic pain that prevents performance of activities of daily living

Example 13-35
25% to 35% Impairment Due to Postherpetic Neuralgia

Subject: 70-year-old woman.

History: Left-handed; episode of herpes zoster rash in left V_1 distribution.

Current Symptoms: Severe, nonstop burning and itching in this area. She cannot comb her hair or wash this area since touching makes it worse.

Physical Exam: White scars of herpes eruption and diminished discrimination of pain and light touch over the left upper face.

Clinical Studies: None.

Diagnosis: Postherpetic neuralgia.

Impairment Rating: 25% impairment of the whole person.

Comment: This condition occurs in 30% of individuals with ophthalmic herpes. Pain may last for years and is associated with a high suicide risk because of severe uncontrolled neuralgic pain preventing normal usual activities.

13.4e Cranial Nerve VII—the Facial Nerve

The facial nerve is a nerve with both motor and sensory components. The motor part innervates the facial muscles of expression and accessory muscles for chewing and swallowing. The sensory fibers carry tactile sensations from a part of the external auditory canal, ear, tympanic membrane, soft palate and adjacent pharynx, and taste to the anterior two thirds of the tongue. Special fibers innervate the lacrimal and salivary glands.

Sensory loss related to facial nerve impairment does not interfere with activities of daily living. Loss of taste usually is not considered to be a major impairment. See Table 13-12 for impairment criteria. Unilateral motor impairment poses a risk of vision impairment because of blinking loss and corneal injury. Eating and speaking also can be affected.

Table 13-12 Criteria for Rating Impairment of Cranial Nerve VII (Facial Nerve)

Class 1 1%–4% Impairment of the Whole Person	Class 2 5%–19% Impairment of the Whole Person	Class 3 20%–45% Impairment of the Whole Person
Complete loss of taste of anterior tongue *or* mild unilateral facial weakness	Mild to moderate bilateral facial weakness *or* severe unilateral facial paralysis with 75% or greater facial involvement and with inability to control eyelid closure	Severe bilateral facial paralysis with 75% or greater facial involvement and with inability to control eyelid closure

Class 2
5%-19% Impairment of the Whole Person
Mild to moderate bilateral facial weakness
or
severe unilateral facial paralysis with 75% or greater facial involvement and with inability to control eyelid closure

Example 13-36
5% to 19% Impairment Due to Bell's Palsy

Subject: 40-year-old woman.

History: Right-handed; 4 months ago, individual developed a "numbness sensation" of the forehead and right side of the face over the course of 2 to 3 days. She also noted drooling from the right side of her mouth when drinking coffee and occasionally bit the right side of her tongue.

Current Symptoms: Total loss of movement of the right side of the face with persistent elevation of the right eyelid without voluntary control of closure. Increased sensitivity to sound in the right ear.

Physical Exam: Mild to moderate loss of motility of the forehead on the right and complete loss of motility of the lower right side of the face and eyelid elevation. No reportable perception of vinegar on the right side of the tongue. No other cranial nerve or long tract signs. Congestion of the conjunctiva of the right eye and apparent irritation.

Clinical Studies: Electromyogram (EMG) of the facial muscle may be considered.

Diagnosis: Bell's palsy, unilateral.

Impairment Rating: 19% impairment of the whole person.

Comment: Corticosteroids may be considered in the first days of Bell's palsy to shorten the course. Most but not all affected individuals lose taste on the anterior two thirds of the tongue. The major problem is to protect the cornea from drying, since the eyelid does not close spontaneously or voluntarily. EMG may be helpful when consideration for innervation is under way.

13.4f Cranial Nerve VIII—the Vestibulocochlear Nerve

Cranial nerve VIII is composed of nerves from two adjacent nuclei. The cochlear portion of the nerve is concerned with hearing, and the vestibular portion of the nerve is concerned with vertigo and position and orientation in space. See Chapter 11 for evaluation of hearing impairment without known nerve dysfunction.

Tinnitus in the presence of unilateral hearing loss may impair speech discrimination and adversely influence the ability to carry out daily activities, especially in crowds or noisy places. Therefore, add up to 5% to the impairment evaluation for severe unilateral hearing loss due to tinnitus when ADL are affected.

Dysfunction of the vestibular part of the eighth nerve may be unilateral or bilateral. The impaired person may or may not be able to compensate for a unilateral loss. With bilateral loss of vestibular function, equilibrium and station are dependent on other systems, such as those for visual cues and kinesthetic senses; however, those systems may be inadequate for normal movement or ambulation.

Vertigo is the most disturbing symptom of vestibular dysfunction and is seldom, if ever, minor. Associated symptoms include nausea, vomiting, headache, fear of movement, ataxia, and nystagmus. Movement or environmental object movement may worsen these uncomfortable symptoms. Vertigo as a single entity is evaluated in Chapter 11. Equilibrium and balance impairment is significant if daily activities are limited. See Table 13-13 for criteria for rating impairment of the vestibulocochlear nerve. Criteria of vestibular impairment are detailed in the section discussing equilibrium in Chapter 11, Ear, Nose, Throat, and Related Structures.

Chapter 13

Table 13-13 Criteria for Rating Impairment of Cranial Nerve VIII (Vestibulocochlear Nerve)

Class 1 1%-9% Impairment of the Whole Person	Class 2 10%-29% Impairment of the Whole Person	Class 3 30%-49% Impairment of the Whole Person	Class 4 50%-70% Impairment of the Whole Person
Minimal equilibrium impairment; limitation required only of activities in hazardous surroundings	Moderate equilibrium impairment; limitation required of all daily activities except simple ones for self-care	Moderately severe equilibrium impairment; limitation required of all daily activities, including those for self-care	Severe equilibrium impairment; limitation of daily activities such that assistance is required for self-care and ambulation, and confinement may be needed

13.4g Cranial Nerves IX and X—the Glossopharyngeal and Vagus Nerves

These are mixed nerves that supply sensory fibers chiefly to the posterior one third of the tongue and to the pharynx, larynx, and trachea. Involvement of the glossopharyngeal nerve by neuralgia usually is self-limiting or treatable and not permanent; the nerve's involvement may cause a condition similar to trigeminal (V) nerve tic or neuralgia. If the neuralgia persists uncontrolled for a period of months, the physician may be justified in assigning a percentage of impairment that is similar to trigeminal nerve impairment (use Table 13-11). Sensory impairments may contribute to difficulties with breathing, swallowing, speaking, and visceral functions.

13.4h Cranial Nerve XI—the Spinal Accessory Nerve

This nerve assists the vagus nerve in supplying some of the muscles of the larynx and innervates the cervical parts of the sternocleidomastoid and trapezius muscles. Impairment of this nerve is judged according to the effects on swallowing and speech, which are considered in Chapter 11, Ear, Nose, Throat, and Related Structures. This nerve also can affect head turning and shoulder motion; related impairments are evaluated according to criteria in *Guides* Chapters 15, The Spine, and 16, The Upper Extremities.

13.4i Cranial Nerve XII—the Hypoglossal Nerve

This is a motor nerve that innervates the musculature of the tongue. Unilateral loss of function is not considered to be impairment. Bilateral loss may result in impaired swallowing, breathing, and speech articulation (see Table 13-14). Speech articulation and swallowing are considered in Chapter 11.

Table 13-14 Criteria for Rating Impairment of Cranial Nerves IX, X, and XII (Glossopharyngeal, Vagus, and Hypoglossal Nerves)

Class 1 1%-14% Impairment of the Whole Person	Class 2 15%-39% Impairment of the Whole Person	Class 3 40%-60% Impairment of the Whole Person
Mild dysarthria, dystonia, or dysphagia with choking on liquids or semisolid food	Moderately severe dysarthria or dysphagia with hoarseness, nasal regurgitation, and aspiration of liquids or semisolid foods	Severe inability to swallow or handle oral secretions without choking, with need for assistance and suctioning

Class 2
15%-39% Impairment of the Whole Person
Moderately severe dysarthria or dysphagia with hoarseness, nasal regurgitation, and aspiration of liquids or semisolid foods

Class 3
40%-60% Impairment of the Whole Person
Severe inability to swallow or handle oral secretions without choking, with need for assistance and suctioning

Example 13-37
15% to 39% Impairment Due to Amyotrophic Lateral Sclerosis

Subject: 45-year-old man.

History: Right-handed; individual has developed progressive weakness of the hands and legs with wasting of the musculature over the past 6 months.

Current Symptoms: Choking and frequent coughing during meals. Difficulty swallowing, with occasional nasal regurgitation of fluids and choking during meals. Voice has become hoarse and difficult to understand. He has lost 9.0 kg (20 lb).

Physical Exam: Severe wasting of the musculature of both hands; however, he can lift his arms and legs against gravity with difficulty. He was drooling from his mouth with a tenacious saliva, which he caught in a handkerchief. Speech was soft with poor articulation, and tongue showed wormlike fasciculations. He also had fasciculations of the hands, arms, and thighs. The deep-tendon reflexes were diminished in the arms and increased at the knee with up-going toes. No sensory impairments.

Clinical Studies: EMG: evidence of denervation by fibrillations, positive sharp waves, and increased insertional activity in all limbs. Neuroimaging and swallowing studies may be appropriate.

Diagnosis: Amyotrophic lateral sclerosis (ALS).

Impairment Rating: 39% impairment due to swallowing disorder associated with amyotrophic lateral sclerosis; combine with appropriate ratings due to other neurologic impairments to determine whole person impairment (see Combined Values Chart, p. 604).

Comment: The most disturbing and potentially dangerous symptom of this terrible condition is the individual's inability to control his secretions, putting him at risk for aspiration.

Example 13-38
40% to 60% Impairment Due to Nondominant-Side Hemiplegia and Hemianopia

Subject: 65-year-old woman.

History: Right-handed; 4 months ago, this hypertensive diabetic woman developed transient episodes of weakness and numbness of the left side of her face, arm, and leg, which progressed to a complete loss of motility and sensation on the left side.

Current Symptoms: Left-sided weakness, with inability to move the left arm or leg and loss of some movement of the left lower face. Difficulty controlling fluids, with frequent nasal regurgitation and aspiration, particularly of liquids or semisolids. Bedridden and requires assistance in all activities of daily living.

Physical Exam: Flaccid left hemiplegia; unable to elevate left arm or leg. Mild to moderate weakness of the left lower face, with drooling. Frequent choking and nasal regurgitation with liquids and semisolids. Confrontation fields show a dense left homonymous hemianopia. Decreased sensation to pin, cold, and vibration of the left arm and leg. Up-going toe on the left.

Clinical Studies: CT scan: large intracranial hemorrhage in the right basal ganglia thalamic area. Swallowing studies: unable to control secretions and aspiration of the dye.

Diagnosis: Late effect of CVA with nondominant side hemiplegia and hemianopia.

Impairment Rating: 60% impairment due to inability to swallow or handle oral secretions without choking due to nondominant-side hemiplegia; combine with appropriate ratings for other neurologic impairments to determine whole person impairment (see Combined Values Chart, p. 604).

Comment: This severe CVA has not improved and has left this woman completely dependent on others, bedridden, with frequent aspirations of her meals and medications.

13.5 Criteria for Rating Impairments of Station, Gait, and Movement Disorders

13.5a Station and Gait Disorders

Problems maintaining balance and a stable gait can develop from a CNS or peripheral neurologic impairment. On physical examination, the physician may observe loss of equal arm or leg movement, falling or staggering to one or the other side, inability to control starting or stopping, and arrhythmic body or extremity movements. Increased tone in the lower extremities from a CNS lesion such as traumatic brain injury, stroke, or multiple sclerosis may result in a spastic paraparesis or spasticity in one limb. Loss of station or Romberg sign (falling with eyes closed) may indicate dysfunction in the peripheral nerves or their ascending pathways to the brain. Peripheral neuropathy, identified by examination and electrodiagnostic tests, is frequently associated with complaints of imbalance or stumbling, since information from sensory receptors is altered.

Impairment ratings for station and gait disorders are determined according to the effect on ambulation (see Table 13-15). Other anatomic or functional changes from other body systems, such as the musculoskeletal system, are combined with the neurologic assessment for station and gait.

Table 13-15 Criteria for Rating Impairments Due to Station and Gait Disorders

Class 1 1%-9% Impairment of the Whole Person	Class 2 10%-19% Impairment of the Whole Person	Class 3 20%-39% Impairment of the Whole Person	Class 4 40%-60% Impairment of the Whole Person
Rises to standing position; walks, but has difficulty with elevations, grades, stairs, deep chairs, and long distances	Rises to standing position; walks some distance with difficulty and without assistance, but is limited to level surfaces	Rises and maintains standing position with difficulty; cannot walk without assistance	Cannot stand without help, mechanical support, and/or an assistive device

Chapter 13

Class 3
20%-39% Impairment of the Whole Person

Rises and maintains standing position with difficulty; cannot walk without assistance

Example 13-39
20% to 39% Impairment Due to Station and Gait Disorders

Subject: 50-year-old woman.

History: Right-handed; 6-month history of progressive weakness of arms and legs, with unsteady and falling gait.

Current Symptoms: Unable to walk without assistance; has difficulty rising from a chair.

Physical Exam: Wasting and loss of muscle mass, mainly in the distal extremities, with diminished deep-tendon reflexes in the arms and increased deep-tendon reflexes in the legs, with up-going toes. No sensory impairment. Unable to get out of a chair without assistance or to walk unaided without falling.

Clinical Studies: EMG: confirmed the motor neuron defect. CT myelogram of the cervical spine: negative for myelopathy secondary to spondylosis.

Diagnosis: Motor neuron disease, probable ALS.

Impairment Rating: 39% station and gait impairment due to motor neuron disease; combine with appropriate ratings due to other neurologic impairments to determine whole person impairment (see Combined Values Chart, p. 604).

Comment: The major impairment rating is based on the gait disorder, to be combined with the other neurologic impairments.

Class 4
40%-60% Impairment of the Whole Person

Cannot stand without help, mechanical support, and/or an assistive device

Example 13-40
40% to 60% Impairment Due to Station and Gait Disorders

Subject: 60-year-old man.

History: Right-handed; sudden onset of inability to use right arm and leg 4 months ago; subsequently wheelchair bound.

Current Symptoms: Able to ambulate only with assistance and needs help standing up.

Physical Exam: Spastic right hemiplegia with increased resistance to passive stretch. Distal weakness in the right hand and foot against gravity. Diminished rapid rhythmical alternating movements and hyperreflexia, with up-going toe. Hemisensory defect present. Uses a walker.

Clinical Studies: CT scan of the brain: left cerebral infarct without hemorrhage.

Diagnosis: Late effect of CVA with dominant-side hemiplegia.

Impairment Rating: 55% whole person station and gait impairment due to dominant-side hemiplegia; combine with appropriate ratings due to other neurologic impairments to determine whole person impairment (see Combined Values Chart, p. 604).

Comment: The cerebral functional loss needs to be combined with the dominant hemispheric hand problems and hemisensory defect (see Table 13-16).

13.5b Movement Disorders

Movement disturbances resulting from cerebral dysfunction are impairments that may affect activities of daily living. Mild tics may have no impact on daily activities, while other involuntary movements, such as tremors (resting, postural, and intention), chorea, athetosis, hemiballismus, and dystonia tone may prevent meaningful use of the extremity. Besides abnormal movements, difficulty with coordination for dexterous or precise movements may interfere with activity; these difficulties can develop from lesions in the basal ganglia or cerebellum. Coordinated movements include gait that may manifest as ataxia requiring use of an ancillary device. Movement disorders, therefore, are assessed for their interference with ADL as described in Tables 13-15, 13-16, and 13-17. For movement disorders affecting the lower extremities, use the station and gait section.

Chapter 13

13.6 Criteria for Rating Impairments of Upper Extremities Related to Central Impairment

The basic tasks of everyday living depend on dexterous use of the **dominant** upper **extremity.** Loss of use of that extremity results, in most instances, in greater impairment than would be the case with impairment of the limb on the nondominant side. Tables 13-16 and 13-17 are used to rate upper extremity dysfunction from any lesion in the brain. Use these tables for rating upper extremity dysfunction, manifested by weakness, tremor, or pain, that affects ADL. The upper extremity impairment may result from, but is not limited to, traumatic brain injury, stroke, neurodegenerative diseases (eg, Parkinson's disease, progressive supranuclear palsy), multiple sclerosis, and sequelae of CNS infection.

When the spinal cord disorder affects both upper extremities, the individual's impairment is greater than indicated by a simple combination of impairments of the dominant and nondominant extremities. For these cases, Chapter 15, which covers neurologic impairment from spinal cord disorders, and other sections in this chapter should be used.

The impairment ratings given in Tables 13-16 and 13-17 are determined from neurologic examination of motor strength, coordination, and dexterity. Functional activities such as buttoning a shirt, lacing shoes, writing, and performing a pegboard task can assess abilities needed for daily activities.

Table 13-16 Criteria for Rating Impairment of One Upper Extremity

Class 1		Class 2		Class 3		Class 4	
Dominant Extremity 1%-9% Impairment of the Whole Person	Nondominant Extremity 1%-4% Impairment of the Whole Person	Dominant Extremity 10%-24% Impairment of the Whole Person	Nondominant Extremity 5%-14% Impairment of the Whole Person	Dominant Extremity 25%-39% Impairment of the Whole Person	Nondominant Extremity 15%-29% Impairment of the Whole Person	Dominant Extremity 40%-60% Impairment of the Whole Person	Nondominant Extremity 30%-45% Impairment of the Whole Person
Individual can use the involved extremity for self-care, daily activities, and holding, but has difficulty with digital dexterity		Individual can use the involved extremity for self-care, can grasp and hold objects with difficulty, but has no digital dexterity		Individual can use the involved extremity but has difficulty with self-care activities		Individual cannot use the involved extremity for self-care or daily activities	

Class 3 Dominant Extremity: 25%-39% Impairment of the Whole Person
Individual can use the involved extremity but has difficulty with self-care activities

Class 4 Dominant Extremity: 40%-60% Impairment of the Whole Person
Individual cannot use the involved extremity for self-care or daily activities

Example 13-41
39% Impairment Due to Dominant-Side Hemiplegia

Subject: 60-year-old man.

History: Right-handed; sudden onset of inability to use right arm and leg 4 months ago; subsequently wheelchair bound.

Current Symptoms: Able to ambulate only with assistance and needs help standing up.

Physical Exam: Spastic right hemiplegia with increased resistance to passive stretch. Distal weakness in the right hand and foot against gravity. Diminished rapid rhythmical alternating movements and hyperreflexia with up-going toe. Hemisensory defect present. Uses a walker and has difficulties with many activities of daily living.

Clinical Studies: CT scan of the brain: left cerebral infarct without hemorrhage.

Diagnosis: Late effects of CVA with dominant-side hemiplegia.

Impairment Rating: 39% impairment due to dominant-side upper limb hemiplegia; combine with appropriate ratings due to other neurologic impairments to determine whole person impairment (see Combined Values Chart, p. 604).

Comment: This individual also had a 55% impairment for gait that, when combined with the 39% impairment for hemiplegia, equals 73% whole person impairment.

Example 13-42
60% Impairment Due to Dominant-Side Hemiplegia

Subject: 55-year-old man.

History: Right-handed; severe sudden onset of right hemiplegia, hemisensory defect, and hemianopia 5 months ago. Minimal improvement in orientation, in communication, and of lateral neurologic impairments.

Current Symptoms: Dependent on others for ADL, including feeding, toileting care, and dressing. Unable to clearly express himself and profess needs. Generalized weakness, in addition to hemiplegia, make individual wheelchair bound with the need for transfer aids.

Physical Exam: Paresis and flaccidity of right arm and leg with persistence of sensory loss and hemianopia. Total dependence on others for all ADL.

Clinical Studies: CT scan: massive intracerebral hemorrhage, bilateral with effacement on ventricles. EEG: bilateral delta slow waves without discharges.

Diagnosis: Late effect of CVA with dysphasia, dominant-side hemiplegia, and homonymous hemianopia.

Impairment Rating: 60% impairment due to dominant-side hemiplegia; combine with appropriate ratings due to other neurologic impairments to determine whole person impairment (see Combined Values Chart, p. 604).

Comment: Involvement of the extremity secondary to a central lesion needs to be combined with ratings from the other tables, including dysphasia (Table 13-7), gait (Table 13-15), and vision impairments (Tables 13-9 and 13-10).

Chapter 13

Table 13-17 Criteria for Rating Impairments of Two Upper Extremities

Class 1 1%-19% Impairment of the Whole Person	Class 2 20%-39% Impairment of the Whole Person	Class 3 40%-79% Impairment of the Whole Person	Class 4 80%+ Impairment of the Whole Person
Individual can use both upper extremities for self-care, grasping, and holding, but has difficulty with digital dexterity	Individual can use both upper extremities for self-care, can grasp and hold objects with difficulty, but has no digital dexterity	Individual can use both upper extremities but has difficulty with self-care activities	Individual cannot use upper extremities

Class 4 80%+ Impairment of the Whole Person
Individual cannot use upper extremities

Example 13-43
80% Impairment of Both Upper Extremities

Subject: 50-year-old woman.

History: Right-handed; 6-month history of progressive weakness of arms and legs, with unsteady and falling gait.

Current Symptoms: Unable to walk without assistance; has difficulty rising from a chair.

Physical Exam: Wasting and loss of muscle mass, mainly in the distal extremities, with diminished deep-tendon reflexes in the arms and increased deep-tendon reflexes in the legs, with up-going toes. No sensory impairment. Unable to get out of a chair without assistance or to walk unaided without falling. Unable to perform activities of daily living.

Clinical Studies: EMG: confirmed the motor neuron defect. CT myelogram of the cervical spine: negative for myelopathy secondary to spondylosis.

Diagnosis: Motor neuron disease, probable ALS.

Impairment Rating: 80% whole person bilateral upper extremity severe impairment due to motor neuron disease; combine with appropriate ratings due to other neurologic impairments to determine whole person impairment (see the Combined Values Chart, p. 604; 80% and 39% for gait impairment = 88% whole person impairment).

Comment: The major impairment rating is based on the gait disorder, to be combined with the other neurologic impairments.

13.7 Criteria for Rating Spinal Cord and Related Impairments

The spinal cord conveys nerve impulses for motor, sensory, and visceral functions. Disorders of impulse transmission can result in permanent impairment. The magnitude of the impairment is estimated according to the effects on the ability to perform activities of daily living and the results of neurologic examination and testing. See Chapter 15, The Spine, for spine impairment rating by neurologic level of involvement.

Impairments resulting from spinal cord injuries and other adverse conditions include those relating to station and gait, use of the upper extremities, respiration, urinary bladder function, anorectal function, sexual function, and pain.

Sensory disturbances, including the loss of sense of touch, sense of pain, temperature perception, and sense of vibration and joint position, and paresthesias, dysesthesias, and phantom limb sensations may indicate spinal cord dysfunction. Autonomic system disorders, including disturbances in sweating patterns, regulation of circulation, and regulation of temperature, may occur. Impairment is determined according to the amount of functional impairment and the level of involvement.

When an individual with a spinal cord injury has impairments of several functions or systems, for instance, those of station and gait (Table 13-15), as with hemiparesis and ataxia; of dexterity in using the upper extremity (Tables 13-16 and 13-17); and of bladder, bowel, or sexual functioning, the Combined Values Chart (p. 604) should be used to combine the whole person impairment estimates for the several functions.

Accompanying disorders, such as trophic lesions, urinary calculi, osteoporosis, nutritional disturbances, infections, and reactive psychological states, may occur. The degree to which any of these conditions augments spinal cord impairment should be based on the criteria given in the *Guides* chapters dealing with those disorders.

13.7a Respiratory System Neurologic Impairments

Neurologic impairment of one's ability to breathe is considered in Table 13-18 only in terms of neurologic limitations. Other aspects of respiratory function are covered in Chapter 5, The Respiratory System.

Table 13-18 Criteria for Rating Neurologic Impairment of Respiration

Class 1 5%-19% Impairment of the Whole Person	Class 2 20%-49% Impairment of the Whole Person	Class 3 50%-89% Impairment of the Whole Person	Class 4 90%+ Impairment of the Whole Person
Individual can breathe spontaneously but has difficulty performing activities of daily living that require exertion	Individual is capable of spontaneous respiration but is restricted to sitting, standing, or limited ambulation	Individual is capable of spontaneous respiration but to such a limited degree that he or she is confined to bed	Individual has no capacity for spontaneous respiration

13.7b Urinary System Neurologic Impairments

The ability to control bladder emptying provides the criterion for evaluating permanent bladder impairment resulting from spinal cord and central nervous system disorders (see Table 13-19). Documentation by cystometric or other tests may be necessary.

When evaluating impairments of the bladder, the physician also must consider the status of the upper urinary tract. Refer to Chapter 7, The Urinary and Reproductive Systems, and apply the Combined Values Chart (p. 604) if impairments of several organ systems are present.

Table 13-19 Criteria for Rating Neurologic Impairment of the Bladder

Class 1 1%-9% Impairment of the Whole Person	Class 2 10%-24% Impairment of the Whole Person	Class 3 25%-39% Impairment of the Whole Person	Class 4 40%-60% Impairment of the Whole Person
Individual has some degree of voluntary control but is impaired by urgency or intermittent incontinence	Individual has good bladder reflex activity, limited capacity, and intermittent emptying without voluntary control	Individual has poor bladder reflex activity, intermittent dribbling, and no voluntary control	Individual has no reflex or voluntary control of bladder

13.7c Anorectal System Neurologic Impairments

The ability to control emptying provides the criterion for evaluating permanent impairment of the anus and rectum due to spinal cord or other neurologic dysfunction (see Table 13-20).

Table 13-20 Criteria for Rating Neurologic Anorectal Impairment

Class 1 1%-19% Impairment of the Whole Person	Class 2 20%-39% Impairment of the Whole Person	Class 3 40%-50% Impairment of the Whole Person
Individual has reflex regulation but only limited voluntary control	Individual has reflex regulation but no voluntary control	Individual has no reflex regulation or voluntary control

13.7d Sexual System Neurologic Impairments

Awareness and capability of having an orgasm are the criteria for evaluating permanent impairment of sexual functioning that may result from spinal cord or other neurologic system disorders (see Table 13-21). The individual's previous sexual functioning should be considered by the physician; age is only one criterion for evaluating previous sexual functioning. Adjust for age according to criteria outlined in Chapter 7, The Urinary and Reproductive Systems.

Table 13-21 Criteria for Rating Neurologic Sexual Impairment

Class 1 1%-9% Impairment of the Whole Person	Class 2 10%-19% Impairment of the Whole Person	Class 3 20% Impairment of the Whole Person
Sexual functioning is possible, but with difficulty of erection or ejaculation in men or lack of awareness, excitement, or lubrication in either sex	Reflex sexual functioning is possible, but there is no awareness	No sexual functioning

13.8 Criteria for Rating Impairments Related to Chronic Pain

Impairment due primarily to intractable pain may greatly influence an individual's ability to function. Psychological factors can influence the degree and perception of pain: different individuals in similar circumstances may be impaired by pain to different degrees. A chronic pain syndrome may follow thalamic lesions, but this is rare. Chronic pain in this section covers the diagnoses of causalgia, posttraumatic neuralgia, and reflex sympathetic dystrophy. The new term *complex regional pain syndrome,* type I and type II, is not used here since it does not represent a single diagnostic criterion.[16]

Causalgia is burning pain that develops in a distal extremity following trauma to a peripheral nerve. The burning pain is triggered by movement, light mechanical stimuli to the skin, and strong emotion. Other features include distal extremity swelling and skin that is smooth, mottled, cold, and sweaty. Sympathetic block frequently relieves the pain. In posttraumatic neuralgia, the burning pain in the distribution of a nerve does not have the other clinical features and does not spread.

Reflex sympathetic dystrophy (RSD) occurs without known nerve lesions and is precipitated by minor soft tissue trauma. Burning spontaneous pain and stimulus-evoked pain are most pronounced in the distal limb (allodynia, hyperpathia, and hyperalgesia). The affected limb is usually warmer acutely (less than 6 months) and then is colder. It is now generally believed that a central nervous system abnormality is present based on the autonomic changes of abnormal sweating and skin blood flow. The acute distal swelling usually responds to sympathetic block. In the chronic stage, trophic changes include alteration in nail and hair growth, thin shiny skin, osteoporosis, and restriction of passive movement. Postural or action tremor is not uncommon, while an associated movement disorder is relatively rare.

To rate these conditions for impairment, diagnosis is key and is based on clinical criteria. Besides the clinical findings previously described, a three-phase bone scan may show increased uptake in the acute and subacute periods. This study is known to have low sensitivity, 50%,[17] and therefore cannot be used as a required criterion for the diagnosis. Plain x-rays may show patchy demineralization, particularly in a periarticular distribution, within months of the onset of RSD. Altered blood flow by laser Doppler flowmetry and abnormal function in the sudomotor reflex also support the diagnosis. It is difficult to examine individuals who are experiencing these symptoms; therefore, once the criteria for the diagnosis have been met, the impact on ADL is determined.

To rate an impairment for causalgia, posttraumatic neuralgia, and RSD in an upper extremity, use Table 13-22. If a lower extremity needs to be rated for casualgia, posttraumatic neuralgia, or RSD, use the station and gait impairment criteria given in Table 13-15.

Table 13-22 Criteria for Rating Impairment Related to Chronic Pain in One Upper Extremity

Class 1		Class 2		Class 3		Class 4	
Dominant Extremity 1%-9% Impairment of the Whole Person	**Nondominant Extremity 1%-4% Impairment of the Whole Person**	**Dominant Extremity 10%-24% Impairment of the Whole Person**	**Nondominant Extremity 5%-14% Impairment of the Whole Person**	**Dominant Extremity 25%-39% Impairment of the Whole Person**	**Nondominant Extremity 15%-29% Impairment of the Whole Person**	**Dominant Extremity 40%-60% Impairment of the Whole Person**	**Nondominant Extremity 30%-45% Impairment of the Whole Person**
Individual can use the involved extremity for self-care, daily activities, and holding, but is limited in digital dexterity		Individual can use the involved extremity for self-care and can grasp and hold objects with difficulty, but has no digital dexterity		Individual can use the involved extremity but has difficulty with self-care activities		Individual cannot use the involved extremity for self-care or daily activities	

> **Class 3**
> **Dominant Extremity: 25%-39% Impairment of the Whole Person**
>
> Individual can use the involved extremity but has difficulty with self-care activities

Example 13-44
25% to 39% Impairment Due to Posttraumatic Neuralgia of the Superficial Radial Nerve

Subject: 45-year-old man.

History: Right-handed; developed burning pain in the distribution of the right superficial radial nerve following a routine venipuncture. Use of a transcutaneous electrical nerve stimulation (TENS) unit provided some relief.

Current Symptoms: Pain increases with attempts to grip or pinch the right hand. Pain is limited to the distribution of the superficial radial nerve. Difficulty using the right hand for bathing, dressing, combing hair, and writing.

Physical Exam: Right hand is cold, edematous, with trophic changes and hyperesthesia over the radial distribution.

Diagnosis: Posttraumatic neuralgia of the superficial radial nerve secondary to injury.

Impairment Rating: 25% impairment of the whole person.

Comment: Because of its location, damage to the superficial radial nerve occurs from glass, knives, power saws, and surgeries, especially de Quervain's tenosynovectomy. This condition can be so severe that some ADL are not possible.

> **Class 4**
> **Dominant Extremity: 40%-60% Impairment of the Whole Person**
>
> Individual cannot use the involved extremity for self-care or daily activities

Example 13-45
40% to 60% Impairment Due to Reflex Sympathetic Dystrophy

Subject: 30-year-old woman.

History: Right-handed; right carpal tunnel release 1 year ago. While recovering from the surgery, she developed diffuse burning pain in the hand, extending to the forearm, accompanied by swelling of the right hand. Several stellate ganglion blocks temporarily relieved the pain and reduced the swelling. Over time, she noted color changes and increased sweating; the hand was always cold, and movement of the fingers and wrist was limited. A TENS unit was used constantly, along with medication, to control the pain.

Current Symptoms: Deep burning pain, increased sweating, right arm weakness, and inability to use the hand for any daily activities.

Physical Exam: Right arm held close to the body in a protected fashion. The hand is dusky with a sweaty palm, and the skin is thinned. Fingers are tightly adducted and cannot be separated. Attempts to move the wrist produce allodynia (occurrence of pain from a painless stimulus, eg, touch). Proximal muscles have poor tone and disuse atrophy.

Clinical Studies: Three-phase bone scan: unremarkable; plain radiograph: diffuse demineralization.

Diagnosis: Reflex sympathetic dystrophy (RSD).

Impairment Rating: 40% impairment of the whole person.

Comment: RSD does not have a preexisting psychological substrate; sufferers may become anxious and depressed because of failed therapies.

13.9 Criteria for Rating Impairments of the Peripheral Nervous System, Neuromuscular Junction, and Muscular System

Evaluating the peripheral nervous system requires documentation of the extent of loss of function due to sensory deficit, pain, or discomfort; loss of muscular strength and control of specific muscles or groups of muscles; and alteration of autonomic nervous system (ANS) control. Documentation of these deficiencies should include, if possible, descriptions of the abnormal finding on examinations of the spinal root(s), portion of the plexus, and/or peripheral nerve(s) that are involved. The mechanism or cause of the abnormality assists in determining the impairment duration and probable prognosis. Ancillary testing by neuroimaging (CT scans, MRIs, radiographs) and physiologic (EMG, nerve conduction velocity [NCV], and evoked responses) tests, may assist in reaching final conclusions.

Neurologic evaluation of pain is based first on the individual's description of the character, location, intensity, duration, and persistence of the discomfort and on verification of the anatomic distribution of the neurologic defect. A description of the ways and the degrees to which the pain interferes with the individual's performance of activities of daily living and the factors that augment the discomfort should be included. Anatomic descriptions should be made according to the usual distributions of the roots, plexuses, and nerves of the nervous system when the distal digital nerves are being evaluated, especially in the hand, as indicated in Chapters 15 and 16.

Grading procedures for sensory and motor impairments in single distal digital nerves of the hand are found in Chapter 16, The Upper Extremities. For evaluations of neurologic problems of the peripheral neuromuscular system, the standard techniques of neurologic examination are used (see Tables 13-23 and 13-24). The muscle strength grading system (Table 13-24) is similar to the system recommended by the Medical Research Council of the United Kingdom. Involvement of peripheral nerves or roots may lead to paralysis or weakness of the muscles supplied by them, as well as to characteristic sensory changes. The system of the Medical Research Council[18] is the one recommended in the *Guides* for evaluating muscle function and testing impairments (Table 13-23). In this system, movement of the part is tested against the examiner's resistance plus gravity, without the effect of gravity, against gravity, and for slight or no movement. The contralateral extremity is tested also, and the results are compared with those in the affected limb.

Symptoms of sensory deficits and pain in peripheral nerves as described in Chapter 16, The Upper Extremities, include anesthesia, hypesthesia, dysesthesia, paresthesia, hyperesthesia, cold intolerance, and an intense, burning pain. Sensory dysfunction associated with peripheral nerve disorders is evaluated according to the following criteria: (1) How does the pain or sensory deficit interfere with the individual's performance of daily activities? (2) To what extent does the pain or sensory deficit follow the defined anatomic pathways of the root, plexus, or peripheral nerve? (3) To what extent does the description of the

pain or sensory deficit indicate that it is caused by a peripheral nerve abnormality? (4) To what extent does the pain or sensory deficit correspond to other disturbances of the involved nerve structure? *Only persistent pain or discomfort that leads to permanent loss of function, in spite of maximum effort toward medical rehabilitation and allowing an optimal period of time for physiologic adjustment, should be evaluated as a permanent impairment. Pain that does not meet more than one of the above criteria is not considered to be within the scope of this section.*

Pain is defined in Chapter 18 as "an unpleasant sensory and emotional experience associated with actual or potential tissue damage or described in terms of such damage." Pain is a subjective symptom and is difficult to evaluate, but its presence, anatomic background, and intensity may be verified with a thorough examination. Chronic pain for causalgia, posttraumatic neuralgia, and RSD is evaluated in Table 13-22.

Motivation and malingering as they may relate to the presence or absence of an impairment or a supposed impairment are considered in Chapter 14, Mental and Behavioral Disorders.

Sensory dysfunction, to be rated, must be considered permanent. The methodology used for spinal nerves, brachial plexus, and individual nerves is described below. Terms used to describe sensory impairment that may not be readily apparent to all readers are defined. *Sensation* refers to the sensory perception of the primary sensory modalities, pain, heat, cold, and touch, those involved in protective sensation. *Sensibility* refers to the discriminative features of sensation such as graphesthesia, stereognosis, or two-point discrimination. The issue of sensibility is important to the normal function of the hand. This is why sensory loss in the digits is focused on impaired two-point discrimination (see Table 16-10).

Grading procedures for sensory and/or motor impairments in all peripheral nerves (except sensory loss in the digits (Table 16-10) is found in Tables 13-23 and 13-24. The maximum impairment for spinal roots, brachial plexus, and individual nerves is noted under the respective sections below.

13.9a Roots of Spinal Nerves

Spinal nerves are evaluated by loss of function in the peripheral nerve that receives contribution from the involved spinal root. If two or more spinal roots are involved, the increased loss of function from the contribution of two spinal roots to a peripheral nerve necessitates that the impairment be rated according to the brachial plexus (see Section 13.8b).

Table 16-13 provides the maximum upper extremity impairment due to unilateral sensory or motor deficits of individual spinal roots C5 through T1. Once the sensory deficit or pain is estimated according to Table 13-23 and motor deficit according to 13-24, these percent deficits in the upper extremity are multiplied by the respective maximum sensory and/or motor impairments of the spinal nerve in question, Table 16-18. The sensory and motor impairments are combined using the Combined Values Chart, p. 604, for the total upper extremity impairment, which is then converted to whole person impairment (Table 16-3). If deficits are bilateral, the whole person impairment is found for each extremity and then combined using the Combined Values Chart.

For the spinal roots in the lower extremity, L3 through S1, use Table 15-18 to determine the maximum lower

extremity impairment due to unilateral sensory or motor deficits. Follow the same procedure already outlined for the upper extremity with regard to grading the impairment; use Tables 13-23 and 13-24, then multiply by the maximum loss of function for the nerve root in question and combine sensory and motor impairment and convert to whole person impairment.

13.9b Brachial Plexus

The anatomy of the brachial plexus and clinical presentation resulting from lesions that involve the upper and lower trunk are presented in Section 16.5b. Table 16-14 provides the maximum impairment due to unilateral sensory or motor deficits of the brachial plexus by the entire brachial plexus and the upper, middle, and lower trunks. If there is partial recovery, individual muscles are graded according to Table 13-24. This value is multiplied by the maximum upper extremity impairment for the nerve innervating

Table 13-23 Classification and Procedure for Determining Impairment Due to Pain or Sensory Deficit Resulting From Peripheral Nerve Disorders

Classification			
Class 1 **0% Sensory Impairment**	**Class 2** **1%-10% Sensory Impairment**	**Class 3** **11%-25% Sensory Impairment**	**Class 4** **26%-60% Sensory Impairment**
No loss of sensation, abnormal sensation, or pain	Normal sensation except for pain, or decreased sensation with or without pain, forgotten during activity	Normal sensation except for pain, or decreased sensation with or without pain, present during activity	Decreased sensation with or without pain, interfering with activity

Procedure

1. Identify the area of involvement using the dermatome charts in Chapter 16 (Figures 16-48 and 16-49).

2. Identify the nerve, part of plexus, or root that innervates the area.

3. Find the value for maximum loss of function of the specific nerve or root due to pain or loss of sensation using the appropriate table in Chapter 16, The Upper Extremities, and Chapter 17, The Lower Extremities. Use Table 16-13 for the cervical roots; Table 16-14 for the brachial plexus; Table 16-15 for upper extremity nerves; Table 15-20 for the lumbosacral roots; and Table 17-37 for the lower extremity nerves.

4. Grade the degree of decreased sensation or pain according to the classification given in Table 13-23.

5. Multiply the percentage associated with the nerve identified in step 3 above by the percentage associated with the decreased sensation.

6. Determine other nerve impairments using the same procedure; combine the impairments using the Combined Values Chart (p. 604) to determine whole person impairment of the nervous system.

the muscle listed in Table 16-15. Results from all the muscles are combined using the Combined Values Chart, p. 604, and the total upper extremity impairment converted to a whole person impairment, Table 16-3. A very useful diagram that demonstrates the motor innervation of all muscles in the upper extremity by spinal roots, peripheral nerve, and anatomical proximal-distal location in the upper extremity is found on Figure 16-47.

13.9c Peripheral Nerve Impairments

This section is used to rate sensory and motor impairments from individual nerve lesions or multiple nerve disorders such as polyneuropathy or mononeuritis multiplex. Grading procedures for sensory and motor impairments resulting from peripheral nerve disorders in the upper and lower extremities are found in Tables 13-23 and 13-24. This percent impairment is multiplied by the appropriate maximum loss of function for the nerve in

question due to sensory deficit and pain or motor deficit, Table 16-15 for the upper extremity and Table 17-37 for the lower extremity. Sensory and motor impairments of the upper extremity are combined using the Combined Values Chart, page 604. The result is converted to a whole person impairment, Table 16-3.

If multiple nerves are involved in one extremity, the same procedure is followed for each nerve. Once the sensory and motor impairments for each nerve have been combined using the Combined Values Chart, all the nerves rated in one extremity are combined, again using the Combined Values Chart to determine the total impairment in the affected limb. If more than one limb is involved, each total extremity impairment is converted to a whole person impairment (Table 16-3), and these values are again combined using the Combined Values Chart.

Class 5 61%-80% Sensory Impairment	Class 6 81%-95% Sensory Impairment
Decreased sensation with or without pain or minor causalgia that may prevent activity	Decreased sensation with severe pain or major causalgia that prevents activity

Chapter 13

Table 13-24 Classification and Procedure for Determining Nervous System Impairment Due to Loss of Muscle Power and Motor Function Resulting From Peripheral Nerve Disorders

Classification

Class 1 0% Motor Deficit	Class 2 1%-25% Motor Deficit	Class 3 26%-50% Motor Deficit	Class 4 51%-75% Motor Deficit
Active movement against gravity with full resistance	Active movement against gravity with some resistance	Active movement against gravity only, without resistance	Active movement with gravity eliminated

Procedure

1. Identify the motion involved, such as flexion or extension.

2. Identify the muscle(s) performing the motion and the motor nerve(s) involved.

3. Grade the severity of motor deficit of the individual muscles according to the classification given above.

4. Find the maximum impairment due to the motor deficit for each nerve structure involved, as listed in Chapter 16, The Upper Extremities, and Chapter 17, The Lower Extremities: (Table 16-15), brachial plexus (Table 16-14), lower extremity nerves (Table 17-37), and lumbosacral nerves (Table 15-20).

5. Multiply the severity of the motor deficit by the percentage associated with the nerve(s) identified in step 4 above to obtain the estimated impairment from strength deficit for each structure involved.

Example 13-46
5% Impairment Due to Mononeuropathy in the Lower Extremity

Subject: 60-year-old woman.

History: Individual has diabetes mellitus; developed a persistent and painful numbness of the right lower extremity over a 6-month period.

Current Symptoms: Dysesthesias involve the lateral aspect of the lower leg and extend in a more severe fashion down to the dorsum of the foot.

Physical Exam: Decreased perception of pinpoint, cold, and light touch on the dorsum of the foot extending to the upper lateral calf area; painful paresthesias and dysesthesias of the foot; and mild weakness of dorsiflexion of the foot with a mild foot drop, characteristic of a peroneal nerve neuropathy. Able to ambulate without a cane.

Clinical Studies: Nerve conduction studies: abnormal right peroneal nerve indicated focal slowing of the motor conduction velocity across the head of the fibula.

Diagnosis: Mononeuropathy of the peroneal nerve secondary to diabetes mellitus.

Impairment Rating: 5% impairment of the whole person.

Comment: Method used to arrive at impairment rating:

Loss of function due to motor involvement of the common peroneal nerve (strength): Maximum motor loss in the peroneal nerve is 15% whole person impairment (Table 17-37) × 25% motor deficit, grade 4 (Table 13-24) = 4% whole person impairment.

Loss of function due to sensory involvement of common peroneal nerve: 25% representing sensory loss (Table 13-23) × 2% representing sensory function of common peroneal nerve (Table 17-37) = 0.5%, or 1% whole person impairment (rounded).

A 4% whole person impairment combined with a 1% whole person impairment is a 5% whole person impairment (see the Combined Values Chart, p. 604).

Class 5 76%-99% Motor Deficit	Class 6 100% Motor Deficit
Slight contraction and no movement	No contraction

Example 13-47
31% Impairment Due to Sensorimotor Polyneuropathy

Subject: 35-year-old man.

History: Prolonged episode of severe nausea, vomiting, and diarrhea, followed by onset of intense paresthesias, burning pain, and muscle tenderness.

Current Symptoms: Paresthesias in extremities with weakness in the feet and—less so—in the hands. Gait is unsteady

Physical Exam: Weakness more profound distally than proximally in the limb. Reflexes diminished in the upper extremities and difficult to obtain at the knees and ankles. Sensory examination intact for pin but diminished for vibration and joint position in the feet and hands. Mees' lines in the fingernails and toenails; desquamating brown rash on the palms and soles.

Clinical Studies: Nerve conduction studies 2 months after the onset of symptoms: no motor or sensory responses. Needle EMG: spontaneous activity (denervation potentials) in the distal muscles with impaired recruitment. Pancytopenia with basophilic stippling of the red blood cells. Elevated arsenic levels present in the hair and nails.

Diagnosis: Arsenic neuropathy involving motor and sensory fibers.

Impairment Rating: 31% impairment due to sensorimotor polyneuropathy; combine with appropriate ratings due to other neurologic impairments to determine whole person impairment. See method used to arrive at impairment rating below.

Comment: The presentation of a distal dying-back neuropathy, as in this case of arsenic neuropathy, is typical of the majority of toxic neuropathies. Removal from exposure is associated with improvement of findings in the peripheral nervous system, but the amount of recovery is related to the severity of the initial insult. As in this case, significant distal weakness in the intrinsic muscles of the hands and feet and moderate weakness in the dorsiflexors and plantar flexors were present 1 year later. Diminished vibration in a stocking-glove distribution and position sense continued to interfere with gait and the performance of dexterous activities with the hands. The individual complained of ongoing dysesthesia in the soles and cramping in the calves. Before rating an impairment following neurotoxic exposure, adequate time must pass to allow for recovery to a relatively stable plateau.

Chapter 13

Method:
1. *Loss of motor function in the distal muscles of the tibial nerve and peroneal nerve in the feet.* The maximum motor loss (Table 17-37) for the medial plantar is 2% whole person impairment and for the lateral plantar is 2% whole person impairment × 25% = grade 4 motor loss (Table 13-24) = 1% for the medial plantar and 1% for the lateral plantar. The maximum motor loss (Table 17-37) for the peroneal nerve in the foot of 5% whole person impairment (5% maximum motor loss is attributed to the foot since the entire common peroneal motor impairment is 15% in Table 17-37) × 25% = grade 4 motor loss (Table 13-24) = 1%. The total motor impairment in the distal muscles of one lower extremity is 1% and 1% and 1% = 3% whole person impairment.

2. *Loss of function due to sensory involvement of the medial and lateral plantar nerves, sural nerve, and superficial peroneal nerves.* The maximum sensory loss (Table 17-37) is 2% for the medial plantar and 2% for the lateral plantar is 2% × 40% = class 4 sensory loss (Table 13-23) = 1% for the medial plantar and 1% for the lateral plantar. The maximum sensory loss (Table 17-37) for the sural nerve is 1% × 40% = class 4 sensory loss (Table 13-23) = 0.4%, which is equal to 0% for the sural nerve. The maximum sensory loss (Table 17-37) for the superficial peroneal nerve is 2% × 40% = class 4 sensory loss (Table 13-24) = 1% for the superficial peroneal nerve. The total sensory impairment in the foot is 1% and 1% + 0% and 1% = 3% whole person impairment (see the Combined Values Chart, p. 604).

3. *Loss of motor function in the hand from median and ulnar nerve dysfunction.* The maximum motor loss for the median nerve is 10% (Table 16-15) × 15% from grade 4 motor loss (Table 13-24) = 1.5% or 2% of the upper extremity impairment. The maximum motor loss for the ulnar nerve is 35% (Table 16-15) × 15% from grade 4 motor loss (Table 13-24) = 5%. The total motor impairment in the hand is 2% and 5% = 7% whole person impairment (see the Combined Values Chart, p. 604).

4. *Loss of sensory function in the hand from median and ulnar nerve dysfunction.* The maximum sensory loss for the median nerve of 38% (Table 16-15) × 15% from class 3 sensory loss (Table 13-23) = 6% of the upper extremity or 4% whole person impairment (Table 16-3). The maximum sensory loss for the ulnar nerve of 7% (Table 16-15) × 15% from class 3 sensory loss (Table 13-23) = 1% of the upper extremity or 1% whole person impairment. The total sensory impairment in the hand is 4% and 1% = 5% whole person impairment.

5. Using the Combined Values Chart (p. 604), the motor and sensory impairment for the foot is 3% and 3% = 6% whole person impairment. The motor and sensory impairment in the hand is 7% and 5% = 12% whole person impairment. Since a sensorimotor polyneuropathy is a symmetric lesion, the 6% and 12% = 17% for one side is doubled to 17% and 17% = 31% whole person impairment.

13.9d Neuromuscular Impairments

Neuromuscular impairment as present in long-standing myasthenia gravis or myasthenic syndromes is accompanied by proximal weakness; impairment is rated by the impact on activities of daily living. For the lower extremities, station and gait are rated as described in activities of Table 13-15. The upper extremities are rated using Tables 13-16 and 13-17, which provide criteria for functional loss in one or both upper extremities.

13.9e Muscular Impairments

This is a varied group of disorders that includes muscular dystrophy, metabolic myopathy, abnormal potassium metabolism and muscle disease, endocrine myopathies, and inflammatory muscle disease. The unifying clinical feature is proximal weakness that, in some cases, may involve the neck and face. The proximal weakness is best rated by its effect on the activities of daily living. See Table 13-15 for the lower extremities and Tables 13-16 and 13-17 for functional loss in one or both upper extremities.

Neuromuscular and muscular impairments for the lower extremities are rated using Tables 17-6 and 17-8 (Chapter 17). Also, Table 13-15 is useful when gait is the most significant impairment from the neuromuscular or muscular disorder.

13.9f The Autonomic Nervous System

The autonomic nervous system (ANS) influences the functioning of many organ systems; thus, failure of the system can increase impairment. Neurologic conditions that have ANS involvement include polyneuropathy of various causes, familial dysautonomia, Landry-Guillain-Barré syndrome, syringomyelia, porphyria, cord and brain tumors, and myelopathy.

Lack of control of blood pressure, body thermal regulation, and bladder and bowel elimination are prominent signs of ANS failure. Impairments related to transient loss of awareness or consciousness after a period of cerebral ischemia may be due to various mechanisms, including orthostasis, reflex actions, or cardiopulmonary disorders, and may be estimated by means of Table 13-2. Referring to other *Guides* chapters also may be necessary to estimate the magnitudes of the impairments (Chapters 3 through 5).

Impairments of spinal nerves, roots, plexuses, or peripheral nerves by various diseases or injuries may be partial or complete, unilateral or bilateral, related to motor or sensory functions, with or without pain. Each of these attributes or characteristics should be evaluated. When there is bilateral involvement, the two unilateral impairments should be determined; then the Combined Values Chart (p. 604) should be used to estimate whole person impairment.

Chapter 13

13.10 Nervous System Impairment Evaluation Summary

See Table 13-25 for an evaluation summary for the assessment of nervous system impairments.

Table 13-25 Nervous System Impairment Evaluation Summary

Disorder	History, Including Selected Relevant Symptoms	Examination Record	Assessment of Neurologic Function
General	Neurologic symptoms may include: alterations in level of consciousness, confusion, memory loss, difficulties with language, headache, visual blurring, double vision, fatigue, facial pain and weakness, ringing in the ears, dizziness, vertigo, difficulty swallowing or speaking, weakness of one or multiple limbs, difficulty walking or climbing stairs, shooting pain, numbness and tingling in the extremities, tremor, loss of coordination, loss of bladder or rectal control, and sexual dysfunction Impact of symptoms on function and ability to do daily activities Review medical history	Constitutional; measure vital signs: blood pressure sitting or standing, supine blood pressure, pulse rate and regularity, respiration, temperature, height; examine visual, cardiovascular, musculoskeletal systems; assess gait and station, motor function, including muscle strength and tone in upper and lower extremities Evaluate higher integrative functions, orientation, recent and remote memory, attention span and concentration, language, fund of knowledge, cranial nerves II-XII Examine sensation (eg, touch, pinprick, vibration, proprioception), deep tendon reflexes, note pathologic reflexes Test coordination	Data derived from relevant studies (eg, EEG, lumbar puncture, neuropsychological assessment, evoked potentials, cartoid duplex examination, CT scan, MRI, MRA, PET, SPECT, NCV, EMG, quantitative sensory tests, automatic function assessment
Central Nervous System: **1. Consciousness Disorders** **2. Arousal Disorders** **3. Cognitive Impairments** **4. Language Disorders** **5. Behavioral or Emotional Disorders** **6. Cranial Nerve Disorders** **7. Station, Gait, and Movement Disorders** **8. Disorders of the Extremities** **9. Spinal Cord Disorders**	Discuss relevant symptoms and any resulting limitation of daily activities	See above physical exam Expand upon relevant areas	CT scan, MRI, EEG, etc
Neurologic Impairment With Chronic Pain	Discuss relevant symptoms and any resulting limitation of daily activities	See above physical exam See Chapter 18, Pain	Expand upon relevant areas Radiographs; bone scan; Doppler
Peripheral Nervous System: **1. Neuromuscular Junction Disorders** **2. Muscular System Disorders**	Discuss relevant symptoms and any resulting limitation of daily activities	See above physical exam Expand upon relevant areas	EMG; NCV

End-Organ Damage	Diagnosis	Degree of Impairment
Include assessment of sequelae, including end-organ damage and impairment	Record all pertinent diagnosis(es); note if they are at MMI; if not, discuss under what conditions and when stability is expected	Criteria outlined in this chapter
Assess relevant systems (eg, mental and behavioral, upper and lower extremities)	Epilepsy; seizures; syncope/dizziness; loss of awareness, sleep apnea; narcolepsy: periodic limb movements; dementia; traumatic brain injury; aphasia; dysphasia; cranial nerve disorders II-XII	See Tables 13-2 through 13-9, 13-14 through 13-18, and 13-21 through 13-24
Assess relevant systems (eg, mental and behavioral, pain)	Reflex sympathetic dystrophy; causalgia; posttraumatic neuralgia	See Table 13-22
Assess relevant systems (eg, upper and lower extremities)	Spinal root; brachial plexus; peripheral nerve; autonomic nervous system disorders	See Tables 13-23 and 13-24

References

1. Practice parameter: assessment and management of patients in the persistent vegetative state. In: *Practice Handbook*. St Paul, Minn: American Academy of Neurology; 1999:229-237.

2. Johns MW. A new method for measuring daytime sleepiness: the Epworth sleepiness scale. *Sleep.* 1991;14:540-545.

3. Katzman R, Brown T, Fuld P, Peck A, Schechter R, Schimmel H. Validation of a short orientation-memory-concentration test of cognitive impairment. *Am J Psychiatry.* 1983;140:734-739.

4. Kiernan RJ, Mueller J, Langston JW, et al. The Neurobehavioral Cognitive Status Examination: a brief but differentiated approach to cognitive assessment. *Ann Intern Med.* 1987;107:481-485.

5. Folstein M, Folstein S, McHugh P. "Mini-mental state"—a practical method for grading the cognitive state of patients for the clinician. *J Psychiatr Res.* 1975;12:189-198.

6. Wade DT, Collins C. The Barthel ADL index: a standard measure of physical disability? *Int Disability Stud.* 1988;10:64-67.

7. Blessed G, Tomlinson BE, Roth M. The association between quantitative measures of dementia and senile change in the cerebral grey matter of elderly subjects. *Br J Psychiatry.* 1968;114:797-811.

8. Berg L. Clinical dementia rating (CDR). *Psychopharmacol Bull.* 1988;24:637-639.

9. Hughes C, Berg L, Danizger W, Doben L, Martin R. A new clinical scale for the staging of dementia. *Br J Psychiatry.* 1982;140:566-572.

10. Morris JC, Heyman A, Mohs RC, et al. The Consortium to Establish a Registry for Alzheimer's Disease (CERAD). Part 1. Clinical and neuropsychological assessment of Alzheimer's disease. *Neurology.* 1989;39:1159-1165.

11. NIH Consensus Development Panel on Rehabilitation of Persons With Traumatic Brain Injury. Rehabilitation of persons with traumatic brain injury. NIH Consensus Statement 1998;16:1-41.

12. Strub RL, Black FW. *The Mental Status Examination in Neurology.* Philadelphia, Pa: FA Davis Company; 1983.

13. Holland A. *The Communicative Abilities in Daily Living* [manual]. Austin, Tex: Pro-Ed; 1980.

14. Cummings J, Mega M, Gary K, Rosenberg-Thompson S, Carusi D, Gornbein J. The neuropsychiatric inventory: comprehensive assessment of psychopathology in dementia. *Neurology.* 1994;44:2308-2314.

15. Doty RL. *The Smell Identification Test Administration Manual.* 3rd ed. Haddon Heights, NJ: Sensonics, Inc; 1995.

16. Baron R, Levine JD, Fields HL. Causalgia and reflex sympathetic dystrophy: does the sympathetic nervous system contribute to the generation of pain? *Muscle Nerve.* 1999;22:678-695.

17. Werner R, Davidoff G, Jackson D, Cremer S, Ventocilla C, Wolf L. Factors affecting the sensitivity and specificity of the three-phase technetium bone scan in the diagnosis of reflex sympathetic dystrophy syndrome in the upper extremity. *J Hand Surg.* 1989;14A:520-523.

18. Walton J, Gilliatt RW, Hutchinson M, et al, eds. *Aids to the Examination of the Peripheral Nervous System.* London, England: Bailliere Tindall; 1988.

Bibliography

General Neurology Techniques, and Autonomic Nervous System and Conditions

Adams RD, Victor M, Ropper AH. *Principles of Neurology.* 6th ed. New York, NY: McGraw-Hill; 1997.

Another good standard textbook of neurology.

Baker AB, Joynt RJ, eds. *Clinical Neurology.* Philadelphia, Pa: JB Lippincott Co; 1999.

A very good, continually edited four-volume text of neurology.

Bennett JC, Plum F, eds. *Cecil's Textbook of Medicine.* 20th ed. Philadelphia, Pa: WB Saunders Co; 1996.

A standard textbook of medicine with an excellent outline of the techniques of neurologic examinations and additional testing and an excellent summary of the autonomic nervous system.

Bleeker ML. *Occupational Neurology and Clinical Neurotoxicology.* Baltimore, Md: Williams & Wilkins; 1994.

A good textbook that covers occupational neurology. It focuses on all aspects related to neurologic outcomes associated with neurotoxic and ergonomic exposure.

Bradley WG, Daroff RB, Fenichel GM, Marsden CD, eds. *Neurology in Clinical Practice.* Vol 2. 3rd ed. Boston, Mass: Butterworth-Heinemann; 2000.

A newer textbook of neurology with an excellent section on autonomic nervous system evaluation.

Dawson DM, Hallett M, Wilbourn AJ. *Entrapment Neuropathies.* 3rd ed. Philadelphia, Pa: Lippincott-Raven; 1998.

An excellent reading book for the entrapment neuropathies, along with the standard textbook of neurology.

Goetz CG, Pappert EJ. *Textbook of Clinical Neurology.* Philadelphia, Pa: WB Saunders Company; 1999:70-80.

A good new textbook with CD-ROM examples of some neurologic situations.

Rowland LP, ed. *Merritt's Neurology.* 10th ed. New York, NY: Lippincott, Williams & Wilkins; 2000.

A very good, well-established, and current standard textbook of neurology.

Spencer PS, Schaumberg HH. *Experimental and Clinical Neurotoxicology.* New York, NY: Oxford University Press; 2000.

This is an excellent compendium of neurotoxic compounds and all their clinical manifestations. It also provides an in-depth discussion of pathophysiologic mechanisms.

Walton J, Gilliatt RW, Hutchinson M, et al, eds. *Aids to the Examination of the Peripheral Nervous System.* London, England: Bailliere Tindall; 1988.

The Medical Research Council post–World War II, which summarized the practical demonstrations of motor and sensory examinations only on CD-ROM.

Musculoskeletal/Orthopedic Reading Texts on Examination Techniques

Clark GL, Shaw Wilgis EF, Aiello B, Eckhaus D, Eddington LV. *Hand Rehabilitation, a Practical Guide.* New York, NY: Churchill Livingstone; 1993.

A very good orthopedic outline of the musculoskeletal techniques of neurologic evaluations of distal nerves and injuries.

Lister G. Reconstruction. In: *The Hand: Diagnosis and Indications.* 3rd ed. New York, NY: Churchill Livingstone; 1993:155-281.

Sunderland S. *Nerve Injuries and Their Repair.* New York, NY: Churchill Livingstone; 1991:305-329.

Organized Neuroanatomy in Segmental, Suprasegmental Orientation

Hausman L. *Clinical Neuroanatomy, Neurophysiology, and Neurology.* Springfield, Ill: CC Thomas; 1958.

A very comprehensive and practical outline. Hausman divides the nervous system into segments, intersegments, and suprasegments, contrary to the "ball and chain" methods of anatomy.

Multiple Sclerosis

Haber A, LaRocca N, eds. *Minimal Record of Disability for Multiple Sclerosis.* New York, NY: National Multiple Sclerosis Society; 1985.

Developed by International Federation of Multiple Sclerosis Societies.

Scheinberg L. Quantitative techniques in the assessment of multiple sclerosis: the problem and current solutions. In: Munsat T, ed. *Quantification of Neurologic Deficit.* Boston, Mass: Butterworth Publishers; 1989.

Traumatic Brain Injury

Cardenas AD. Institute of Medicine model of disability. NIH Consensus Development Conference, Bethesda, Md, October 26-28, 1998:97-99.

Entire Consensus Panel conclusions in publication.

Cooper PR. *Head Injury.* 3rd ed. Baltimore, Md: Williams & Wilkins; 1993.

Dobkin BH. Neurologic rehabilitation. In: *Contemporary Neurology Series #47.* Philadelphia, Pa: FA Davis; 1996.

Fraser RT, Clemmons DC. *Traumatic Brain Injury Rehabilitation: Practical Vocational, Neuropsychological, and Psychotherapy Interventions.* Boca Raton, Fla: CRC Press; 2000.

Autonomic Nervous System Reading in Addition to Neurologic Texts

Johnson RH, Lambie DG, Spalding JMK. The autonomic nervous system. In: Joynt RJ, ed. *Clinical Neurology.* Vol 4. Philadelphia, Pa: JB Lippincott Co; 1989.

Mathias CJ. Autonomic disorders and their recognition. *N Engl J Med.* 1997;336:721-724.

A brief summary of the ANS with 16 references.

Chapter 13

Pain

Dalessio DJ. *Wolff's Headache and Other Head Pain*. New York, NY: Oxford University Press; 1993.

A standard on headache edited by a previous resident of Dr Wolff's who has continued working with head pain patients.

Osterweis M, Kleinman A, Mechanic D, eds. *Pain and Disability: Clinical, Behavioral, and Public Policy Perspectives*. Washington, DC: National Academy Press; 1987.

Raskin NH. *Headache*. 2nd ed. New York, NY: Churchill Livingstone; 1988.

A very practical text by an experienced neurologist on the clinical aspects of headache.

Stereopsis

McKee S, Levi D, Bowne S. The importance of stereopsis. *Vision Res.* 1990;30:1763-1779

Describes a series of very scientific tests to measure the accuracy of stereopsis. The authors conclude that stereopsis can be very good in judging small differences in the plane of fixation, but that it is many times worse than monocular cues in judging depth differences beyond the plane of fixation and is also time-consuming. Stereopsis is most useful to guide fine hand movements.

Sheedy J, Bailey I, Buri M, Bass E. Binocular vs monocular task performance. *Am J Optom Physiol Opt.* 1986;63:839-846.

In this study, subjects were timed as they performed various tasks monocularly and binocularly. The findings confirm the fact that stereopsis is useful for fine hand coordination but not for tasks at greater distances.

Chapter 14

Mental and Behavioral Disorders

Introduction

This chapter discusses impairments due to mental disorders and considers behavioral impairment of function that may complicate any condition. As did Chapter 13 (The Central and Peripheral Nervous System), this chapter assesses the brain; however, here the emphasis is on evaluating brain function and its effect on behavior for mental disorders. Unlike the other chapters in the *Guides,* this chapter focuses more on the *process* of performing a mental and behavioral impairment assessment. Numerical impairment ratings are not included; however, instructions are given for how to assess an individual's abilities to perform activities of daily living.

The following revisions have been made for the fifth edition:

1. The importance of following the ***Diagnostic and Statistical Manual of Mental Disorders, Fourth Edition (DSM-IV)*** criteria for determining a mental impairment is emphasized.[1]

2. The section on social security disability assessment has been removed. The Social Security Administration criteria focus on disability and work disability assessment, which is not the purpose of the AMA *Guides.* However, some of the

material in this chapter is taken directly from Social Security Administration (SSA) regulations.[2-4]

3. Additional case examples exemplify the relationship between diagnosis, typical symptoms and signs of the disorder, and the impact on the ability to perform activities of daily living. Examples are included for depression, personality disorder, and posttraumatic stress disorder (PTSD). The case examples, together with Table 14-1, should help clarify how, in common psychiatric disorders, one can provide a nonnumerical impairment rating. Some states have chosen to assign numerical percentages to these categories.

4. A summary template of factors to be included in a psychiatric assessment has been added.

14.1 Principles of Assessment

Before using the information in this chapter, the *Guides* user should become familiar with Chapters 1 and 2 and the Glossary. Chapters 1 and 2 discuss the *Guides'* purpose, applications, and methods for performing and reporting impairment evaluations. The Glossary provides definitions of common terms used by many specialties in impairment evaluations.

Several principles, described below, are central to assessing mental impairment. A clear diagnosis is required to assess permanent mental or behavioral impairment. This diagnosis needs to be established according to *DSM-IV* criteria. The diagnosis is among the factors to be considered in assessing the severity and possible duration of the impairment, but it is not the sole criterion to be used.

Motivation for improvement may be a key factor in the severity and extent of an individual's impairment, whether that impairment is physical or mental. The examiner needs to assess changes in motivation and whether problems in motivation are due to the illness or to secondary gains. Motivation is influenced by multiple factors, including the illness, as well as the individual's personality, coping style, self-esteem, and self-confidence. These factors may change over time. The loss of motivation for even purely pleasurable activities may be a sign or symptom of an illness such as depression or schizophrenia. However, some individuals may be demoralized or in some way unmotivated to improve by external circumstances (such as fiscal incentives to stay ill and maintain health insurance).

Assessing impairment requires a thorough review of the history of the mental disorder, the history of the individual's ability to function over time, and his or her response to treatment and rehabilitation.

14.1a Interpretations of Symptoms and Signs

The individual's own description of his or her functioning and limitations is an important source of information. Information from nonmedical sources, such as family members and others who have knowledge of the person, may be useful in indicating the level of functioning and the severity of the impairment.

Information concerning the individual's behavior while performing activities of daily living is particularly useful in determining his or her ability to function. Results of work evaluations and rehabilitation programs, as well as information from day programs, are also useful in assessing level of functioning.

Information from both medical and nonmedical sources may be used to obtain detailed descriptions of the individual's activities of daily living, social functioning, concentration, persistence, pace, and ability to tolerate increased mental demands (stress). This information may be available from professionals in community mental health centers, daycare centers, and sheltered workshops, and it also can be provided by family members. If the descriptions from these sources are insufficiently detailed or in conflict with the observed clinical picture or the reports of others, it is necessary to resolve the inconsistencies. Any gaps in the history should also be explained.

An individual's level of functioning may vary considerably over time. The level of functioning at a specific time may seem relatively adequate or, conversely, rather poor. Proper evaluation of an impairment must take into account variations in the level of functioning over time to arrive at a determination of severity. Thus, it is important to obtain evidence over a sufficiently long period of time before the date of examination. This evidence should include treatment notes, hospital discharge summaries, work evaluations, and rehabilitation progress notes if they are available.

14.1b Description of Clinical Studies

The use of well-standardized psychological tests, such as the Wechsler Adult Intelligence Scale (WAIS) and the Minnesota Multiphasic Personality Inventory-2 (MMPI-2) may improve diagnostic acumen and help establish the existence of a mental disorder. For example, the WAIS is useful in documenting mental retardation. Broad-based neuropsychological assessments using, for example, the Halstead-Reitan or the Luria-Nebraska batteries may be useful in determining deficiencies in brain functioning, particularly in individuals with subtle signs such as those that may be seen in traumatic brain injuries.

Taking a standardized test requires concentration, persistence, and pacing; thus, observing individuals during the testing process may yield useful information. The summary of test results should include the objective findings, a description of what occurred during the testing, and the test results. A report of intellectual assessment should include a discussion of whether the obtained intelligence quotient (IQ) score is considered to be valid and consistent with the individual's impairment and degree of functional limitation.

14.2 Psychiatric Diagnosis and Impairment

In general, the history, signs, and symptoms of a mental disorder should justify the diagnosis, which should be made according to *DSM-IV* criteria. If there is uncertainty about the exact diagnosis, the differential diagnosis should be discussed. Document adequate descriptions of impairments and functional limitations from the reports of professional sources, such as psychiatrists, psychologists, psychiatric nurses, psychiatric social workers, and health professionals in hospitals and clinics. Data gathered over a period of years are particularly useful.

The *Diagnostic and Statistical Manual of Mental Disorders, Fourth Edition,* commonly known as *DSM-IV,* is a widely accepted classification system for mental disorders. It is similar to another system, the *International Classification of Diseases (ICD),* which also is in widespread use.[5] The criteria for mental disorders include a wide range of signs, symptoms, and impairments. Many mental disorders are characterized by impairments in a number of

areas. *DSM-IV* calls for a multiaxial evaluation. Each of five axes refers to a different class of information. The first three axes constitute the major diagnostic categories. These include the major clinical syndromes and the conditions that are the focus of treatment (axis I), the personality and developmental disorders (axis II), and the physical disorders and conditions that may be relevant to understanding and managing the care of the individual (axis III). Axis IV, referring to psychosocial stressors, and axis V, referring to adaptive functioning, may be particularly important for assessing impairment severity. In particular, axis V is a rating of the individual's global functional capacity and, like disability, is related directly to the effects of impairments.

In some individuals it is not possible to make a determination on the basis of the available information. Under these circumstances, the examiner should not feel obligated to provide an opinion about which he or she is uncertain but should seek and review relevant information from additional sources, such as medical and employment records, before rendering an opinion. The examiner must also consider the effects that medication, motivation, and rehabilitation may have on the individual's signs, symptoms, and ability to function. A detailed discussion of these factors follows.

14.2a Effects of Medication

Attention must be given to the **effects of medication** on the individual's signs, symptoms, and ability to function. Although psychoactive medications may control certain signs or symptoms, such as hallucinations, impaired attention span, restlessness, or hyperactivity, such treatment may not affect all impairments and limitations imposed by the mental disorder. If an individual's symptoms are attenuated by psychoactive medications, the evaluator should focus particular attention on limitations that may persist. Those limitations should be used as measures of the impairment's severity.

Psychoactive medications used to treat some mental illnesses may cause drowsiness, blunted affect, or unwanted effects involving various body systems. Moreover, medications necessary to control such symptoms as hallucinations may result in decreased motivation and level of activity. These side effects should be considered in evaluating the overall severity of the individual's impairment and ability to function. As explained in Chapter 2, the evaluator may need to provide an impairment estimate for the drug's side effects.

14.2b Effects of Motivation

Assessing motivation is difficult because lack of motivation may be hard to distinguish from mental impairment and is, in fact, a classic symptom of schizophrenia. When is an individual lacking energy, concentration, and initiative depressed or autistically preoccupied, and when is the individual unmotivated? Ultimately, making this distinction requires a clinical judgment, which should be aided by careful investigation of the individual's efforts and accomplishments before the onset of the alleged impairment and a search for associated signs and symptoms of common mental disorders.

Motivation is a difficult issue for assessment since it is mutifactorial in nature, involving the following potential factors: (1) lack of motivation as a sign of illness such as depression or schizophrenia; (2) fear of losing entitlement or other benefits of being ill; (3) a side effect of some neuroleptic medications; (4) conscious malingering; (5) a consequence of demoralization of persons with any chronic illness; (6) social network support for illness; and others. Thus, the determination of motivation is often non-empirical, and conclusions are all too often drawn on the basis of prejudice. Many times, an individual's motivation is not well understood even after careful assessment.

Nevertheless, motivation is a link between impairment and disability. For some people, poor motivation is a major cause of poor functioning. An individual's underlying character may be important in determining whether he or she is motivated to benefit from rehabilitation. Personality characteristics usually remain unchanged throughout life. However, internal events and psychological reactions can influence the course of illness. An individual who tends to be dependent, for example, may become even more dependent as his or her illness proceeds.

14.2c Effects of Rehabilitation

Frequently, the degree of vocational limitation of the individual with impairment of function is of paramount importance to the evaluator. This limitation may range from minimal to total. In addition, the severity of functional impairment may change with the course of the illness. When the individual needs less medical care, vocational skills may be intact, or the individual may have limitations that may or may not be reversible. The evaluator should judge the possible duration of the impairment that remains, whether remission is likely to be fast or slow, whether it will be partial or total, and whether the

impairment is likely to remain stable or to change. These considerations should contribute to the examiner's judgment about the degree of impairment.

Rehabilitation is a sine qua non in the treatment of most people who have recovered or are recovering from the acute phase of a mental disorder, especially a major mental disorder. Even if it is not possible to effect total remission, an outcome may be considered worthwhile if it has been possible to move the individual's functional impairment to a lesser degree.

While for some persons lack of motivation appears to be a major feature of continuing impairment and may be a major feature of an ongoing mental disorder, many individuals who undergo proper rehabilitative measures, including some who have organic illnesses, achieve improvements in functioning. Determining whether impaired functioning will persist is sometimes an imprecise science, and some degree of uncertainty about this prediction often exists. The use of the impairment label can be seen as pessimistic, providing an adverse prediction that may be self-fulfilling. However, the tendency for physicians and others to minimize psychiatric impairments must also be considered; this tendency may lead to failure to refer individuals for potentially helpful rehabilitative measures.

An important aspect of rehabilitation is the recognition that an individual who is taking certain types of medication may be able to sustain a satisfactory degree of functioning, whereas without medication he or she might fail to do so. For instance, there may be only a slight problem in the thinking process while the person is taking a suitable medication but a severe one if he or she is not taking medication. The physician should note the individual's performance with and without medication.

Another consideration is providing an employer the assurance that a worker who is taking the proper medication and is in an appropriate job can avoid injury both to himself or herself and to coworkers. An analogy is seen in the care and treatment of a worker who has seizures: in such an instance, informing and educating the worker, as well as his or her family, employer, and coworkers, are vital steps and should be a part of the rehabilitation process.

Just as there are degrees of impairment, total rehabilitation may not be possible, as is the case in the great majority of individuals afflicted with schizophrenia. To use an analogy from physical medicine, it is essentially impossible for an amputated leg to be replaced, and the affected individual cannot hope to regain perfect ambulation. However, a well-fitted prosthesis, accompanied by practice and training, can greatly improve the individual's ability to walk. If, in addition, the individual obtains suitable transportation, he or she may be restored to full gainful employment. If normal ambulation is a job requirement, an employer may be able to provide an alternative position or to modify existing tasks so that they can be performed by an amputee making skillful use of a prosthesis.

Although the analogy between the loss of a limb and the loss of capability resulting from a mental disorder has limitations, impairment from a mental disorder can be just as real and severe as the impairment resulting from an injury or other illness. The link between motivation and recovery may need strengthening in individuals who are impaired by either physical or mental illness. This task falls primarily to rehabilitationists and psychiatrists, but others can assist. An employer's providing alternative tasks or modifying existing work conditions may be as much a part of restoring vocational possibilities to an individual with mental illness as it is to one recovering from an injury or to one who has elements of both mental and physical illness.

14.3 A Method of Evaluating Psychiatric Impairment

Percentages are not provided to estimate mental impairment in this edition of the *Guides*. Unlike cases with some organ systems, there are no precise measures of impairment in mental disorders. The use of percentages implies a certainty that does not exist. Percentages are likely to be used inflexibly by adjudicators, who then are less likely to take into account the many factors that influence mental and behavioral impairment. In addition, the authors are unaware of data that show the reliability of the impairment percentages. After considering this difficult matter, the Committee on Disability and Rehabilitation of the American Psychiatric Association advised *Guides* contributors against the use of percentages in the chapter on mental and behavioral disorders of the fourth edition, and that remains the opinion of the authors of the present chapter.

No available empirical evidence supports any method for assigning a percentage of impairment of the whole person; however, the following approach may be helpful in estimating the extent of mental impairments. Not everyone who has a mental or behavioral disorder is limited in the ability to perform activities of daily living; however, there are individuals with less than chronic, but still unremitting, impairments who are severely limited in some areas of function.[6]

Translating specific impairments directly and precisely into functional limitations is a complex and poorly understood process. Current research finds little relationship between such psychiatric signs and symptoms as those identified during a mental status examination and the ability to perform competitive work. However, four main categories exist that assess many areas of function: (1) ability to perform activities of daily living; (2) social functioning; (3) concentration, persistence, and pace; and (4) deterioration or decompensation in work or worklike settings. Independence, appropriateness, and effectiveness of activities should also be considered. The four aspects of functional limitation are discussed below and can be linked, or causally related, to specific impairments as described in Table 14-1. The examiner should assess and record the extent of function in all these categories.

14.3a Activities of Daily Living

Activities of daily living, as indicated in Table 1-2, include such activities as self-care, personal hygiene, communication, ambulation, travel, sexual function, and sleep. Any limitations in these activities of daily living should be related to the mental disorder rather than to such factors as lack of money or transportation. In the context of the individual's overall situation, the quality of these activities is judged by their independence, appropriateness, effectiveness, and sustainability. It is necessary to define the extent to which the individual is capable of initiating and participating in these activities independent of supervision or direction.

The examiner must assess not simply the number of activities that are restricted but the overall degree of restriction or combination of restrictions. For example, a person who is able to cook and clean might be considered to have marked restriction of daily activities if he or she were too fearful to leave home to shop or go to the physician's office.

14.3b Social Functioning

Social functioning refers to an individual's capacity to interact appropriately and communicate effectively with other individuals. Social functioning includes the ability to get along with others, such as family members, friends, neighbors, grocery clerks, landlords, or bus drivers. Impaired social functioning may be demonstrated by a history of altercations, evictions, firings, fear of strangers, avoidance of interpersonal relationships, social isolation, or similar events or characteristics. It is helpful to give specific examples illustrating the individual's impaired social functioning.

Strength in social functioning may be documented by an individual's ability to initiate social contact with others, communicate clearly with others, and interact and actively participate in group activities. Cooperative behavior, consideration for others, awareness of others' sensitivities, and social maturity also need to be considered. Social functioning in work situations may involve interactions with the public, responding to persons in authority such as supervisors, or being part of a team.

The overall degree of interference with a particular aspect or combination of aspects is as significant as the number of aspects in which social functioning is impaired. For example, a hostile, uncooperative person who is tolerated by local storekeepers and neighbors may have marked restriction in overall functioning because antagonism and hostility are not acceptable in the workplace or in social contexts.

14.3c Concentration, Persistence, and Pace

Concentration, persistence, and pace are needed to perform many activities of daily living, including task completion. Task completion refers to the ability to sustain focused attention long enough to permit the timely completion of tasks commonly found in activities of daily living or work settings. Deficiencies in concentration, persistence, and pace are best noted from previous work attempts or from observations in worklike settings, such as day-treatment centers and incentive work programs. Describing specific examples of the individual's capabilities is useful. Major impairments of these abilities can often be assessed through direct psychiatric examinations or psychological testing. However, mental status examinations or psychological test data alone should not be considered adequate to fully describe the individual's concentration and sustained ability to perform work tasks.

Concentration and mental status may be assessed by having the individual perform such tasks as subtracting 7s serially from 100. In psychological tests of intelligence or memory, concentration is assessed through tasks requiring short-term memory or tasks that must be completed within established time limits. Strengths and weaknesses in mental concentration may be described in terms of frequency of errors, the time it takes to complete the task, and the extent to which assistance is required to complete the task. A person who appears to concentrate adequately during a mental status examination or a psychological test may not do so in a setting more like one common to the working world.

14.3d Deterioration or Decompensation in Complex or Worklike Settings

Deterioration or **decompensation** in complex or worklike settings refers to an individual's repeated failure to adapt to stressful circumstances. In the face of such circumstances, the individual may withdraw from the situation or experience exacerbation of signs and symptoms of a mental disorder; that is, he or she may decompensate and have difficulty maintaining performance of activities of daily living, continuing social relationships, and completing tasks. Stresses common to the work environment include attendance, making decisions, scheduling, completing tasks, and interacting with supervisors and peers. It is useful to give examples of the individual's decompensation and the stresses that might have brought it about.

In assessing the individual's stress tolerance, the examiner should be mindful of the following issues. First, *stress* may be defined in reference to a "reasonable man" standard in some systems and to other standards in other systems. Second, the circumstances of a given case might suggest a prophylactic preclusion from certain types of tasks or work settings. For example, a person with symptoms of posttraumatic stress disorder that date from a robbery and assault might require a prophylactic preclusion from jobs involving contact with the general public or handling large sums of money. In contrast, a stressful personality clash between the individual and his or her supervisor might require only that the individual be precluded from working with that particular supervisor.

14.3e Classes of Impairment Due to Mental and Behavioral Disorders

Table 14-1 provides a guide for rating mental impairment in each of the four areas of functional limitation on a five-category scale that ranges from no impairment to extreme impairment. The following are recommended as anchors for the categories of the scale.

1. None means no impairment is noted in the function.
2. Mild implies that any discerned impairment is compatible with most useful functioning.
3. Moderate means that the identified impairments are compatible with some, but not all, useful functioning.
4. Marked is a level of impairment that significantly impedes useful functioning. Taken alone, a marked impairment would not completely preclude functioning, but together with marked limitation in another class, it might limit useful functioning.
5. Extreme means that the impairment or limitation is not compatible with useful function. Extreme

impairment in carrying out activities of daily living implies complete dependency on another person for care. In the sphere of social functioning, extreme impairment implies that the individual engages in no meaningful social contact, as with a person who is in a withdrawn, catatonic state. An extreme limitation in concentration, persistence, and pace means that the individual cannot attend to conversation or any productive task; this might be seen in a person who is in an acute confusional state or in a person with a complete loss of short-term memory.

A person who cannot tolerate any change at all in routines or in the environment, or one who cannot function and who decompensates when schedules change in an otherwise structured environment, has an extreme limitation of adaptive functioning and an extreme psychiatric impairment. Such an individual might, for example, experience a psychotic episode if a meal is not served on time or might have a panic attack if left without a companion in any situation.

Table 14-1 Classes of Impairment Due to Mental and Behavioral Disorders

Area or Aspect of Functioning	Class 1 No Impairment	Class 2 Mild Impairment	Class 3 Moderate Impairment	Class 4 Marked Impairment	Class 5 Extreme Impairment
Activities of daily living Social functioning Concentration Adaptation	No impairment noted	Impairment levels are compatible with most useful functioning	Impairment levels are compatible with some, but not all, useful functioning	Impairment levels significantly impede useful functioning	Impairment levels preclude useful functioning

In the ordinary individual, extreme impairment in only one area or marked limitation in two or more spheres would be likely to preclude the performance of any complex task, such as one involving recreation or work, without special support or assistance, such as that provided in a sheltered environment.

An individual impaired to a moderate degree in all four categories of functioning would be limited in the ability to carry out many, but not all, complex tasks. Mild and moderate limitations reduce overall performance but do not preclude some performance. Table 14-2 links specific impairments to potential associated disabilities.

Translating these guidelines for rating individual impairment on ordinal scales into a method for assigning percentage of impairments, as if valid estimates could be made on precisely measured interval scales, cannot be done reliably. One cannot be certain that the difference in impairment between a rating of mild and moderate is of the same magnitude as the difference between moderate and marked. Furthermore, a moderate impairment does not imply a 50% limitation in useful functioning, and an estimate of moderate impairment in all four categories does not imply a 50% impairment of the whole person.

Eventually, research may disclose direct relationships between medical findings and percentages of mental impairment. Until that time, the medical profession must refine its concepts of mental and physical impairment, improve its ability to measure limitations, and continue to make clinical judgments.

14.4 Assessing Impairment Severity

The following factors, discussed below, must be considered when assessing severity of an individual's impairment: (1) the effects of treatment; (2) the effects of structured settings; (3) the variability of mental disorders; (4) an assessment of workplace function; and (5) the effects of common mental and behavioral conditions.

14.4a Effects of Treatment
Problems often arise in evaluating mental impairments of individuals who have long histories of repeated hospitalizations or prolonged outpatient care with supportive therapy and medication. Individuals with

chronic psychotic disorders commonly have their lives structured in such a way as to minimize stress and reduce their signs and symptoms. Such individuals may therefore be more impaired in terms of work capability than their signs and symptoms indicate. The results of a single examination may not adequately describe the ability of such a person to function in a sustained way. Thus, it is necessary to review information pertaining to the individual's functioning at times of increased stress, such as in a worklike setting.

14.4b Effects of Structured Settings
In cases involving long-standing mental disorders, overt symptoms may be particularly controlled or attenuated by psychosocial factors, such as placement in a hospital, halfway house, board and care facility, or similar environment. These highly structured and supportive settings may greatly reduce the mental demands placed on an individual. Although overt signs and symptoms of the underlying mental disorder may be minimized with lowered mental demands, the individual's ability to function outside of the structured setting may not have changed. The evaluator of an individual whose symptoms are controlled in a structured setting must consider such factors as the individual's response to past attempts to function successfully at work or in other unstructured environments.

14.4c Variability of Mental Disorders
In judging the degree of mental impairment, it is important to recognize that there are various types of mental disorders, each of which, like a physical disorder, has its own natural course and unique characteristics. In addition, degrees of impairment may vary considerably among individuals with the same diagnosis.

It is apparent that some serious mental disorders are chronic. The term *remission,* rather than *cure,* is therefore used to indicate an individual's improvement. The remission may be intermittent, long term, or short term, and it may occur in stages rather than all at once. For example, an episode of depression that follows a stressful life event may turn out to be an adjustment disorder with depressed mood, which often is a short-term, self-limiting illness that clears up when the stressful situation is relieved. Other affective disorders have their own patterns of recurrence and chronicity that often, but not always, respond well to therapeutic interventions. Thus, an individual with a medication-resistant major depressive episode may remain unable to sleep, eat, concentrate, etc, for months or even years.

14.4d Assessment of Workplace Function

Assessment of the ability to perform activities at work requires evaluation of similar abilities, along with unique skills, particular to the workplace. To assess the ability of an individual to function in the workplace, the evaluator may obtain additional information by using a multidimensional description of remaining work-related abilities. Four capacities, indicated below, have been used by SSA regulations to characterize residual functional capacity.

1. *Understanding and memory* relate to the individual's ability to remember procedures related to work; to understand and remember short, simple instructions; and to understand and remember detailed instructions.

2. *Sustained concentration and persistence* relate to the individual's ability to carry out short, simple instructions; carry out detailed instructions; maintain attention and concentration for extended periods of time; perform activities within a given schedule; maintain regular attendance and be punctual within customary tolerances; sustain an ordinary routine without special supervision; work with or near others without being distracted; make simple work-related decisions; complete a normal workday and workweek without interruptions from psychologically based symptoms; and perform at a consistent pace without an unreasonable number of and unreasonably long rest periods.

3. *Social interaction* involves the individual's ability to interact appropriately with the general public; ask simple questions or request assistance; accept instructions and respond appropriately to criticism from supervisors; get along with coworkers and peers without distracting them or exhibiting behavioral extremes; maintain socially appropriate behavior; and adhere to basic standards of neatness and cleanliness.

4. *Adaptation* is the ability to respond appropriately to changes in the work setting; to be aware of normal hazards and take appropriate precautions; to use public transportation and travel to and within unfamiliar places; to set realistic goals; and to make plans independently of others.

14.4e Effects of Common Mental and Behavioral Conditions

Some categories of mental and behavioral conditions, including substance-dependence disorders, personality disorders (especially antisocial personality disorders), and adjustment disorders, are characterized by abnormal emotional responses to stressful life events, which resolve in a short time when the stressor is removed. The behavior during both controlled intervals and times of exacerbation should be noted.

The schizophrenias are usually chronic disorders; the onset may be insidious and recognized only in retrospect. Certain organic disorders, such as traumatic brain injury and lifelong mental retardation, are persistent and chronic, and treatment consists of minimizing the functional loss inherent to the pathophysiologic changes. Evaluation of mental retardation and autism for social security considers the presence of mental incapacity evidenced by (1) dependence on others for personal needs, such as toileting, eating, dressing, or bathing; and (2) an inability to follow directions, which precludes tests of intellectual functioning; or (3) a valid verbal performance or full-scale IQ of 59 or less, or a score of 60 through 69 along with physical or mental impairment affecting daily activities, social functioning, or concentration, persistence, and pace. Common psychiatric diagnoses, associated impairments in the form of demonstrable signs and symptoms, and commonly seen areas of decreased performance are discussed below and in Table 14-2 .

14.4e.1 Substance Abuse and Personality Disorders

Chronic substance abuse and personality disorders can coincide. The effects of chronic substance abuse include impairments in concentration, attention, impulse control, judgment, etc, which often last for the duration of the dependency. These behaviors can also occur with personality disorders. To evaluate the severity of the impairment, the examiner needs to assess whether there are (1) restrictions in activities of daily living; (2) difficulties in maintaining social functioning; (3) difficulties in completing tasks in a timely manner because of deficiencies in concentration, persistence, and pace; and (4) repeated episodes of decompensation and loss of adaptive functioning, averaging three times per year, with each episode lasting 2 or more weeks.

14.4e.2 Somatoform Pain Disorders

Pain that accompanies a medical impairment is generally taken into account in the impairment ratings throughout the *Guides.* Chronic pain and pain exceeding the anticipated amount are discussed in Chapter 18. Mental illness may distort the perception of pain. Pain may be part of a somatic delusion in an individual with a major depression or a psychotic disorder. Pain may become the object of an obsessive preoccupation, or it may be the chief complaint in a conversion disorder. A frequent problem in pain assessment is the failure of physicians to agree on whether there is an adequate physical explanation for the pain. It would be useful for the examining psychiatrist to understand whether other professionals treating the individual feel that his or her symptoms are out of proportion with the physical findings. If they are, the psychiatrist should consider this finding in making a differential diagnosis and should recognize the possibility of the presence of somatoform or other mental disorders.

The essential feature of **somatoform pain disorder** in *DSM-IV* is preoccupation with pain in the absence of physical findings that adequately account for the pain and its intensity, as well as the presence of psychological factors that are judged to have a major role in the onset, severity, exacerbation, and maintenance of pain. In the past, this syndrome has been called psychogenic pain disorder or idiopathic pain disorder, but these terms are often used more loosely to describe any complaint of pain that is greater than the physician expects for the average person who has the same physical findings. The physician should recognize that anxiety and depression almost always magnify pain, and vice versa.

The following guidelines may be useful in determining whether pain is a symptom of a mental impairment: (1) All possible somatic causes of the pain have been eliminated by careful, comprehensive medical examinations; (2) some significant emotional stressor has occurred in the individual's life that may have acted as a triggering agent, and the stressor and the pain have occurred in a reasonable sequence; and (3) evidence exists of a mental disorder other than a conversion-related one, and the pain may be a symptom of nonconversion-related mental disorders. For example, delusional pain may occur in an individual who has a subtle paranoid disorder such as might be the case with someone who believes Martians are irradiating his head, producing constant headaches, and where the belief antedated the pain.

14.4e.3 Malingering

Malingering may arise with mental disorders as well as with nonpsychiatric conditions. Examiners should be aware of this possibility when evaluating impairments. The possibility of obtaining monetary awards and avoiding work increases the likelihood of malingering. Certain symptoms, such as headache, low-back pain, peripheral neuralgia, and vertigo, are difficult to objectively assess. Conditions that have more of an apparent organic basis, such as appendicitis, a fracture, or pregnancy, tend to be more amenable to objective diagnostic studies than are some psychiatric and neurologic complaints. Malingerers with supposed psychiatric conditions may be seen in circumstances involving the avoidance of an unpleasant duty or requirement, such as going to jail or entering military service, and may be seen seeking insurance or entitlement benefits.

Rather than giving outright fabrications, individuals may consciously or unconsciously exaggerate the symptoms of a disorder in the clinical or impairment evaluation setting. Malingering may be suspected when the individual's symptoms are vague, ill defined, overdramatized, inconsistent, or not in conformity with signs and symptoms known to occur. In this situation, results of the physical and mental status examinations and other data and information of the evaluation may be inconsistent with the nature and intensity of the person's complaints.

Circumstances in which an unusual number of ill-defined complaints occur in a circumscribed group, perhaps in a setting of poor morale or conflict, also may be viewed with suspicion. But the most appropriate approach for the examining physician is one of clinical neutrality, the application of standard interview and diagnostic procedures, and, if warning signs appear, a careful investigation that includes multidisciplinary evaluation and psychological testing as appropriate. For a more elaborate discussion of malingering, a text may be useful.[7,8]

Table 14-2 Selected Impairments and Common Limitations in Ability

Impairment	Signs and Symptoms	Limitations in Ability
Schizophrenia	Loosening of associations	Social, vocational, and activities of daily living*
	Delusions and hallucinations	Social, vocational, and activities of daily living
	Flat affect	Social
	Inappropriate affect	Social, vocational, and activities of daily living
	Bizarre behavior	Social and vocational
	Disorganized behavior	Social, vocational, and activities of daily living
Schizophrenia or depression	Social withdrawal; autism	Social and vocational
Schizophrenia, depression, or anxiety disorder	Impaired concentration and attention	Social, vocational, and activities of daily living
Posttraumatic stress disorder	Decreased concentration	Vocational
	Explosive outbursts	Social and vocational
Borderline personality disorder	Impulsivity	Social and vocational
	Affective lability	Social and vocational
Panic disorder with agoraphobia	Social withdrawal	Social and vocational

* Activites of daily living are listed in Table 1-2.

14.5 Examples of Impairment Due to Mental and Behavioral Disorders

The following cases indicate the information needed to accurately assess impairment and residual function.

Example 14-1
Impairment Due to Major Depressive Episode and Associated Anxiety

Subject: 47-year-old man.

History: Cardiologist; lives with his wife and two teenage children in the suburbs. Well until 4 months ago, when he developed acute chest pain due to a myocardial infarction (MI) involving the anterior descending coronary artery. He was in shock when sent to the cardiac ICU with a BP of 78/40 mm Hg. He underwent angioplasy and stent placement with good results, and was placed on Coumadin. He recovered without complications and was discharged to cardiac rehabilitation. On follow-up with his cardiologist, he appeared frightened, telling the cardiologist that this was the first time he'd been out of his home except for his rehab appointments and that he was afraid to travel alone. When the cardiologist informed him that he could safely return to work on a limited

basis and engage in all normal activities, including slowly resuming sexual intercourse with his wife, he seemed relieved. The remainder of the exam was normal, with his ECG charges consistent with an MI.

The man was fearful of a recurrence and became anxious, returning home when attempting to go to work. His father and two paternal uncles had all died of heart disease in their 50s and 60s. He and his wife did not resume their sex life. He said he was afraid the "strain will kill me." At the fourth follow-up visit at 6 months he reported no improvement in his anxiety; avoidance of work, sex, and playing with his children; and spending his time "trying to read and watch TV"; the cardiologist referred him to a psychiatrist.

Current Symptoms: His fears of dying young have immobilized him. He describes frequent awakenings with anxiety at night but cannot remember any dreams. He describes continual preoccupation with his somatic sensations, particularly of the chest. He feels hopeless and pessimistic all the time and, while not crying, feels sad and unable to enjoy anything.

Physical Exam: He has lost 9 kg (20 lb) since the hospitalization. On mental status evaluation, he appeared to be a thin, somewhat agitated man, both sad and anxious. He denied suicidal feelings but added, "I guess I feel I'll die soon anyway." He described feeling a "failure" because "I'm not earning for my family and I'm such a coward."

His concentration was poor; he lost his train of thought when asked to do serial 7s and spell *world* backwards. He showed little insight, although there were no psychotic features.

Clinical Studies: No additional diagnostic tests were performed.

Diagnosis: Axis I: Depressive episode, major, with associated anxiety precipitated by MI but not secondary to medical condition.
Axis II: Deferred.
Axis III: Status post-MI, healed. Surgical stent of anterior descending coronary artery. Normal cholesterol on Lipacor and Coumadin.
Axis IV: Stressors include his cardiac illness and early death of male relatives from heart disease.
Axis V: GAF of 50.

Impairment Rating: At the time of the examination, the man was assessed a class 3 on social function, class 5 on concentration, class 1 on activities of daily living, and class 4 to 5 on adaptation.

Comment: An antidepressant once a day was begun, as was twice-weekly focal dynamic therapy with a time frame of 2 months. The man talked of his guilt about surviving all his male relatives (he had one older sister) and particularly his father, who had died when he was 14, leaving him "the stag in the house." He resented his father's dominant personality and his father's push for him to be a scholar/athlete just like he had been. His father was a general surgeon. He envied and resented his father and was ambivalent about his death. He experienced his own MI as punishment for his resentment of his father and for his own success. As the antidepressant took effect and therapy elucidated his anger at his father, the guilt, as well as his fear of punishment and anxiety, diminished. He resumed working a few hours a day, eventually returned to full practice, and resumed his sexual life as well. He stopped psychotherapy after 2 months but was to continue the antidepressant for 1 year to help prevent recurrence of the depression.

Example 14-2
Impairment Due to Borderline Personality Disorder

Subject: 32-year-old woman.

History: Twice-divorced woman, living alone in an apartment, and working as a legal secretary. She was briefly hospitalized after slashing her wrists in an apparent suicidal gesture several weeks prior to the evaluation.

Her illness began as a teenager, when she began using alcohol and recreational drugs, became promiscuous, and would become depressed in response to parental attempts to restrict her behavior or when she was rejected by a boyfriend or lover. During her teens, she was seen in the emergency room for overdoses and cutting herself— once superficially, once requiring stitches— following rejections by lovers. Her schoolwork, however, remained good. She graduated from high school and college with Bs and Cs despite continuation of the above-noted behaviors. During college she married twice, at age 19 for 3 months and at age 21 for 6 months. Each relationship was characterized by adoration of her lover, quickly followed by disappointment and denigration of their characters and abilities as men. Each time she broke off the relationship, but the men were already alienated by her critical, clinging, and jealous behavior.

Following college, she trained as a legal secretary. She has not held a job for more than 6 months in the 10 years she has been working. Each time she begins by idolizing her boss and the firm she works for and finds some male attorney she attempts to seduce or simply ingratiate herself with. When this fails, she becomes enraged, truculent, depressed, and critical to the point where she is fired or leaves of her own accord.

Her recent wrist slashing was precipitated by her having experienced two rejections within the same week. Her most recent job was terminated because of her seeming inability to tolerate relationships with the male attorneys in her firm. Also, her most recent lover (of only a month) decided to relocate to another city for a job opportunity. She quickly grew depressed and developed some insomnia, anorexia, and feelings of "deadness," worthlessness, and hopelessness. She cut both wrists and took 30 Tylenol and 20 fluoxetine tablets.

After having her wrist lacerations stitched and gastric lavage in the ER, she was transferred to the psychiatric unit of the hospital. On the unit, she quickly reconstituted a good mood, became active, flirted with patients and staff, and developed a crush on her physician while reviling the other staff. She was discharged after 5 days and had one appointment with a private psychiatrist, who began her on weekly psychotherapy and prescribed an antidepressant twice a day.

Current Symptoms: The woman describes current feelings of some regret at her suicidal behavior. She does, however, still feel dead, numb, and bored, all of which she says she always experiences when she is uninvolved with a man sexually, at work in a mentoring relationship, or both. She admits to using occasional cocaine by snorting, as well as alcohol to "feel better or feel something," and to occasional superficial cutting of her skin to achieve the same end. She states that she has been advised by her therapists to avoid a relationship or a job at least until the therapy and medication have helped her with her quick tendency to depressed and suicidal feelings and her now obvious pattern of losing jobs due to her uncontrollable anger.

Physical Exam: On examination, she is a well-groomed, well-dressed, attractive young woman who is cooperative and dramatically gives her history, which corroborates that obtained from the hospital records. She has bandages on both wrists, which she fails to cover with her short-sleeved blouse. Her speech is logical and coherent, as well as goal directed. There is no evidence of delusions, hallucinations, or suspiciousness. As she talks of former bosses or lovers, however, they are uniformly and angrily described in demonizing, denigrating, and debasing terms. Her sensorium is clear, and her ability to abstract is intact. Physical examination is within normal limits except for the wrists.

Clinical Studies: Psychological testing, including IQ and projective, done on the inpatient service demonstrated an overall IQ of 123 and a "borderline personality structure" with "tendencies to affective instability, splitting (idealizing or denigrating significant others), and impulsivity," as well as "dissociative states and defensive numbness of affect to deal with her rage and dependency."

Diagnosis: Axis I: Rule out depressive disorder not otherwise specified; cocaine and alcohol use.
Axis II: Borderline personality disorder.
Axis III: Status postsurgical suture of cuts to both wrists.
Axis IV: Rejection by job and boyfriend.
Axis V: GAF of 50 to 60.

Impairment Rating: This woman would be rated as having no impairment noted on activities of daily living in Table 14-1. However, her social functioning is class 3, as is her concentration, and her adaptation would be considered class 5.

Comment: The class 5 adaptation rating is based on the woman's inability to hold a job for longer than a few months due to her affective dyscontrol and impulsivity, as well as her inability to sustain any long-term relationships.

Example 14-3
Impairment Due to Personality Disorder

Subject: 28-year-old man.

History: Lives with his parents in the family home; unemployed since his parents sold the family business 4 years ago. He describes himself—and school records and school psychological testing concur—as a fearful and isolated child. Based on school and home records, when he was 4 and was to begin nursery school, he refused to allow his mother to leave him, growing intensely frightened as she was about to leave him with the teacher and classmates. He was tremulous, crying, and clung to his mother's coat. This lasted for several months; he later would allow her to leave but would cling to the teacher and refuse to play with other children. This pattern continued until he graduated from high school. He developed fear of the dark and required a light to be on in order to go to sleep. He also refused to go to other children's houses to play and made few, if any, friends.

In adolescence, his peers would occasionally tease him, but "mainly they left me alone, which was okay with me." Upon graduation from high school, he refused to go to college despite having earned As and Bs in school. He was taken on in the family's small grocery store as a clerk and delivery boy. He avoided conversations with customers, who would occasionally comment to his parents on his normal appearance but behavioral "strangeness." He refused other employment by family members and friends. He spends his time reading or watching TV.

Current Symptoms: The man shops for his mother, engages in household chores, answers the phone, dresses himself appropriately, and accompanies his parents to family gatherings and outings. He will go to the movies by himself. He has refused multiple attempts to take him for counseling and/or psychiatric treatment, saying "nothing is wrong with me except my parents want me to work and have friends. Well, maybe I should and even want to, but you can't help me." He states that he is interested in women and masturbates regularly. He has never been on a date, fearing rejection and not knowing "what would I do or talk about."

Physical Exam: A well-dressed, well-groomed young man who appears his stated age. Though superficially pleasant, he is monosyllabic and resistant to any spontaneous conversation. Although his isolation from social relationships "is voluntary, I don't need people except my family," he does admit to wishing he had a "girl-friend" and a "job to keep me busy and get my family off my back." His speech and thoughts are logical and goal directed, without evidence of delusions, although he does report, "I feel like people think I'm strange and talk about me when I'm in a group, but maybe that's true or I just imagine it. I don't really hear them talking, but I worry about it." He denies hallucinations, obsessions, compulsions, or any episodes of severe depression or mania. He does feel anxiety in social situations, accompanied by sweating and palpitations and a wish "to scram out of there," but denies symptoms of panic attacks or specific phobias. His sensorium is clear in regard to orientation and both short-term and long-term memory, and his ability to abstract is intact. He has some insight but no motivation for treatment, which he describes as "another relationship I don't want." Examination is otherwise normal.

Clinical Studies: Psychological testing was done—IQ, projective, and MMPI—at age 11 and again 2 years ago. They revealed an intelligence in the low normal range (105) and "pronounced tendencies toward avoidant, anxious, phobic traits in the absence of any psychotic features" and concluded he was suffering from "severe avoidant, schizoid, and dependent personality traits" with a past history of "school phobia."

Diagnosis: Axis I: None.
Axis II: Personality disorder, mixed, with avoidant, dependent, and schizoid features.
Axis III: None.
Axis IV: Separation from family.
Axis V: GAF of 50 to 60.

Impairment Rating: Using Table 14-1, this person would be rated as class 1 on activities of daily living, class 4 on social functioning, class 1 or possibly 2 on concentration, and class 5 on adaptation.

14.6 Format of the Impairment Report

The following general format for impairment reports has been adapted from that recommended by the Social Security Administration.[4] The content of the report may vary, depending on the system for which the report is being prepared. An impairment report based on the *Guides* also should include the main features of the Report of Medical Evaluation form shown in Chapter 2.

A. **Introduction:** The psychiatric or psychological examination report should show not only the individual's signs, symptoms, laboratory findings (psychological test results), and diagnosis but also the effect of the emotional or mental disorder on his or her ability to function at the usual and customary level of personal, social, and occupational adjustment.
   1. **Specialty:** The exam should be performed by a psychiatrist.
   2. **General Observations:** Include in the report general observations of the following:
      a. How the individual came to the examination.
         (1) Alone or accompanied.
         (2) Distance and mode of transportation.
         (3) If by automobile, who drove?
      b. General appearance:
         (1) Dress.
         (2) Grooming.
         (3) Appearance of invalidism.
      c. Attitude and degree of cooperation.
      d. Posture and gait.
      e. Involuntary movements.
   3. **Informant:** The psychiatrist should identify the person providing the history (usually the examinee) and should provide an estimate of the reliability of the history.
   4. **Chief Complaint:** This should include a detailed chronological account of the onset and progression of the current mental/emotional condition with special reference to the individual's concerns.
      a. Date and circumstances of onset of the condition.
      b. Date the individual reported that the condition began to interfere with work, and how it interfered.
      c. Date the individual reported inability to work because of the condition and the circumstances.
      d. Attempts to return to work and the results.

e. Outpatient evaluations and treatment for mental/emotional problems, including:
  (1) Name of treating sources.
  (2) Dates of treatment.
  (3) Type of treatment (name and dosage of medications, if prescribed).
  (4) Response to treatment.

f. Hospitalizations for mental disorders, including:
  (1) Names of hospitals.
  (2) Dates of hospitalizations.
  (3) Treatment and response.

g. Information concerning the individual's:
  (1) Activities of daily living.
  (2) Social functioning.
  (3) Ability to complete tasks timely and appropriately.
  (4) Episodes of decompensation and their resulting effects.

5. **Past History:** This should include a longitudinal account of the individual's personal life, including:
  a. Relevant educational, medical, social, legal, military, marital, and occupational data and any associated problems in adjustment.
  b. Details (dates, places, etc) of any past history of outpatient treatment and hospitalizations for mental/emotional problems.
  c. History, if any, of substance abuse and/or treatment in detoxification and rehabilitation centers.

6. **Mental Status:** The individual case facts will determine the specific areas of mental status that need to be emphasized during the examination, but generally the report should include a detailed description of the individual's:
  a. Appearance, behavior, and speech (if not already described).
  b. Thought process (eg, loosening of association).
  c. Thought content (eg, delusion).
  d. Perceptual abnormalities (eg, hallucinations).
  e. Mood and affect (eg, depression, mania).
  f. Sensorium and cognition (eg, orientation, recall, memory, concentration, scope of information, and intelligence).
  g. Judgment and insight.

7. **Diagnosis:** American Psychiatric Association standard nomenclature as set forth in the current *Diagnostic and Statistical Manual of Mental Disorders.*

8. **Prognosis:** Prognosis and recommendations for treatment, if indicated; also recommendations for any other medical evaluation (eg, neurologic, general physical) if indicated.

B. **Policy—Additional Requirements by Impairment**
  1. **Schizophrenic, Delusional (Paranoid) Schizo-affective, and Other Psychotic Disorders:** The report should reflect:
    a. Periods of residence in structured settings such as halfway houses and group homes.
    b. Frequency and duration of episodes of illness and periods of remission.
    c. Side effects of medications.
  2. **Organic Mental Disorders:** The report should reflect:
    a. The source of the disorder, if known, the prognosis, and:
      (1) Whether there is an acute or chronic process.
      (2) Whether stable or progressive.
      (3) Changes at various points in time.
    b. The results of any psychological or neuropsychological testing that could serve to further document an organic process and its severity.
    c. Information regarding the results of any neurologic evaluations.
    d. Information about any neurologic testing (eg, EEG, CT scan) that may have been performed and the results, if available.
  3. **Mental Retardation**
    a. Current documentation of IQ by a standardized, well-recognized measure. Acceptable instruments will have a representative normative sample, a mean of approximately 100, and a standard deviation of approximately 15 in the general population, and will cover a broad range of cognitive and perceptual-motor functions (eg, the Wechsler scales).
    b. Verbal performance and full-scale IQ scores, together with the individual subtest scores.
    c. Interpretation of the scores and assessment of the validity of the obtained scores, indicating any factors that may have influenced the results, such as the individual's attitude and degree of cooperation; the presence of visual, hearing, or other physical problems; and recent prior exposure to the same or a similar test.
    d. Consistency of the obtained test results with the individual's education, vocational background, and social adjustment, especially in the area of personal self-sufficiency.

References

1. American Psychiatric Association, Committee on Nomenclature and Statistics. *Diagnostic and Statistical Manual of Mental Disorders, Revised Third Edition.* Washington, DC: American Psychiatric Association; 1987. *Diagnostic and Statistical Manual of Mental Disorders, Fourth Edition.* Washington, DC: American Psychiatric Association; 1994.

2. Social Security Administration. Federal Old-Age, Survivors and Disability Insurance. *Listing of Impairments, Mental Disorders: Final Rule (Listing).* 20 CFR Part 404 (Reg No. 4) 50(167), *Federal Register* 1985:35038-35070. The *Listing* and other guidance appear also in: *Disability Evaluation Under Social Security.* Baltimore, Md: Social Security Administration; February 1986. Publication No. 64-039.

3. Social Security Administration. Federal Old-Age, Survivors and Disability Insurance. *Listing of Impairments, Mental Disorders in Adults: Proposed Rules. Federal Register,* July 18, 1991, vol 56, No. 138.

4. Social Security Administration. *Consultative Examinations—Guide for Physicians.* Baltimore, Md: Social Security Administration; 1985. Publication No. 64-025.

5. World Health Organization. *Manual of the International Statistical Classification of Diseases, Injuries, and Causes of Death: International Classification of Diseases (ICD).* Geneva, Switzerland: World Health Organization; 1978.

6. Meyerson A, Fine T. *Psychiatric Disability: Clinical, Legal, and Administrative Dimensions.* Washington, DC: American Psychiatric Press; 1987.

7. Meyerson A. Malingering. In: Kaplan H, Sadock B, eds. *Textbook of Psychiatry.* 5th ed. New York, NY: Williams & Wilkins; 1989.

8. Rogers R, ed. *Clinical Assessment of Malingering and Deception.* 2nd ed. New York, NY: Guilford Publications; 1997.

Chapter 14

Chapter 15

The Spine

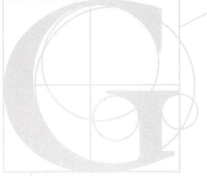

Introduction

This chapter provides criteria for evaluating permanent impairments of the spine, including how they affect an individual's ability to perform activities of daily living (ADL). The spine consists of four regions: the cervical, thoracic, lumbar and sacral vertebrae, and associated soft tissues including muscles, ligaments, disks, and neural elements. Impairments of the spine discussed in this chapter include lumbar, thoracic, cervical, spinal cord, and pelvic impairments.

The following revisions have been made for the fifth edition: (1) The use of the diagnosis-related estimate (DRE) and range-of-motion (ROM) methods has been modified, and applications are described in greater detail; (2) impairment is rated only when the individual has reached maximal medical improvement (MMI); (3) impairments within a DRE category encompass a range, with adjustments of up to 3%; (4) spinal cord injury is evaluated according to the functional approach in the nervous system chapter; (5) the "differentiators" in the fourth edition have been replaced by "objective findings" and are more specifically defined; and (6) alterations of motion segment integrity have been redefined to reflect current scientific knowledge.

As in the fourth edition,[1] *the DRE method is the primary method used to evaluate individuals with an injury. Use the ROM method when the impairment is not caused by an injury or when an individual's condition is not well represented by a DRE category. The ROM method is also now used to evaluate individuals with an injury at more than one level in the same spinal region and in certain individuals with recurrent pathology.* This approach addresses the difficulty of assigning these individuals to an appropriate DRE category. An exception, however, is individuals with corticospinal involvement who have been treated with decompression and multilevel fusions within the same region; they should be rated by the DRE method because assessing ROM in paralyzed individuals is difficult. Finally, the range-of-motion method should be used if statutorily mandated in a particular jurisdiction. A more detailed description of the applications of either method is provided in Section 15.2.

As stated in this edition, an individual with a spinal condition is rated only when the condition is stable (unlikely to change within the next year regardless of treatment), ie, when MMI has been reached (Chapter 1 and Glossary). The individual is evaluated based on medical findings that are present when MMI has been reached.

15.1 Principles of Assessment

Before using the information in this chapter, the *Guides* user should become familiar with Chapters 1 and 2 and the Glossary. Chapters 1 and 2 discuss the *Guides'* purpose, applications, and methods for performing and reporting impairment evaluations. The Glossary provides definitions of common terms used by many specialties in impairment evaluation.

The evaluation should include a comprehensive, accurate medical history; a review of all pertinent records; a comprehensive description of the individual's current symptoms and their relationship to daily activities; a careful and thorough physical examination; and all findings of relevant laboratory, radiologic (imaging), electrodiagnostic, and ancillary tests. It is also essential that the rater include in the report a description of how the impairment was calculated. Because many ratings are reviewed by other physicians and nonmedical personnel, the explanation of the calculation will lead to a better understanding of the method used and the report will be considered more reliable and complete.

15.1a Interpretation of Symptoms and Signs

History
The history should be based primarily on the individual's own statements rather than secondhand information. While the medical history should consider information from others, the physician should be cautious about using subjective information from medical records. It is not appropriate to question the individual's integrity. If information from the individual is inconsistent with what is known about the medical condition, circumstances, or written records, the physician should report and comment on the inconsistencies.

The history must describe in detail the chief complaint and the quality, severity, anatomic location, frequency, and duration of symptoms, including pain, numbness, paresthesias, and weakness. Document exacerbating and alleviating factors and the way in which the condition interferes with daily activities. The physician should elicit the history of when and how the condition started, any precipitating events or factors, and the relationship to any previous spine problems.[2-4]

The history should include the individual's description, in his or her own words, of how the symptoms developed and the assumed cause. In addition, the response to treatment and the results of special studies that have been performed should be described. The physician should either review available roentgenograms and other imaging studies personally or report the findings as being those of another reviewer (based on reports). A review of organ systems and of the general medical history can provide potentially helpful information, including complicating medical problems that can affect the diagnosis, treatment plan, prognosis, disability, etc.

Examination
Physical examination of nonmusculoskeletal areas (eg, nervous system) is discussed in other parts of the *Guides*. Since a targeted neurologic assessment is needed for individuals with back or neck problems, the physician must have a good grasp of basic neurologic examination techniques and principles. Guided by the history, the physician should focus on spine-related physical findings, such as range of motion, reflexes, muscle strength and atrophy, sensory deficits, root tension signs, gait, and the need for assistive devices (Table 15-1). Range-of-motion measurements are discussed later in this chapter.

Table 15-1 Physical Examination

Lumbar Spine

Individual Position	Examination

Standing	Posture
	  Scoliosis
	  Lordosis
	  Kyphosis

	Palpation
	  Muscles
	  Tenderness

	Gait
	Range of motion

	Muscle strength screening
	  Heel-toe walk
	  Squatting

Sitting	Neurologic
	  Reflexes (ankle, knee)
	  Strength
	  Sensation

	Nerve tension Straight leg raising (or similar)

Recumbent
  Supine
	Neurologic
	  Reflexes
	  Strength
	  Sensation
	  Straight leg raising (or similar)

	Other
	  Pulses
	  Hip range of motion

Recumbent
  Prone
	Nerve tension
	  Femoral stretch test

	Palpation
	  Muscles
	  Spinous processes

Thoracic Spine

Individual Position	Examination

Standing	Posture
	  Scoliosis
	  Kyphosis

	Palpation
	  Muscles
	  Tenderness

	Range of motion

Cervical Spine

Individual Position	Examination

Standing or sitting	Posture
	  Scoliosis
	  Kyphosis
	  Lordosis

	Palpation
	  Muscles
	  Tenderness

	Range of motion

	Other
	  Shoulder motion
	  Cervical compression
	  Foraminal compression
	    (Spurling test)

	Neurologic
	  Reflexes (biceps, triceps,
	    brachioradialis, finger)
	  Motor
	  Sensory

The physical examination of the spine must be placed in the context of the individual's general health and condition. For findings such as atrophy, consider other possible explanations besides spine impairment, such as previous joint surgery or hypertrophy of the contralateral side from overuse. Other physical conditions may be present that influence motor and sensory function, ranges of motion, and sciatic nerve tension. Examination of associated systems (vascular, nervous) and follow-up of any possibly significant information from the history and physical examination will allow the physician to distinguish between spine-related findings and other abnormalities.[2-4]

The physician should record and discuss any physical findings that are inconsistent with the history. Many physical findings are subjective, ie, potentially under the influence of the individual. It is important to appreciate this and not confuse such observations with truly objective findings.

It is not the purpose of this text to discuss in detail how the physical examination is performed; textbooks are available to cover that subject. A few aspects of particular value to the impairment evaluation will be discussed subsequently.

Evaluation of Sciatic Nerve Tension Signs

Sciatic nerve tension signs are important indicators of irritation of the lumbosacral nerve roots. While most commonly seen in individuals with a herniated lumbar disk, this is not always the case. In chronic nerve root compression due to spinal stenosis, tension signs are often absent. A variety of nerve tension signs have been described. The most commonly used is the straight leg raising test (SLR). When performed in the supine position, the hip is flexed with the knee extended. In the sitting position, with the hip flexed 90°, the knee is extended. The test is positive when thigh and/or leg pain along the appropriate dermatomal distribution is reproduced. The degree of elevation at which pain occurs is recorded.

Research indicates that the maximum movement of nerve roots occurs when the leg is at an angle of 20° to 70° relative to the trunk. However, this may vary depending on the individual's anatomy. Further, the L4, L5, and S1 nerve roots are those that primarily change their length when straight leg raising is performed. Thus, pathology at higher levels of the lumbar spine is often associated with a negative SLR. Root tension signs are most reliable when the pain is elicited in a dermatomal distribution. Back pain on

SLR is not a positive test. Hamstring tightness must also be differentiated from posterior thigh pain due to root tension.

With time, spine-related symptoms usually improve, and a positive root tension (SLR) test is elicited only at the extremes of hip flexion (leg raising). While straight leg raising in disk herniation is a relatively sensitive test (72% to 97%), it is nonspecific (11% to 45%).[5] Straight leg raising of the asymptomatic limb (eg, crossed SLR) that produces **sciatica** in the limb with symptoms (crossed positive) is a specific (85% to 100%) but less sensitive (23% to 42%) test.

Results of supine SLR can be further validated by recording the individual's response to gentle dorsiflexion and plantar flexion of the ankle, and to internal and external rotation of the hip when the straightened leg is raised to the point where symptoms begin. Normally, ankle dorsiflexion and hip internal rotation increase the pain, and ankle plantar flexion and hip external rotation decrease the sciatica. Since sitting knee extension and supine hip flexion culminate in essentially identical positions, symptomatic responses to the two types of SLR should be similar, although the angle at which pain is elicited may vary.

The reverse SLR or femoral stretch test causes root tension of L2, L3, and L4 and may be a sign of disk herniations at the higher levels. This test has low sensitivity and specificity.

Neurologic Tests

Neurologic examination of the lower extremity should include measurement of knee and ankle reflexes and motor and sensory functions. Because over 90% of all nerve-related pathology in the lumbar spine occurs at the L3-4, L4-5, and L5-S1 levels, it is especially important to recognize the functions of the L4, L5, and S1 nerves (Table 15-2). The knee reflex is primarily a test of L4 nerve root function. Individuals with pathology at the L3-4 level may also have sensory changes in the L4 dermatome (Figure 15-1) and quadriceps weakness. L5 nerve root compression will often influence the strength of the extensor hallucis longus muscle, but other foot and ankle muscles can be affected as well, resulting in weakness in foot dorsiflexion and difficulty walking on the heels. The ankle reflex is primarily mediated by the S1 nerve root. Weakness in foot plantar flexion and difficulty with toe walking can also occur with S1 root compression. The Babinski sign and the presence of clonus and hyperreflexia are important indicators of corticospinal tract involvement.

Table 15-2 Common Radicular Syndromes

Disk Level	Nerve Root	Motor Deficit	Sensory Deficit	Reflex Compromise
Lumbar				
L3-4	L4	Quadriceps	Anterolateral thigh Anterior knee Medial leg and foot	Knee
L4-5	L5	Extensor hallucis longus	Lateral thigh Anterolateral leg Middorsal foot	Medial hamstrings
L5-S1	S1	Ankle plantar flexors	Posterior leg Lateral foot	Ankle
Cervical				
C4-5	C5	Deltoid Biceps	Anterolateral shoulder and arm	Biceps
C5-6	C6	Wrist extensors Biceps	Lateral forearm and hand Thumb	Brachioradialis Pronator teres
C6-7	C7	Wrist flexors Triceps Finger extensors	Middle finger	Triceps
C7-T1	C8	Finger flexors Hand intrinsics	Medial forearm and hand, ring and little fingers	None
T1-T2	T1	Hand intrinsics	Medial forearm	None

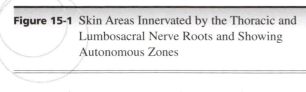

Figure 15-1 Skin Areas Innervated by the Thoracic and Lumbosacral Nerve Roots and Showing Autonomous Zones

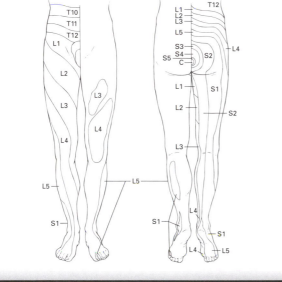

Changes in balance and gait pattern may also signify myelopathy.

A systematic neurologic examination can also localize the affected cervical nerve root (Table 15-2). The upper spine and extremity sensory dermatomes appear in Figure 15-2. The biceps (C5, partially C6), brachioradialis (C6), and triceps (C7) reflexes should be elicited. Weakness of the deltoid and biceps muscles implicates C5; wrist extensors C6; triceps, wrist flexors, and finger extensors C7; finger flexors C8; and intrinsics C8 and T1. Sensation can be grossly evaluated by touch and more precisely determined by pinprick, light touch, and a vibrating fork. Dermatomal overlap is common.

Reflexes should always be compared between extremities and elicited several times to determine reproducibility. Importantly, reflexes once "lost" due to previous injury or disease rarely return. Strength should also be compared between extremities and may need repeat testing to determine effort and reproducibility.

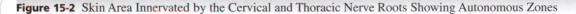

Figure 15-2 Skin Area Innervated by the Cervical and Thoracic Nerve Roots Showing Autonomous Zones

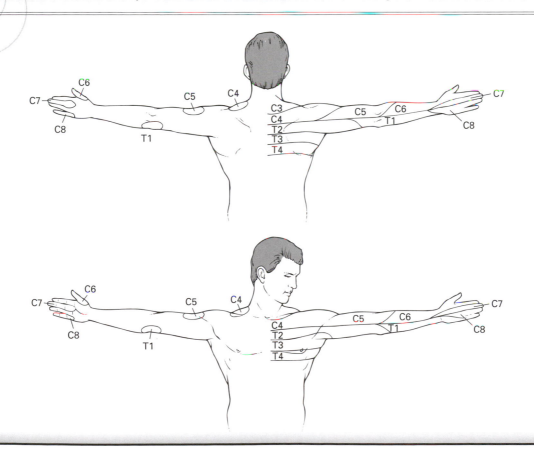

15.1b Description of Clinical Studies

General

The individual may have undergone a variety of special tests including electromyographic, cystometric, roentgenographic studies with or without dye, CT scans, and MRI studies with or without contrast. The physician should determine when, where, and by whom the studies were done, the findings, and who interpreted them. Whenever possible, the physician should personally review the studies and report agreement or disagreement with previous interpretations. A summary of the studies should be included as a separate paragraph or section.

While imaging and other studies may assist physicians in making a diagnosis, it is important to note that a positive imaging study in and of itself does not make the diagnosis. Several reports indicate approximately 30% of persons who have never had back pain will have an imaging study that can be interpreted as positive for a herniated disk, and 50% or more will have bulging disks. Further, the prevalence of degeneration changes, bulges, and herniations increases with advancing age.[6-11] To be of diagnostic value, clinical symptoms and signs must agree with the imaging findings. In other words, an imaging test is useful to confirm a diagnosis, but an imaging result alone is insufficient to qualify for a DRE category. Individuals with electromyography (EMG) studies that are clearly positive support a diagnosis of radiculopathy and therefore qualify for at least DRE category III.[14]

Motion Segment Integrity

A motion segment of the spine is defined as two adjacent vertebrae, the intervertebral disk, the apophyseal or facet joints, and ligamentous structures between the vertebrae. The range of motion from segment to segment varies. In the upper cervical spine (occiput to C2), there is little flexion-extension, while the lower cervical spine permits increasing flexion-extension movements from about 10° at C2 to C3 to about 20° at C5 to C6 and C6 to C7. Flexion-extension movements are about 4° in the upper thoracic spine, 6° in the midthoracic spine, and 12° in the lower thoracic spine segments. In the lumbar spine there is a gradual increase from about 12° at L1 to L2 to 20° at the L5 to S1 level.[13]

Lateral bending is 5° to 6° in the lower cervical spine and about 6° in the upper thoracic spine. In the lumbar spine, lateral bending is greatest at L3 to L4, where it is about 8° to 9°. Axial rotation is 30° to 40° in each direction in the upper cervical spine, 5° to 6° in the lower cervical and upper thoracic spine, and minimal in the lumbar spine.

Throughout the spine, movements are coupled; this means that the primary motion in one direction always is accompanied by a secondary motion in another direction. For example, rotation is almost always combined with side bending. The dominant motions at both the lower cervical and entire lumbar spine, where most clinical pathology occurs, are flexion-extension.

Alteration of motion segment integrity can be either loss of motion segment integrity (increased translational or angular motion) or decreased motion resulting mainly from developmental changes, fusion, fracture healing, healed infection, or surgical arthrodesis. An attempt at arthrodesis may not necessarily result in a solid fusion, but it may significantly limit motion at a motion segment and qualify for alteration of motion segment integrity.

Figure 15-3a Loss of Motion Segment Integrity, Translation

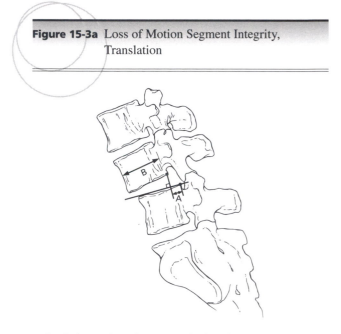

A line is drawn along the posterior bodies of the vertebrae below and above the motion segment in question on dynamic (flexion and extension), lateral roentgenograms of the spine. The distance between lines A and B and the distance between lines B and C at the level of the posteroinferior corner of the upper vertebral body are summed. A value greater than 2.5 mm in the thoracic spine, greater than 4.5 mm in the lumbar spine, and greater than 3.5 mm in the cervical spine qualifies as loss of structural integrity.

Motion of the individual spine segments cannot be determined by a physical examination but is evaluated with flexion and extension roentgenograms (see Figures 15-3a through 15-3c).[13,14] Loss of motion segment integrity is defined as an anteroposterior motion of one vertebra over another that is greater than 3.5 mm in the cervical spine, greater than 2.5 mm in the thoracic spine, and greater than 4.5 mm in the lumbar spine (Figure 15-3a). Loss of motion segment integrity is also defined as a difference in the angular motion of two adjacent motion segments greater than 15° at L1-2, L2-3, and L3-4 and greater than 20° at L4 to L5. Loss of integrity of the lumbosacral joint is defined as angular motion between L5 and S1 that is greater than 25°. In the cervical spine, loss of motion segment integrity is defined as motion at the level in question that is more than 11° greater than at either adjacent level.

When routine x-rays are normal and severe trauma is absent, motion segment alteration is rare; thus, flexion and extension x-rays are indicated *only* when the physician suspects motion segment alteration from history or findings on routine x-rays.[14]

15.2 Determining the Appropriate Method for Assessment

Spinal impairment rating is performed using one of two methods: the diagnosis-related estimate (DRE) or range-of-motion (ROM) method.

The DRE method is the principal methodology used to evaluate an individual who has had a distinct injury. When the cause of the impairment is not easily determined and if the impairment can be well characterized by the DRE method, the evaluator should use the DRE method.

The ROM method is used in several situations:
1. When an impairment is not caused by an injury, if the cause of the condition is uncertain and the DRE method does not apply, or an individual cannot be easily categorized in a DRE class. It is acknowledged that the cause of impairment (injury, illness, or aging) cannot always be determined. The reason for using the ROM method under these circumstances must be carefully supported in writing.

Figure 15-3b Loss of Motion Segment Integrity, Angular Motion (Sagittal Rotation), Lumbar Spine

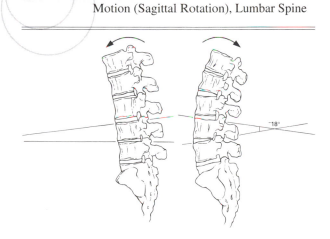

Lines are drawn along the superior border of the vertebral body of the lower vertebrae and the superior border of the body of the upper vertebrae and the lines extended until they join. The angles are measured and subtracted. Note that lordosis (extension) is represented by a negative angle and kyphosis (flexion) by a positive angle. Loss of motion segment integrity is defined as motion greater than 15° at L1-2, L2-3, and L3-4 and greater than 20° at L4 to L5. Loss of integrity of the lumbosacral joint is defined as angular motion between L5 and S1 that is greater than 25°. The flexion angle is +8° and the extension angle is −18°. Therefore (+8) − (−18) = +26° and would qualify for loss of structural integrity at any lumbar level.

Figure 15-3c Loss of Motion Segment Integrity, Cervical Spine

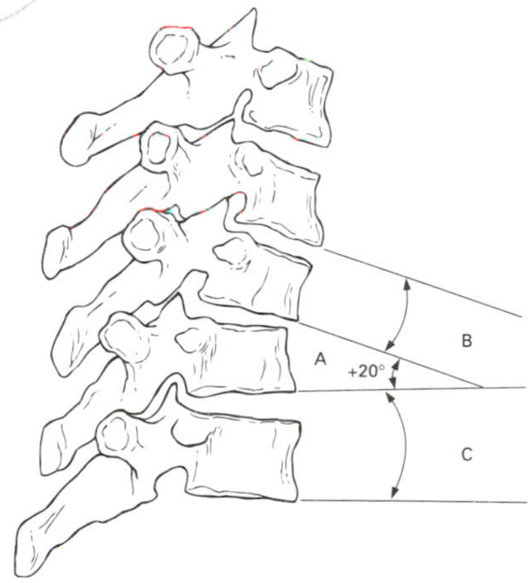

Lines are drawn along the inferior borders of the two vertebral bodies adjacent to the level in question and of the vertebral bodies above and below those two vertebrae. Angles A, B, and C are measured on both flexion and extension x-rays and the measurements subtracted from one another. Note that lordosis (extension) is represented by a negative angle and kyphosis (flexion) is represented by a positive angle. Loss of motion segment integrity is defined as motion at the level in question that is more than 11° greater than at either adjacent level.

2. When there is multilevel involvement in the same spinal region (eg, fractures at multiple levels, disk herniations, or stenosis with radiculopathy at multiple levels or bilaterally).
3. Where there is alteration of motion segment integrity (eg, fusions) at multiple levels in the same spinal region, unless there is involvement of the corticospinal tract (then use the DRE method for corticospinal tract involvement).
4. Where there is recurrent radiculopathy caused by a new (recurrent) disk herniation or a recurrent injury in the same spinal region.
5. Where there are multiple episodes of other pathology producing alteration of motion segment integrity and/or radiculopathy.

The ROM method can also be used if statutorily mandated in a particular jurisdiction.

In the small number of instances in which the ROM and DRE methods can both be used, evaluate the individual with both methods and award the higher rating.

All spine impairment ratings shown in Tables 15-3 to 15-5 estimate whole person impairment. With both the DRE method and the ROM method, whole person function is regarded as 100%. For converting whole person to regional spine impairments, see Section 15.13. When two or more regions are impaired and rated by either the DRE or ROM method, the ratings should be combined using the Combined Values Chart, p. 604.

A flowchart of the spine impairment evaluation process is provided in Figure 15-4.

15.2a Summary of Specific Procedures and Directions

1. Take a careful history, perform a thorough medical examination, and review all pertinent records and studies. This is helpful in determining the presence or absence of structural abnormalities, nerve root or cord involvement, and motion segment integrity.
2. Consider the permanency of the impairment, referring to *Guides* Chapter 1 and the Glossary for definitions as needed. If the impairment is resolving, changing, unstable, or expected to change significantly with or without medical treatment within 12 months, it is not considered a permanent (stable) impairment and should not be rated under the *Guides* criteria.

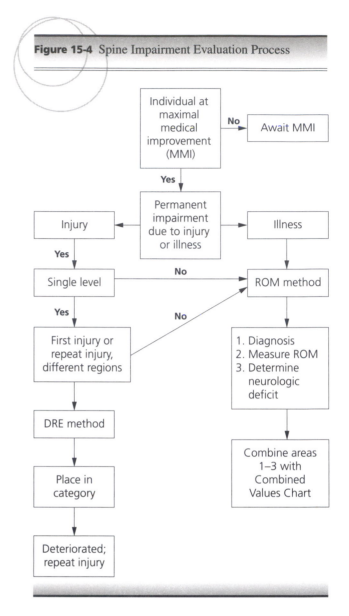

Figure 15-4 Spine Impairment Evaluation Process

3. Select the region that is primarily involved (ie, the lumbar, cervical, or thoracic spine) and identify the individual's most serious objective findings.
4. Determine whether the individual has multilevel involvement or multiple recurrences/occasions within the same region of the spine. Use the ROM method if:
   a. there are fractures at more than one level in a spinal region,
   b. there is radiculopathy bilaterally or at multiple levels in the same spinal region,
   c. there is multilevel motion segment alteration (such as a multilevel fusion) in the same spinal region, or
   d. there is recurrent disk herniation or stenosis with radiculopathy at the same or a different level in the same spinal region; in this case, combine the ratings using the ROM method.

5. If the individual does not have multilevel involvement or multiple recurrences/occasions and an injury occurred, determine the proper DRE category. Most ratings will fall into categories I, II, or III. A corticospinal tract injury is evaluated according to Section 15.7.

6. If the individual has been treated with surgery or another modality, evaluate the results, extent of improvement, and impact on the ability to perform activities of daily living. If residual symptoms or objective findings impact the ability to perform ADL despite treatment, the higher percentage in each range should be assigned. If an individual had a prior condition, was asymptomatic, and now—at MMI—has symptoms that impact the ability to perform activities of daily living, the higher rating within a range may also be used. If ratings are increased, explicit documentation of the reasons for the increase should be included in the report.

7. If more than one spine region is impaired, determine the impairment of the other region(s) with the DRE method. Combine the regional impairments using the Combined Values Chart (p. 604) to express the individual's total spine impairment.

8. From historical information and previously compiled medical data, determine if there was a preexisting impairment. Congenital, developmental, and other preexisting conditions may be differentiated from those attributable to the injury or illness by examining preinjury roentgenograms or by performing a bone scan after the onset of the condition.

9. If requested, apportion findings to the current or prior condition, following jurisdiction practices and assuming adequate information is available on the prior condition. In some instances, to apportion ratings, the percent impairment due to previous findings can simply be subtracted from the percent based on the current findings. Ideally, use the same method to compare the individual's prior and present conditions. If the ROM method has been used previously, it must be used again. If the previous evaluation was based on the DRE method and the individual now is evaluated with the ROM method, and prior ROM measurements do not exist to calculate a ROM impairment rating, the previous DRE percent can be subtracted from the ROM ratings. Because there are two methods and complete data may not exist on an earlier assessment, the apportionment calculation may be a less than ideal estimate.

10. For individuals with corticospinal tract involvement, refer to Table 15-6 for the appropriate impairment rating.

15.3 Diagnosis-Related Estimates Method

The DRE method has eight diagnosis-related categories for each of the three spinal regions. In assigning the individual to the correct DRE category, one of two approaches is used. The first is based on symptoms, signs, and appropriate diagnostic test results. The second is based on the presence of fractures and/or dislocations with or without clinical symptoms. If a fracture is present that places the individual into a DRE category, no other verification is required. The symptoms, signs other than fractures, and tests used to assist correct categorization of an individual are defined in Box 15-1.

Box 15-1 Definitions of Clinical Findings Used to Place an Individual in a DRE Category

Muscle Spasm

Muscle spasm is a sudden, involuntary contraction of a muscle or group of muscles. Paravertebral muscle spasm is common after acute spinal injury but is rare in chronic back pain. It is occasionally visible as a contracted paraspinal muscle but is more often diagnosed by palpation (a hard muscle). To differentiate true muscle spasm from voluntary muscle contraction, the individual should not be able to relax the contractions. The spasm should be present standing as well as in the supine position and frequently causes a scoliosis. The physician can sometimes differentiate spasm from voluntary contraction by asking the individual to place all his or her weight first on one foot and then the other while the physician gently palpates the paraspinous muscles. With this maneuver, the individual normally relaxes the paraspinal muscles on the weight-bearing side. If the examiner witnesses this relaxation, it usually means that true muscle spasm is not present.

Muscle Guarding

Guarding is a contraction of muscle to minimize motion or agitation of the injured or diseased tissue. It is not true muscle spasm because the contraction can be relaxed. In the lumbar spine, the contraction frequently results in loss of the normal lumbar lordosis, and it may be associated with reproducible loss of spinal motion.

Asymmetry of Spinal Motion

Asymmetric motion of the spine in one of the three principal planes is sometimes caused by muscle spasm or guarding. That is, if an individual attempts to flex the spine, he or she is unable to do so moving symmetrically; rather, the head or trunk leans to one side. To qualify as true asymmetric motion, the finding must be reproducible and consistent and the examiner must be convinced that the individual is cooperative and giving full effort.

Nonverifiable Radicular Root Pain

Nonverifiable pain is pain that is in the distribution of a nerve root but has no identifiable origin; ie, there are no objective physical, imaging, or electromyographic findings. For dermatomal distributions, see Figures 15-1 and 15-2.

Reflexes

Reflexes may be normal, increased, reduced, or absent. For reflex abnormalities to be considered valid, the involved and normal limb(s) should show marked asymmetry between arms or legs on repeated testing. Once lost because of previous radiculopathy, a reflex rarely returns. Abnormal reflexes such as Babinski signs or clonus may be signs of corticospinal tract involvement.

Weakness and Loss of Sensation

To be valid, the sensory findings must be in a strict anatomic distribution, ie, follow dermatomal patterns (see Figures 15-1 and 15-2). Motor findings should also be consistent with the affected nerve structure(s). Significant, long-standing weakness is usually accompanied by atrophy.

Atrophy

Atrophy is measured with a tape measure at identical levels on both limbs. For reasons of reproducibility, the difference in circumference should be 2 cm or greater in the thigh and 1 cm or greater in the arm, forearm, or leg. The evaluator can address asymmetry due to extremity dominance in the report.

Radiculopathy

Radiculopathy for the purposes of the *Guides* is defined as significant alteration in the function of a nerve root or nerve roots and is usually caused by pressure on one or several nerve roots. The diagnosis requires a dermatomal distribution of pain, numbness, and/or paresthesias in a dermatomal distribution. A root tension sign is usually positive. The diagnosis of herniated disk must be substantiated by an appropriate finding on an imaging study. The presence of findings on an imaging study in and of itself does not make the diagnosis of radiculopathy. There must also be clinical evidence as described above.

Electrodiagnostic Verification of Radiculopathy

Unequivocal electrodiagnostic evidence of acute nerve root pathology includes the presence of multiple positive sharp waves or fibrillation potentials in muscles innervated by one nerve root. However, the quality of the person performing and interpreting the study is critical. Electromyography should be performed only by a licensed physician qualified by reason of education, training, and experience in these procedures. Electromyography does not detect all compressive radiculopathies and cannot determine the cause of the nerve root pathology. On the other hand, electromyography can detect noncompressive radiculopathies, which are not identified by imaging studies.

Alteration of Motion Segment Integrity

Motion segment alteration can be either loss of motion segment integrity (increased translational or angular motion) or decreased motion secondary to developmental fusion, fracture healing, healed infection, or surgical arthrodesis. An attempt at arthrodesis may not necessarily result in a solid fusion but may significantly limit motion at a motion segment. Motion of the individual spine segments cannot be determined by a physical examination but is evaluated with flexion and extension roentgenograms. The loss of motion segment integrity is defined in Section 15.1b.

Cauda Equina Syndrome

Cauda equina syndrome is manifested by bowel or bladder dysfunction, saddle anesthesia, and variable loss of motor and sensory function in the lower extremities. Individuals with cauda equina syndrome usually have loss of sphincter tone on rectal examination and diminished or absent bladder, bowel, and lower limb reflexes.

Urodynamic Tests

Cystometrograms are useful in individuals where a cauda equina syndrome is possible but not certain. A normal cystometrogram makes the presence of a nerve-related bladder dysfunction unlikely. Occasionally, more extensive urodynamic testing is necessary.

To use the DRE method, obtain an individual's history, examine the individual, review the results of appropriate diagnostic studies, and place the individual in the appropriate category. Although there are eight categories, almost all individuals will fall into one of the first three DRE categories. Altered motion segment integrity (ie, increased motion or loss of motion) qualifies the individual for category IV or V. A fracture and/or dislocation, with or without clinical symptoms, permits placement of the individual into a DRE category with no additional verification. If there are impairments in different spinal regions, rate each spinal region separately using the DRE method; then combine the ratings using the Combined Values Chart on page 604. As stated previously, fractures at more than one level in the same spinal region should be rated using the ROM method.

In most cases, using the definitions provided in Box 15-1, the physician can assign an individual to DRE category I, II, or III. An individual in category I has only subjective findings. In category II, the individual has objective findings but no radiculopathy or alteration of structural integrity, while in category III, radiculopathy with objective verification must be present. Since an individual is evaluated after having reached MMI, a previous history of objective findings may not define the current, ratable condition but is important in determining the course and whether MMI has been reached. *The impairment rating is based on the condition once MMI is reached, not on prior symptoms or signs.*

If the individual had a radiculopathy caused by a herniated disk or lateral spinal stenosis that responded to conservative treatment and currently has no radicular symptoms or signs, he or she is placed in category II, since at MMI there is no radiculopathy. Category III is for individuals with a symptomatic radiculopathy, either after medical or surgical treatment, or for individuals who have a history of previous radiculopathy caused by disk herniation or lateral spinal stenosis but have improved or become asymptomatic following surgery.

The DRE method recommends that physicians document physiologic and structural impairments relating to injuries or diseases other than common developmental findings, such as (1) spondylolysis, found normally in 7% of adults; (2) spondylolisthesis, found in 3% of adults; (3) herniated disk without radiculopathy, found in approximately 30% of individuals by age 40 years; and (4) aging changes, present in 40% of adults after age 35 years and in almost all individuals after age 50.[6,12] As previously noted, the presence of these abnormalities on imaging studies does not necessarily mean the individual has an impairment due to an injury.

In cases where the abnormalities discussed above are present on imaging studies and are known or assumed to have preexisted an injury being rated, physicians should acknowledge these antecedent conditions. If requested, physicians may need to assess whether the condition was previously symptomatic and whether any aggravation occurred as a result of the injury. Physicians should be aware of the statutory definition in the involved jurisdiction pertaining to *aggravation* to ensure their use of the term is consistent with their state's legal interpretation.

DRE categories are discussed in the following three sections.

15.4 DRE: Lumbar Spine

The lumbar spine DRE categories are summarized in Table 15-3. Apart from category I, each category includes a range to account for the resolution or continuation of symptoms and their impact on the ability to perform ADL.

Table 15-3 Criteria for Rating Impairment Due to Lumbar Spine Injury

DRE Lumbar Category I 0% Impairment of the Whole Person	DRE Lumbar Category II 5%- 8% Impairment of the Whole Person	DRE Lumbar Category III 10%-13% Impairment of the Whole Person	DRE Lumbar Category IV 20%-23% Impairment of the Whole Person	DRE Lumbar Category V 25%-28% Impairment of the Whole Person
No significant clinical findings, no observed muscle guarding or spasm, no documentable neurologic impairment, no documented alteration in structural integrity, and no other indication of impairment related to injury or illness; no fractures	Clinical history and examination findings are compatible with a specific injury; findings may include significant muscle guarding or spasm observed at the time of the examination, asymmetric loss of range of motion, or nonverifiable radicular complaints, defined as complaints of radicular pain without objective findings; no alteration of the structural integrity and no significant radiculopathy **or** individual had a clinically significant radiculopathy and has an imaging study that demonstrates a herniated disk at the level and on the side that would be expected based on the previous radiculopathy, but no longer has the radiculopathy following conservative treatment **or** fractures: (1) less than 25% compression of one vertebral body; (2) posterior element fracture without dislocation (not developmental spondylolysis) that has healed without alteration of motion segment integrity; (3) a spinous or transverse process fracture with displacement without a vertebral body fracture, which does not disrupt the spinal canal	Significant signs of radiculopathy, such as dermatomal pain and/or in a dermatomal distribution, sensory loss, loss of relevant reflex(es), loss of muscle strength or measured unilateral atrophy above or below the knee compared to measurements on the contralateral side at the same location; impairment may be verified by electrodiagnostic findings **or** history of a herniated disk at the level and on the side that would be expected from objective clinical findings, associated with radiculopathy, or individuals who had surgery for radiculopathy but are now asymptomatic **or** fractures: (1) 25% to 50% compression of one vertebral body; (2) posterior element fracture with displacement disrupting the spinal canal; in both cases, the fracture has healed without alteration of structural integrity	Loss of motion segment integrity defined from flexion and extension radiographs as at least 4.5 mm of translation of one vertebra on another or angular motion greater than 15° at L1-2, L2-3, and L3-4, greater than 20° at L4-5, and greater than 25° at L5-S1 (Figure 15-3); may have complete or near complete loss of motion of a motion segment due to developmental fusion, or successful or unsuccessful attempt at surgical arthrodesis **or** fractures: (1) greater than 50% compression of one vertebral body without residual neurologic compromise	Meets the criteria of DRE lumbosacral categories III and IV; that is, both radiculopathy and alteration of motion segment integrity are present; significant lower extremity impairment is present as indicated by atrophy or loss of reflex(es), pain, and/or sensory changes within an anatomic distribution (dermatomal), or electromyographic findings as stated in lumbosacral category III and alteration of spine motion segment integrity as defined in lumbosacral category IV **or** fractures: (1) greater than 50% compression of one vertebral body with unilateral neurologic compromise

<table>
<tr><td>

DRE Lumbar Category I
0% Impairment of the Whole Person

No significant clinical findings, no observed muscle guarding or spasm, no documentable neurologic impairment, no documented alteration in structural integrity, and no other indication of impairment related to injury or illness; no fractures

</td></tr>
</table>

Example 15-1
0% Impairment Due to Lumbar Injury

Subject: 24-year-old man.

History: Hurt his back while lifting a large, heavy box; described the pain as being in the lumbosacral region. Examination shortly after the injury was normal, except for a slight decrease in lumbar motion due to pain. No muscle spasm or weakness. The individual was treated with an analgesic. He was off work for 3 days and then returned and has continued to work.

Current Symptoms: Occasional soreness in the low back with heavy lifting; denies leg pain or numbness.

Physical Exam: No positive finding was present, including a negative SLR, normal strength, range of motion, and normal neurologic examination. No atrophy.

Clinical Studies: None.

Diagnosis: Minor lumbar strain.

Impairment Rating: 0% impairment of the whole person.

Comment: Since there are no objective findings at the time of the impairment evaluation, the individual is assigned to lumbar DRE category I.

<table>
<tr><td>

DRE Lumbar Category II
5%- 8% Impairment of the Whole Person

Clinical history and examination findings are compatible with a specific injury; findings may include significant muscle guarding or spasm observed at the time of the examination, asymmetric loss of range of motion, or nonverifiable radicular complaints, defined as complaints of radicular pain without objective findings; no alteration of the structural integrity and no significant radiculopathy

or

individual had a clinically significant radiculopathy and has an imaging study that demonstrates a herniated disk at the level and on the side that would be expected based on the previous radiculopathy, but no longer has the radiculopathy following conservative treatment

or

fractures: (1) less than 25% compression of one vertebral body; (2) posterior element fracture without dislocation (not developmental spondylolysis) that has healed without alteration of motion segment integrity; (3) a spinous or transverse process fracture with displacement without a vertebral body fracture, which does not disrupt the spinal canal

</td></tr>
</table>

Example 15-2
5% to 8% Impairment Due to Lumbar Injury

Subject: 25-year-old man.

History: Onset of low back and left thigh pain while lifting on the job. Examination revealed muscle spasm, a positive SLR on the left at 60°, a positive crossed SLR at 70°, and an absent left Achilles tendon reflex. Treated with physical therapy, improved, and returned to work after 6 weeks.

Current Symptoms: No pain at rest or numbness in the lower extremities 1 year after onset. Able to perform all ADL; some back pain with heavy activity.

Physical Exam: Full range of motion of the lumbar spine. SLR: negative. Motor and sensory functions are normal.

Clinical Studies: MRI: left posterolateral disk herniation L5-S1.

Diagnosis: Left posterolateral disk herniation L5-S1 with left S1 radiculopathy, resolved.

Impairment Rating: 5% impairment of the whole person.

Comment: This individual had a radiographically confirmed herniated disk, at the level and side expected from the physical examination. Most symptoms resolved with conservative treatment. At the time of evaluation, the individual was doing well, with no evidence of residual radiculopathy.

> **DRE Lumbar Category III**
> **10%-13% Impairment of the Whole Person**
>
> Significant signs of radiculopathy, such as dermatomal pain and/or in a dermatomal distribution, sensory loss, loss of relevant reflex(es), loss of muscle strength or measured unilateral atrophy above or below the knee compared to measurements on the contralateral side at the same location; impairment may be verified by electrodiagnostic findings
>
> *or*
>
> history of a herniated disk at the level and on the side that would be expected from objective clinical findings, associated with radiculopathy, or individuals who had surgery for radiculopathy but are now asymptomatic
>
> *or*
>
> fractures: (1) 25% to 50% compression of one vertebral body; (2) posterior element fracture with displacement disrupting the spinal canal; in both cases, the fracture has healed without alteration of structural integrity

Example 15-3
10% to 13% Impairment Due to Surgically Treated Herniated Disk

Subject: 25-year-old man.

History: Onset of back and left posterior thigh and leg pain while twisting in a flexed position when lifting a moderately heavy package. Initially presented with muscle spasm, a positive SLR on the side at 60°, a positive crossed SLR at 70°, and an absent left Achilles tendon reflex. Treatment with physical therapy did not produce significant improvement. Underwent surgical diskectomy 3 months after the injury. Improved and returned to work without restrictions after 4 months of rehabilitation.

Current Symptoms: No pain at rest or numbness in the lower extremities 8 months after injury. Able to do most ADL but complains of back pain with heavy activity.

Physical Exam: Full range of motion of the lumbar spine. Loss of the Achilles reflex but normal motor and sensory functions. SLR: negative.

Clinical Studies: Original MRI: herniated disk at L5-S1. No additional studies have been done.

Diagnosis: Left posterolateral herniated disk at L5-S1 with left S1 radiculopathy, partially resolved status postdiskectomy.

Impairment Rating: 10% impairment of the whole person.

Comment: Symptoms, physical findings, and imaging studies are all consistent with a symptomatic herniated disk. Most symptoms and signs resolved with surgical treatment.

Example 15-4
10% to 13% Impairment Due to Radiculopathy

Subject: 25-year-old man.

History: New onset of back and left leg pain while lifting on the job. Initially presented with muscle spasm, a positive SLR on the left side at 60°, a positive crossed SLR at 70°, and an absent left Achilles tendon reflex. An MRI revealed a left posterolateral disk herniation at L5-S1. Was treated with analgesics and physical therapy but did not improve. Underwent surgical diskectomy 3 months after the injury. Some improvement in the symptoms after 9 months of rehabilitation.

Current Symptoms: Persistent back and thigh pain and numbness along the lateral side of the foot at rest. Unable to do his usual recreational and some household activities.

Physical Exam: Restricted lumbar motion. Loss of the Achilles reflex, numbness in the S1 nerve root distribution, and pain in the posterior thigh and leg on SLR.

Clinical Studies: Original MRI: herniated disk at L5-S1. Postoperative MRI with gadolinium: fibrosis but no residual or recurrent herniation.

Diagnosis: Chronic low back pain and radiculopathy.

Impairment Rating: 13% impairment of the whole person.

Comment: Symptoms, physical findings, and imaging studies are all consistent with a symptomatic herniated disk. Symptoms did not completely resolve after surgical treatment, with subjective and objective signs of persistent radiculopathy. Individual therefore qualifies for DRE lumbar category III. Because of significant persistent symptoms that limit the ability to perform ADL and continued objective findings, the impairment rating is increased to 13%.

DRE Lumbar Category IV
20%-23% Impairment of the Whole Person

Loss of motion segment integrity defined from flexion and extension radiographs as at least 4.5 mm of translation of one vertebra on another or angular motion greater than 15° at L1-2,
L2-3, and L3-4, greater than 20° at L4-5, and greater than 25°
at L5-S1 (Figure 15-3); may have complete or near complete loss
of motion of a motion segment due to developmental fusion,
or successful or unsuccessful attempt at surgical arthrodesis

or

fractures: (1) greater than 50% compression of one vertebral
body without residual neurologic compromise

DRE Lumbar Category V
25%-28% Impairment of the Whole Person

Meets the criteria of DRE lumbosacral categories III and IV; that
is, both radiculopathy and alteration of motion segment integrity
are present; significant lower extremity impairment is present as
indicated by atrophy or loss of reflex(es), pain, and/or sensory
changes within an anatomic distribution (dermatomal), or electromyographic findings as stated in lumbosacral category III and
alteration of spine motion segment integrity as defined in lumbosacral category IV

or

fractures: (1) greater than 50% compression of one vertebral
body with unilateral neurologic compromise

Example 15-5
20% to 23% Impairment Due to Fracture With Greater Than 50% Compression of Vertebrae

Subject: 54-year-old woman.

History: Fell from a ladder and sustained a burst fracture of L2 with a 55% loss of height, without neurologic findings. Treated with bracing, the fracture healed; returned to most ADL 6 months after the injury.

Current Symptoms: No neurologic complaints, but has back pain after heavy activity or with weather changes.

Physical Exam: Mild tenderness to palpation at the fracture site. Neurologic examination and SLR: negative. Range of motion is mildly decreased.

Clinical Studies: Radiograph: fracture healed with 60% loss of height.

Diagnosis: Burst fracture L2 > 50%.

Impairment Rating: 20% impairment of the whole person.

Comment: Individual qualifies for lumbar DRE cat-egory IV based on the fracture. Neurologic deficit, if present, would warrant category V or Section 15.7. If she had multiple compression fractures in the same or different spinal regions, use the ROM method for rating.

Example 15-6
25% to 28% Impairment Due to Radiculopathy and Alteration of Motion Segment Integrity

Subject: 25-year-old man.

History: Onset of back and left leg pain after a fall on a concrete surface while carrying a box. Initially presented with muscle spasm, an SLR on the left side at 60°, a positive crossed SLR at 70°, and an absent left Achilles tendon reflex. Treated with physical therapy but did not improve. Underwent surgical diskectomy and arthrodesis of L5-S1 3 months after the injury. After 9 months of rehabilitation, leg and back symptoms were diminished but persistent.

Current Symptoms: Back and thigh pain at rest and persistent numbness along the lateral side of the foot 1 year after the onset of symptoms. Pain and numbness prevent individual from maintaining a constant position, prolonged standing or walking, or performing his prior work, recreational, and some household activities.

Physical Exam: Severely restricted range of motion. Loss of the Achilles reflex. Numbness in the S1 nerve root distribution and dermatomal pain in the leg on SLR.

Clinical Studies: Original MRI: a severely degener-ated L5-S1 disk with a herniation on the left side. Postoperative MRI with gadolinium: fibrosis, but no residual or recurrent herniation. Fusion appears solid.

Diagnosis: Left posterolateral disk herniation L5-S1 with S1 radiculopathy and severe disk degenera-tion, unresolved status postdiskectomy and L5-S1 fusion.

Impairment Rating: 28% impairment of the whole person.

Comment: Symptoms, physical findings, and imaging studies are all consistent with a symptomatic herniated disk. Excision of the offending disk and a single-level fusion did not relieve all symptoms, which are supported by signs of a persistent radiculopathy. Individual qualifies for lumbar DRE category V because he has persistent radiculopathy as well as single-level alteration of motion segment integrity.

15.5 DRE: Thoracic Spine

Thoracic problems are evaluated as follows:

For thoracic spine problems localized to the thoracic region, use Table 15-4. If the thoracic pathology also leads to isolated bowel or bladder dysfunction not due to corticospinal damage, obtain the appropriate estimates for bowel and bladder dysfunction listed in the gastrointestional and urology chapters and combine these with the thoracic spine DRE category (I-V) listed in Table 15-4. If the thoracic spine problem is due to corticospinal tract involvement, use Section 15.7. If thoracic injury–related bowel or bladder symptoms exist without verifiable lower extremity involvement, then appropriate estimates for bowel and bladder impairments from the *Guides* chapters on the urinary and reproductive and digestive systems should be combined (Combined Values Chart, p. 604) with an impairment percent from one of the thoracic categories II through V.

The thoracic spine impairment DRE categories are summarized in Table 15-4.

Table 15-4 Criteria for Rating Impairment Due to Thoracic Spine Injury

DRE Thoracic Category I 0% Impairment of the Whole Person	DRE Thoracic Category II 5%-8% Impairment of the Whole Person	DRE Thoracic Category III 15%-18% Impairment of the Whole Person	DRE Thoracic Category IV 20%-23% Impairment of the Whole Person	DRE Thoracic Category V 25%-28% Impairment of the Whole Person
No significant clinical findings, no observed muscle guarding, no documentable neurologic impairment, no documented changes in structural integrity, and no other indication of impairment related to injury or illness; no fractures	History and examination findings are compatible with a specific injury or illness; findings may include significant muscle guarding or spasm observed at the time of the examination, asymmetric loss of range of motion (dysmetria), or nonverifiable radicular complaints, defined as complaints of radicular pain without objective findings; no alteration of motion segment integrity *or* herniated disk at the level and on the side that would be expected from objective clinical findings, but without radicular signs following conservative treatment *or* fractures: (1) less than 25% compression of one vertebral body; (2) posterior element fracture without dislocation that has healed without alteration of motion segment integrity or radiculopathy; (3) a spinous or transverse process fracture with displacement, but without a vertebral body fracture	Ongoing neurologic impairment of the lower extremity related to a thoracolumbar injury, documented by examination of motor and sensory functions, reflexes, or findings of unilateral atrophy above or below the knee related to no other condition; impairment may be verified by electrodiagnostic testing *or* clinically significant radiculopathy, verified by an imaging study that demonstrates a herniated disk at the level and on the side that would be expected from objective clinical findings; history of radiculopathy, which has improved following surgical treatment *or* fractures: (1) 25% to 50% compression fracture of one vertebral body; (2) posterior element fracture with mild displacement disrupting the canal; in both cases the fracture has healed without alteration of structural integrity; differentiation from a congenital or developmental condition should be accomplished, if possible, by examining preinjury roentgenograms, if available, or by a bone scan performed after the onset of the condition	Alteration of motion segment integrity or bilateral or multilevel radiculopathy; alteration of motion segment integrity is defined from flexion and extension radiographs as translation of one vertebra on another of more than 2.5 mm; radiculopathy as defined in thoracic category III need not be present if there is alteration of motion segment integrity; if an individual is to be placed in DRE thoracic category IV due to radiculopathy, the latter must be bilateral or involve more than one level *or* fractures: (1) more than 50% compression of one vertebral body without residual neural compromise	Impairment of the lower extremity as defined in thoracolumbar category III and loss of structural integrity as defined in thoracic category IV *or* fractures: (1) greater than 50% compression of one vertebral body with neural motor compromise but not bilateral involvement that would qualify the individual for corticospinal tract evaluation

DRE Thoracic Category I 0% Impairment of the Whole Person
No significant clinical findings, no observed muscle guarding, no documentable neurologic impairment, no documented changes in structural integrity, and no other indication of impairment related to injury or illness; no fractures

Example 15-7
0% Impairment Due to Thoracic Injury

Subject: 44-year-old man.

History: Working from home spending many hours on the phone and computer.

Current Symptoms: Chronic, bilateral, upper back discomfort under the scapula area worsened 3 to 4 months ago, but unchanged since. Feels better when not working at the computer.

Physical Exam: Hunched posture. Minimal tenderness to deep palpation over the descending trapezius muscles and the periscapular area, right side more pronounced. Otherwise normal examination.

Clinical Studies: None.

Diagnosis: Upper back pain.

Impairment Rating: 0% impairment of the whole person.

Chapter 15

Comment: The individual was educated concerning the importance of proper posture, an appropriate workstation, and the need for stretching and strengthening exercises to alleviate the temporary discomfort.

DRE Thoracic Category II
5%-8% Impairment of the Whole Person

History and examination findings are compatible with a specific injury or illness; findings may include significant muscle guarding or spasm observed at the time of the examination, asymmetric loss of range of motion (dysmetria), or nonverifiable radicular complaints, defined as complaints of radicular pain without objective findings; no alteration of motion segment integrity

or

herniated disk at the level and on the side that would be expected from objective clinical findings, but without radicular signs following conservative treatment

or

fractures: (1) less than 25% compression of one vertebral body; (2) posterior element fracture without dislocation that has healed without alteration of motion segment integrity or radiculopathy; (3) a spinous or transverse process fracture with displacement, but without a vertebral body fracture

---

Example 15-8
5% to 8% Impairment Due to Thoracic Injury

Subject: 56-year-old man.

History: Laborer with prior history of multiple musculoskeletal injuries during college football, from which he had fully recovered. Developed severe right-sided, radiating arm pain with tingling along the chest and the underside of the right arm while moving a refrigerator. Most of the pain has disappeared, but individual still has some discomfort when lifting the right arm above shoulder level.

Current Symptoms: Persistent numbness along the medial right arm.

Physical Exam: Numbness along a T1-3 dermatomal area in chest, not clearly defined.

Clinical Studies: MRI: degenerative disk changes at T1-2. Radiographs: osteophyte T1, T2 levels.

Diagnosis: Degenerative disk disease T1.

Impairment Rating: 5% impairment of the whole person.

Comment: Impairment rating would increase by up to 3% if individual was unable to do ADL as indicated in Table 1-2.

DRE Thoracic Category III
15%-18% Impairment of the Whole Person

Ongoing neurologic impairment of the lower extremity related to a thoracolumbar injury, documented by examination of motor and sensory functions, reflexes, or findings of unilateral atrophy above or below the knee related to no other condition; impairment may be verified by electrodiagnostic testing

or

clinically significant radiculopathy, verified by an imaging study that demonstrates a herniated disk at the level and on the side that would be expected from objective clinical findings; history of radiculopathy, which has improved following surgical treatment

or

fractures: (1) 25% to 50% compression fracture of one vertebral body; (2) posterior element fracture with mild displacement disrupting the canal; in both cases the fracture has healed without alteration of structural integrity; differentiation from a congenital or developmental condition should be accomplished, if possible, by examining preinjury roentgenograms, if available, or by a bone scan performed after the onset of the condition

---

Example 15-9
15% to 18% Impairment Due to Thoracic Injury

Subject: 35-year-old man.

History: Individual fell from the second floor of a building on which he was working and sustained a compression fracture of T8. After conservative treatment, able to perform most ADL and walk without braces or crutches.

Current Symptoms: Minor back pain with heavy physical activity. Left lower extremity weakness and numbness in the left leg.

Physical Exam: Spotty numbness in the left leg and grade 4/5 left leg weakness. Measurable atrophy of left thigh and leg. Left leg reflexes are slightly hypoactive.

Clinical Studies: Compression fracture of T8 with loss of height of the vertebral body of about 30%.

Diagnosis: Compression fracture T8 with residual left lower extremity neurologic involvement.

Impairment Rating: 15% impairment of the whole person.

Comment: This individual qualifies for DRE thoracic category III because of his ongoing neurologic deficits and structural inclusion of a compression fracture with 25% to 50% loss of height.

<table>
<tr><td>

DRE Thoracic Category IV
20%–23% Impairment of the Whole Person

Alteration of motion segment integrity or bilateral or multilevel radiculopathy; alteration of motion segment integrity is defined from flexion and extension radiographs as translation of one vertebra on another of more than 2.5 mm; radiculopathy as defined in thoracic category III need not be present if there is alteration of motion segment integrity; if an individual is to be placed in DRE thoracic category IV due to radiculopathy, the latter must be bilateral or involve more than one level

or

fractures: (1) more than 50% compression of one vertebral body without residual neural compromise

</td></tr>
</table>

Example 15-10
20% to 23% Impairment Due to Compression Fracture of T1

Subject: 56-year-old-man.

History: Truck driver in motor vehicle accident was unconscious and had a seizure. Improved with physical therapy. Able to drive again and do usual ADL. No further seizures; off medication.

Current Symptoms: Bilateral upper extremity heaviness and weakness.

Physical Exam: Numbness over T1 distribution bilaterally; weakness of the intrinsic hand muscles.

Clinical Studies: 65% compression fracture of T1.

Diagnosis: Compression fracture of T1 with bilateral radiculopathy. New onset seizure disorder.

Impairment Rating: 20% impairment due to musculoskeletal disorder; combine with appropriate rating due to the seizure disorder to determine whole person impairment (see Combined Values Chart, p. 604).

Comment: No additional impairment since he is doing well.

<table>
<tr><td>

DRE Thoracic Category V
25%–28% Impairment of the Whole Person

Impairment of the lower extremity as defined in thoracolumbar category III and loss of structural integrity as defined in thoracic category IV

or

fractures: (1) greater than 50% compression of one vertebral body with neural motor compromise but not bilateral involvement that would qualify the individual for corticospinal tract evaluation

</td></tr>
</table>

Example 15-11
25% to 28% Impairment Due to Radiculopathy and Alteration of Motion Segment Integrity

Subject: 35-year-old man.

History: Individual fell from the second floor of a building on which he was working and sustained a compression fracture of T8. He had minor right lower extremity weakness and numbness. After anterior surgical decompression and instrumented fusion from T7 through T9 he improved and was able to return to most ADL and walk without braces or crutches, but he still had weakness and patchy numbness in the right lower extremity.

Current Symptoms: Minor pain on heavy activity.

Physical Exam: Neurologically, spotty numbness in the right lower extremity with 4/5 weakness and mild atrophy of the right thigh and leg muscles. Right lower extremity reflexes are slightly hyperactive.

Clinical Studies: MRI: compression fracture T8 without canal compromise. Radiograph: treated fracture with fusion.

Diagnosis: Compression fracture T8 treated surgically with mild residual right lower extremity neurologic involvement.

Impairment Rating: 25% impairment of the whole person by DRE method; another option is to use the ROM method.

Comment: This individual qualifies for DRE thoracic category V because he has mild right lower extremity neurologic deficits (category III) and alteration of motion segment integrity given the fusion (category IV). A combination of categories III and IV in the thoracic region means that the individual qualifies for category V. Because he has alteration of motion segment integrity of more than one level (multilevel fusion), he could also be rated by the ROM method. The best approach would be to rate the individual by both methods and award the higher rating.

15.6 DRE: Cervical Spine

15.6a Criteria for Rating Impairment Due to Cervical Disorders

For cervical problems localized to the cervical or cervicothoracic region, use Table 15-5. If the cervical spine problem also leads to isolated bowel and/or bladder dysfunction not due to corticospinal damage, obtain the appropriate estimates for bowel and

bladder dysfunction from the gastrointestinal and urology chapters (Chapters 6 and 7) and combine these with the appropriate cervical spine DRE category from DRE I to V, listed in Table 15-5. If the cervical spine problem is due to corticospinal tract involvement, use Table 15-6 alone.

The DRE cervical categories are summarized in Table 15-5.

Table 15-5 Criteria for Rating Impairment Due to Cervical Disorders

DRE Cervical Category I 0% Impairment of the Whole Person	DRE Cervical Category II 5%-8% Impairment of the Whole Person	DRE Cervical Category III 15%-18% Impairment of the Whole Person	DRE Cervical Category IV 25%-28% Impairment of the Whole Person	DRE Cervical Category V 35%-38% Impairment of the Whole Person
No significant clinical findings, no muscular guarding, no documentable neurologic impairment, no significant loss of motion segment integrity, and no other indication of impairment related to injury or illness; no fractures	Clinical history and examination findings are compatible with a specific injury; findings may include muscle guarding or spasm observed at the time of the examination by a physician, asymmetric loss of range of motion or nonverifiable radicular complaints, defined as complaints of radicular pain without objective findings; no alteration of the structural integrity *or* individual had clinically significant radiculopathy and an imaging study that demonstrated a herniated disk at the level and on the side that would be expected based on the radiculopathy, but has improved following nonoperative treatment *or* fractures: (1) less than 25% compression of one vertebral body; (2) posterior element fracture without dislocation that has healed without loss of structural integrity or radiculopathy; (3) a spinous or transverse process fracture with displacement	Significant signs of radiculopathy, such as pain and/or sensory loss in a dermatomal distribution, loss of relevant reflex(es), loss of muscle strength, or unilateral atrophy compared with the unaffected side, measured at the same distance above or below the elbow; the neurologic impairment may be verified by electrodiagnostic findings *or* individual had clinically significant radiculopathy, verified by an imaging study that demonstrates a herniated disk at the level and on the side expected from objective clinical findings with radiculopathy or with improvement of radiculopathy following surgery *or* fractures: (1) 25% to 50% compression of one vertebral body; (2) posterior element fracture with displacement disrupting the spinal canal; in both cases the fracture is healed without loss of structural integrity; radiculopathy may or may not be present; differentiation from congenital and developmental conditions may be accomplished, if possible, by examining preinjury roentgenograms or a bone scan performed after the onset of the condition	Alteration of motion segment integrity or bilateral or multilevel radiculopathy; alteration of motion segment integrity is defined from flexion and extension radiographs as at least 3.5 mm of translation of one vertebra on another, or angular motion of more than 11° greater than at each adjacent level (Figures 15-3a and 15-3b); alternatively, the individual may have loss of motion of a motion segment due to a developmental fusion or successful or unsuccessful attempt at surgical arthrodesis; radiculopathy as defined in cervical category III need not be present if there is alteration of motion segment integrity *or* fractures: (1) more than 50% compression of one vertebral body without residual neural compromise	Significant upper extremity impairment requiring the use of upper extremity external functional or adaptive device(s); there may be total neurologic loss at a single level or severe, multilevel neurologic dysfunction *or* fractures: structural compromise of the spinal canal is present with severe upper extremity motor and sensory deficits but without lower extremity involvement

DRE Cervical Category I
0% Impairment of the Whole Person

No significant clinical findings, no muscular guarding, no documentable neurologic impairment, no significant loss of motion segment integrity, and no other indication of impairment related to injury or illness; no fractures

Example 15-12
0% Impairment Due to Cervical Injury

Subject: 37-year-old man.

History: Complaints of neck discomfort when painting.

Current Symptoms: Intermittent neck pain, occasionally extending into upper back bilaterally, moreso on the left side.

Physical Exam: Full neck motion, but pain at the extremes; some tenderness over the trapezius muscles; no spasm; no neurologic findings.

Clinical Studies: Radiographs: normal cervical spine.

Diagnosis: Intermittent cervical neck strain.

Impairment Rating: 0% impairment of the whole person.

Comment: No evidence of permanent impairment, without objective signs. Advised to do appropriate stretching and neck exercises regularly, before and after vigorous activity.

DRE Cervical Category II
5%-8% Impairment of the Whole Person

Clinical history and examination findings are compatible with a specific injury; findings may include muscle guarding or spasm observed at the time of the examination by a physician, asymmetric loss of range of motion or nonverifiable radicular complaints, defined as complaints of radicular pain without objective findings; no alteration of the structural integrity

or

individual had clinically significant radiculopathy and an imaging study that demonstrated a herniated disk at the level and on the side that would be expected based on the radiculopathy, but has improved following nonoperative treatment

or

fractures: (1) less than 25% compression of one vertebral body; (2) posterior element fracture without dislocation that has healed without loss of structural integrity or radiculopathy; (3) a spinous or transverse process fracture with displacement

Example 15-13
5% to 8% Impairment Due to Cervical Injury

Subject: 37-year-old woman.

History: Pain in the neck and lateral right upper extremity extending to the thumb following a rear-end auto collision. An MRI showed a herniated disk at C6. She elected nonoperative treatment and recovered after 18 months.

Current Symptoms: Some residual neck pain with physical activity; upper limb symptoms have resolved.

Physical Exam: Slight loss of motion of the cervical spine. Neurologic examination is normal.

Clinical Studies: Initial MRI: right posterolateral disk herniation at C5. No additional imaging studies were done.

Diagnosis: Herniated disk C5-6 with resolved right C6 radiculopathy.

Impairment Rating: 5% impairment of the whole person.

Comment: The individual qualifies for DRE cervical category II because she had a radiculopathy caused by a herniated disk that responded to treatment. She has no significant residual signs.

DRE Cervical Category III
15%-18% Impairment of the Whole Person

Significant signs of radiculopathy, such as pain and/or sensory loss in a dermatomal distribution, loss of relevant reflex(es), loss of muscle strength, or unilateral atrophy compared with the unaffected side, measured at the same distance above or below the elbow; the neurologic impairment may be verified by electro-diagnostic findings

or

individual had clinically significant radiculopathy, verified by an imaging study that demonstrates a herniated disk at the level and on the side expected from objective clinical findings with radiculopathy or with improvement of radiculopathy following surgery

or

fractures: (1) 25% to 50% compression of one vertebral body; (2) posterior element fracture with displacement disrupting the spinal canal; in both cases the fracture is healed without loss of structural integrity; radiculopathy may or may not be present; differentiation from congenital and developmental conditions may be accomplished, if possible, by examining preinjury roentgenograms or by bone scans performed after the onset of the condition

---

Example 15-14
15% to 18% Impairment Due to Radiculopathy

Subject: 44-year-old man.

History: Sustained a blow to his posterior neck from a machine support that slipped. Unable to use his dominant left hand for ADL without considerable pain in neck, left upper back, and ulnar left upper limb. No discomfort in the lower extremities. Refuses surgery.

Current Symptoms: Neck pain, radiating to the ulnar hand with numbness of the ring and little fingers.

Physical Exam: Decreased range of motion in the neck with severe radiating pain to the left arm in a C6 distribution.

Clinical Studies: MRI: left posterolateral disk herniation C7-8.

Diagnosis: Radiculopathy due to disk herniation C6.

Impairment Rating: 18% impairment of the whole person.

Comment: Residual symptoms and functional limitations to perform ADL.

DRE Cervical Category IV
25%-28% Impairment of the Whole Person

Alteration of motion segment integrity or bilateral or multilevel radiculopathy; alteration of motion segment integrity is defined from flexion and extension radiographs as at least 3.5 mm of translation of one vertebra on another, or angular motion of more than 11° greater than at each adjacent level (Figures 15-3a and 15-3b); alternatively, the individual may have loss of motion of a motion segment due to a developmental fusion or successful or unsuccessful attempt at surgical arthrodesis; radiculopathy as defined in cervical category III need not be present if there is alteration of motion segment integrity

or

fractures: (1) more than 50% compression of one vertebral body without residual neural compromise

---

Example 15-15
25% to 28% Impairment Due to Alterations of Motion Segment Integrity

Subject: 37-year-old woman.

History: Onset of pain in the neck and right arm along the radial aspect and into the thumb following a medium-speed rear-end auto collision. Individual failed conservative treatment, and an MRI showed a herniated disk at C6-7. Underwent a diskectomy of the sixth cervical disk and fusion of C6 to C7. Healed uneventfully and returned to work 4 months after the injury.

Current Symptoms: Occasional neck pain with physical activity. Upper extremity pain resolved.

Physical Exam: Slight loss of cervical spine motion. Neurologic examination is normal.

Clinical Studies: Radiographs: healed C6-7 fusion.

Diagnosis: Herniated disk C6-7 with C7 radiculopathy resolved following anterior cervical diskectomy and C6-7 fusion.

Impairment Rating: 25% impairment of the whole person.

Comment: This individual meets criteria for DRE cervical category IV because of alteration of motion segment integrity due to fusion.

> **DRE Cervical Category V**
> **35%–38% Impairment of the Whole Person**
>
> Significant upper extremity impairment requiring the use of upper extremity external functional or adaptive device(s); there may be total neurologic loss at a single level or severe, multilevel neurologic dysfunction
>
> *or*
>
> fractures: structural compromise of the spinal canal is present with severe upper extremity motor and sensory deficits but without lower extremity involvement

Example 15-16
35% to 38% Impairment Due to Herniated Cervical Disk Postdiskectomy and Fusion

Subject: 37-year-old woman.

History: Individual fell and struck her posterior head and neck on a conveyor machine while working on an assembly line. She had severe and persistent pain in the neck and lateral right upper limb extending into the thumb. An MRI showed a herniated disk at C5-6. She failed nonoperative treatment and underwent a diskectomy of the sixth cervical disk and fusion of C6 to C7. She has continued neck and bilateral upper extremity pain. Unable to perform most ADL and uses assistive devices for gripping and turning objects.

Current Symptoms: Severe neck and bilateral upper extremity pain aggravated by movements of the neck and use of the upper extremities. Persistent numbness in the radial forearm, hand, and digits on both sides.

Physical Exam: Slight loss of cervical motion. Neurologic examination reveals decreased sensation in the thumb and index finger and weakness of the biceps and wrist extensors bilaterally. Diminished brachioradialis reflexes, right worse than left.

Clinical Studies: Radiographs: healed fusion.

Diagnosis: Herniated C5-6 disk treated with residual bilateral C6 radiculopathy.

Impairment Rating: 38% impairment of the whole person.

Comment: This individual meets criteria for both DRE cervical category III, with a surgically treated radiculopathy, and DRE cervical category IV, because of alteration of motion segment integrity due to the fusion, and is placed in DRE category V because of objective findings supportive of significant upper extremity impairment requiring the use of adaptive devices.

15.7 Rating Corticospinal Tract Damage

The neurologic level of involvement is determined by identifying the level of cord involvement, not necessarily the same level as a fracture, because the root function at the fracture level frequently returns with time. The level of cord involvement is determined by identifying the lowest normally functioning nerve root. Identifying the level of nerve root function helps to determine the degree of residual function. Figure 15-5 illustrates the relationship of nerve roots to the vertebral level.

Figure 15-5 Relationship of Spinal Nerves to Vertebrae

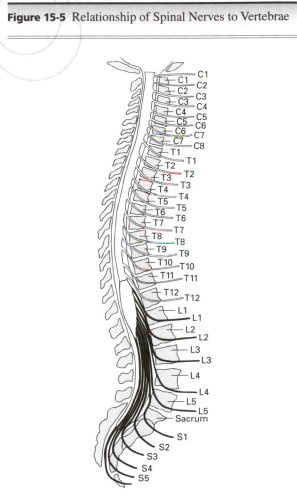

The level at which nerve roots exit the spine relative to the vertebrae. The neurologic level of involvement is determined by identifying the lowest normally functioning nerve root.

Table 15-6 Rating Corticospinal Tract Impairment

a. Impairment of One Upper Extremity Due to Corticospinal Tract Impairment

Class 1		Class 2		Class 3		Class 4	
Dominant Extremity 1%-9% Impairment of the Whole Person	Nondominant Extremity 1%-4% Impairment of the Whole Person	Dominant Extremity 10%-24% Impairment of the Whole Person	Nondominant Extremity 5%-14% Impairment of the Whole Person	Dominant Extremity 25%-39% Impairment of the Whole Person	Nondominant Extremity 15%-29% Impairment of the Whole Person	Dominant Extremity 40%-60% Impairment of the Whole Person	Nondominant Extremity 30%-45% Impairment of the Whole Person
Individual can use the involved extremity for self-care, daily activities, and holding, but has difficulty with digital dexterity		Individual can use the involved extremity for self-care, can grasp and hold objects with difficulty, but has no digital dexterity		Individual can use the involved extremity but has difficulty with self-care activities		Individual cannot use the involved extremity for self-care or daily activities	

b. Criteria for Rating Impairments of Two Upper Extremities

Class 1 1%-19% Impairment of the Whole Person	Class 2 20%-39% Impairment of the Whole Person	Class 3 40%-79% Impairment of the Whole Person	Class 4 80%+ Impairment of the Whole Person
Individual can use both upper extremities for self-care, grasping, and holding, but has difficulty with digital dexterity	Individual can use both upper extremities for self-care, can grasp and hold objects with difficulty, but has no digital dexterity	Individual can use both upper extremities but has difficulty with self-care activities	Individual cannot use upper extremities

c. Criteria for Rating Impairments Due to Station and Gait Disorders

Class 1 1%-9% Impairment of the Whole Person	Class 2 10%-19% Impairment of the Whole Person	Class 3 20%-39% Impairment of the Whole Person	Class 4 40%-60% Impairment of the Whole Person
Rises to standing position; walks, but has difficulty with elevations, grades, stairs, deep chairs, and long distances	Rises to standing position; walks some distance with difficulty and without assistance, but is limited to level surfaces	Rises and maintains standing position with difficulty; cannot walk without assistance	Cannot stand without help, mechanical support, and/or an assistive device

In prior editions of the *Guides*, rating spinal cord injury was done either through a combination of DRE categories or in the nervous system chapter. It was decided in this edition to evaluate spinal cord injuries based on the criteria in the nervous system chapter (Chapter 13). These criteria are repeated in this section. For bilateral neurologic or corticospinal tract damage, consultation with a spinal cord injury specialist and review of Chapter 13, The Central and Peripheral Nervous System, is recommended. Thus, for an individual with a spinal cord injury affecting the upper extremities, use Table 15-6 and the appropriate impairment rating for impairment of one or both upper extremities. For impairments involving loss of use of the lower extremities, use the section in Table 15-6 pertaining to station and gait impairment. If there is additional bowel or bladder dysfunction, combine the upper extremity or lower extremity loss with impairments in bladder, anorectal, and/or neurologic sexual impairment as warranted.

Once a class has been selected, the exact value is obtained by combining the value with the corresponding additional impairment from DRE categories II through V for cervical and lumbar impairment and DRE categories II through IV for thoracic impairment. An exact value is determined based on the degree of impairment of ADL. Table 15-6 and the following examples illustrate the method for impairment rating of spinal cord injury.

Example 15-17
69% Impairment Due to Compression Fracture With Corticospinal Tract Damage

Subject: 28-year-old man.

History: Sustained a C6 vertebral body fracture with almost 40% compression after a fall from a scaffold. Had loss of bladder control and weakness of both lower extremities. He also had numbness and

d. Criteria for Rating Neurologic Impairment of the Bladder

Class 1 1%-9% Impairment of the Whole Person	Class 2 10%-24% Impairment of the Whole Person	Class 3 25%-39% Impairment of the Whole Person	Class 4 40%-60% Impairment of the Whole Person
Individual has some degree of voluntary control but is impaired by urgency or intermittent incontinence	Individual has good bladder reflex activity, limited capacity, and intermittent emptying without voluntary control	Individual has poor bladder reflex activity, intermittent dribbling, and no voluntary control	Individual has no reflex or voluntary control of bladder

e. Criteria for Rating Neurologic Anorectal Impairment

Class 1 1%-19% Impairment of the Whole Person	Class 2 20%-39% Impairment of the Whole Person	Class 3 40%-50% Impairment of the Whole Person
Individual has reflex regulation but only limited voluntary control	Individual has reflex regulation but no voluntary control	Individual has no reflex regulation or voluntary control

f. Criteria for Rating Neurologic Sexual Impairment

Class 1 1%-9% Impairment of the Whole Person	Class 2 10%-19% Impairment of the Whole Person	Class 3 20% Impairment of the Whole Person
Sexual functioning is possible, but with difficulty of erection or ejaculation in men or lack of awareness, excitement, or lubrication in either sex	Reflex sexual functioning is possible, but there is no awareness	No sexual functioning

g. Criteria for Rating Neurologic Impairment of Respiration

Class 1 5%-19% Impairment of the Whole Person	Class 2 20%-49% Impairment of the Whole Person	Class 3 50%-89% Impairment of the Whole Person	Class 4 90%+ Impairment of the Whole Person
Individual can breathe spontaneously but has difficulty performing activities of daily living that require exertion	Individual is capable of spontaneous respiration but is restricted to sitting, standing, or limited ambulation	Individual is capable of spontaneous respiration but to such a limited degree that he or she is confined to bed	Individual has no capacity for spontaneous respiration

weakness of both upper extremities, which was verified as a C7-level radiculopathy by positive sharp waves on the electromyogram in three arm muscles 4 weeks after the injury. Underwent corpectomy of C6 and a fusion from C5 to C7.

Current Symptoms: Pain free with numbness and weakness of upper extremities; no remaining bladder symptoms. Unable to walk without leg braces (orthoses).

Physical Exam: Mild sensory changes from C7 distally. C6-innervated muscles function normally, but he had weakness of muscles innervated by C7 and lower nerve roots.

Clinical Studies: Neurodiagnostic studies: see above; radiographs show a solid fusion from C5 through C7.

Diagnosis: C6 compression fracture with corticospinal tract damage.

Impairment Rating: 69% impairment of the whole person.

Comment: Although this man has a vertebral fracture, his corticospinal tract involvement indicates he should be rated using the neurology tables. His numbness, weakness, and difficulty with dexterity movements of both upper extremities warrant a 39% WPI. He is unable to walk without braces, indicating a class 3 WPI of 39%. He has no bowel or bladder dysfunction. His vertebral fracture results in a DRE III, or 15% impairment. Combining 39%, 39%, and 15% WPI using the Combined Values Chart results in a 69% WPI.

Example 15-18
78% Impairment Due to Burst Fracture With Cauda Equina Syndrome

Subject: 54-year-old woman.

History: Fell from a ladder and sustained a burst fracture of L2 with a loss of height of 35%. In addition to numbness and weakness of both lower extremities, she was unable to empty her bladder and required catheterization. Following anterior decompression of the cauda equina and fusion from L1 to L3, the fractures healed, and she regained partial function in the muscles innervated by the L2 and lower nerve roots.

Current Symptoms: Persistent weakness of both lower extremities requiring the use of ankle-foot orthoses. Walks using two crutches. Requires intermittent catheterization of her bladder. She has occasional bowel incontinence.

Physical Exam: Mild tenderness to palpation at the fracture site. Neurologic examination reveals weakness of L2 to S1 innervated muscle and numbness and atrophy of both lower extremities. Decreased rectal tone. Knee and ankle reflexes are absent.

Clinical Studies: Repeat x-rays of the region: solid fusion from L1 to L3.

Diagnosis: Burst fracture L2 with cauda equina syndrome.

Impairment Rating: 78% impairment of the whole person.

Comment: Her lower extremity weakness and use of orthoses and crutches indicate a class 3, or 39%, WPI. The bladder impairment, requiring intermittent catheterization, indicates a class 4, or 50%, WPI. Her rectal tone is deceased, with occasional bowel incontinence, indicating a class 2 anorectal impairment of 20%. The burst fracture receives a DRE lumbar category III rating of 10%. Combining 50%, 39%, 20%, and 10% results in a combined whole person impairment of 78%.

15.8 Range-of-Motion Method

Although called the range-of-motion method, this evaluation method actually consists of three elements that need to be assessed: (1) the range of motion of the impaired spine region; (2) accompanying diagnoses (Table 15-7); and (3) any spinal nerve deficit, which is described in this chapter and in Chapter 13 (The Central and Peripheral Nervous System). Mobility, diagnoses, and nerve root deficits all provide important clinical information about function of an individual's spine.[15-21] An impairment rating based on loss of motion is valid only if there is medical evidence of a documented injury or illness with a permanent anatomic and/or physiologic residual dysfunction. The whole person impairment rating is obtained by combining ratings from all three components, using the Combined Values Chart (p. 604).

All impairment estimates shown in the tables of this section are expressed as whole person impairments. Section 15.13 explains how to express a whole person spine impairment as a regional spine impairment. Tables 15-8 through 15-14 provide estimates for rating ankylosis and range of motion, while neurologic impairments are rated based on Tables 15-15 through 15-18. The data on standards and normal functioning described in this section are based on both medical studies and consensus judgments.[15,18-27]

As previously stated (Section 15.2) the ROM method should be used only (1) if the DRE method is not applicable (no verifiable injury); (2) if, after obtaining the history and performing the examination, the physician cannot place the individual within a multilevel DRE category; (3) if multilevel involvement and/or alteration of motion segment integrity has occurred in the same spinal region; (4) if there is recurrent radiculopathy caused by a new (recurrent) disk herniation or a recurrent injury in the same spinal region; (5) if there are multiple episodes of other pathology producing alteration of motion segment integrity and/or radiculopathy; or (6) if statutorily mandated by the involved jurisdiction.

Concerns have been raised by users of the *Guides* regarding perceived age- and gender-related variations in the normal population, which may bias impairments in favor of males or older individuals, both of whom are perceived to be less flexible and therefore may be judged "impaired" even under normal circumstances. Since preparation of the fourth edition, some scientific evidence has accumulated and several relevant articles have been identified.[27-45]

Regarding gender, the scientific evidence is inconsistent. The majority of studies actually show a nonsignificant trend toward greater motion for male normal individuals in each age group. The only movement showing any statistically significant gender difference is cervical extension, and then only in younger women. This finding is inconsistent among various studies, however, and the difference disappears with advancing age.[35,41]

There is a decrease in normal motion with advancing age, but the effect is not linear. Most studies examining a wide spectrum of age groups find greater alterations in mobility below 20 and above 60 years of age. Several studies suggest that lifestyle factors may influence flexibility far more than inherent factors, as the variability of overall motion between individuals increases with advancing years. However, the evidence is inconsistent, and the changes in normative data too small for the most relevant age groups 20 to 59, to warrant age adjustment in this edition of the *Guides*.

15.8a General ROM Method Measurement Principles

Impairment should be evaluated when the condition has stabilized after completion of all necessary medical, surgical, and rehabilitative treatment. This principle precludes rating an acute illness or injury. For example, if acute muscle spasm is present, this should be noted in the examiner's report; however, the mobility measurements would not be valid for estimating permanent impairment. Because the *Guides* only considers permanent impairment, rating should be deferred until after any acute exacerbation of the chronic condition has subsided, ie, when the individual is at MMI (see Chapter 1 and the Glossary).

Pain, fear of injury, disuse, or neuromuscular inhibition may limit mobility by diminishing the individual's effort, leading to inaccurately low and inconsistent measurements. *The physician should seek consistency when testing active motion, strength, and sensation. Tests with inconsistent results should be repeated. Results that remain inconsistent should be disregarded. When the physiologic measurements fail to match known pathology, they should be repeated and, if still inconsistent, disallowed until documented evidence is provided for the abnormalities noted on the physical examination.*

The reproducibility (precision) of an individual's performance is one (but not the sole) indicator of optimum effort. When measuring range of motion, the examiner should obtain at least three consecutive measurements and calculate the mean (average) of the three. Measurements should not change substantially with repeated efforts. If the average is less than 50°, three consecutive measurements must fall within 5° of the mean; if the average is greater than 50°, three consecutive measurements must fall within 10% of the mean. Motion testing may be repeated up to six times to obtain three consecutive measurements that meet these criteria. If after six measurements inconsistency persists, the spinal motions are considered invalid. The measurements and accompanying impairment estimates may then be disallowed, in part or in their entirety.

There are multiple potential *sources of error* in a quantitative physical examination.[17,20,21] The greatest source of error that occurs is due to test administrator inexperience or lack of knowledge. The evaluator should also ensure adequate warm-up movements have been performed.[16] When possible, the individual being evaluated should warm up prior to the ROM measurements: flexion and extension twice, left and right rotation twice, left and right lateral bending twice, and one additional flexion and extension. The warm-up movements do not need to be repeated before each subsequent test of motions of the same spinal region.

The physician also needs to ensure the anatomical landmarks are accurate, the body part is stabilized, the measurement device is properly stabilized on the spine, and appropriate instructions are provided to the individual.[17,20,21] If these principles are followed, errors due to examination technique, the measurement device itself, or normal human variability will be minimized.

15.8b Principles of Inclinometry and Spine Motion Measurement

Since spinal motion is compound, it is essential to measure simultaneously motion of both the upper and lower extremes of the spine region being examined. Because the small joints of the spine do not lend themselves readily to two-arm goniometric measurements and measuring a spine segment's mobility is confounded by motion above and below the assessed points, an inclinometer is the preferred device for obtaining accurate, reproducible measurements in a simple, practical, and inexpensive way. The subcutaneous bony structures that mark the upper and lower ends of the three spine regions can be palpated readily.

Inclinometers, also called angle finders or level indicators, are small angle-measuring devices traditionally used by carpenters, mechanics, and tradespeople. Recently, physicians, therapists, and veterinarians have used them to measure angles and ranges of motion in humans and animals. Inclinometers work like a plumb line, operating on the principle of gravity, which is a constant. An inclinometer used by a physician should be marked off in 2° increments or less and in good operating condition (Figure15-6). A mechanical inclinometer has a starting or 0° position indicated by a weighted needle or pendulum. A fluid level can cause errors in reading the meniscus. A fluid-filled inclinometer should allow rotation of its inclinometer face so any number on the face can be set as the initial position. Electronic inclinometers use gravity sensors to determine an angle from the vertical, and then perform internal calculations.[21]

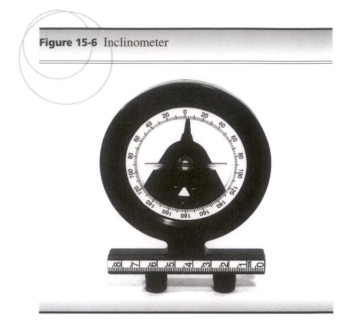

Figure 15-6 Inclinometer

Features of a properly designed inclinometer for medical use include a dial large enough to allow easy reading of 2° increments but small enough to enable application on the spine and all joints of the body; features to enable repeated, accurate application and stabilization of the instrument on the body; and a dial that can both display the 0° gravity position and be set by the examiner to a 0° starting position when the body part cannot be placed in a 0° gravity or neutral position.

Box 15-2 offers a partial list of companies that produce or distribute inclinometers. The American Medical Association does not endorse or recommend any particular type or brand of inclinometer.

Box 15-2 Inclinometer Distributors

The following companies distribute inclinometers. To receive information about their products, *Guides* users should contact the company.

Acumar Technology
1314 SW 57th Ave
Portland, OR 97221
503 292-7137
www.acumar.com

ISOMED, Inc
975 SE Sandy Blvd
Portland, OR 97214
503 233-0051
503 233-5128 (fax)
www.isomedinc.com
isomedinc@heaven.com (e-mail)

McMaster Carr
600 County Line Rd
Elmhurst, IL 60126
630 834-9600
www.mcmaster.com

The Saunders Group, Inc
4250 Norex Dr
Chaska, MN 55318
612 944-1656; 800 654-8357 (toll-free)
www.thesaundersgroup.com

Techmaster
11855 SW Ridge Crest Dr
Beaverton, OR 97008
503 671-9317
503 671-0168 (fax)
techmaster@transport.com (e-mail)

The following principles, discussed in greater detail by Mayer,[17] by Gerhardt et al,[20,21] and in forthcoming AMA educational material, are important to follow to obtain accurate measurements.

Gravitational plane. An inclinometer works only in the vertical position because only that plane allows the pointer or sensor to move freely in response to gravity. An inclinometer will not operate properly if tilted or at all when horizontal. Therefore, the individual being examined must be in a position that permits motion of the part being tested in a vertical plane. For spinal measurements in the sagittal and frontal (coronal) planes the individual should be standing or sitting, with the spine vertical (Figure 15-7). Measurements in the transverse or axial plane must be made with the individual in the supine, prone, or flexed hip position.

Measure spinal ROM in three principal planes: sagittal (extension-flexion), frontal or coronal, and transverse or axial (rotation) (Figure 15-7). If a spinal region has two or more impaired motions, the ratings for each range of motion impairment are *added*. Impairments of two or more regions of the spine are *combined* using the Combined Values Chart (p. 604).

Stabilization. If the caudad (superior), or lower, part of a spine region can be stabilized so it does not move when the superior, or upper, part moves, a single mechanical inclinometer may be used, as with measuring cervical rotation (see Figure 15-17). However, two inclinometers are usually needed to measure most movements of the spine. Single electronic inclinometers use microprocessors to duplicate functions of mechanical inclinometers. Their use will not be described in detail here as information is available from the manufacturer. The user should ensure that the features described above are addressed.

Figure 15-7 Body Planes for Measuring Motion

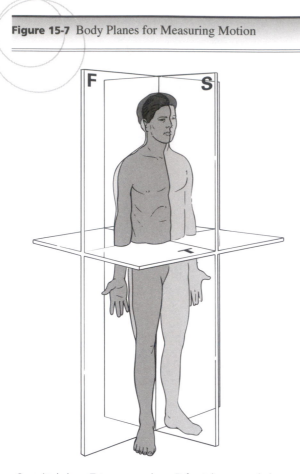

S: sagittal plane, T: transverse plane, F: frontal or coronal plane.

Manual pressure during use. The inclinometer should be held so it remains firmly applied to the subcutaneous skeletal structure while the spine is moving through the entire range of motion. It must not deviate from the original position because of skin movement or uneven pressure on the skin overlying the bony landmark, which might occur with an obese individual. The inclinometer design is important to allow proper application and avoid slippage on subcutaneous bony prominences. Firm contact of two points of the instrument with the structure is essential, especially if a convex surface such as the sacrum or calvarium (top of the head) is involved.

Recording ROM Measurements

ROM measurements can be recorded on the summary sheets (Figures 15-10, 15-15, and 15-18).

15.8c Ankylosis and Motion With Ankylosis

Ankylosis is defined as the complete absence of joint motion and is expressed as a fixed position. In the spine, which has multiple motion segments in each region with vertebrae moving together and separately, complete absence of regional motion is rare. For spine impairment evaluation only, when an individual cannot reach the neutral (0°) position, the position or angle of restriction closest to neutral is considered the position of ankylosis or end-restricted movement.

If the individual has end-restricted movement, this value, taken as the ankylosis value, is used to determine impairment instead of the ROM. If the motion crosses the neutral position in any plane, the examiner should use the abnormal motion section of the appropriate table to determine the impairment for that plane.

In determining ankylosis impairments, the examiner should *add* the ankylosis impairments in several planes within a single region or *combine* the ankylosis impairments of two or more regions (Combined Values Chart, p. 604). If a spinal region has several range-of-motion impairments and an ankylosis impairment, the ROM impairments are added and the total is combined with the ankylosis impairment. Impairments of two or more regions are always combined (Combined Values Chart).

15.8d Estimating Whole Person Impairment Using the ROM Method

1. Determine whether the individual has reached MMI and the impairment is stable. If the condition is changing or likely to improve substantially with medical treatment, the impairment is not permanent and should not be rated. If it is permanent, proceed to step 2.
2. Select the impaired region: cervical, thoracic, or lumbar.
3. Use Table 15-7 to determine the percentage impairment for the part of the ROM diagnosis–based method. If there are two or more diagnoses within a spinal region, use that which is most significant. This percent will be combined with those for the impaired range(s) of motion and the whole person neurologic deficit (steps 7-9 below).

4. Measure the range of motion in the relevant sagittal, frontal (coronal), and transverse planes (Figure 15-7), and determine any angle of ankylosis or any restricted motion that is present.
5. Perform at least three measurements of each motion. Determine which measurements meet reproducibility criteria described under general measurement principles described in Section 15.8b. Calculate the average of each set of three measurements and determine whether the three measurements in each set fall within 5° or 10% of the mean, whichever is larger.
6. If the measurements do not meet the consistency requirements described in step 5, perform additional tests until the reproducibility criteria are satisfied, up to a maximum of six. If the test results remain inconsistent after six measurements, repeat the tests at a later date or disallow impairment related to that motion.
7. Use the maximum motion from a reproducible set of measurements to determine any impairment rating from the appropriate tables, based on the spinal region and type of movement. Refer to Section 15.8c, Ankylosis and Motion With Ankylosis, if there are several range-of-motion or ankylosis impairments in a region. For example, an individual who can flex the cervical spine from 30° to 60° but who lacks 30° of motion in reaching the neutral 0° position has restricted end motion and the same estimated impairment as if he or she had fixed ankylosis at 30° of cervical flexion. According to Table 15-12, the individual's impairment is 30% of the whole person. If there are impairments due to loss of motion in more than one plane in the same spinal region (extension, flexion, or rotation), the impairments are added to determine total impairment due to loss of motion in a spinal region.
8. Determine any impairments due to neurologic deficits, such as radiculopathy or spinal nerve injury. Refer to Table 15-15 for the procedure to evaluate the sensory deficit. Use Table 15-16 to determine the procedure for estimating loss of strength. Apply these tables to Table 15-17 (cervical and thoracic nerve roots) or Table 15-18 (lumbar and sacral nerve roots) as needed. Convert the neurologic impairments, initially calculated as upper or lower extremity, into a whole person impairment.
9. Combine the diagnosis-based (Table 15-7) and physical examination–based (mobility and neurologic) impairment percents using the Combined Values Chart (p. 604).
10. Repeat steps 1 through 9 for either of the other two spinal regions with significant involvement related to the primary diagnosis.
11. Combine the regional impairments into a single whole person impairment using the Combined Values Chart (p. 604).
12. Combine the whole person spine impairment with whole person ratings for any other organ system using the Combined Values Chart, if indicated.
13. Record the results of the evaluation on the Spine Impairment Summary form (see Table 15-20).

Instructions for Using Table 15-7

1. Use this table only when the ROM method is used.
2. Identify the most significant (impairing) diagnosis of the primarily involved region (lumbar, thoracic, or cervical).
3. The diagnosis-based impairment percent should be combined with range-of-motion impairment estimates and whole person impairment estimates involving sensation, weakness, and other conditions of the musculoskeletal, nervous, or other organ systems.
4. Combine the diagnosis-based, range-of-motion, and other whole person impairment estimates using the Spine Impairment Summary form (Table 15-20).
5. Repeat for other involved spine regions and combined regional impairments if those exist.

Table 15-7 Criteria for Rating Whole Person Impairment Percent Due to Specific Spine Disorders to Be Used as Part of the ROM Method*

Disorder	% Impairment of the Whole Person		
	Cervical	Thoracic	Lumbar
I. Fractures			
A. Compression of one vertebral body.			
0%-25%	4	2	5
26%-50%	6	3	7
> 50%	10	5	12
B. Fracture of posterior element (pedicle, lamina, articular process, transverse process).	4	2	5
Note: An impairment due to compression of a vertebra and one due to fracture of a posterior element are combined using the Combined Values Chart (p. 604). Fractures or compressions of several vertebrae are combined using the Combined Values Chart.			
C. Reduced dislocation of one vertebra.	5	3	6
If two or more vertebrae are dislocated and reduced, combine the estimates using the Combined Values Chart.			
An unreduced dislocation causes impairment until it is reduced; the physician should then evaluate the impairment on the basis of the individual's condition with the dislocation reduced.			
If no reduction is possible, the physician should evaluate the impairment on the basis of the range-of-motion and neurologic findings according to criteria in this chapter and Chapter 13, The Central and Peripheral Nervous System.			
II. Intervertebral disk or other soft-tissue lesion			
Diagnosis must be based on clinical symptoms and signs and imaging information.			
A. Unoperated on, with no residual signs or symptoms.	0	0	0
B. Unoperated on, with medically documented injury, pain, and rigidity* associated with none to minimal degenerative changes on structural tests.†	4	2	5
C. Unoperated on, stable, with medically documented injury, pain, and rigidity* associated with moderate to severe degenerative changes on structural tests;† includes herniated nucleus pulposus with or without radiculopathy.	6	3	7
D. Surgically treated disk lesion without residual signs or symptoms; includes disk injection.	7	4	8
E. Surgically treated disk lesion with residual, medically documented pain and rigidity.	9	5	10
F. Multiple levels, with or without operations and with or without residual signs or symptoms.	Add 1% per level		
G. Multiple operations *with* or without residual signs or symptoms			
1. Second operation	Add 2%		
2. Third or subsequent operation	Add 1% per operation		
III. Spondylolysis and spondylolisthesis, not operated on			
A. Spondylolysis or grade I (1%-25% slippage) or grade II (26%-50% slippage) spondylolisthesis, accompanied by medically documented injury that is stable, and medically documented pain and rigidity with or without muscle spasm.	6	3	7
B. Grade III (51%-75% slippage) or grade IV (76%-100% slippage) spondylolisthesis, accompanied by medically documented injury that is stable, and medically documented pain and rigidity with or without muscle spasm.	8	4	9
IV. Spinal stenosis, segmental instability, spondylolisthesis, fracture, or dislocation, operated on			
A. Single-level decompression without spinal fusion and without residual signs or symptoms	7	4	8
B. Single-level decompression without spinal fusion with residual signs or symptoms	9	5	10
C. Single-level spinal fusion with or without decompression without residual signs or symptoms	8	4	9
D. Single-level spinal fusion with or without decompression with residual signs and symptoms	10	5	12
E. Multiple levels, operated on, with residual, medically documented pain and rigidity.	Add 1% per level		
1. Second operation	Add 2%		
2. Third or subsequent operation	Add 1% per operation		

* The phrase "medically documented injury, pain, and rigidity" implies not only that an injury or illness has occurred but also that the condition is stable, as shown by the evaluator's history, examination, and other diagnostic data, and that a permanent impairment exists, which is at least partially due to the condition being evaluated.

† Structural tests include radiographs, myelograms with and without CT scan, CT scan and MRI with and without contrast, and diskogram with and without CT scan.

15.9 ROM: Lumbar Spine

15.9a Flexion and Extension

Two-Inclinometer Technique

1. Provide information about the test and allow warm-up within pain tolerance. Warm-up exercises, as described in Section 15.8a, are done as tolerated by the individual, based on physician judgment.
2. The individual should be standing with knees extended and weight balanced on both feet, ideally with hands on hips for support to permit greater motion. The spine should be in the neutral position while the inclinometers are set at 0° (See Figure 15-8a). Locate and place horizontal skin marks over the T12 spinous process and the sacrum. Center the first inclinometer aligned in the sagittal plane, over the mark for the T12 spinous process. Center the second inclinometer over the sacral horizontal mark. It is generally best to place the sacral mark at the midpoint of the posterior superior iliac spine because if the mark is placed too high on the sacral convexity, the inclinometer may be displaced during extension. Be certain of the bony landmarks.
3. Instruct the individual to flex the trunk as far as possible (Figure 15-8b), again recording both inclinometer angles and subtracting the sacral (hip) from the T12 inclinometer angle to obtain true lumbar flexion angle. Ask the individual to return the trunk to the neutral position.

Figure 15-8 Two-Inclinometer Technique for Measuring Lumbar Flexion and Extension

The inclinometers are placed over T12 and the sacrum (S1), the anatomical landmarks.

a. neutral position

b. flexion

c. extension

d. straight leg raising (used for validation purposes)

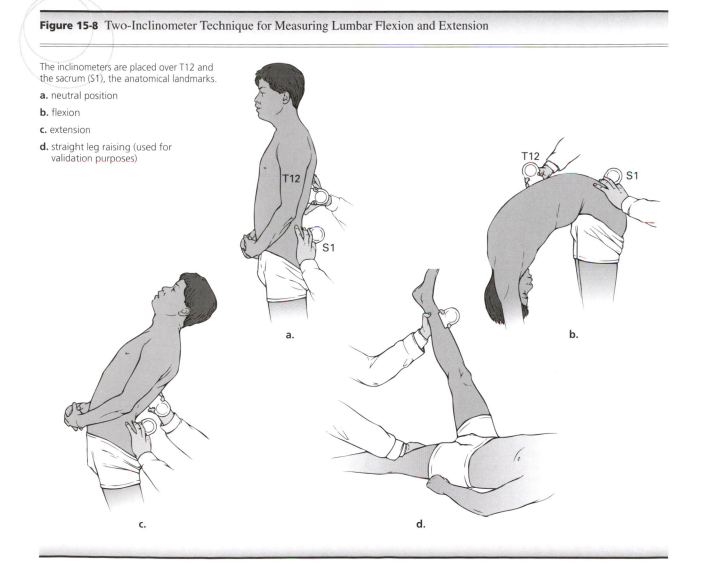

4. Ask the individual to extend maximally while holding the inclinometers firmly, and record both angles (Figure 15-8c). Subtract the sacral (hip) inclination from the T12 inclinometer angle to obtain the true lumbar extension angle. Return the trunk to the neutral position (verify that the inclinometers are still at 0°).

5. Repeat the procedure at least three times and at most six times for flexion and extension to obtain a valid measurement set (three consecutive, reproducible measurements). Only the true lumbar spine flexion and extension angles need to be consistently measured within 5° if the average is less than 50°, or within 10° if the average is greater than 50°. The impairment is based on the maximum true extension and flexion angles from within the three measurements. The average of the three is only used to determine consistency.

6. An accessory validity test can be performed for lumbosacral flexion and extension.[35] In this test, record the straight-leg-raising angle of the supine individual by placing an inclinometer on each tibial crest with the knees extended and the hip flexed (Figure 15-8d). Compare the straight-leg-raising angle to the sum of the sacral flexion and extension (sacral or hip motion) angles (Figures 15-9a and 15-9c). If the straight-leg-raising angle exceeds the sum of sacral flexion and extension angles by more than 15°, the lumbosacral flexion test is invalid. Normally, the straight-leg-raising angle is about the same as the sum of the sacral flexion-extension angle. If the individual resists passive SLR without other evidence of radiculopathy, the accessory test is also invalid. If invalid, the examiner should either repeat the flexion-extension test or disallow impairment for lumbosacral spine flexion and extension.

Tightest SLR – [sacral flexion + sacral extension] ≤ 15° for validity (assumes sacral flexion and extension are less than normal).

Note: This accessory validity test is useful only when sacral flexion plus extension is less than the average for normal individuals (ie, 65° for women and 55° for men). At these levels or above, the difference between sacral motion and supine straight leg raising will usually exceed 15° because the hamstring and gluteal muscles are contracted in the standing flexed position and relaxed in the supine position. However, below the threshold of 65° for women and 55° for men, the tightest supine straight-leg-raising angle should not be more than 15° greater than the combined sacral (hip) flexion and extension angle in the standing position.

Example of the accessory validity test: A 40-year-old man has a lumbar extension and flexion of 10° and 60°, respectively, with a sacral extension angle of 10° and sacral flexion measurement of 20°. Total sacral motion is 20° + 10°, or 30°. The straight-leg-raising angle is 70°. The measured left straight-leg-raising angle is the tighter one, 70°. The difference between 70° and 30° is greater than 15°, which indicates the results are invalid. The validity test is applicable because the individual's total sacral motion, 30°, is less than the normal 55°. The examiner has the choice of either encouraging the individual to repeat the test with greater effort or invalidating (disallowing) any finding of lumbar spine ROM impairment in the sagittal plane.

7. Once obtaining the lumbar flexion and extension, use Table 15-8 to determine impairment of the whole person. Notice that when interpreting Table 15-8, the physician must take into account the sacral (hip) flexion angle when assessing impairment due to limited lumbar spine flexion because individuals with limited hip flexion have increased impairment with limited lumbar flexion.

Table 15-8 Impairment Due to Abnormal Motion of the Lumbar Region: Flexion and Extension*

The proportion of flexion and extension of total lumbosacral motion is 75%.

Sacral (Hip) Flexion Angle (°)	True Lumbar Spine Flexion Angle (°)	% Impairment of the Whole Person
45+	60+	0
	45	2
	30	4
	15	7
	0	10
30-45	40+	4
	20	7
	0	10
0-29	30+	5
	15	8
	0	11

True Lumbar Spine Extension From Neutral Position (0°) to:	Degrees of Lumbosacral Spine Motion		% Impairment of the Whole Person
	Lost	Retained	
0	25	0	7
10	15	10	5
15	10	15	3
20	5	20	2
25	0	25	0

* Use this table only if the sum of sacral (hip) flexion and sacral (hip) extension is within 15° of the straight-leg-raising test on the tighter side; see text.

Ankylosis

Ankylosis in the lumbosacral spine is rare. It is important mainly if immobility occurs in both the hips and lumbar spine, so the neutral position cannot be attained in the sagittal plane.

Isolated fusion of either a hip or two or more lumbar vertebrae places larger stresses on adjacent segments but does not lead to mechanical failure of the lumbosacral region. Ankylosis impairments related to fusion of the hip or part of the hip motion complex should be evaluated according to Table 15-8 on abnormal motion of the lumbosacral region.

Lateral Bending (Flexion): Two-Inclinometer Technique

1. Provide information to the individual about the procedure and allow for the appropriate warm-up exercises.
2. With the individual standing erect with knees extended, locate and place horizontal skin marks over the T12 spinous process and the sacrum. Verify with the inclinometer that the skin marks are truly horizontal; do not rely solely on visual assessment. Place the first inclinometer aligned in the frontal (coronal) plane over the T12 spinous process and hold the second over the sacrum (Figure 15-9a). The trunk should be in the neutral position while the inclinometers show gravity at 0°.
3. Instruct the individual to bend the trunk laterally to the left and record both angles. Subtract the sacral (hip) inclination angle from the T12 inclination angle to determine the lumbar left lateral angle. Ask the individual to return to the neutral position.

Figure 15-9 Two-Inclinometer Technique for Measuring Lumbosacral Lateral Bend

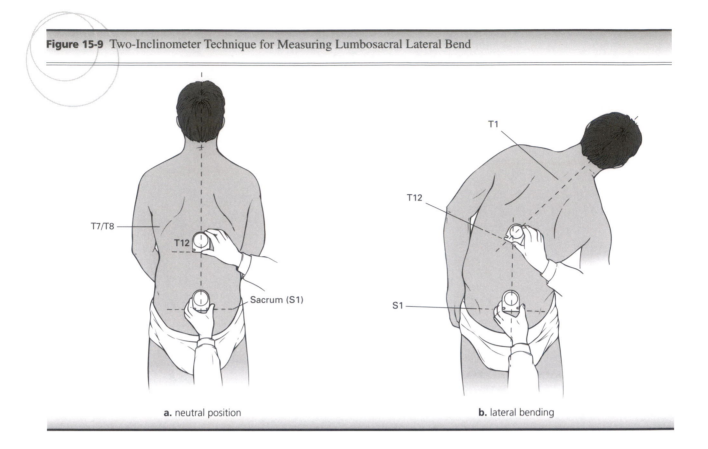

a. neutral position   **b.** lateral bending

4. Instruct the individual to bend the trunk to the right as far as possible (Figure 15-9b), again recording both inclinometer angles and subtracting the sacral (hip) angle from the T12 inclinometer angle to obtain the lumbar right lateral bending angle. Ask the individual to return to the neutral position.

5. Repeat the procedure at least three times per side. To be valid, three of six consecutive measurements must lie within 5° or 10% of the mean, whichever is greater. The impairment estimate is based on the highest (least impairing) angle of a valid set. The mean is used only for a test of reproducibility.

With measurements for left and right lateral bending and any ankylosis, use Table 15-9 to determine the whole person impairment.

Add the impairments within the lumbar region. If other regions are impaired, the lumbar impairment should be *combined* with the other region impairment using the Combined Values Chart (p. 604).

Table 15-9 Impairment Due to Abnormal Motion and Ankylosis of the Lumbar Region: Lateral Bending

Abnormal Motion
Average range of left and right lateral bending is 50°; the proportion of total lumbosacral motion is 40% of the total spine.

a.	Left Lateral Bending From Neutral Position (0°) to:	Degrees of Lumbosacral Motion		% Impairment of the Whole Person
		Lost	Retained	
	0	25	0	5
	10	15	10	3
	15	10	15	2
	20	5	20	1
	25	0	25	0

b.	Right Lateral Bending From Neutral Position (°) to:	Degrees of Lumbosacral Motion		% Impairment of the Whole Person
		Lost	Retained	
	0	25	0	5
	10	15	10	3
	15	10	15	2
	20	5	20	1
	25	0	25	0

c.	Ankylosis Region Ankylosed at (°):	
	0 (neutral position)	10
	30	20
	45	30
	60	40
	75 (full flexion)	50

Example 15-19
1% Impairment Due to Loss of Left Lateral Bending

Subject: 55-year-old man.

History: Persisting back pain, worse over the last year; no specific injury identified.

Current Symptoms: Lumbar pain increases with standing or walking for more than 1 hour.

Physical Exam: Measured T12 angles for left lateral bending are 20°, 20°, 30°, and 25°. Corresponding sacral (hip) lateral flexion measurements to the right are 15°, 5°, 10°, and 10°. Subtracting the sacral bending measurements, the true lumbosacral left lateral flexion angles are 5°, 15°, 20°, and 15°, respectively. The first measurement is discarded, being more than 5° less than the mean of 13.75°, but the next three measurements fulfill reproducibility criteria. The best left lateral bending angle is 20°.

Diagnosis: Chronic low back pain.

Impairment Rating: 1% impairment due to loss of left lateral bending (Table 15-9). Obtain the other ROM measurements for the lumbar spine and add the ROM impairments.

Ankylosis

Ankylosis in lumbar spine lateral bending (flexion) is generally associated with a scoliosis and usually produces only limited impairment. Mark the T12 and spinous process and sacrum, and ask the individual to stand in the most erect position possible that corrects the deformity. Using measurements made in the frontal (coronal) plane, subtract the sacral (hip) inclination from the T12 inclination and record the ankylosis angle or the angle of restriction (closest to the 0° neutral position). Consult Table 15-9 for the impairment rating.

Figure 15-10 provides a measurement template for lumbar impairment evaluation using the ROM method.

Figure 15-10 Lumbar Range of Motion (ROM)*

Name _____   Soc. Sec. No. _____   Date _____

Movement	Description	Range					
Lumbar flexion	T12 ROM						
	Sacral ROM						
	True lumbar flexion angle						
	±10% or 5°	Yes	No				
	Maximum true lumbar flexion angle	_____					
	% Impairment						
Lumbar extension	T12 ROM						
	Sacral ROM						
	True lumbar extension angle						
	±10% or 5°	Yes	No				
	Maximum true lumbar extension angle	_____	(Add sacral flexion and extension ROM and compare to tightest straight-leg-raising angle)				
	% Impairment						
Straight leg raising (SLR), left	Left SLR						
	±10% or 5°	Yes	No	(If tightest SLR ROM exceeds sum of sacral flexion and extension by more than 15%, lumbar ROM test is invalid)			
	Maximum SLR Left						
Straight leg raising (SLR), right	Right SLR						
	±10% or 5°	Yes	No	(If tightest SLR ROM exceeds sum of sacral flexion and extension by more than 15%, lumbar ROM test is invalid)			
	Maximum SLR right						
Lumbar left lateral bending	T12 ROM						
	Sacral ROM						
	Lumbar left lateral bending angle						
	±10% or 5°	Yes	No				
	Maximum lumbar left lateral bending angle	_____					
	% Impairment						
Lumbar right lateral bending	T12 ROM						
	Sacral ROM						
	Lumbar right lateral bending angle						
	±10% or 5°	Yes	No				
	Maximum lumbar right lateral bending angle	_____					
	% Impairment						
Lumbar ankylosis in lateral bending	Position	_____	(Excludes any impairment for abnormal flexion or extension motion)				
	% Impairment						

Total lumbar range-of-motion and ankylosis* impairment_____ %

* If ankylosis is present, combine the ankylosis impairment with the range-of-motion impairment (Combined Values Chart, p. 604).

  If ankyloses in several planes are present, combine the ankylosis estimates (Combined Values Chart), then combine the result with the range-of-motion impairment.

Chapter 15

Example 15-20
15% Impairment Due to Limitation (Ankylosis) of Lateral Bending

Subject: 40-year-old man.

History: Fell from a ladder, landed on his buttocks, and fractured L3 and L4 vertebrae with wedging toward the left side.

Current Symptoms: Low back pain after heavy lifting, with radiating pain to the knee.

Physical Exam: Leaning to the left; cannot straighten his back to a neutral position.

Clinical Studies: Inclinometric measurements show his starting position is at 20° of left lateral bending with further motion to 30°. The 20° is closest to the neutral position and is considered an ankylosis of 20° for rating purposes. Use the Ankylosis section of Table 15-9.

Diagnosis: Compression fractures of L3 and L4 with apex left lateral wedging.

Impairment Rating: 15% impairment of the whole person due to limitation (ankylosis) of lateral bending.

Comment: Add to this any impairments for other ROM deficits in the lumbar spine, then combine the total ROM impairment with those for the compression fractures (Table 15-7) and neurologic deficits, if any.

15.10 ROM: Thoracic Spine

15.10a Flexion and Extension

Thoracic flexion and extension are relatively limited motions. The amount of extension is determined mainly by the individual's posture and the degree of fixed kyphosis or curvature of the thoracic spine. To determine the ranges of motion of this region, the individual is measured in the military brace posture to obtain the angle of extension or minimum kyphosis. Then, with the individual fully flexing the thoracic spine, the flexion angle is determined. The angle of minimum kyphosis is actually a measure of ankylosis, and impairment resulting from deformity corresponding to this angle is found in the Ankylosis part of Table 15-10.

Table 15-10 Impairment Due to Abnormal Motion (Flexion) and Ankylosis of the Thoracic Region

Average range of flexion and extension is 50°; the proportion of all thoracic motion is 60% of the total spine.

Abnormal Motion

Flexion From Erect Position (Angle of Thoracic Flexion) to:	Degrees of Thoracic Motion		% Impairment of the Whole Person
	Lost	Retained	
0	50	0	4
15	35	15	2
30	20	30	1
60	0	50	0

Ankylosis
Angle of Minimum Kyphosis (°)

−30 (Extension thoracic lordosis)	20
0 (neutral)	0
60	5
80	20
100	40

Two-Inclinometer Technique

1. Provide information to the individual, and allow for the appropriate warm-up exercises. Measurements are obtained with the individual standing or sitting.

2. Locate and place horizontal skin marks over the T1 and T12 spinous processes. Place both inclinometers, which do not show gravity 0 automatically against a true vertical surface, such as a wall, and set the neutral 0° positions. Place the inclinometers over the T1 and T12 spinous processes while instructing the individual to maintain the maximally extended military brace posture position (Figures 15-11a and 15-11c). Subtract the T12 inclinometer reading from the T1 inclinometer reading (if both are inclined in the same direction from the vertical) to obtain the angle of minimum kyphosis. If T12 and T1 are inclined in opposite directions from the vertical, add the angles. Find the impairment percent in the Ankylosis part of Table 15-10.

3. Set the inclinometers to 0° with the individual standing in the erect military brace posture. Then ask the individual to fully flex the thoracic spine. Flexing at the hips is permitted. Subtract the T12 inclinometer reading from the T1 reading obtained in step 1 above to obtain the angle of thoracic flexion (Figures 15-11b and 15-11d).

4. Repeat either the sitting or the standing test up to six times to obtain three measurements within 5° of the mean or 10%, whichever is greater.

5. A reproducibility test is done after a positional change, having the standing individual sit or vice versa. If the initial measurements were made standing, seat the individual on a stool, record the neutral 0° position, and ask him or her to flex the thoracic spine maximally from the military brace position. The thoracic flexion sitting angle should be nearly identical to the flexion angle obtained in the erect position.

6. Consult the Abnormal Motion part of Table 15-10 to determine the whole person impairment.

Figure 15-11 Two-Inclinometer Technique for Measuring Angles of Minimum Kyphosis and Thoracic Flexion

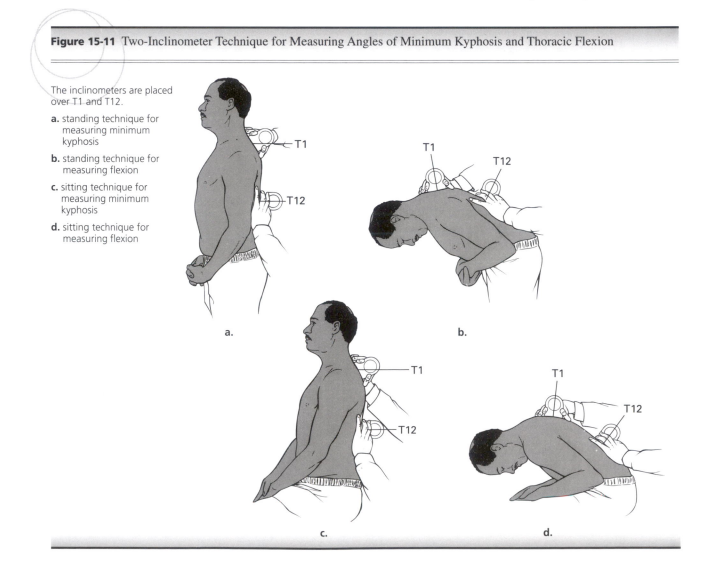

The inclinometers are placed over T1 and T12.

a. standing technique for measuring minimum kyphosis

b. standing technique for measuring flexion

c. sitting technique for measuring minimum kyphosis

d. sitting technique for measuring flexion

Ankylosis

The angle of minimum kyphosis of the thoracic spine may be considered equal to the angle of ankylosis. Excessive kyphosis or thoracic lordosis is evaluated as an impairment according to Table 15-10.

Example 15-21
5% Impairment Due to Ankylosing Spondylitis and Low Back Pain

Subject: 47-year-old man.

History: Ankylosing spondylitis.

Current Symptoms: Chronic low back pain.

Physical Examination: Attempts to extend his thoracic spine fully demonstrate an angle of minimum kyphosis of 60°. With maximum flexion, T1 readings of 35°, 45°, and 55° are recorded, which are matched with T12 flexion angles of 25°, 30°, and 40°, respectively. The angles of thoracic flexion, derived by subtracting the T12 from the T1 angles, are 10°, 15°, and 15°. These three measurements meet validity criteria.

Clinical Studies: Radiographs: consistent with ankylosing spondylitis.

Diagnosis: Ankylosing spondylitis and low back pain.

Impairment Rating: According to Table 15-10, the impairment due to a 60° ankylosis (angle of minimum kyphosis) is 5% whole person impairment. The maximum flexion of 15° is 2% whole person impairment. The total impairment is the greater of the ankylosis and abnormal motion percentages, in this instance, 5%.

Comment: Combine this with impairments from the diagnosis table (Table 15-7).

15.10b Rotation

Two-Inclinometer Technique

1. Provide information to the individual about the procedure and allow for appropriate warm-up exercises.
2. The individual should be seated or standing, whichever is more comfortable, and in a forward flexed position, with the thoracic spine in as horizontal a position as can be achieved (Figure 15-12a). Locate and place horizontal skin marks over the T1 and T12 spinous processes. The trunk should be in the neutral position for rotation. The inclinometers are set to 0 by placement against a flat, horizontal table or floor if they do not automatically indicate gravity 0°. Place the first inclinometer aligned vertically in the transverse (axial) plane over the T1 spinous process while holding the second over the T12 spinous process.
3. Ask the individual to rotate the trunk maximally to the left and record both angles (Figure 15-12b). Subtract the T12 angle from the T1 angle to obtain the thoracic left rotation angle. Return the trunk to the neutral position (Figure 15-12a).
4. Instruct the individual to rotate the trunk maximally to the right, again recording both inclinometer angles; subtract the T12 angle from the T1 angle to obtain the thoracic right rotation angle.
5. Repeat the procedure three to six times per side to obtain a valid set of three consecutive measurements. The angles of a valid set should be within 5° or 10% of the mean of the set, whichever is greater. The final impairment percent is based on the best (least impairing) angle measured.

Using the best angle of rotation and Table 15-11, determine the whole person impairment.

Figure 15-12 Two-Inclinometer Technique for Measuring Left Thoracic Rotation

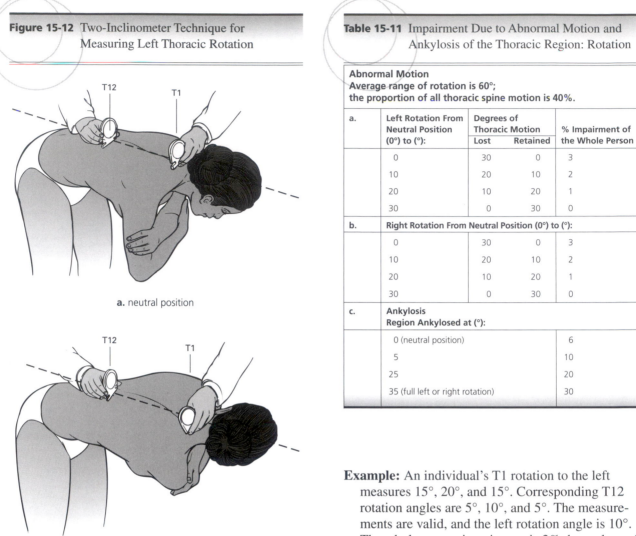

a. neutral position

b. rotation

The figure shows the individual standing. The inclinometers are placed at T1 and T12 and aligned in the vertical plane.

Table 15-11 Impairment Due to Abnormal Motion and Ankylosis of the Thoracic Region: Rotation

Abnormal Motion
Average range of rotation is 60°;
the proportion of all thoracic spine motion is 40%.

a.	Left Rotation From Neutral Position (0°) to (°):	Degrees of Thoracic Motion		% Impairment of the Whole Person
		Lost	Retained	
	0	30	0	3
	10	20	10	2
	20	10	20	1
	30	0	30	0
b.	Right Rotation From Neutral Position (0°) to (°):			
	0	30	0	3
	10	20	10	2
	20	10	20	1
	30	0	30	0
c.	Ankylosis Region Ankylosed at (°):			
	0 (neutral position)			6
	5			10
	25			20
	35 (full left or right rotation)			30

Example: An individual's T1 rotation to the left measures 15°, 20°, and 15°. Corresponding T12 rotation angles are 5°, 10°, and 5°. The measurements are valid, and the left rotation angle is 10°. The whole person impairment is 2% due to loss of rotation (Table 15-11).

15.10c Alternative Thoracic Rotation Technique

1. The individual lies supine on the exam table. Stabilize the hips and pelvis. Place the inclinometer across the manubrium, just below the sternal notch. The trunk should be in the neutral position and the inclinometer set at 0° gravity if it is not automatically set to 0 (Figure 15-13a).
2. Ask the individual to rotate the trunk maximally to the left and record the angle on the sternum inclinometer, making certain an assistant holds the pelvis to the table without permitting rotation. Because the angle actually measures left thoracolumbar rotation, subtract 5°, the average lumbar rotation, to obtain the estimated thoracic rotation.

3. Instruct the individual to rotate the trunk maximally to the right (Figure 15-13b), again maintaining pelvic stabilization. Read the sternal inclinometer angle and subtract 5° to obtain the right thoracic rotation angle.

Ankylosis

Rotational ankylosis of the thoracic spine is generally a component of a scoliosis deformity and by itself creates only limited impairment. To evaluate this type of ankylosis, use the same posture as for measuring abnormal motion in the thoracic spine, and ask the individual to achieve maximum correction of the rotation deformity. Then subtract the T12 rotation angle from the T1 rotation angle and determine the ankylosis angle or angle of restricted motion. Refer to the Ankylosis part of Table 15-11 to determine the impairment percent.

Figure 15-14 provides a measurement template for thoracic impairment evaluation using the ROM method.

Figure 15-13 Alternative Technique for Measuring Thoracic Spine Rotation

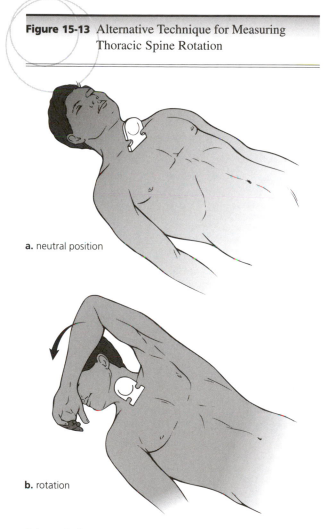

a. neutral position

b. rotation

Only one inclinometer is used. The individual is supine on the exam table with the thoracolumbar spine and pelvis in neutral position. The inclinometer is placed on the manubrium, just below the sternal notch. Stabilize the pelvis.

Chapter 15

Figure 15-14 Thoracic Range of Motion (ROM)*

Name _____   Soc. Sec. No. _____   Date _____

Movement	Description	Range							
Angle of minimum kyphosis (thoracic ankylosis in extension)	T1 reading			XXXX	XXXX	XXXX	XXXX	XXXX	
	T12 reading			XXXX	XXXX	XXXX	XXXX	XXXX	
	Angle of minimum kyphosis			XXXX	XXXX	XXXX	XXXX	XXXX	
	% Impairment due to thoracic ankylosis	(Use larger of either ankylosis or flexion impairment)							
Thoracic flexion	T1 ROM								
	T12 ROM								
	Thoracic flexion angle								
	10% or 5°	Yes	No						
	Maximum thoracic flexion angle								
	% Impairment								
Thoracic left rotation	T1 ROM								
	T12 ROM								
	Thoracic left rotation angle								
	10% or 5°	Yes	No						
	Maximum thoracic left rotation angle								
	% Impairment								
Thoracic right rotation	T1 ROM								
	T12 ROM								
	Thoracic right rotation angle								
	10% or 5°	Yes	No						
	Maximum thoracic right rotation angle								
	% Impairment								
Thoracic ankylosis in rotation	Position		(Excludes any impairment for abnormal flexion or extension motion)						
	% Impairment								

Total thoracic range of motion and ankylosis* impairment _____ %

*If ankylosis is present, combine the ankylosis impairment with the range-of-motion impairment (Combined Values Chart, p. 604).

If ankyloses in several planes are present, combine the ankylosis estimates (Combined Values Chart), then combine the result with the range-of-motion impairment.

Figure 15-15 Two-Inclinometer Technique for Measuring Cervical Flexion and Extension

The individual is sitting and the inclinometers placed over the calvarium and at T1.

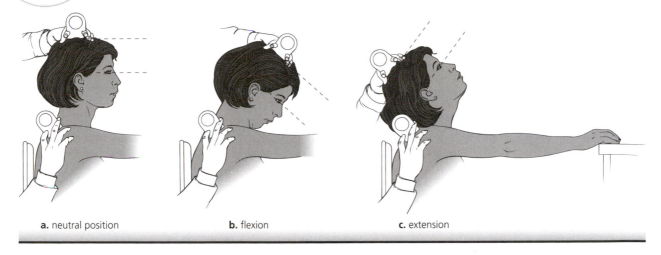

a. neutral position   **b.** flexion   **c.** extension

15.11 ROM: Cervical Spine

15.11a Flexion and Extension

Two-Inclinometer Technique

1. Provide information to the individual about the procedure, and allow for appropriate warm-up exercises.
2. Locate and place a horizontal skin mark over the T1 spinous process. With the individual seated, place the first inclinometer, aligned in the sagittal plane, over the T1 spinous process. Place the second inclinometer at the side of the face, from the corner of the eye to the ear, along a parallel line where the temple of eyeglasses would sit (Figure 15-15a). From this position, set the inclinometer to 0. This represents the 0° true neutral position. Move the second inclinometer to the calvarium, and set the head to the neutral position in both the sagittal and frontal planes, where the inclinometer again reads 0 (Figure 15-15a).

3. Ask the individual to flex maximally and record both angles. Subtract the T1 angle from the calvarium angle to obtain the cervical flexion angle (Figure 15-15b) and record it. Return the head to the neutral position so both inclinometers read 0° again.
4. Instruct the individual to extend the neck as far as possible, keeping the chin close to the sternum, again recording both inclinometer angles. Subtract the T1 angle from the calvarium angle to obtain the cervical extension angle (Figure 15-15c). Ask the individual to return the head to the neutral position.
5. Repeat the procedure three times. The cervical flexion and extension angles should be consistently measured within 5° or 10%, whichever is greater. The impairment rating is based on the greatest angle of a valid set of three consecutive measurements.
6. Using the largest valid cervical flexion and extension measurements, obtain the whole person impairment rating for cervical flexion and extension using Table 15-12.
7. *Add* the cervical flexion and extension impairment ratings and *combine* the sum with any ratings for diagnostic criteria (Table 15-7) and/or neural impairment.

Ankylosis

1. Note whether there is motion of the cervical spine in the sagittal plane or whether the spine is unable either to flex or extend beyond the neutral point. Determine if the ankylosis or restricted motion is in flexion or extension. If some motion is possible in the sagittal plane, ask the individual to hold the position closest to the neutral point.
2. Place the inclinometer's base against a vertical surface to set the inclinometer to the neutral 0 position. Then place it at the side of the face, from the corner of the eye to the ear, along a parallel line where eyeglass temples would lie (Figure 15-15b). Move the inclinometer to the calvarium and set the head to the neutral position in both the sagittal and frontal planes, where the inclinometer again reads 0 (Figure 15-15b).
3. Place the second inclinometer at T1 and record the angle. Subtract or add the T1 angle from the first-read angle to obtain the angle of ankylosis in either flexion or extension.
4. Consult the Ankylosis section of Table 15-12 to determine the whole person impairment.
5. Add the impairment percent for left rotation and right rotation. Their sum is the whole person impairment contributed by abnormal rotation of the cervical region.

Table 15-12 Cervical Region Impairment From Abnormal Flexion or Extension or Ankylosis

Abnormal Motion
Average range of flexion and extension is 110°; the proportion of all cervical motions is 40%.

a.	Flexion From Neutral Position (0°) to (°):	Degrees of Cervical Motion Lost	Retained	% Impairment of the Whole Person
	0	50	0	5
	15	35	15	4
	30	30	20	2
	50	0	50	0
b.	Extension From Neutral Position (0°) to (°):	Degrees of Cervical Motion Lost	Retained	% Impairment of the Whole Person
	0	60	0	6
	20	40	20	4
	40	20	40	2
	60	0	60+	0
c.	Region Ankylosed at (°):			
	0 (neutral position)			12
	15			20
	30			30
	50 (full flexion)			40
d.	Region Ankylosed at (°):			
	0 (neutral position)			12
	20			20
	40			30
	60 (full extension)			40

Example: A 55-year-old man has an extension deformity on attempted flexion. Inclinometer reading from the calvarium is 15° extension from the neutral 0° position. The T1 angle is 5° of flexion from neutral 0°. In this case, because the angles are in different directions from the neutral position, they are *added*, and the cervical spine thus is ankylosed at 20° extension. This is considered a 20% whole person impairment (Table 15-12).

Figure 15-16 Two-Inclinometer Technique for Measuring Cervical Lateral Flexion

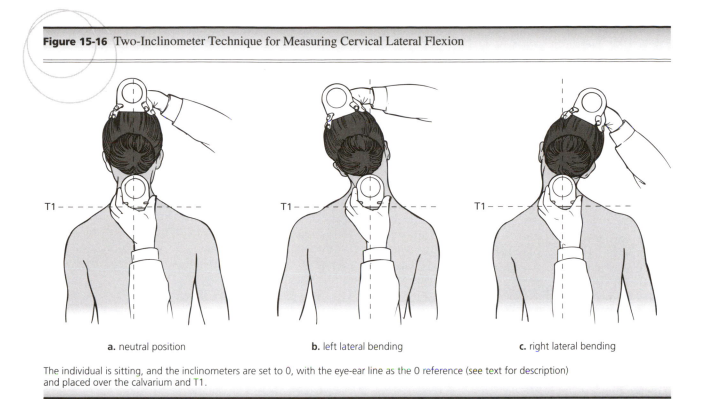

a. neutral position   **b.** left lateral bending   **c.** right lateral bending

The individual is sitting, and the inclinometers are set to 0, with the eye-ear line as the 0 reference (see text for description) and placed over the calvarium and T1.

15.11b Lateral Bending

Two-Inclinometer Technique

1. Provide information to the individual about the procedure and allow for appropriate warm-up exercises.
2. Place a skin mark over the T1 spinous process. With the individual in the seated position, place the first inclinometer aligned in the coronal plane over the T1 spinous process while holding the second inclinometer over the calvarium (Figure 15-16a). The head should be in the neutral position while the inclinometers are set at 0°.
3. Ask the individual to tilt the head maximally to the left and record both angles (Figure 15-16b). Subtract the T1 angle from the calvarium angle to determine the degrees of left lateral bending. Return the head to the neutral position.
4. Instruct the individual to tilt the head maximally to the right as far as possible, recording both inclinometer angles. Subtract the T1 angle from the calvarium angle to determine cervical right lateral bending (Figure 15-16c).
5. Repeat the above procedure at least three times. The angles measured should be within 5° or 10% of the mean of the three measurements, whichever is greater. The measurement used for impairment rating is the greatest angle of a valid set of three consecutive measurements.
6. Consult Table 15-13 to determine the whole-person impairment related to abnormal lateral flexion of the cervical region.

Add the impairment percent from left lateral bending and right lateral bending. Their sum represents the whole person impairment related to abnormal lateral bending of the cervical region.

Table 15-13 Impairment Due to Abnormal Motion and Ankylosis of the Cervical Region: Lateral Bending

Abnormal Motion
The average range of lateral bending is 90°; the proportion of all cervical motions is 25%.

a.	Left Lateral Bending From Neutral Position (0°) to (°):	Degrees of Cervical Motion		% Impairment of the Whole Person
		Lost	Retained	
	0	45	0	4
	15	30	15	2
	30	15	30	1
	45	0	45	0
b.	Right Lateral Bending From Neutral Position (0°) to (°):	Degrees of Cervical Motion		% Impairment of the Whole Person
		Lost	Retained	
	0	45	0	4
	15	30	15	2
	30	15	30	1
	45	0	45	0
c.	**Ankylosis** Region Ankylosed at (°):			
	0 (neutral position)			8
	15			20
	30			30
	45 (full left or right rotation)			40

Example: The left bending flexion angles measured from the calvarium are 20°, 35°, 35,° and 40°. The corresponding T1 measurements are 5°, 5°, 10°, and 10°. The true left lateral degrees of bending are 15°, 20°, 25°, and 30°. The 15° is discarded. The other three measurements fulfill the validation criteria, being more than 5° from the mean of 25°. The greatest left lateral bending angle of the three trials is 30°, and the impairment rating due to left lateral bending limitation is 1% (Table 15-13).

Ankylosis

1. Place both inclinometer bases against a desk or tabletop and adjust until they read 0°, or the neutral position.

2. Place one inclinometer in the frontal plane at T1 (Figure 15-16b) and the second inclinometer over the calvarium.

3. Determine whether the individual has cervical lateral motion or is unable to attain the neutral position. If there is motion and the individual cannot reach the neutral position, read the angle closest to neutral 0. This is the angle of ankylosis used for rating (Figure 15-16b).

Consult the Ankylosis section of Table 15-13 to determine the whole person impairment.

15.11c Cervical Rotation

Because the technique for cervical evaluation stabilizes the trunk in the supine position, with the shoulders on the table, only one inclinometer is required for measurement of rotation.

1. Provide information to the individual about the procedure, and allow for appropriate warm-up exercises. Set the inclinometer to 0° or the gravity position.

2. Have the individual lie supine on a flat exam table with shoulders exposed to permit observation of any truncal (thoracolumbar) rotation. Stand at the head of the table and place the inclinometer in the transverse plane with the base applied to the forehead (Figure 15-17a). Record the neutral 0° position with the individual's nose pointing to the ceiling.

3. Ask the individual to rotate the head maximally to the left, and record the cervical left rotation angle.

4. Ask the individual to rotate the head maximally to the right, and record the cervical right rotation angle (Figure 15-17b).

5. Repeat the procedure three to six times to obtain a valid set of three consecutive measurements. The left and right cervical rotation angles should be within 5° or 10% of the mean of a valid set, whichever is greater. The impairment rating is based on the greatest angle of a valid set.

Example: Left cervical rotation is 15°, 35°, 55°, 60°, and 55°. The initial two measurements are discarded, while the others are close enough to be valid. The largest measurement, 60°, is used and corresponds to a whole person impairment estimate for abnormal left cervical rotation of 1% (Table 15-14).

Figure 15-17 Measuring Cervical Rotation

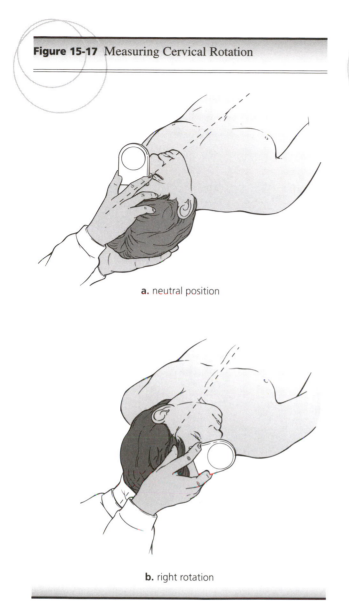

a. neutral position

b. right rotation

Table 15-14 Impairment Due to Abnormal Motion and Ankylosis of the Cervical Region: Rotation

Abnormal Motion
Average range of rotation is 160°;
the proportion of all cervical motion is 35%.

a.	Left Rotation From Neutral Position (0°) to (°):	Degrees of Cervical Motion		% Impairment of the Whole Person
		Lost	Retained	
	0	80	0	6
	20	60	20	4
	40	40	40	2
	60	20	60	1
	80	0	80+	0

b.	Right Rotation From Neutral Position (0°) to (°):	Degrees of Cervical Motion		% Impairment of the Whole Person
		Lost	Retained	
	0	80	0	6
	20	60	20	4
	40	40	40	2
	60	20	60	1
	80	0	80+	0

c.	Ankylosis Region Ankylosed at (°):	
	0 (neutral position)	12
	20	20
	40	30
	60	40
	80 (full right or left rotation)	50

Ankylosis

1. Determine whether the individual has cervical axial motion and is unable to attain the neutral position. If the individual has some motion, ask him or her to maintain the position closest to neutral and record the ankylosis angle closest to neutral (Figure 15-17).
2. Place the inclinometer on the calvarium with the cervical region in the ankylosis position, and record the ankylosis angle.
3. Consult the Ankylosis part of Table 15-14 to determine the whole person impairment.

Figure 15-18 provides a template for evaluating cervical impairment using the ROM method.

Figure 15-18   Cervical Range of Motion (ROM)*

Name _____   Soc. Sec. No. _____   Date _____

Movement	Description	Range						
Cervical flexion	Calvarium angle							
	T1 ROM							
	Cervical flexion angle							
	±10% or 5°	Yes	No					
	Maximum cervical flexion angle							
	% Impairment							
Cervical extension	Calvarium angle							
	T1 ROM							
	Cervical extension angle							
	±10% or 5°	Yes	No					
	Maximum cervical extension angle							
	% Impairment							
Cervical ankylosis in flexion/extension	Position							
	% Impairment	_____ (Excludes any impairment for abnormal flexion or extension motion)						
Cervical left lateral bending	Calvarium angle							
	T1 ROM							
	Cervical left lateral flexion angle							
	±10% or 5°	Yes	No					
	Maximum cervical right lateral flexion angle							
	% Impairment							
Cervical right lateral bending	Calvarium angle							
	T1 ROM							
	Cervical right lateral flexion angle							
	±10% or 5°	Yes	No					
	Maximum cervical right lateral flexion angle							
	% Impairment							
Cervical ankylosis in lateral bending	Position							
	% Impairment	_____ (Excludes any impairment for abnormal lateral flexion or extension motion)						
Cervical left rotation	Cervical left rotation angle							
	±10% or 5°	Yes	No					
	Maximum cervical left rotation angle							
	% Impairment							
Cervical right rotation	Cervical right rotation angle							
	±10% or 5°	Yes	No					
	Maximum cervical right rotation angle							
	% Impairment							
Cervical ankylosis in rotation	Position							
	% Impairment	_____ (Excludes any impairment for abnormal rotation)						

Total cervical range of motion and ankylosis* impairment _____ %

Total cervical range of motion = % impairments of flexion + extension + left lateral bending + right lateral bending + left rotation + right rotation

* If ankylosis is present, combine the ankylosis impairment with the range-of-motion impairment (Combined Values Chart, p. 604). If ankyloses in several planes are present, combine the estimates (Combined Values Chart), then combine the result with the range-of-motion impairment.

15.12 Nerve Root and/or Spinal Cord

When using the ROM method, it is important to consider any nerve root or spinal cord impairment. Injury or illness to the cervical spine may produce nerve root compression manifested by sensory or motor loss in the upper extremities, as well as long tract signs from spinal cord compression. In the thoracic spine, spinal cord compression or injury may produce long tract signs, but nerve roots are uncommonly compressed. In the lumbosacral spine, spinal cord involvement is rare because the cord typically ends at L1, although nerve root compression (cauda equina or isolated root[s]) affecting the lower extremities is common. If any neural impairment is identified, proceed with the following evaluation:

1. Identify the nerve(s) involved, based on the clinical evaluation and the dermatome distribution charts for the lower (Figure 15-1) and upper extremity (Figure 15-2).
2. Determine the extent of any sensory and motor loss due to nerve impairment, based on Tables 15-15 and 15-16.
3. Find the maximum impairment due to nerve dysfunction in Table 15-17 for the upper extremity and Table 15-18 for the lower extremity.
4. Multiply the severity of the sensory or motor deficit by the maximum value of the relevant nerve (Tables 15-17, 15-18). If there is both sensory and motor impairment of a nerve root, the impairment percents are combined (Combined Values Chart, p. 604) to determine the extremity impairment. If both extremities are impaired, the impairment percent for each extremity is determined, converted to whole person impairment, and the two impairment ratings combined using the Combined Values Chart.

5. Convert to whole person impairment by multiplying the upper extremity impairment by 0.6 and the lower extremity impairment by 0.4. To convert any regional ROM spine impairment to whole person impairment, multiply the specific spinal nerve impairment by the regional weight: 0.80 for the cervical spine, 0.40 for the thoracic spine, and 0.90 for the lumbosacral spine. Impairment ratings above 100% are rounded down to 100% since a whole person impairment rating cannot exceed 100%. This is described further in Section 15.14.

If there is bilateral spinal nerve impairment or spinal cord involvement, especially if in conjunction with head injury, consultation with a neurologist and/or neurosurgeon and review of the diagnostic criteria in the neurology chapter (Chapter 13) is advisable. The physician should decide whether evaluation by the spine or neurology chapter criteria is most appropriate.

Table 15-15 Determining Impairment Due to Sensory Loss

a. Classification

Grade	Description of Sensory Deficit	% Sensory Deficit
5	No loss of sensibility, abnormal sensation, or pain	0
4	Distorted superficial tactile sensibility (diminished light touch), with or without minimal abnormal sensations or pain, that is forgotten during activity	1-25
3	Distorted superficial tactile sensibility (diminished light touch and two-point discrimination), with some abnormal sensations or slight pain, that interferes with some activities	26-60
2	Decreased superficial cutaneous pain and tactile sensibility (decreased protective sensibility), with abnormal sensations or moderate pain, that may prevent some activities	61-80
1	Deep cutaneous pain sensibility present; absent superficial pain and tactile sensibility (absent protective sensibility), with abnormal sensations or severe pain, that prevents most activity	81-99
0	Absent sensibility, abnormal sensations, or severe pain that prevents all activity	100

b. Procedure

1.	Identify the area of involvement using the dermatome charts (Figures 15-1 and 15-2).
2.	Identify the nerve(s) that innervate the area(s) (Table 16-12 and Figure 16-48).
3.	Grade the severity of the sensory deficit or pain according to the classification above.
4.	Find the maximum impairment of the extremity(ies) due to sensory deficit or pain for each: spinal nerves (Table 15-8) and brachial plexus (Table 16-14).
5.	Multiply the severity of the sensory deficit by the maximum impairment value to obtain the extremity impairment for each spinal nerve involved.

Table 15-16 Determining Impairment Due to Loss of Power and Motor Deficits

a. Classification

Grade	Description of Muscle Function	% Motor Deficit
5	Active movement against gravity with full resistance	0
4	Active movement against gravity with some resistance	1–25
3	Active movement against gravity only, without resistance	26–50
2	Active movement with gravity eliminated	51–75
1	Slight contraction and no movement	76–99
0	No contraction	100

b. Procedure

1.	Identify the motion involved, such as flexion, extension, etc.
2.	Identify the muscle(s) performing the motion and the spinal nerve(s) involved.
3.	Grade the severity of motor deficit of individual muscles according to the classification given above.
4.	Find the maximum impairment of the extremity due to motor deficit for each spinal nerve structure involved (Tables 15-18, 16-11, 16-13, and 17-37).
5.	Multiply the severity of the motor deficit by the maximum impairment value to obtain the extremity impairment for each spinal nerve involved.

* Adapted from Medical Research Council. [16]

Table 15-17 Unilateral Spinal Nerve Root Impairment Affecting the Upper Extremity*

Nerve Root Impaired	Maximum % Loss of Function Due to Sensory Deficit or Pain	Maximum % Loss of Function Due to Strength
C5	5	30
C6	8	35
C7	5	35
C8	5	45
T1	5	20

* For description of the process of determining impairment percent, see text.

Table 15-18 Unilateral Spinal Nerve Root Impairment Affecting the Lower Extremity*

Nerve Root Impaired	Maximum % Loss of Function Due to Sensory Deficit or Pain	Maximum % Loss of Function Due to Strength
L3	5	20
L4	5	34
L5	5	37
S1	5	20

* For description of the process of determining impairment percent, see text.

15.12a Examples Using the ROM Method

Example 15-22
23% Impairment Due to Herniated Disk
With Radiculopathy

Subject: 55-year-old man.

History: Developed low back pain and right sciatica after lifting furniture at home. A herniated lumbar disk was treated surgically, with near complete relief of pain. About 15 months ago postoperatively, he reinjured his lumbar spine while lifting on the job. An MRI showed a recurrent herniated disk at the same level and side as before. He underwent a second diskectomy, but this time was unrelieved of pain.

Current Symptoms: Back and unilateral, radiating right leg pain, unchanged for many months.

Physical Exam: Healed scar on the back. Straight leg raising caused pain along the lateral leg and foot at 30°. The right Achilles reflex was absent. Numbness in the right S1 nerve root distribution range of motion and straight-leg-raising testing using the double-inclinometer technique resulted in the following measurements: true lumbar extension 20°; true lumbar flexion 30°; left lateral flexion 25°; right lateral flexion 20°.

The sensory changes in S1 nerve distribution were judged to be grade 4 according to Table 15-15, and weakness in the S1-innervated muscles was judged to be grade 4 according to Table 15-16.

Clinical Studies: MRI after the second injury: recurrent herniated disk. Repeat MRI with gadolinium after surgery and failure to improve: only perineural scarring. Repeat routine x-rays: slight disk space narrowing at the involved level.

Diagnosis: Recurrent herniated disk with radiculopathy.

Impairment Rating: 23% impairment of the whole person.

Comment: Individual has a 12% whole person impairment according to Table 15-7, 10% due to "surgically treated disk lesion with residual, medically documented pain and rigidity," added to 2% for the second operation. He has an impairment of 2% impairment due to loss of lumbar extension and 4% due to loss of flexion, with at least 45° of sacral (hip) motion (Table 15-8) and 6% loss due to extension and flexion. He has 0% impairment due to loss of left lateral lumbar flexion, 1% loss of right lateral flexion (Table 15-9), and 1% loss of lateral movement. He therefore has 7% impairment due to loss of lumbar motion. From Table 15-15 we see that he has a grade 4 sensory loss of S1. Multiplying 25% (the maximum percentage in this case) by the 5% for maximum loss of S1 sensation from Table 15-18 results in a rating of 1% due to sensory loss. We also see that he has a grade 4 motor loss according to Table 15-16. Multiplying 25% (the maximum in this case) by the 20% from Table 15-18 for S1 motor loss results in 5% impairment due to motor loss of S1. Combining the 1% for sensory loss and the 5% for motor loss results in a 6% impairment due to neurologic loss. Using the Combined Values Chart to combine the impairment from Table 15-7, (12%) with the impairments due to loss of motion (7%) and neurologic involvement (6%) results in a whole person impairment of 23%. In some cases, the physician may be asked to apportion the findings. One approach is to subtract 10% from the latest impairment rating due to the first injury, assuming it was a DRE III without ROM data after the first operation and the radiculopathy had resolved after the first surgery.

Example 15-23
7% Impairment Due to Ankylosing Spondylitis

Subject: 56-year-old man.

History: Individual with known ankylosing spondylitis has become unable to work because of pain and is considering retirement, depending on his impairment rating.

Current Symptoms: Moderate pain; cannot straighten up completely.

Physical Exam: Measurement of the motion and ankylosis in the thoracic spine demonstrates an angle of minimum kyphosis of 60°. With maximum flexion, T1 readings of 35°, 45°, and 55° are recorded, which are matched with T12 flexion angles of 25°, 30°, and 40°, respectively. The angles of thoracic flexion, which are derived by subtracting the T1 angles from the T12 angles, are 10°, 15°, and 15°. These meet validity criteria. T1 rotation to the right measures 15°, 20°, and 15°. Corresponding T12 rotation angles measure 5°, 10°, and 5°. The measurements are valid, and the left rotation angle is 10°. The right thoracic rotation angles are the same as the right.

Diagnosis: Ankylosing spondylitis.

Impairment Rating: 7% impairment of the whole person.

Comment: According to Table 15-10, the impairment due to ankylosis (angle of minimum kyphosis) of 60° is 5% of the whole person and, considering maximum flexion, the impairment due to abnormal motion of 15° is 2%. The total impairment is the greater of the ankylosis and abnormal motion percentages, in this instance, 5%. The impairment due to loss of right thoracic rotation is, according to Table 15-11, 1%. Impairment due to loss of left thoracic rotation is the same. Adding these impairments results in a whole person impairment of 7%. Because there has been no injury or surgery, the individual does not meet any of the other diagnostic criteria in Table 15-7, and there is no neurologic involvement, the whole person impairment is derived solely from the loss of motion and is 7%. If there was loss of motion in any other spinal region, each region would be rated separately and the ratings combined using the Combined Values Chart (p. 604).

Example 15-24
23% Impairment Due to Compression Fractures

Subject: 54-year-old woman.

History: Fell from a ladder and sustained burst fractures of L2 with loss of height of 55% and L3 with loss of height of 20%. Treated with bracing and the fractures healed. Returned to work as a customer service agent 6 months after the injury.

Current Symptoms: No neurologic findings, but she has back pain after heavy activity.

Physical Exam: Mild tenderness to palpation at the fracture site. Neurologic examination is negative. Straight leg raising is negative. True lumbar extension is 10°, flexion is 30°, and left and right lateral bending are each 10°. There is normal hip motion.

Clinical Studies: Repeat x-rays of the area: healed fractures with persistent loss of height of greater than 50% at L2 and 20% at L3.

Diagnosis: Compression fractures L2 and L3.

Impairment Rating: 23% impairment of the whole person.

Comment: Injuries at two vertebrae within the same region, with a 55% compression of L2, according to Table 15-7, results in an impairment of 7%. The compression fracture of L3 results in an impairment of 5%, according to Table 15-7. The instructions are to combine these two impairment ratings; doing so results in an impairment rating of 12%.

The woman has true lumbar extension of 10° which, according to Table 15-8, results in an impairment of 5%, a lumbar flexion of 30°, which results in an impairment of 4% (Table 15-8), and left and right lateral bending of 10°, which results in an impairment of 2% for each (Table 15-9). Adding these four impairments due to loss of motion results in an impairment of 13%. Combining the impairment of 12% from Table 15-7 and the 13% from Tables 15-8 and 15-9 results in a whole person impairment of 23%.

15.13 Criteria for Converting Whole Person Impairment to Regional Spine Impairment

In some instances, the evaluator may be asked to express an impairment rating in terms of the involved spine region rather than the whole person. This is done by dividing the whole person impairment estimate by the percent of spine function that has been assigned to that region. Under the DRE method, a whole person estimate being converted to a regional estimate would be divided by 0.35 for the cervical spine, 0.20 for the thoracic spine, and 0.75 for the lumbar and sacral spines. Under the ROM method, a whole person estimate being converted to a regional estimate should be divided by 0.80 for the cervical spine, 0.40 for the thoracic spine, or 0.90 for the lumbosacral spine (Figure 15-19). For example, a 24-year-old female office worker sustained a cervical injury that, after it was healed and stable, resulted in a whole body impairment, estimated by the DRE method, of 20%. Dividing the 20% by 0.35 results in 57% impairment of the cervical spine. An individual with multiple lumbar compression fractures was rated 25% whole body impairment by the ROM method. To obtain an estimate of lumbar spine impairment, the physician should divide the 25% by 0.9, resulting in a 27.7% rounded up to 28% lumbar spine impairment. Any values that exceed 100% are rounded down to 100% regional impairment.

Figure 15-19 Side View of Spinal Column

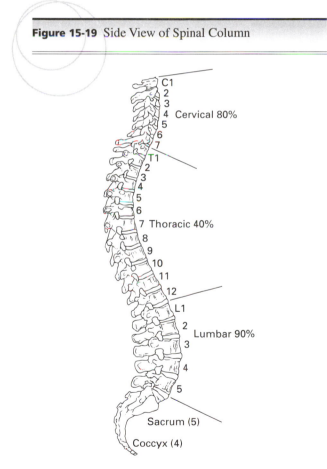

C1
2
3
4 Cervical 80%
5
6
7
T1
2
3
4
5
6
7 Thoracic 40%
8
9
10
11
12
L1
2
3 Lumbar 90%
4
5
Sacrum (5)
Coccyx (4)

The whole spine divided into regions indicating the maximum whole person impairment represented by a total impairment of one region of the spine. Lumbar 90%, thoracic 40%, cervical 80%.

15.14 The Pelvis

Criteria for Rating Impairment Due to Pelvic Injury

The pelvis is composed bilaterally of three bones: the ilium, the ischium, and the pubis, forming a ringlike structure. Each ilium is attached to the sacrum via the sacroiliac synchondrosis. The pelvis, including the symphysis pubis, assists in transfer of body weight to the lower extremities. In females, the pelvic structure and function are also of paramount importance in pregnancy and delivery.

Pelvic disorders are evaluated using Table 15-19. When necessary, these disorders may be combined with impairment ratings from either the DRE or ROM methods for spine impairment.

Table 15-19 Whole Person Impairment Due to Selected Disorders of the Pelvis

Disorder	% Impairment of the Whole Person
1. Healed fracture without displacement or residual sign(s)	0
2. Healed fracture with displacement and without residual sign(s) involving:	
a. Single ramus	0
b. Rami, bilateral	0
c. Ilium	0
d. Ischium	0
e. Symphysis pubis, without separation	5
f. Sacrum	5
g. Coccyx	0
3. Healed fracture(s) with displacement, deformity, and residual sign(s) involving:	
a. Single ramus	0
b. Rami, bilateral	5
c. Ilium	2
d. Ischium, displaced 1 inch or more	10
e. Symphysis pubis, displaced or separated	15
f. Sacrum, into sacroiliac joint	10
g. Coccyx, nonunion or excision	5
h. Fracture into acetabulum	Evaluate on basis of restricted motion of hip joint

The impairment estimate for hemipelvectomy is 50% of the whole person (Table 17-32).

Example 15-25
5% Impairment Due to Pelvic Stress Fracture

Subject: 22-year-old man.

History: Military intensive training involving running with a backpack of 40 lbs over extended time and distance. Difficulty standing up because of pain in the pelvis and in the right upper thigh. Pain was enhanced by walking and running. Felt challenged not to report the pain, which he felt while jumping over a boulder 2 weeks prior to the time of the medical exam. The pain was intensified with further running.

Current Symptoms: Pain in the right groin and medial upper thigh aggravated by standing and walking; improved in the supine position.

Physical Exam: Acute tenderness to palpation and pressure on the right pubic bone and the right adductor and hamstrings origin at the inferior ischiopubic junction.

Clinical Studies: Pelvic x-rays: transverse fissure in the upper border of the obturator foramen; there is already a callus development in the area.

Diagnosis: Stress fracture at the right ischiopubic junction.

Impairment Rating: 5% whole person impairment due to delayed union with deformity and residual signs after achieving MMI.

Comment: The callus formation continued and grew, producing a delayed union. He continued to have right groin and medial upper thigh pain, increasing with walking and running, and stabilizing after 9 months. Stress fractures of the pelvis, especially of the inferior branch of the pubic bone, need to be investigated and treated in a timely manner. Delay in investigation and diagnosis may result in massive callus formation and abnormal union, as well as continued pain, especially with standing and running.

15.15 Spine Evaluation Summary

See Table 15-20 for a spine evaluation summary form.

Table 15-20 Spine Evaluation Summary

Name _____   Soc. Sec. No. _____   Date _____

Impairment	Cervical	Thoracic	Lumbar
1. DRE Method (Tables 15-3 through 15-5)			
2. Range-of-Motion Method (and Table 15-8)			
3. Nerve root: Loss of sensation with or without pain Loss of strength			
4. Other (From Section 15.14)			
5. Regional impairment total (combine impairments in each column using the Combined Values Chart, p. 604)			
6. Spine impairment total (combine all regional totals using the Combined Values Chart)			

7. Impairment(s) of other organ systems: for each impairment list condition, page number in *Guides,* and percentage of impairment.

Impaired System	% Impairment	*Guides* Page Number
a.		
b.		
c.		
d.		
e.		

8. Impairment of the whole person: Use Combined Values Chart to combine spine impairment with the impairment(s) listed in 7 above. If several impairments are listed, combine spine impairments with the larger or largest value, then combine the resulting percentage with any other value(s), until all the listed impairments have been accounted for.

   Total whole person impairment: _____

References

1. *Guides to the Evaluation of Permanent Impairment.* Fourth ed. Chicago, Ill: American Medical Association; 1993.

2. Andersson GBJ. Diagnostic considerations in individuals with back pain. *Phys Med Rehabil Clin North Am.* 1998;9:2.

3. Andersson GBJ, Frymoyer JW. Joint systems: lumbar and thoracic spine in disability evaluation. In: Demeter SL, Andersson GBJ, Smith GM, eds. *Disability Evaluation.* St Louis, Mo: Mosby, Inc; 1996:277-299.

4. Andersson GBJ, Deyo R. History and physical examination in individuals with herniated lumbar disks. *Spine.* 1996;2:24.

5. Andersson GBJ, Deyo RA. Sensitivity, specificity, and predictive value: a general issue in screening for disease in interpretation of diagnostic studies in spinal disorders. In: Frymoyer JW, ed. *The Adult Spine: Principles and Practice.* 2nd ed. Philadelphia, Pa: Lippincott Raven; 1997:305-317.

6. Valkenburg HA, Haanen HCN. The epidemiology of low back pain. In: White AA III, Gordan SL. *Symposium on Idiopathic Low Back Pain.* St Louis, Mo: CV Mosby Co; 1982:9-22.

7. Boden SD, Davis DO, Dina TS, et al. Abnormal magnetic-resonance imaging scans of the lumbar spine in asymptomatic subjects. *J Bone Joint Surg Am.* 1990;72:403-408.

8. Hitselberger WE, Witten RM. Abnormal myelograms in asymptomatic individuals. *J Neurosurg.* 1968;28:204-208.

9. Jensen MC, Brant-Zawdski MN, Obuchwki N, et al. Magnetic resonance imaging of the lumbar spine in people without back pain. *N Engl J Med.* 1994;331:69-73.

10. Symmons DPM, van Hemert AM, Vandenbroucke JP, Valkenburg HA. A longitudinal study of back pain and radiological changes in the lumbar spines of middle aged women, II: radiographic findings. *Ann Rheum Dis.* 1991;50:161-165.

11. Andersson GBJ. The epidemiology of spinal disorders. In: Frymeyer JW, ed. *The Adult Spine: Principles and Practice.* 2nd ed. Philadelphia, Pa: Lippincott-Raven; 1997:93-141.

12. Nardin RA, Patel MR, Gidas TF, Rutkov SB, Raynor EM. Electromyography and magnetic resonance imaging in the evaluation of radiculopathy. *Muscle Nerve.* 1999;22:151-155.

13. White AW, Punjabi MM. *Clinical Biomechanics of the Spine.* 2nd ed. Philadelphia, Pa: JB Lippincott; 1990.

14. Shaffer WO, Spratt KF, Weinstein J, Lehmann TR. The consistency and accuracy of roentgenograms for measuring sagittal translation in the lumbar vertebral motion segment: an experimental model. *Spine.* 1990;15:741-750.

15. Battle MC, Bigos SJ, Fisher LD, et al. The role of spinal flexibility in back pain complaints within industry: a prospective study. *Spine.* 1989;15:768-773.

16. Waddell G, Sommerville D, Henderson I, Newton M. Objective clinical evaluation of physical impairment in chronic low back pain. *Spine.* 1992;17:617-628.

17. Mayer T, Kondraske G, Beals S, Gatchel R. Spinal range of motion: accuracy and sources of error with inclinometric measurement. *Spine.* 1997;22:1976-1984.

18. Fitzgerald G, Wynveen K, Rheauit W, Rothschild B. Objective assessment with establishment of normal values for lumbar spinal range of motion. *Phys Ther.* 1983; 63:1776-1781.

19. Gerhardt JJ. *Documentation of Joint Motion.* Rev 3rd ed. Portland, Ore: Oregon Medical Association; 1992.

20. Gerhardt JJ. Rippstein JR. *Measuring and Recording of Joint Motion: Instrumentation and Techniques (International SFTR Method of Measuring and Recording Joint Motion.* Bern, Switzerland: Hans Huber; 1989.

21. Lea RD, Gerhardt JJ. Current concepts review range of motion measurement. *Bone Joint Surg* 1995;77:784-798.

22. Keeley J, Mayer T, Cox R, et al. Quantification of lumbar function: reliability of range of motion measures in the sagittal plane and in vivo torso rotation measurement techniques. *Spine.* 1986;11:31-35.

23. Mellin G. Measurement of thoracolumbar posture and mobility with myrin inclinometer. *Spine.* 1986; 11:759-776.

24. Helliwell P, Moll J, Wright V. Measurements of spinal movement and function. In: Jayson M, ed. *The Lumbar Spine and Low Back Pain.* 4th ed. New York, NY: Churchill Livingstone; 1992:173-206.

25. Pedrics M, Portek I, Sheperd J. The effect of low back pain on lumbar spinal movements measured by three dimensional x-ray analysis. *Spine.* 1985;10:150-153.

26. Reynolds P. Measurement of spinal mobility: a comparison of three methods. *Rheum Rehabil.* 1975;14:180-185.

27. Alaranta H, Hurri H, Heliovaara M, et al. Flexibility of the spine: normative values of goniometric and tape measurements. *Scand J Rehab Med.* 1994;26:147-154.

28. Loebl W. Measurements of spinal posture and range in spinal movements. *Am Phys Med.* 1967;9:103.

29. Mayer T, Gatchel R, Polatin P, eds. *Occupational Musculoskeletal Disorders.* Philadelphia, Pa: Lippincott; 1999.

30. Chen J, Solinger A, Poncet J, Lantz A. Meta-analysis of normative cervical motion. *Spine*. 1999;24:1571-1578.

31. Dvorak J, Antinnes J, Panjabi M, Loustalot D, Bonomo M. Age and gender related normal motion of the cervical spine. *Spine*. 1992;17:S393-S398.

32. Dvorak J, Vajda E, Grob D, Panjabi H. Normal motion of the lumbar spine as related to age and gender. *Eur Sp J*. 1994;4:18-23.

33. Kuhlman, K. Cervical range of motion in the elderly. *Arch Phys Med Rehabil*. 1993;74:1071-1079.

34. Lantz C, Chen J, Buch D. Clinical validity and stability of active and passive cervical range of motion with regard to total and unilateral uniplanar motion. *Spine*. 1999;24:1082-1089.

35. Mayer T, Brady S, Bovasso E, Pope P, Gatchel R. Noninvasive measurement of cervical tri-planar notion in normal subjects. *Spine*. 1993;18:2191-2195.

36. Mellin G. Method and instrument for non-invasive measurements of thoracolumbar rotation. *Spine*. 1987;12:28-31.

37. Petersen BP, White AA, Panjabi MP. In: Mayer TG, Gatchel RJ, Polatin PB, eds. *Occupational Musculoskeletal Disorders, Function, Outcomes and Evidence*. Philadelphia, Pa: Lippincott Williams & Wilkins; 1999.

38. White AA, Johnson RM, Panjabi MM, Southwick WA. Biomechanical analysis of clinical stability in the cervical spine. *Clin Orthop*. 1975;109:85-96.

39. McGregor A, McCarthy I, Hughes S. Motion characteristics of the lumbar spine in the normal population. *Spine*. 1995;20:2421-2428.

40. Netzer O, Payne V. Effects of age and gender on functional restoration and lateral movements of the neck and back. *Gerontology*. 1993;39:320-326.

41. Nilsson N, Hartvigsen J, Christensen H. Normal ranges of passive cervical motion for women and men 20-60 years old. *J Manipulative Physiol Ther*. 1996;19:306-309.

42. Sullivan M, Dickinson C, Troup J. The influence of age and gender on lumbar spine sagittal plane range of motion: a study of 1126 healthy subjects. *Spine*. 1994;19:662-686.

43. Youdas J, Garrett T, Suman V, Bogard C, Hallman H, Carey J. Normal range of motion of the cervical spine: an initial goniometric study. *Phys Ther*. 1992;72:770-780.

44. Adams M, Dolan P, Marks C, et al. An electroinclinometer technique for measuring lumbar curvature. *Clin Biomech*. 1986;1:130-134.

45. Mayer T, Tencer A, Kristoferson S, Mooney V. Use of noninvasive techniques for quantification of spinal range of motion in normal subjects and chronic low back dysfunction individuals. *Spine*. 1984;9:588-595.

46. Oxorn B, Foote WR. *Human Labor and Birth*. New York, NY: Appleton;1975.

Chapter 16

The Upper Extremities

Introduction

This chapter provides criteria for evaluating permanent impairments due to anatomic impairments of the hand and the upper extremity. The methods discussed in this chapter for evaluation of upper extremity impairment due to amputation, sensory loss, and abnormal motion or ankylosis were based on A. B. Swanson's work and adapted from the fourth edition and updated with input from many of the specialty societies listed in the preface.

The following revisions have been made for the fifth edition: (1) basic principles of assessment have been clarified, (2) updates of the latest scientific information in assessment of upper extremity impairments have been provided, (3) measurement of range of motion of the fingers has been clarified to also detect limited motion due to limited excursion of tendons, (4) impairment determination for nerve entrapment syndromes has been clarified, (5) the criteria for diagnosis of complex regional pain syndrome are discussed and consistent throughout the book, (6) criteria for diagnosis and rating of carpal instability have been clarified, and (7) criteria for diagnosis and rating of weakness not due to other ratable conditions have been clarified.

16.1 Principles of Assessment

16.1a Principles of Impairment Evaluation

Before using the information in this chapter, the *Guides* user should become familiar with Chapters 1 and 2 and the Glossary. Chapters 1 and 2 discuss the *Guides'* purpose, applications, and methods for performing and reporting impairment evaluations. The Glossary provides definitions of common terms used by many specialties in impairment evaluation.

Methods for evaluating impairments of the upper extremities may be described as having anatomic, cosmetic, or functional bases. The physical evaluation determines the *anatomic impairment* and is based on the history and a detailed examination of the individual and the upper extremity(ies). The *cosmetic evaluation* concerns both the individual's and society's reaction to the individual's condition. The *functional evaluation* measures the individual's motor performance of activities of daily living or of a specific task within a set time frame. Functional studies are increasingly sophisticated and can complement the evaluation process. However, the necessary level of standardization in precision and reproducibility to assess function has not yet been developed to derive a numeric impairment rating. Therefore, evaluation of anatomic impairment forms the basis for upper extremity assessment. The impairment ratings originally developed and retained in this chapter were developed to reflect the degree of impairment and its impact on the ability of the individual to perform activities of daily living.

The most practical and useful approach to evaluating impairment of a digit is to compare the current loss of function with the loss resulting from amputation. Total loss of motion and sensibility of a digit, or ankylosis with severe malposition that renders the digit essentially useless, is considered to be about the same as amputation of the part. Ankylosis of a digit or joint in the optimal functional position is given the least motion impairment of the part. Impairment due to total transverse sensory loss of a digit corresponds to 50% of the amputation impairment at the same length or level of involvement (Figures 16-6 and 16-7). Impairment values derived from amputation, loss of motion or ankylosis, and sensibility loss are *combined* using the Combined Values Chart (p. 604).

16.1b Impairment Evaluation: Documentation and Recording

The medical evaluation is the basis for determination of permanent anatomic impairment of the upper extremities. It must be accurate, objective, and well documented. Evaluation of the upper extremities requires a sound knowledge of the normal functional anatomy and would be incomplete without assessment of the general condition of the whole person. It must be thorough and should include several elements: status of activities of daily living; careful observations; both local and general physical examinations; appropriate imaging evaluation; laboratory tests; and, preferably, a photographic record.

An impairment evaluation is based on the examiner's actual findings. A prior injury or illness is considered during assessment of causation and apportionment, as discussed in Chapters 1 and 2. Impairment ratings in this chapter have not been adjusted for hand dominance, as is done in Chapter 13, The Central and Peripheral Nervous System. Hand dominance is difficult to objectively measure and is not accounted for in these impairment ratings. Hand dominance may be right or left and may be marked or slight, or the individual may be completely ambidextrous. Hand dominance should be considered in the determination of disability. If the examiner believes that hand dominance has a significant impact on the ability to perform activities of daily living, this can be discussed in the impairment evaluation report along with the resulting impairment rating. Hand dominance may, of course, be significant when assessing disability.

A complete and detailed examination of the upper extremities is necessary for accurate impairment evaluation. One method for recording results from a systematic examination is the use of the Upper Extremity Impairment Evaluation Record (Figures 16-1a and 16-1b). Part 1 of the evaluation record addresses the hand region and lists impairments due to abnormal motion or ankylosis, amputation, and sensory loss resulting from digital nerve lesions and to other disorders. Part 2 is designed to assist impairment evaluation of the wrist, elbow, and shoulder due to abnormal motion or ankylosis, amputation, and "other" disorders, as well as those related to the peripheral nerve system, peripheral vascular system, and other disorders not included in regional impairments (eg, grip strength). Table 16-1 gives conversions from digit to hand impairment, and Table 16-2 gives those from hand to upper extremity impairment. Regional impairments resulting from the hand, wrist, elbow, and shoulder regions are *combined* to provide the upper extremity impairment (see Section 1.4, Philosophy and Use of the Combined Values Chart, and the Combined Values Chart, p. 604). The upper extremity impairment is then converted to a whole person impairment by means of Table 16-3. When to *add* as opposed to *combine* impairments is discussed in Sections 16.1c and 16.1d and noted in Figure 16-1.

The impairment evaluation record form is designed for use with unilateral upper extremity impairments. Cases of *bilateral involvement* require completion of a separate record form for each upper extremity. The whole person impairment values derived for each upper extremity are then *combined* using the Combined Values Chart (p. 604) to derive the total whole person impairment. If the total *combined* whole person impairment does not seem to adequately reflect the actual extent of alteration in the individual's ability to perform activities of daily living, this should be noted.

Figure 16-1a Upper Extremity Impairment Evaluation Record–**Part 1 (Hand)**　　　Side ☐ R ☐ L

Name_____ Age_____ Sex ☐ M ☐ F　Dominant hand ☐ R ☐ L　Date_____

Occupation_____ Diagnosis_____

	Abnormal Motion					Amputation	Sensory Loss	Other Disorders	Hand Impairment%
	Record motion or ankylosis angles and digit impairment %					Mark level & impairment %	Mark type, level, & impairment %	List type & impairment %	●Combine digit imp % ★Convert to hand imp %

Thumb

		Flexion	Extension	Ankylosis	Imp %
IP	Angle°				
	Imp %				
MP	Angle°				
	Imp %				

			Motion	Ankylosis	Imp %
CMC	Radial abduction	Angle°			
		Imp %			
	Adduction	Cm			
		Imp %			
	Opposition	Cm			
		Imp %			

Amputation: [2]　‡UE IMP % = [5]

Hand Impairment	
Abnormal motion [1]	
Amputation [2]	
Sensory loss [3]	
Other disorders [4]	
Total digit imp % ●Combine 1, 2, 3, 4	

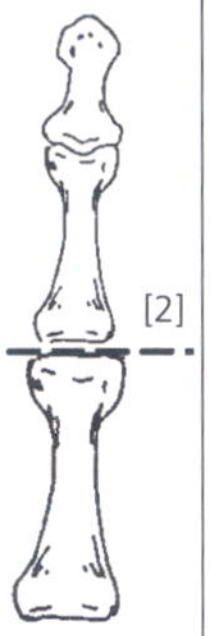

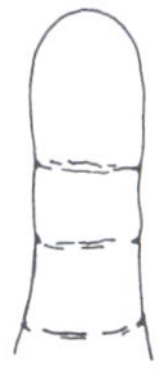

Add digit impairment %　CMC + MP + IP = [1]　**Digit** [2] **IMP % =**　**Digit** [3] **IMP % =**　**Digit** [4] **IMP % =**　**Hand impairment % ★Convert above**

Index

		Flexion	Extension	Ankylosis	Imp %
DIP	Angle°				
	Imp %				
PIP	Angle°				
	Imp %				
MP	Angle°				
	Imp %				

Hand Impairment	
Abnormal motion [1]	
Amputation [2]	
Sensory loss [3]	
Other disorders [4]	
Total digit imp % ●Combine 1, 2, 3, 4	

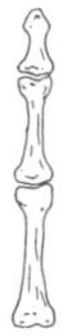

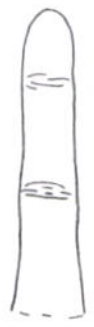

●Combine digit impairment %　MP, PIP, DIP = [1]　**Digit** [2] **IMP % =**　**Digit** [3] **IMP % =**　**Digit** [4] **IMP % =**　**Hand impairment % ★Convert above**

Middle

DIP	Angle°				
	Imp %				
PIP	Angle°				
	Imp %				
MP	Angle°				
	Imp %				

Hand Impairment	
Abnormal motion [1]	
Amputation [2]	
Sensory loss [3]	
Other disorders [4]	
Total digit imp % ●Combine 1, 2, 3, 4	

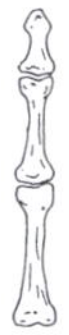

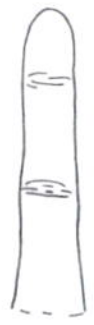

●Combine digit impairment %　MP, PIP, DIP = [1]　**Digit** [2] **IMP % =**　**Digit** [3] **IMP % =**　**Digit** [4] **IMP % =**　**Hand impairment % ★Convert above**

Ring

DIP	Angle°				
	Imp %				
PIP	Angle°				
	Imp %				
MP	Angle°				
	Imp %				

Hand Impairment	
Abnormal motion [1]	
Amputation [2]	
Sensory loss [3]	
Other disorders [4]	
Total digit imp % ●Combine 1, 2, 3, 4	

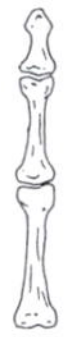

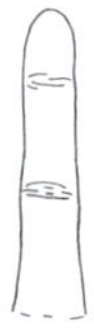

●Combine digit impairment %　MP, PIP, DIP = [1]　**Digit** [2] **IMP % =**　**Digit** [3] **IMP % =**　**Digit** [4] **IMP % =**　**Hand impairment % ★Convert above**

Little

DIP	Angle°				
	Imp %				
PIP	Angle°				
	Imp %				
MP	Angle°				
	Imp %				

Hand Impairment	
Abnormal motion [1]	
Amputation [2]	
Sensory loss [3]	
Other disorders [4]	
Total digit imp % ●Combine 1, 2, 3, 4	

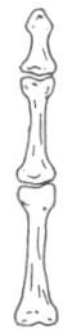

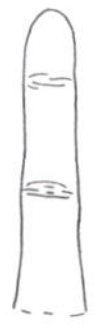

●Combine digit impairment %　MP, PIP, DIP = [1]　**Digit** [2] **IMP % =**　**Digit** [3] **IMP % =**　**Digit** [4] **IMP % =**　**Hand impairment % ★Convert above**

Total hand impairment: Add hand impairment % for thumb + index + middle + ring + little finger =	%
Convert total hand impairment to upper extremity impairment† (if thumb metacarpal intact, enter on Part 2, line II) =	%
‡Add thumb ray upper extremity amputation imp [5] ____ % + hand upper extremity imp ____ % =	%
If hand region impairment is only impairment, convert upper extremity impairment to whole person impairment§ =	%

● Combined Values Chart (p. 604).　　★Use Table 16-1 (digits to hand).　　†Use Table 16-2 (hand to upper extremity).　　§Use Table 16-3.
Courtesy of G. de Groot Swanson, MD, Grand Rapids, Michigan.

Figure 16-1b Upper Extremity Impairment Evaluation Record–**Part 2 (Wrist, elbow, and shoulder)**   Side ☐R ☐L

Name_____   Age_____   Sex ☐M ☐F   Dominant hand ☐R ☐L   Date _____

Occupation_____   Diagnosis_____

	Abnormal Motion					Other Disorders	Regional Impairment %	Amputation
	Record motion or ankylosis angles and impairment %					List type & impairment %	●Combine [1] + [2]	Mark level & impairment %
Wrist		Flexion	Extension	Ankylosis	Imp %			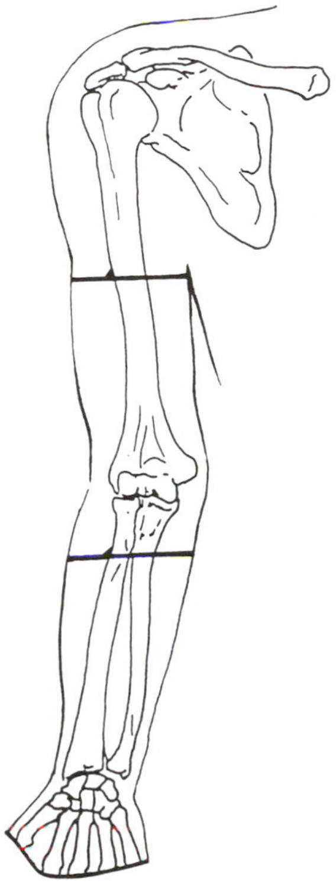
	Angle°							
	Imp %							
		RD	UD	Ankylosis	Imp %			
	Angle°							
	Imp %							
	Add Imp % Flex/Ext + RD/UD =				[1]	Imp % =	[2]	
Elbow		Flexion	Extension	Ankylosis	Imp %			
	Angle°							
	Imp %							
		Pronation	Supination	Ankylosis	Imp %			
	Angle°							
	Imp %							
	Add Imp % Flex/Ext + Pro/Sup =				[1]	Imp % =	[2]	
Shoulder		Flexion	Extension	Ankylosis	Imp %			
	Angle°							
	Imp %							
		Adduction	Abduction	Ankylosis	Imp %			
	Angle°							
	Imp %							
		Int Rot	Ext Rot	Ankylosis	Imp %			
	Angle°							
	Imp %							
	Add Imp % Flex/Ext + Add/Abd + Int Rot/Ext Rot =				[1]	Imp % =	[2]	Imp % =

I. Amputation impairment (other than digits)	=	%
II. Regional impairment of upper extremity ●(Combine hand_____ % + wrist _____% + elbow _____ % + shoulder _____%)	=	%
III. Peripheral nerve system impairment	=	%
IV. Peripheral vascular system impairment	=	%
V. Other disorders (not included in regional impairment)	=	%

Total upper extremity impairment (●Combine I, II, III, IV, and V)	=	%
Impairment of the whole person (Use Table 16-3)	=	%

● Combined Values Chart (p. 604).

If both limbs are involved, calculate the whole person impairment for each on a separate chart and *combine* the percents (Combined Values Chart).

Table 16-1 Conversion of Impairment of the Digits to Impairment of the Hand*

% Impairment of		% Impairment of		% Impairment of	
Thumb	Hand	Index or Middle Finger	Hand	Ring or Little Finger	Hand
0 - 1 =	0	0 - 2 =	0	0 - 4 =	0
2 - 3 =	1	3 - 7 =	1	5 - 14 =	1
4 - 6 =	2	8 - 12 =	2	15 - 24 =	2
7 - 8 =	3	13 - 17 =	3	25 - 34 =	3
9 - 11 =	4	18 - 22 =	4	35 - 44 =	4
12 - 13 =	5	23 - 27 =	5	45 - 54 =	5
14 - 16 =	6	28 - 32 =	6	55 - 64 =	6
17 - 18 =	7	33 - 37 =	7	65 - 74 =	7
19 - 21 =	8	38 - 42 =	8	75 - 84 =	8
22 - 23 =	9	43 - 47 =	9	85 - 94 =	9
24 - 26 =	10	48 - 52 =	10	95 -100 =	10
27 - 28 =	11	53 - 57 =	11		
29 - 31 =	12	58 - 62 =	12		
32 - 33 =	13	63 - 67 =	13		
34 - 36 =	14	68 - 72 =	14		
37 - 38 =	15	73 - 77 =	15		
39 - 41 =	16	78 - 82 =	16		
42 - 43 =	17	83 - 87 =	17		
44 - 46 =	18	88 - 92 =	18		
47 - 48 =	19	93 - 97 =	19		
49 - 51 =	20	98 -100 =	20		
52 - 53 =	21				
54 - 56 =	22				
57 - 58 =	23				
59 - 61 =	24				
62 - 63 =	25				
64 - 66 =	26				
67 - 68 =	27				
69 - 71 =	28				
72 - 73 =	29				
74 - 76 =	30				
77 - 78 =	31				
79 - 81 =	32				
82 - 83 =	33				
84 - 86 =	34				
87 - 88 =	35				
89 - 91 =	36				
92 - 93 =	37				
94 - 96 =	38				
97 - 98 =	39				
99 -100 =	40				

* See Table 16-2 for converting hand impairment to upper extremity impairment.

16.1c Combining Impairment Ratings

The method for combining various impairments is based on the principle that a second and each succeeding impairment do not apply to the whole unit (eg, whole finger) but only to the part or value that remains (eg, proximal phalanx) after the preceding impairment (eg, amputation through the proximal interphalangeal joint) has been applied.

When a given unit has more than one type of impairment (eg, abnormal motion, sensory loss, and partial amputation of a finger), the various impairments are *combined* to determine the total impairment of the unit (eg, finger) before conversion to the next larger unit (eg, hand). Similarly, multiple regional impairments, such as those of the hand, wrist, elbow, and shoulder, are first expressed individually as upper extremity impairments and then *combined* to determine the total upper extremity impairment. The latter is finally converted to whole person impairment (Table 16-3). The combined value determination is based on the following formula: A% + B% (100% − A%) = the combined value of A% and B%.

The Combined Values Chart (p. 604) is used to determine the combined value of two impairment percentages. *All percentages being combined must be expressed on a common denominator or same unit relative value.* If three or more values are to be combined, the two lowest values are first selected and their combined value is found. The combined value and the third value are then combined to give the total value. This procedure can be repeated indefinitely, with the value obtained in each case being a combination of all the previous values.

Table 16-2 Conversion of Impairment of the Hand to Impairment of the Upper Extremity*

% Impairment of		% Impairment of		% Impairment of		% Impairment of		% Impairment of		% Impairment of	
Hand	Upper Extremity	Hand	Upper Extremity	Hand	Upper Extremity	Hand	Upper Extremity	Hand	Upper Extremity	Hand	Upper Extremity
0 = 0		18 = 16		36 = 32		54 = 49		72 = 65		90 = 81	
1 = 1		19 = 17		37 = 33				73 = 66		91 = 82	
2 = 2		20 = 18		38 = 34		55 = 50		74 = 67		92 = 83	
3 = 3				39 = 35		56 = 50				93 = 84	
4 = 4		21 = 19				57 = 51		75 = 68		94 = 85	
		22 = 20		40 = 36		58 = 52		76 = 68			
5 = 5		23 = 21		41 = 37		59 = 53		77 = 69		95 = 86	
6 = 5		24 = 22		42 = 38				78 = 70		96 = 86	
7 = 6				43 = 39		60 = 54		79 = 71		97 = 87	
8 = 7		25 = 23		44 = 40		61 = 55				98 = 88	
9 = 8		26 = 23				62 = 56		80 = 72		99 = 89	
		27 = 24		45 = 41		63 = 57		81 = 73		100 = 90	
10 = 9		28 = 25		46 = 41		64 = 58		82 = 74			
11 = 10		29 = 26		47 = 42				83 = 75			
12 = 11				48 = 43		65 = 59		84 = 76			
13 = 12		30 = 27		49 = 44		66 = 59					
14 = 13		31 = 28				67 = 60		85 = 77			
		32 = 29		50 = 45		68 = 61		86 = 77			
15 = 14		33 = 30		51 = 46		69 = 62		87 = 78			
16 = 14		34 = 31		52 = 47				88 = 79			
17 = 15				53 = 48		70 = 63		89 = 80			
		35 = 32				71 = 64					

* Consult Table 16-3 to convert upper extremity impairment to whole person impairment.

Table 16-3 Conversion of Impairment of the Upper Extremity to Impairment of the Whole Person

% Impairment of		% Impairment of		% Impairment of		% Impairment of		% Impairment of	
Upper Extremity	Whole Person	Upper Extremity	Whole Person	Upper Extremity	Whole Person	Upper Extremity	Whole Person	Upper Extremity	Whole Person
0 = 0		20 = 12		40 = 24		60 = 36		80 = 48	
1 = 1		21 = 13		41 = 25		61 = 37		81 = 49	
2 = 1		22 = 13		42 = 25		62 = 37		82 = 49	
3 = 2		23 = 14		43 = 26		63 = 38		83 = 50	
4 = 2		24 = 14		44 = 26		64 = 38		84 = 50	
5 = 3		25 = 15		45 = 27		65 = 39		85 = 51	
6 = 4		26 = 16		46 = 28		66 = 40		86 = 52	
7 = 4		27 = 16		47 = 28		67 = 40		87 = 52	
8 = 5		28 = 17		48 = 29		68 = 41		88 = 53	
9 = 5		29 = 17		49 = 29		69 = 41		89 = 53	
10 = 6		30 = 18		50 = 30		70 = 42		90 = 54	
11 = 7		31 = 19		51 = 31		71 = 43		91 = 55	
12 = 7		32 = 19		52 = 31		72 = 43		92 = 55	
13 = 8		33 = 20		53 = 32		73 = 44		93 = 56	
14 = 8		34 = 20		54 = 32		74 = 44		94 = 56	
15 = 9		35 = 21		55 = 33		75 = 45		95 = 57	
16 = 10		36 = 22		56 = 34		76 = 46		96 = 58	
17 = 10		37 = 22		57 = 34		77 = 46		97 = 58	
18 = 11		38 = 23		58 = 35		78 = 47		98 = 59	
19 = 11		39 = 23		59 = 35		79 = 47		99 = 59	
								100 = 60	

Example 16-1

Exam: An index finger has an amputation at the distal interphalangeal (DIP) joint (45% digit impairment, Table 16-4) and 90° flexion ankylosis at the PIP joint (75% digit impairment, Figure 16-23).

Analysis: The *combined* impairment is found as follows: 45% + 75% (100% − 45%) = 45% + 41% = 86% digit impairment. This number may be found using the Combined Values Chart (p. 604) at the intersection of the row of the chart for 75% and the column indicated by 45% at the bottom of the chart.

Impairment Rating: Since the index finger represents 20% of the hand, as listed in Table 16-1, the above impairment would represent 20% × 86% impairment of the hand, or 17% (Table 16-1).

16.1d Principles for Adding Impairment Values

When the components of a unit have been assigned a value relative to the whole unit on the same 100% scale, the impairment rating values are *added* rather than combined. Impairment ratings in the hand are *added only* in the following situations:

1. The *total hand impairment rating* is determined by *adding* the hand impairment values contributed by each digit. The hand unit value (100%) is the sum of its component digit values: 40% for the thumb and 20% for the index, 20% for the middle, 10% for the ring, and 10% for the little fingers (Tables 16-1 and 16-4).

2. As shown in Table 16-4, thumb amputations proximal to the MP joint level are expressed in terms of impairment of the upper extremity and receive greater values (37% to 38%, according to level) than amputation of the thumb at the MP joint level (36%). When other hand impairments are present, the total hand impairment value is converted to impairment of the upper extremity and then *added* directly to the upper extremity impairment value resulting from amputation of the thumb ray.

Table 16-4 Impairment Estimates for Upper Limb Amputation at Various Levels

Amputation Levels	Impairment % of			
	Digit	Hand	Upper Extremity	Whole Person
Scapulothoracic (forequarter)	—	—	—	70
Shoulder disarticulation	—	—	100	60
Arm: deltoid insertion and proximally	—	—	100	60
Arm/forearm: from distal to deltoid insertion to bicipital insertion	—	—	95	57
Forearm/hand: from distal to bicipital insertion to transmetacarpophalangeal loss of all digits	—	—	94-90	56-54
Hand: all digits at MP joints	—	100	90	54
Hand: all fingers at MP joints except thumb	—	60	54	32
Thumb ray at/or near:				
CMC joint	—	—	38	23
Distal third of 1st metacarpal	—	—	37	22
Thumb at:				
MP joint	100	40	36	22
IP joint	50	20	18	11
Index or middle finger at:				
MP joint	100	20	18	11
PIP joint	80	16	14	8
DIP joint	45	9	8	5
Ring or little finger at:				
MP joint	100	10	9	5
PIP joint	80	8	7	4
DIP joint	45	5	5	3

Compiled by G. de Groot Swanson, MD, Grand Rapids, Mich.

3. The *thumb ray motion impairment value* is determined by *adding* the motion impairment values contributed by each joint. The thumb functional unit (100%) is the sum of its component joint values: carpometacarpal, 75%; metacarpophalangeal (MP), 10%; and interphalangeal (IP), 15%. However, the finger joint impairment ratings for loss of motion are not added, but *combined*, because their individual values (MP, 100%; PIP, 80%; DIP, 45%) are not assigned on a 100% finger unit scale.

4. For each unit of motion, the *motion impairment value* is found by *adding* together the two impairment values contributed by its components, based on the formula A% = E% + F%. Similarly, for each joint, the total motion impairment rating is found by *adding* the impairment values contributed by each unit of motion. For example, the upper extremity impairment due to abnormal elbow motion is found by *adding* the impairments from the flexion + extension ($I_E\% + I_F\%$) unit to those from the pronation + supination ($I_P\% + I_S\%$) unit, or total motion impairment equals ($I_F\%$ + $I_E\%$) + ($I_P\% + I_S\%$).

5. In Section 16.7, Impairment of the Upper Extremities Due to Other Disorders, the relative value of each joint has been assigned on a 100% digit unit scale: thumb CMC 60%, MP 15%, and IP 25%; and finger MP 50%, PIP 30%, and DIP 20% (Table 16-18). However, the relative value scale used in Table 16-18 is not the same as that assigned for amputations (Table 16-4) and range of motion. Therefore, if more than one joint of a specific digit is affected by other disorders, the impairments are *added* directly together *only* in the absence of amputation and presence of full motion of each joint involved. Otherwise, they are *combined.*

All other upper extremity impairment ratings are combined.

16.2 Amputations

16.2a General Principles
Important factors to consider in evaluating amputations include not only the level of occurrence but also the presence of associated problems relating to the condition of the residual stump (Section 16.2d), to regional or central pain syndromes, and to restriction or loss of motion of existing proximal joints (Section 16.4).

The upper limb is considered as a unit of the whole person and is divided into shoulder, elbow, wrist, and hand regions. The hand is further separated into digits and their parts. From distally to proximally, each anatomic unit is given a relative value to the next larger unit and, eventually, the whole person. By multiplying the appropriate percent, impairment of each unit can be converted sequentially to hand, upper extremity, and whole person impairment as indicated in Tables 16-1, 16-2, 16-3, and 16-4 and Figures 16-2 and 16-3.

It should be noted that, in terms of upper extremity impairment, the functional unit values for the shoulder (60%), elbow (70%), wrist (60%), and digital joints differ from those assigned for amputation at similar levels (Tables 16-4 and 16-18 and Section 16.4).

16.2b Amputation Impairment: Levels Proximal to Digits
The amputation impairment ratings increase with progressively shorter stumps and reach 70% of the whole person for a scapulothoracic (forequarter) amputation, as illustrated in Figure 16-2 and noted in Table 16-4. Amputations through the humerus at or proximal to the deltoid tubercle level (approximately the axillary fold) correspond to 100% loss of the limb, or 60% impairment of the whole person. Amputations occurring between a level just distal to the deltoid tubercle and the bicipital tuberosity

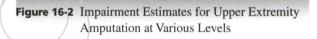

Figure 16-2 Impairment Estimates for Upper Extremity Amputation at Various Levels

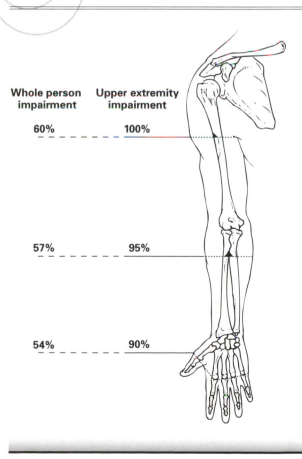

Redrawn with permission from Swanson AB. Evaluation of impairment of function in the hand. *Surg Clin North Am.* 1964;44:925-940.

Figure 16-3 Impairments of the Digits (values outside digits) and the Hand (values inside digits) for Amputations at Various Levels

Transmetacarpophalangeal amputation of all digits represents 100% hand impairment

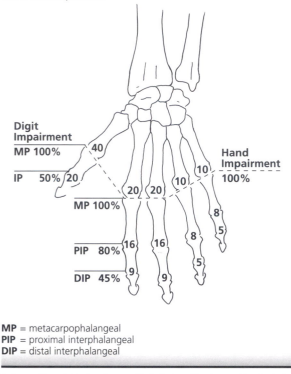

MP = metacarpophalangeal
PIP = proximal interphalangeal
DIP = distal interphalangeal

Redrawn with permission from Swanson AB. Evaluation of impairment of function in the hand. *Surg Clin North Am.* 1964;44:925-940.

upper extremity. Since loss of the entire upper extremity represents 60% impairment of the whole person, this corresponds to 90% × 60%, or 54% impairment of the whole person (Figures 16-2 and 16-3 and Tables 16-1 through 16-4).

Amputation through each joint level of a digit is given a relative value of loss to the entire digit as follows: digit metacarpophalangeal (MP) joint, 100%; thumb interphalangeal (IP) joint, 50%; finger proximal interphalangeal (PIP) joint, 80%; and finger distal interphalangeal (DIP) joint, 45% (Figures 16-3, 16-4, and 16-5; Table 16-4). Digit impairment values for amputation at various levels are shown in Figures 16-4 (thumb) and 16-5 (fingers). Joints should be named rather than numbered.

Amputations of the thumb at levels proximal to the metacarpophalangeal joint are considered to provide a greater severity of impairment than amputation at the MP joint level. Amputation through the thumb MP joint represents a 36% impairment of the upper extremity. Amputation through the distal third of the first metacarpal receives 37% impairment of the upper extremity, and amputation at or near the first carpometacarpal joint is given 38% impairment of the upper extremity (Table 16-4).

The digits represent five coordinated units into which hand function is unequally divided. Each digit is given a relative value to the entire hand as follows: thumb, 40%; index and middle fingers, 20% each; and ring and little fingers, 10% each (Figure 16-3; Tables 16-1 and 16-4). To avoid confusion, digits are named rather than numbered.

By multiplying the appropriate percentages, the impairment rating for each digit, or portion thereof, is converted to an impairment rating of the larger units, the hand, the upper extremity, and, finally, the whole person (Tables 16-1 through 16-4).

(insertion of the biceps brachii on the radius) constitute a 95% impairment of the upper extremity, or 57% impairment of the whole person. Amputations occurring between a level just distal to the bicipital tuberosity and the metacarpophalangeal joints of all digits are estimated to represent 94% to 90% impairment of the upper extremity (56% to 54% of the whole person) according to the functional possibilities afforded by either prosthetic or surgical options (eg, Krukenberg procedure), or simply by the actual length of the residual stump. The evaluator must use clinical judgment to select the appropriate values.

16.2c Amputation Impairment: Digital Levels
Principles
Amputation of all digits (fingers and thumb) through the metacarpophalangeal joints removes the most essential parts of the hand and is considered 100% impairment of the hand, or 90% impairment of the

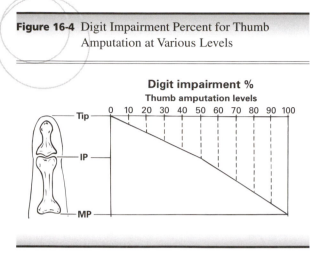

Figure 16-4 Digit Impairment Percent for Thumb Amputation at Various Levels

Redrawn with permission from Swanson AB. Evaluation of impairment of function in the hand. *Surg Clin North Am.* 1964;44:925-940.

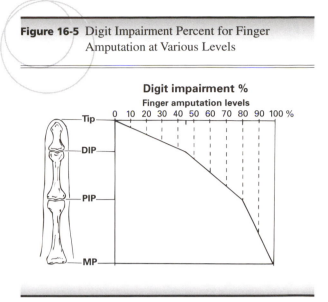

Figure 16-5 Digit Impairment Percent for Finger Amputation at Various Levels

Redrawn with permission from Swanson AB. Evaluation of impairment of function in the hand. *Surg Clin North Am.* 1964;44:925-940.

Example 16-2

Exam: Amputation through the PIP joint of the index finger.

Analysis: A PIP joint amputation represents 80% finger impairment. The relative index finger value to the hand is 20%; therefore, this amputation represents 80% × 20%, or 16% hand impairment (Table 16-1). The relative hand value to the upper extremity is 90%; 16% hand impairment corresponds to 16% × 90%, or 14% upper extremity impairment (Table 16-2).

Impairment Rating: The relative upper extremity value to the whole person is 60%; a 14% upper extremity impairment equals 14% × 60%, or 8% whole person impairment (Table 16-3).

Impairment Rating for Digit Amputation

1. Determine the length of the digit remaining after amputation and evaluate the digit impairment according to Figure 16-4 for the thumb and Figure 16-5 for the fingers. Amputations through the metacarpal are considered to be 100% impairment of the finger. Amputations of the thumb through the first metacarpal receive additional consideration (see 4. below).

2. If *a digit has more than one type of impairment* (eg, sensory, motion, amputation), the *total digit impairment* rating is obtained by *combining* the various digit impairment ratings. The total digit impairment rating is then converted to a hand impairment (Table 16-1).

3. When *multiple digits are involved*, the hand impairment values for each digit are *added* directly to obtain the *total hand impairment*. The total hand impairment is multiplied by 90% to obtain the upper extremity impairment (Table 16-2) and then by 60% to obtain impairment of the whole person (Table 16-3).

4. As shown on Table 16-4, thumb amputations proximal to the MP joint level are expressed in terms of impairment of the upper extremity and receive greater values (37% to 38%, according to level) than amputation of the thumb at the MP joint level (36%). *When other hand impairments are present, the total hand impairment value is converted to impairment of the upper extremity and then added directly to the upper extremity impairment value resulting from amputation of the thumb ray.*

5. Convert the hand impairment rating to the upper extremity and whole person impairment ratings (Tables 16-2 and 16-3).

Example 16-3

Exam: Thumb amputation through the proximal metaphysis of the proximal phalanx.

Analysis: According to Figure 16-4, a proximal metaphysis thumb amputation receives a 90% digit impairment rating. Since the relative value of the thumb to the hand is 40% (Figure 16-3 and Table 16-1), the thumb amputation converts to 36% hand impairment. Using Table 16-2, the 36% hand impairment converts to 32% upper extremity impairment.

Impairment Rating: According to Table 16-3, the 32% upper extremity impairment converts to 19% impairment of the whole person.

Example 16-4

Exam: Amputation of the thumb at the MP joint with amputation through the DIP joint of the index finger.

Analysis: Amputation of the thumb at the MP joint (100% × 40% = 40% hand impairment) with amputation through the DIP joint of the index finger (45% × 20% = 9% hand impairment) corresponds to 40% + 9%, or 49% hand impairment. This is equivalent to 49% × 90%, or 44% impairment of the upper extremity (Table 16-2).

Impairment Rating: The impairment of the whole person is 44% × 60%, or 26% (Table 16-3).

Example 16-5

Exam: Thumb ray amputation at the CMC joint with amputation of the index finger at the MP joint.

Analysis: Thumb amputation at the CMC joint equals 38% impairment of the upper extremity (Table 16-4). Amputation of the index finger at the MP joint equals 20% hand impairment (Table 16-4 and Figure 16-3), or 18% impairment of the upper extremity (Table 16-2). The upper extremity impairment values of 38% for the thumb and 18% for the index finger are *added* directly together, or equal 56%.

Impairment Rating: A 56% impairment of the upper extremity converts to a 34% impairment of the whole person (Table 16-3).

16.2d Conditions Associated With Amputation

Evaluation of the residual stump must assess the status of soft tissue coverage, of the peripheral nerve and vascular systems, and of the bone itself. Unstable *soft tissue coverage* or painful scars are evaluated according to Chapter 8, The Skin. *Peripheral nerve problems,* such as associated neuromas and complex regional pain syndromes, are assessed according to Section 16.5, Impairment of the Upper Extremities Due to Peripheral Nerve Disorders, or Chapter 13, The Central and Peripheral Nervous System. *Phantom pain* is of neurogenic or central origin and is discussed in Chapter 18, Pain. Impairments resulting from *peripheral vascular disorders* are evaluated according to Section 16.6; Chapter 4, The Cardiovascular System: Systemic and Pulmonary Arteries; or Chapter 13. *Bone overgrowth* rarely occurs in other than the long bones of juvenile amputees and receives special consideration according to the problems presented. Any impairment resulting from lost or *restricted motion of proximal joints* is evaluated according to Section 16.4, Evaluating Abnormal Motion.

Impairments related to any of the above associated conditions are rated separately in terms of upper extremity impairment and then *combined* with the total upper extremity impairment due to amputation.

Example 16-6

Exam: Forearm amputation stump at a level just distal to the bicipital tubercle of the radius.

Current Symptoms: Unable to fit elbow prosthesis due to severely restricted elbow motion. Refused surgical shortening of the residual stump.

Analysis: Amputation of the forearm just distal to the bicipital tuberosity corresponds to a 94% impairment of the upper extremity (Table 16-4 and Figure 16-2). The upper extremity impairment rating for decreased elbow motion was calculated as 50%.

Impairment Rating: Use the Combined Values Chart (p. 604) to *combine* the amputation impairment (94%) with the elbow motion impairment (50%) to obtain the total upper extremity impairment of 97%. Convert the 97% upper extremity impairment to 58% impairment of the whole person (Table 16-3).

16.3 Sensory Impairment Due to Digital Nerve Lesions

It has been said that "the hand without feeling is blind." The important difference between "sensation" and "sensibility" was clearly defined by George Omer in 1974. "Sensation is the acceptance and activation of impulses in the afferent nerve fibers of the nervous system. . . . Sensibility is the conscious appreciation and interpretation of the stimulus that produced sensation." The palmar surfaces of the digits have a unique sensibility or capacity for precise interpretation of sensation because of their dense population of specialized receptor organs and free nerve endings. The impairment evaluation of sensibility in the hand, therefore, deserves special attention.

This section addresses the impairment evaluation of sensibility losses in the digits associated with lesions of digital nerves. Sensibility impairment in the hand associated with lesions proximal to digital nerves, painful conditions such as neuromas, and complex regional pain syndromes are considered in Section 16.5 and Chapter 13, The Central and Peripheral Nervous System. Impairment due to neuromas of digital nerves is discussed in Section 16.3c.

16.3a Clinical Evaluation

Evaluation of sensory function in the hand considers all modalities of sensibility, including perception of pain, warmth, cold, and touch-pressure, as well as vibration.

The grading system introduced by the Nerve Injuries Committee of the British Medical Research Council in 1954 describes six levels of sensory recovery after nerve injury. These levels are still used today to describe sensory changes:

S0 Absent sensibility
S1 Recovery of deep cutaneous pain and pressure sensibility (protective sensibility absent)
S2 Return of some degree of superficial cutaneous pain and tactile sensibility, and temperature appreciation (protective sensibility decreased)
S3 Return of superficial cutaneous pain and tactile sensibility (light touch diminished)
S3+ Some recovery of two-point discrimination
S4 Complete sensory recovery

Generally, if an individual has some light touch recognition, the sensory submodalities are assumed to be present.

All clinical tests used to examine the degree of functional loss of sensibility are related to cutaneous touch-pressure sensation. At present, the two-point test for fine discrimination sensibility is most widely used, followed by the monofilament touch-pressure threshold test. The pinprick test can be useful to determine whether pain protective sensation is intact and to identify discrepancies between dermatomal findings and reported symptoms. More accurate assessment is obtained by using the sharp and dull sides of the pin at random. Vibration testing has yet to be associated with functional levels of sensibility.

The Ninhydrin sweat test and wrinkle test may be useful in documenting interruption of digital nerves, especially where questions exist concerning consistency between reported symptoms and neurologic findings. However, these tests have limitations in evaluating a recovering or compressed nerve, because they do not correlate with the presence or absence of sensibility in a regenerating nerve. The Semmes-Weinstein monofilament pressure aesthesiometer measures light-touch and deep-pressure thresholds with sufficient accuracy to quantify returning sensibility levels long before two-point discrimination is measurable. The moving two-point discrimination test may be useful in evaluating recovering nerve function because response to this stimulus returns before response to a static two-point stimulus. Functional isolation of the finger, as noted in the blindfolded picking-up test, can help determine the presence or absence of any useful sensibility in the digit.

The patterns of nerve loss and recovery seen in neuropathy or neuritis from disease or nerve compression are different from those following nerve lacerations. Within the limits of current instruments, two-point discrimination tests have been normal, whereas both the Semmes-Weinstein pressure aesthesiometer and nerve conduction studies have been abnormal in both clinical and induced neuropathies. Two-point discrimination has its widest application for individuals who have sustained nerve lacerations, in whom presence of two-point discrimination usually indicates significant return of function.

The classic Weber static two-point discrimination test is most valuable. Moberg originally described the use of a paper clip opened and bent into a caliper. The Disk-Criminator, DeMayo 2-Point Discrimination Device, and Boley Gauge are some of the currently available testing instruments. Testing is started distally and proceeds proximally. The distance between the tips of the instrument is set first at 5 mm. As the individual being tested closes his or her eyes, the tips of the testing device are applied lightly to the sides of the pulp of the distal segment of the digit in a random sequence, in a longitudinal orientation. Because it is light-touch discrimination that is being tested, the pressure applied should be very light and must not produce a point of blanching or skin indentation. The interval between applications should be no less than 3 to 5 seconds. A series of touches with one or two

points is made, and the individual immediately indicates whether one or two points are felt. Two out of three responses must be accurate for scoring. The distance between the ends is progressively increased until the required accurate responses are elicited, at which time the distance is recorded.

Sensibility assessment is one of the most challenging tasks in impairment evaluation. The subjective nature of sensibility testing can relate to a number of variables involving the testing environment, the individual being tested, the test instruments and methods of administration, and the examiner. Tests should be administered in a quiet environment void of extraneous noises that distract the individual and the tester. Examinee-related variables can include attitude, concentration, anxiety, and the like. Abnormal skin texture, such as calluses, also influences the test results. Instrument-related variables include manufacturing quality control, readjustment of calibration as needed over time, and the weight of various instruments. Important method-related variables include rate and duration of stimulus application, the amount of pressure exerted on the skin, and whether the stimulus is moving or constant. Instruments designed to control the force and velocity of two-point or monofilament application and of other stimuli are not yet available. The examiner's experience, attention to detail, and adherence to methods of administration can minimize the effects of the above variables.

16.3b Digital Nerve Sensory Impairment Evaluation: Principles

Only unequivocal and permanent sensory deficits are given permanent impairment ratings. Sensory impairment is rated according to the sensory quality and the distribution of the sensory loss.

The *sensory quality* is based on the results of the two-point discrimination test carried out over the distal palmar area of the digit, or on the most distal part of the stump in the presence of a partial amputation. Sensibility defects on the dorsal surfaces of the digits are not considered impairing. The sensory quality impairment is classified according to Table 16-5. In total sensory losses (>15 mm), the response to touch, pinprick, pressure, and vibratory stimuli is absent. In partial sensory losses (7-15 mm), there is poor localization and abnormal response to the sensory stimuli.

Table 16-5 Sensory Quality Impairment Classification

Two-Point Discrimination	Sensory Loss	Sensory Quality Impairment (%)
≤ 6 mm	None	0%
7-15 mm	Partial	50%
> 15 mm	Total	100%

The sensory quality impairment ratings derived from Table 16-5 are to be used only for impairment due to lesions of digital nerves. They cannot be used in Table 16-10 as a substitute for selecting the grade of severity of sensory deficits or pain resulting from peripheral nerve disorders. Values from Table 16-5 are not to be used as severity index multipliers in conjunction with assessment of individual spinal nerves (Table 16-13), brachial plexus (Table 16-14), or major peripheral nerves (Table 16-15).

The distribution, or area, of sensory loss is determined by the level of involvement (percentage of digit length affected) of either both digital nerves (transverse sensory loss) or one digital nerve on either the radial or ulnar side of the digit (longitudinal sensory loss). The percentage of digit length involved is derived from the top scale of Figure 16-6 for the thumb and of Figure 16-7 for the fingers.

Total transverse sensory loss represents 100% sensory loss (>15 mm) involving both digital nerves and receives 50% of the digit amputation impairment value for the corresponding level (Figures 16-6 and 16-7, bottom scale, and Tables 16-6 and 16-7).

Partial transverse sensory loss represents 50% sensory loss (7-15 mm) involving both digital nerves and receives 25% of the digit amputation impairment value for the corresponding digit length percentage (Tables 16-6 and 16-7).

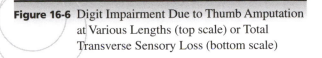

Figure 16-6 Digit Impairment Due to Thumb Amputation at Various Lengths (top scale) or Total Transverse Sensory Loss (bottom scale)

Total transverse sensory loss impairments correspond to 50% of amputation values.

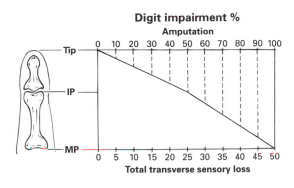

Redrawn with permission from Swanson AB. Evaluation of impairment of function in the hand. *Surg Clin North Am.* 1964;44:925-940.

Figure 16-7 Digit Impairment Due to Finger Amputation at Various Lengths (top scale) or Total Transverse Sensory Loss (bottom scale)

Total transverse sensory loss impairments correspond to 50% of amputation values.

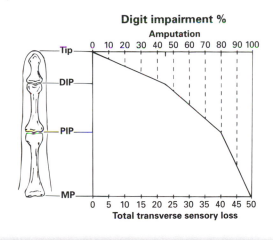

Redrawn with permission from Swanson AB. Evaluation of impairment of function in the hand. *Surg Clin North Am.* 1964;44:925-940.

Table 16-6 Digit Impairment for Transverse and Longitudinal Sensory Losses in *Thumb* and *Little Finger* Based on the Percentage of Digit Length Involved

Percent of Digit Length	Percent of Digit Impairment					
	Tranverse Loss		Longitudinal Loss			
	Both Digital Nerves		Ulnar Digital Nerve		Radial Digital Nerve	
	Total	Partial	Total	Partial	Total	Partial
100	50	25	30	15	20	10
90	45	23	27	14	18	9
80	40	20	24	12	16	8
70	35	18	21	11	14	7
60	30	15	18	9	12	6
50	25	13	15	8	10	5
40	20	10	12	6	8	4
30	15	8	9	5	6	3
20	10	5	6	3	4	2
10	5	3	3	2	2	1

From Swanson AB, de Groot Swanson G, Hagert CG. Evaluation of impairment of hand function. In: Hunter JM, Mackin EJ, Callahan AD, eds. *Rehabilitation of the Hand: Surgery and Therapy.* Fourth ed. St Louis, Mo: CV Mosby; 1995:1858.

Table 16-7 Digit Impairment for Transverse and Longitudinal Sensory Losses in *Index, Middle,* and *Ring Fingers* Based on the Percentage of Digit Length Involved

Percent of Digit Length	Percent of Digit Impairment					
	Tranverse Loss		Longitudinal Loss			
	Both Digital Nerves		Ulnar Digital Nerve		Radial Digital Nerve	
	Total	Partial	Total	Partial	Total	Partial
100	50	25	20	10	30	15
90	45	23	18	9	27	14
80	40	20	16	8	24	12
70	35	18	14	7	21	11
60	30	15	12	6	18	9
50	25	13	10	5	15	8
40	20	10	8	4	12	6
30	15	8	6	3	9	5
20	10	5	4	2	6	3
10	5	3	2	1	3	2

From Swanson AB, de Groot Swanson G, Hagert CG. Evaluation of impairment of hand function. In: Hunter JM, Mackin EJ, Callahan AD, eds. *Rehabilitation of the Hand: Surgery and Therapy.* Fourth ed. St Louis, Mo: CV Mosby; 1995:1858.

Example 16-7

Exam: Total transverse sensory loss (both digital nerves) from the level of the IP joint of the thumb (50% length) distally.

Analysis: Corresponds to 50% (sensory impairment) × 50% (thumb length) = 25% digit impairment (Figure 16-6 and Table 16-6).

Impairment Rating: 25% thumb impairment corresponds to 10% hand impairment (Table 16-2).

Example 16-8

Exam: Partial transverse sensory loss (both digital nerves) from the level of the index PIP joint (80% length) distally.

Analysis: 25% (sensory impairment) × 80% (digit length) = 20% digit impairment (Figure 16-7 and Table 16-7).

Impairment Rating: 20% index impairment corresponds to 4% hand impairment (Table 16-2).

Longitudinal sensory loss impairments are based on the relative importance of the side of the digit for sensory function as follows: thumb and little finger, radial side 40% and ulnar side 60%; index, middle, and ring fingers, radial side 60% and ulnar side 40%. The surfaces used for opposition in various pinch functions and the ulnar aspect of the border finger are rated more highly. If the little finger has been amputated, the relative value of the ulnar side of the ring finger becomes 60% and that of the radial side, 40%. The digit impairment values are calculated similarly as above based on the sensory quality and distribution of the sensory loss.

For ease of determination, digit impairment values for total transverse and longitudinal and partial transverse and longitudinal sensory losses were calculated according to the percentage of digit length involved and are presented in table form. Consult Table 16-6 for the thumb and little finger and Table 16-7 for the index, middle, and ring fingers. Corresponding hand impairment values can be derived from Table 16-1, as shown in Figure 16-8, for total sensory losses involving 100% of the digit length.

Figure 16-8 Hand Impairment Values for Total Transverse Sensory Loss (numbers at tips of digits) and Total Longitudinal Sensory Loss on Radial and Ulnar Sides (numbers at sides of digits) Involving 100% of the Digit Length

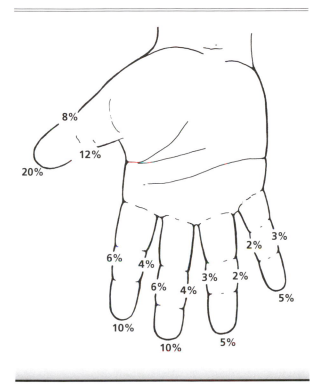

Redrawn with permission from Swanson AB. Evaluation of impairment of function in the hand. *Surg Clin North Am.* 1964;44:925-940.

Relatively small impairment values are given for sensory deficits in areas other than the palmar surfaces of the digits. In the hand region, up to 5% impairment of the hand (5% impairment of the upper extremity) may be given for loss of sensibility in territories innervated by the palmar or dorsal ulnar cutaneous nerve, median palmar cutaneous nerve, or superficial radial nerve (Figure 16-48).

16.3c Rating Impairment Due to Digital Neuromas

The grade of severity of pain and decreased function associated with neuromas of the digital nerves is rated according to Table 16-10a. The severity grade percentage is multiplied by the maximum impairment value of the digital nerve involved (see Table 16-10b, Procedure). The maximum digit impairment values for each digital nerve are found in Table 16-6 for the thumb and little finger and Table 16-7 for the index, middle, and ring fingers under the columns headed Longitudinal Loss, Total (Ulnar or Radial),

100% Digit Length. These values were converted to hand impairment values (Figure 16-8) and upper extremity impairment values (Table 16-15).

If both digital nerves are involved in the same digit, the sensory impairments relating to the ulnar and radial palmar nerves are *added*. Similarly, the percentage of digit impairment due to neuroma formation along one digital nerve is *added* to any sensory deficit impairment due to the contralateral nerve. However, if other impairments of the same digit are present (eg, from amputation, decreased motion, or other disorders), their percentages are *combined* with the percentage due to sensory loss.

16.3d Digital Nerve Sensory Impairment Determination Method

1. Use the two-point discrimination test to identify the sensory quality, or type of sensory loss, as total (>15 mm) or partial (7 through 15 mm) (Table 16-5).
2. Determine the distribution of sensory loss involvement or whether one (longitudinal sensory loss) or both (transverse sensory loss) digital nerves are involved.
3. Identify the level of involvement, or percentage of digit length involved, using the top scale of Figure 16-6 for the thumb and of Figure 16-7 for the fingers.
4. Consult Table 16-6 for the thumb and little finger and Table 16-7 for the index, middle, and ring fingers to determine the digit impairment for either total or partial, transverse or longitudinal (ulnar or radial) sensory loss according to the percentage of digit length involved.
5. If both digital nerves are involved in the same digit, the sensory impairments relating to the ulnar or radial palmar nerves are *added*.
6. Convert the digit impairment to hand, upper extremity, and whole person impairment by using Tables 16-1, 16-2, and 16-3. When a digit has more than one impairment, obtain the total digit impairment value by combining its various impairments before converting the digit values to a hand value.

Example 16-9

Exam: A total transverse sensory loss (>15 mm) over the index finger palmar surface from the level of the PIP joint distally (80% finger length).

Analysis: Equivalent to 40% index impairment (Figure 16-7 and Table 16-7).

Impairment Rating: 8% hand impairment (Table 16-1).

Example 16-10

Exam: A partial transverse sensory loss (7-15 mm) involving the full length of the palmar surface of the thumb from the level of the MP joint distally (100% length).

Analysis: 25% impairment of the thumb (Figure 16-6 and Table 16-6).

Impairment Rating: 10% hand impairment (Table 16-1).

Example 16-11

Exam: A total longitudinal sensory loss (>15 mm) over the distribution of the thumb ulnar digital nerve from the level of the IP joint distally (50% length).

Analysis: Equivalent to 15% thumb impairment (Figure 16-6 and Table 16-6).

Impairment Rating: 6% hand impairment (Table 16-1).

Example 16-12

Exam: A partial longitudinal sensory loss (7-15 mm) over the distribution of the index radial nerve from the level of the MP joint distally (100% length).

Analysis: Equivalent to 15% index impairment (Figure 16-7 and Table 16-7).

Impairment Rating: 3% hand impairment (Table 16-1).

16.4 Evaluating Abnormal Motion

16.4a Clinical Measurements of Motion

Figure 16-9 illustrates the principles of the range of motion (ROM) as measured on the basis of the neutral position of a joint being zero. The "extended anatomic position" is therefore accepted as 0° rather than 180°, and the degrees of joint motion increase in the direction the joint moves from the zero starting point. The term *extension* describes motion opposite to flexion. Incomplete extension from a flexed position to the neutral starting point is defined as *extension lag*. Extension exceeding the zero starting position, as can be seen in normal metacarpophalangeal, elbow, and knee joints, is referred to as *hyperextension*. *Ankylosis* refers to complete absence of motion of a joint. For ease of notation, a plus sign (+) is used to indicate joint hyperextension and a minus sign (−) to indicate extension lag. These signs have no mathematical significance. Using this notation system, a finger joint flexion contracture of 15° with flexion to 45° would be recorded as −15° to 45°. A joint motion with 15° hyperextension and 45 flexion would be recorded as +15° to 45° (Figure 16-9).

The *arc of motion* represents the total number of degrees traced between the two extreme positions of movement in a specific plane of motion, such as from maximum flexion to maximum extension of the PIP joint. When a joint has more than one plane of movement, each type of motion is referred to as a *unit of motion*. For example, the wrist has two units of motion: flexion/extension (anteroposterior plane) and ulnar/radial deviation (lateral plane). The term *functional position* of a joint denotes the optimal or least impairing angle(s) recommended for joint fusion. When a joint has more than one unit of motion, each separate unit is assigned a functional position. For example, the functional position of the elbow is considered to be 80° flexion and 20° pronation.

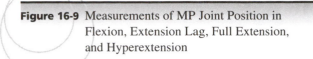

Figure 16-9 Measurements of MP Joint Position in Flexion, Extension Lag, Full Extension, and Hyperextension

Full extension or the neutral position is considered to be 0°.

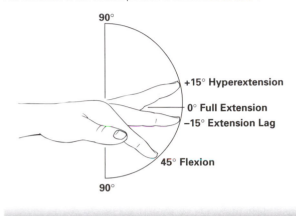

Redrawn with permission from Swanson AB. Evaluation of impairment of function in the hand. *Surg Clin North Am.* 1964;44:925-940.

In assessing motion, the examiner should first observe what an individual can and cannot do by asking him or her to move each joint of the extremity, from the shoulder down, through its full range of motion. *Both extremities should be compared.* Individual joints are then evaluated separately. Similarly, movements of the digits are first evaluated as a unit by having the individual make a complete fist and then extend the digits fully over several repetitions. In determining the range of motion of individual joints, the examiner must evaluate both the active and the passive motion. *Active or voluntary motion* is that performed by the active contraction of the governing muscles and is evaluated first. When a person has full active joint excursion, passive motion values need not to be taken because a joint that has full active excursion will have a full passive range as well. However, if the active arc of motion is incomplete, assisted active and/or passive motion measurements are necessary to evaluate the joint motion. *Passive motion* is that produced by an external force to determine the freedom and range of motion existing at a joint when all muscles are relaxed. An example, is Bunnell's test for intrinsic tightness in the hand. *Assisted active motion* is the result of active muscle contraction and an external force applied to the joint; it allows for stabilization of a segment to improve the mechanical advantage of the muscles that move the joint being measured. In both cases, approximately 0.5 kg of force is applied while a segment of the joint is stabilized. *Measurements of active motion take precedence in the Guides.* The *actual measured goniometer readings or linear measurements* are recorded.

Many different factors can limit the normal range of motion of the joints of the upper extremities. Limitation of active motion can be due to failure of the nerve, muscle, or tendon to execute the motion. Limitation of passive motion can be from involvement of the joint itself, a fixed **contracture,** or the antagonistic muscle or tendon that holds back the motion because it is adherent or too short. Sound clinical knowledge and measurement techniques are necessary for appropriate impairment evaluation and rating.

Digital joints are measured with the wrist held in neutral position and the forearm pronated. To measure the ROM of individual joints, the proximal joint(s) are stabilized in extension, and only the joint being measured is flexed. Note that if all three joints are flexed simultaneously, as in making a fist, active flexion of the metacarpophalangeal joint will be decreased. In some cases of decreased finger motion due to limited excursion of the activating musculotendinous unit or blockage of motion by the antagonistic musculotendinous unit, the measurement of individual joints, as described earlier, can be normal or near normal. In these situations, the *total active range of motion* (TAM) of the digit is measured. Flexion of each joint is measured while all three joints are held in a position of maximum active flexion, or the finger is flexed as a whole unit; similarly, extension of each joint is measured while all three joints are held in maximum extension. The methods used to derive motion impairment of a digit using individual joint measurements and the total active range of motion of a digit are different, as explained on p. 465, Combining Abnormal Motion at More Than One Finger Joint. *The joint measurement technique that best reflects the existing impairment is selected.*

16.4b Principle for Motion Impairment Calculation: A = E + F

The arc of motion is the total number of degrees of excursion measured between the two extreme angles of a plane of motion of a joint, for example, from maximum extension to maximum flexion. When there is complete loss of joint motion, or ankylosis, the total number of degrees of lost motion (A) equals the sum of lost extension degrees (E) and lost flexion degrees (F), or A = E + F. A always equals the total number of degrees of the normal arc of motion.

The symbol V represents the measured angle. The measured angle of extension is represented by V_{ext}, and the measured angle of flexion is represented by V_{flex}. Assuming that a joint, which normally has a range of motion of 0° extension to 90° flexion, has a measured V_{ext} at 0° and V_{flex} at 90°, then there is no loss of motion.

When the joint flexion is decreased, F (lost flexion degrees) equals the theoretically largest V_{flex} minus the measured V_{flex}. For example, if a joint that would normally flex to 90° has a measured V_{flex} at 60°: F = 90° − 60° = 30° flexion loss.

When joint extension is decreased, E (lost extension degrees) equals the measured V_{ext} minus the theoretically smallest V_{ext}. For example, if a joint that would normally extend to 0° has an extension lag measured at V_{ext} 20°: E = 20° − 0° = 20° extension loss.

With decreasing flexion, V_{flex} decreases, and with increasing extension loss, V_{ext} increases; as motion is lost, these values will finally meet at the same point on the arc of motion, or V_{flex} will equal V_{ext}. When this occurs, there is ankylosis, or total loss of the potential arc of motion degrees (A). For example, if a joint that would normally extend to 0° and flex to 90° is ankylosed at 40°: $V_{ext} = V_{flex} = 40°$; E = 40° − 0° = 40°; F = 90° − 40° = 50°; A = 40° (E) + 50° (F), or 90°; and there is total loss of the potential full arc of motion.

Impairment of finger motion may be due to loss of extension (E) with or without loss of flexion (F) or to ankylosis (A). The restricted motion impairment percents are called $I_E\%$, $I_F\%$, and $I_A\%$, respectively, and are functions of the angle (V) measured at examination.

$I_E\%$ = 0% when V_{ext} reaches its smallest theoretical value.
$I_F\%$ = 0% when V_{flex} reaches its largest theoretical value.
$I_A\% = I_E\% + I_F\%$ when $V_{ext} = V_{flex}$.

The formula A% = E% + F% can also be written E% = A% − F%; therefore, impairment values for lack of extension ($I_E\%$) can be derived for any measured extension angle on the basis that $I_E\% = I_A\% − I_F\%$. The derivation of both $I_E\%$ and $I_F\%$ allows estimation of impairment percentages relating not only to the number of degrees of lost motion but, most important, to the location of the loss on the arc of motion.

Motion impairment curves based on the formula A% = E% + F% were derived on a 100% scale for each motion unit of each upper extremity joint, taking into consideration the functional position of each joint as recommended in the literature for fusion (eg, Figure 16-11). The value of A% reaches its maximum, or 100%, at the two extreme positions of the arc of motion and drops to its lowest percent when the angle of ankylosis corresponds to the position of function of the joint. The motion impairment curves plotted on a 100% motion unit scale were converted to pie charts of regional motion impairment (thumb, finger, upper extremity) by applying the relative regional value of each respective motion unit as a conversion factor (eg, Figure 16-12).

For example, wrist functional unit = 60% of upper extremity function. Flexion/extension unit = 70% of wrist function unit, or 70% × 60% = 42% of upper extremity function. Radial/ulnar deviation unit = 30% of wrist functional unit, or 30% × 60% = 18% of upper extremity function. The flexion/extension motion unit impairment curve (Figure 16-27) was multiplied by 42% to derive the pie chart of upper extremity impairment (Figure 16-28) resulting from restricted wrist flexion/extension. The radial/ulnar deviation motion unit impairment curve (Figure 16-30) was multiplied by 18% to obtain the pie chart of upper extremity impairment (Figure 16-31) resulting from restricted wrist lateral deviation.

16.4c Method for Motion Impairment Calculation

The motion impairment pie charts are used for motion impairment calculation of a specific joint. Because the same relative value scale is applied to each motion unit and to its components, the impairment values derived for each are *added* directly together to obtain the total motion impairment of a specific joint. The total impairment value of a motion unit is obtained by *adding* the impairment values contributed by its two component movements (eg, impairment of flexion/extension motion unit = $I_F\%$ + $I_E\%$). Similarly, when a joint has more than one unit of motion (eg, elbow flexion/extension and pronation/supination), its total motion impairment is obtained by *adding* the impairment values contributed by each unit of motion. When a joint that has a single unit of motion (eg, MP joint) is ankylosed, $I_A\%$ represents its motion impairment. When a joint that has more than one unit of motion (eg, the elbow) is ankylosed, the ankylosis impairments ($I_A\%$) derived for each motion unit are *added* to obtain its total motion impairment.

Example 16-13

Exam: Wrist 10° flexion, 10° extension, 0° radial deviation, and 10° ulnar deviation.

Analysis: Motion impairments derived from pie charts:
I_F % at 10° V_{Flex} = 8% (Figure 16-28).
I_E % at 10° V_{Ext} = 8% (Figure 16-28).
I_{RD}% at 0° V_{RD} = 4% (Figure 16-31).
I_{UD}% at 10° V_{UD} = 4% (Figure 16-31).
Wrist motion impairment = (I_F% + I_E%) + (I_{RD}% + I_{UD}%).

Impairment Rating: *Add* contributing motion impairments: (8% + 8%) + (4% + 4%) = 24% impairment of the upper extremity.

Example 16-14

Exam: Wrist ankylosis 0° extension and 0° lateral deviation.

Analysis: Ankylosis impairments derived from pie charts:
I_A% at 0° $V_{Flex/Ext}$ = 21% impairment of upper extremity (Figure 16-28).
I_A% at 0° $V_{RD/UD}$ = 3% impairment of upper extremity (Figure 16-31).

Impairment Rating: *Add* contributing ankylosis impairments: Wrist motion impairment = 21% + 9% = 30% impairment of the upper extremity.

The actual ROM measurements are recorded and applied to the various impairment pie charts. Impairment values for degree measurements falling between those listed may be adjusted or interpolated proportionally in the corresponding interval.

Example 16-15

Exam: A finger MP joint active motion is measured at –25° extension lag and 65° flexion (Figure 16-25).

Analysis: Find listed values and interpolate for actual measurements.
I_E% at –30° V_{Ext} = 12%; I_E% at –20° V_{Ext} = 10%.
The impairment span between 12% and 10% is 2%.
The interpolated value for I_E% at –25° V_{Ext} = 11% finger impairment.
I_F% at 70° V_{Flex} = 11%; I_F% at 60° V_{Flex} = 17%.
The impairment span between 17% and 11% is 6%.
The interpolated value for I_F% at 65° V_{Flex} = 14% finger impairment.

Impairment Rating: 11% (I_E%) + 14% (I_F%) = 25% finger impairment due to abnormal motion at the MP joint.

The measurements reported in the impairment tables and pie charts reflect the accepted average active range(s) of motion for each joint. However, certain people can have either lesser or greater joint flexibility than average. It is therefore most important to always compare measurements of the relevant joint(s) in both extremities.

If a contralateral "normal" joint has a less than average mobility, the impairment value(s) corresponding to the uninvolved joint can serve as a baseline and are subtracted from the calculated impairment for the involved joint. The rationale for this decision should be explained in the report.

Example 16-16

Exam: Active wrist extension is measured at 30° in the involved extremity and at 50° in the contralateral, uninjured extremity (Figure 16-28).

Analysis: I_E% at 30° V_{Ext} = 5% (involved wrist).
I_E% at 50° V_{Ext} = 2% (baseline wrist).

Impairment Rating: The upper extremity impairment value for the involved wrist is adjusted to 5% – 2% = 3%.

If an involved joint has "normal" motion according to the values specified in the *Guides* and *the contralateral uninvolved joint has greater than average motion,* there is a relative loss of motion. However, a loss of motion in a zone beyond the normal values does not as a rule represent a loss of function or impairment. In fact, with the exception of some specialized activities such as gymnastics or Eastern expressive dancing (hyperextension of digits and wrist), an overly flexible joint could be considered an impairment. For example, if the hyperlaxity resulted in subluxation or dislocation, it would be ratable in accordance with Table 16-22 or 16-26. In rare cases, based on the examiner's clinical judgment, an impairment percent not to exceed 2% of the maximum regional impairment value of a unit of motion could be given. The rationale for this decision must be explained in the report.

Example 16-17

Exam: Active wrist extension is measured at 60° in the involved extremity and at 80° in the contralateral, uninjured extremity.

Analysis: The maximum allowable value for unilateral loss of wrist extension beyond the normal 60° would be 42% × 2% = 0.84%.

Impairment Rating: This is rounded up to 1% of the upper extremity (Figure 16-28).

Motion impairment derivation methods are presented in detail for each joint of the upper extremity in the subsections covering thumb ray; finger joints; *combining* digit amputation, sensory loss, and abnormal motion impairment; determining hand impairment from two or more digits; wrist joint; elbow joint; and shoulder joint.

16.4d Thumb Ray Motion Impairment

The thumb ray has three articular units: interphalangeal (IP) joint, metacarpophalangeal (MP) joint, and carpometacarpal (CMC) joint. The five thumb ray functional units of motion have been assigned a relative value to the entire thumb ray on a 100% scale as follows:

IP joint flexion and extension:		15%
MP joint flexion and extension:		10%
CMC joint:		75%
Adduction:	20%	
Radial abduction:	10%	
Opposition:	45%	

Unit-of-motion impairment curves were derived and expressed on a 100% motion unit scale (Figures 16-11, 16-14, 16-18, and 16-19) and then converted to pie charts or tables of thumb ray impairment by applying the relative value of each functional unit of motion as a conversion factor (Figures 16-12 and 16-15 and Tables 16-8a, 16-8b, and 16-9). Because they are expressed on the same relative value denominator, the pie charts and tables of thumb impairment are used to calculate the total thumb ray motion impairment value. The percents contributed by each motion unit are *added* directly.

Thumb IP Joint: Flexion and Extension

The thumb IP joint motion ranges from +30° hyperextension to 80° flexion. The functional position is 20° flexion. The relative value of this functional unit is 15% of the thumb ray.

1. Measure the maximum active flexion and extension and record the *actual* goniometer readings (Figure 16-10).

Figure 16-10 Neutral Position (top) and Flexion (bottom) of Thumb IP joint

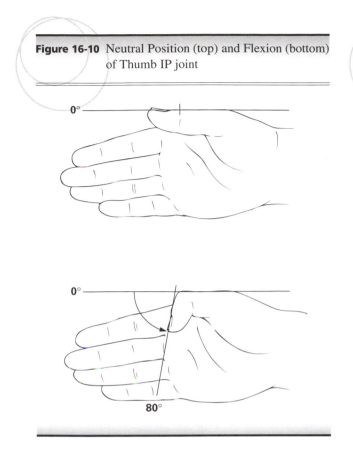

0°

0°

80°

Figure 16-11 Motion Unit Impairment Curves for Ankylosis (I$_A$%), Loss of Flexion (I$_F$%), and Loss of Extension (I$_E$%) of IP Joint of Thumb

Ankylosis in functional position (20° flexion) receives lowest I$_A$% value (50%).

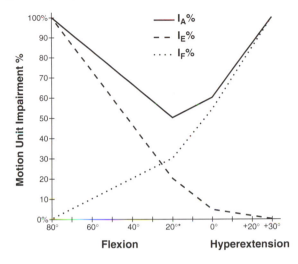

Adapted from Swanson AB, Hagert CG, de Groot Swanson G. Evaluation of impairment of hand function. In: Hunter JM, Schneider LH, Mackin E, Calahan A, eds. *Rehabilitation in the Hand.* St Louis, Mo: CV Mosby Co; 1978:31-69.

2. Using Figure 16-12, match the measured angles of flexion and extension (row headed V) to their corresponding impairments of flexion (row headed I$_F$%) and of extension (row headed I$_E$%). Impairment percents for positions of hyperextension are read above the 0° neutral position. Impairment values for measured angles falling between those listed in Figure 16-12 may be adjusted or interpolated proportionally in the corresponding interval.
3. *Add* I$_F$% and I$_E$% values to obtain thumb impairment for decreased motion of the IP joint.
4. If the IP joint is ankylosed, match the measured angle (row headed V) to its corresponding ankylosis impairment under the row headed I$_A$% (Figure 16-12). Interpolate impairment values for intervening angles. Ankylosis in the functional position (20° flexion) is given the lowest ankylosis impairment value (7%).

Example 16-18

Exam: A thumb IP joint has −10° extension lag and 50° flexion.

Analysis: I$_E$% = 2%; I$_F$% = 2% (Figure 16-12).

Impairment Rating: 2% + 2% = 4% thumb impairment, or 2% hand impairment (Table 16-1).

Example 16-19

Exam: A thumb IP joint has ankylosis in 65° flexion.

Analysis: I$_A$% in 70° flexion = 14%; I$_A$% in 60° flexion = 12%.

Impairment Rating: The interpolated value for I$_A$% in 65° flexion = 13% thumb impairment, or 5% hand impairment.

Figure 16-12 Pie Chart of Thumb Impairments Due to Abnormal Motion at the IP Joint

Relative value of functional unit is 15% of the thumb ray motion.

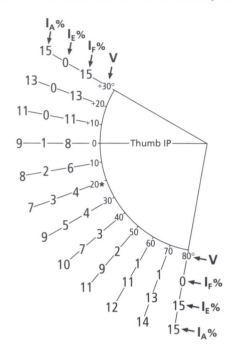

$I_A\%$ = Impairment due to ankylosis
$I_E\%$ = Impairment due to loss of extension
$I_F\%$ = Impairment due to loss of flexion
V   = Measured angles of motion
*   = Position of function

Adapted from Swanson AB, Hagert CG, de Groot Swanson G. Evaluation of impairment of hand function. In: Hunter JM, Schneider LH, Mackin E, Calahan A, eds. *Rehabilitation in the Hand.* St Louis, Mo: CV Mosby Co; 1978:31-69.

Figure 16-13 Neutral Position (top) and Flexion (bottom) of Thumb MP Joint

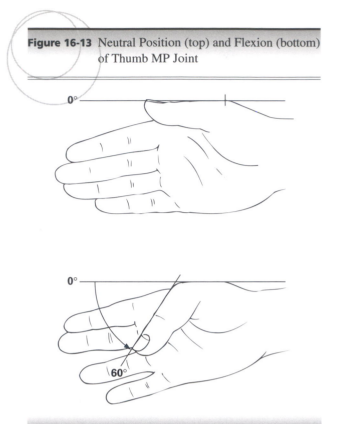

Thumb MP Joint: Flexion and Extension

The thumb MP joint motion ranges from +40° hyperextension to 60° flexion. The functional position is 20° flexion. The relative value of the functional unit is 10% of the thumb ray.

1. Measure the maximum active flexion and extension and record the goniometer readings (Figure 16-13).
2. Using Figure 16-15, match the measured angles of flexion and extension (row headed V) to their corresponding impairments of flexion (row headed $I_F\%$) and of extension (row headed $I_E\%$). Impairment percents for positions of hyperextension are read above the 0° neutral position. Impairment values for measured angles falling between those listed in Figure 16-15 may be adjusted or interpolated to be proportionally in the corresponding interval.

3. *Add* the values for $I_F\%$ and $I_E\%$ to obtain thumb impairment for decreased motion of the MP joint.
4. If the MP joint is ankylosed, match the measured angle (row headed V) to its corresponding ankylosis impairment under the row headed $I_A\%$ (Figure 16-15). Interpolate impairment values for intervening angles. Ankylosis in the functional position (20° flexion) is given the lowest $I_A\%$, or 5%.

Figure 16-14 Motion Unit Impairment Curves for Ankylosis (I_A%), Loss of Flexion (I_F%), and Loss of Extension (I_E%) of Thumb MP Joint

Ankylosis in functional position (20° flexion) receives the lowest I_A% value (50%).

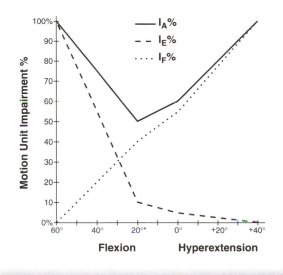

Adapted from Swanson AB, Hagert CG, de Groot Swanson G. Evaluation of impairment of hand function. In: Hunter JM, Schneider LH, Mackin E, Calahan A, eds. *Rehabilitation in the Hand.* St Louis, Mo: CV Mosby Co; 1978:31-69.

Figure 16-15 Pie Chart of Thumb Impairments Due to Abnormal Motion at the MP Joint

Relative value of functional unit is 10% of the thumb ray motion.

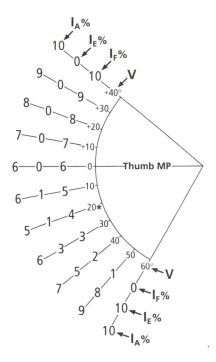

I_A% = Impairment due to ankylosis
I_E% = Impairment due to loss of extension
I_F% = Impairment due to loss of flexion
V   = Measured angles of motion
*   = Position of function

Adapted from Swanson AB, Hagert CG, de Groot Swanson G. Evaluation of impairment of hand function. In: Hunter JM, Schneider LH, Mackin E, Calahan A, eds. *Rehabilitation in the Hand.* St Louis, Mo: CV Mosby Co; 1978:31-69.

Example 16-20

Exam: A thumb MP joint has +10° hyperextension and 40° flexion.

Analysis: I_E% = 0%; I_F% = 2% (Figure 16-15).

Impairment Rating: 0% + 2% = 2% thumb impairment, or 1% hand impairment (Table 16-1).

Example 16-21

Exam: A thumb MP joint has −25° extension and 60° flexion.

Analysis: I_E% = 2% (interpolated value); I_F% = 0%.

Impairment Rating: 2% + 0% = 2% thumb impairment.

Example 16-22

Exam: A thumb MP joint is ankylosed in 60° flexion.

Analysis: I_A% = 10% thumb impairment.

Impairment Rating: 4% hand impairment.

Thumb Radial Abduction

Radial abduction is measured in degrees as the largest angle of separation actively formed between the first and second metacarpals in the coronal plane (Figure 16-16). The stationary arm of the goniometer is aligned over the second metacarpal, and the movable arm over the first metacarpal. The normal angle of radial abduction is 50°. Note that in full radial adduction, the smallest angle of separation is 15° due to anatomic configurations. The relative value of radial abduction is 10% of the thumb ray.

1. Measure and record the goniometer reading for maximum active radial abduction and radial adduction, or the angle of ankylosis.
2. Using Table 16-8a, match the measured angles of radial abduction to their corresponding impairments of radial abduction.
3. If the CMC joint is ankylosed, match the measured angle to its corresponding ankylosis impairment (Table 16-8a) to obtain the thumb impairment due to loss of this function.
4. Convert thumb impairment to hand impairment using Table 16-1.

Example 16-23

Exam: A thumb has complete active radial adduction and 25° radial abduction.

Impairment Rating: 7% thumb impairment for loss of radial abduction (Table 16-8a).

Thumb Adduction

Adduction is measured as the smallest possible distance in centimeters from the flexion crease of the thumb IP joint to the distal palmar crease over the level of the MP joint of the little finger (Figures 16-17 and 16-18). The normal range of motion is from 8 to 0 cm of adduction. The relative value of this functional unit is 20% of the thumb ray.

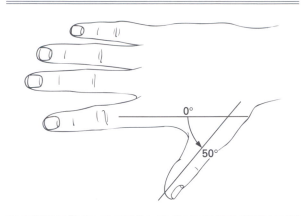

Figure 16-16 Thumb Radial Abduction Measures in Degrees the Angle of Separation Formed Between the First and Second Metacarpal in the Coronal Plane

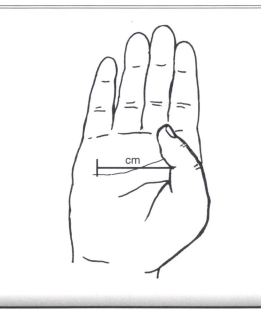

Figure 16-17 Adduction of Thumb, Measured in Centimeters From the Flexion Crease of the Thumb IP Joint to the Distal Palmar Crease Over the Level of the MP Joint of the Little Finger

Figure 16-18 Linear Measurements of Thumb Adduction in Centimeters at Various Positions and Motion Unit Impairment Curve for Lack of Adduction

Adduction of 0 cm gives 0% impairment; 8 cm of adduction lack gives 100% impairment.

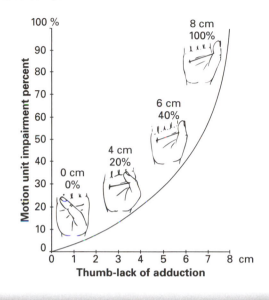

Redrawn from Swanson AB, Hagert CG, de Groot Swanson G. Evaluation of impairment of hand function. In: Hunter JM, Schneider LH, Mackin E, Calahan A, eds. *Rehabilitation in the Hand.* St Louis, Mo: CV Mosby Co; 1978:31-69.

1. Measure and record the *actual* smallest active adduction distance in centimeters.
2. Consult Table 16-8b to determine the percentage of thumb impairment contributed by adduction lack or ankylosis. Impairment values for measured distances falling between those shown in Table 16-8b may be adjusted or interpolated proportionally in the corresponding interval.

Example 16-24

Exam: An individual has a 4-cm thumb adduction lack.

Analysis: This is equivalent to a 20% motion unit impairment (Figure 16-18).

Impairment rating: 4% thumb impairment (Table 16-8b).

Table 16-8a Thumb Impairment Values Due to Lack of Radial Abduction and to Ankylosis

Measured Radial Abduction (°)	% Thumb Impairment Due to		
	Lack of Radial Abduction	Lack of Radial Adduction	Ankylosis
15	10	0	10
20	9	1	10
25	7	1	8
30	5	1	6
35	3	3	6
40	2	5	7
45	0	8	8
50	0	9	9

Relative value of functional unit is 10% of the thumb ray motion. Motion ranges from 15° of radial adduction to 50° of radial abduction.

Adapted from Swanson AB, Hagert CG, de Groot Swanson G. Evaluation of impairment of hand function. In: Hunter JM, Schneider LH, Mackin E, Calahan A, eds. *Rehabilitation in the Hand.* St Louis, Mo: CV Mosby Co; 1978:31-69.

Table 16-8b Thumb Impairment Values Due to Lack of Adduction and to Ankylosis

Measured Lack of Adduction (cm)	% Thumb Impairment Due to	
	Abnormal Motion	Ankylosis
8	20	20
7	13	19
6	8	17
5	6	15
4	4	10
3	3	15
2	1	17
1	0	19
0	0	20

Relative value of functional unit is 20% of the thumb ray motion. Motion ranges from 8 to 0 cm of adduction.

Adapted from Swanson AB, Hagert CG, de Groot Swanson G. Evaluation of impairment of hand function. In: Hunter JM, Schneider LH, Mackin E, Calahan A, eds. *Rehabilitation in the Hand.* St Louis, Mo: CV Mosby Co; 1978:31-69.

Thumb Opposition

Thumb opposition is measured in centimeters as the largest achievable distance between the flexor crease of the thumb IP joint to the distal palmar crease directly over the third MP joint (Figure 16-19). The relative value of this functional unit is 45% of the thumb ray. The normal range of opposition is from 0 to 8 cm. However, in smaller hands, the normal distance of opposition can be slightly smaller. Both sides are measured and compared. If the contralateral "normal" opposition distance is smaller than average, the impairment value corresponding to the uninvolved side serves as a baseline and is subtracted from the calculated impairment for the involved joint. This adjustment should be stated in the report.

Figure 16-19 Linear Measurements of Thumb Opposition (cm) at Various Positions

Motion unit impairment curve for lack of opposition.

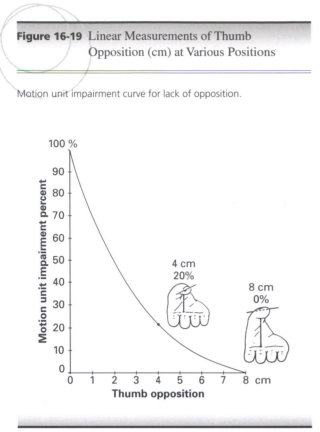

Redrawn from Swanson AB, Hagert CG, de Groot Swanson G. Evaluation of impairment of hand function. In: Hunter JM, Schneider LH, Mackin E, Calahan A, eds. *Rehabilitation in the Hand.* St Louis, Mo: CV Mosby Co; 1978:31-69.

1. Measure and record the *actual* linear distance of maximum active opposition in centimeters.
2. Consult Table 16-9 to determine the percentage of thumb impairment contributed by opposition loss or ankylosis. Impairment values for measured distances falling between those listed in Table 16-9 may be adjusted or interpolated proportionally in the corresponding interval.

Adding Two or More Abnormal Thumb Motions

1. Measure and record the thumb impairments of flexion and extension at the IP and MP joints (Figures 16-12 and 16-15), radial abduction and adduction (Table 16-8a), adduction (Table 16-8b), and opposition (Table 16-9) as described above.
2. *Add* the impairment values contributed by each motion unit to determine the total thumb impairment due to abnormal motion.

Table 16-9 Thumb Impairments Due to Lack of Opposition and to Ankylosis

Measured Opposition (cm)	% Thumb Impairment Due to	
	Abnormal Motion	Ankylosis
0	45	45
1	31	40
2	22	36
3	13	31
4	9	27
5	5	22
6	3	24
7	1	27
8	0	29

Relative value of functional unit is 45% of the thumb ray motion. Motion ranges from 0 to 8 cm of oposition.

Adapted from Swanson AB, Hagert CG, de Groot Swanson G. Evaluation of impairment of hand function. In: Hunter JM, Schneider LH, Mackin E, Calahan A, eds. *Rehabilitation in the Hand..* St Louis, Mo: CV Mosby Co; 1978:31-69.

Because the relative value of each unit of motion to the entire thumb ray was taken into consideration in the thumb impairment charts and tables, the *thumb impairments resulting from abnormal motion are added directly together.* If each thumb unit of motion were impaired to its maximum value, the total thumb motion impairment would add to 100%. Note that when more than one finger joint is involved, the impairment values are combined because the relative value of each finger joint (DIP, PIP, MP) was not assigned on a 100% finger unit scale.

Example 16-25

Exam: Thumb IP joint flexion and extension impairment of 4%, radial adduction and abduction of 0%, and opposition of 10%.

Analysis: *Add* the impairments: 4% + 4% + 0% + 10%.

Impairment Rating: 18% thumb impairment resulting from abnormal motion.

The method for combining multiple digit impairments due to amputation, sensory loss, and abnormal motion is described in Section 16.4f.

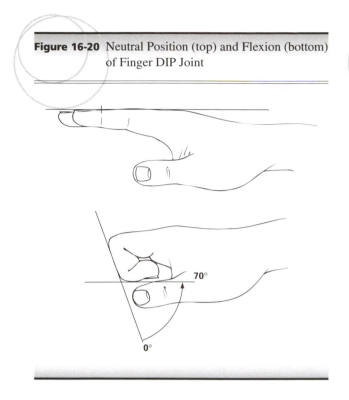

Figure 16-20 Neutral Position (top) and Flexion (bottom) of Finger DIP Joint

70°

0°

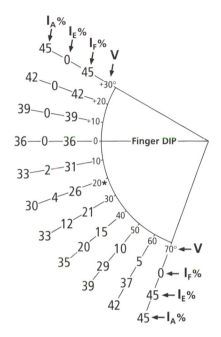

Figure 16-21 Finger Impairments Due to Abnormal Motion at the DIP Joint

Relative value of functional unit is 45% of the finger. Ankylosis in function position (20° flexion) receives lowest I_A% (30%).

I_A% = Impairment due to ankylosis
I_E% = Impairment due to loss of extension
I_F% = Impairment due to loss of flexion
V   = Measured angles of motion
*   = Position of function

Adapted from Swanson AB, Hagert CG, de Groot Swanson G. Evaluation of impairment of hand function. In: Hunter JM, Schneider LH, Mackin E, Calahan A, eds. *Rehabilitation in the Hand.* St Louis, Mo: CV Mosby Co; 1978:31-69.

16.4e Finger Motion Impairment

The fingers have three functional units of motion, each having the same relative functional value as that found in amputation impairment: DIP, 45%; PIP, 80%; and MP, 100% (Table 16-4).

For each joint, unit-of-motion impairment curves were derived according to the basic formula, A = E + F, and converted to pie charts of finger impairment values by applying the relative value of each functional unit as a conversion factor (Figures 16-21, 16-23, and 16-25).

In the normal hand, the MP joint can hyperextend usefully to 20°; a small percentage of extension impairment has been assigned to loss of hyperextension, or I_E% = 5% at 0° extension (Figure 16-25). The PIP and DIP joints normally extend to 0°, and I_E% equals 0% at this angle; between the angles of 0° extension and +30° hyperextension, impairment values are given for lack of flexion and not for hyperextension. Consideration for positions of hyperextension allows one to rate impairment of flexion or ankylosis for angles above the 0° neutral position. For example, ankylosis of the PIP joint in 30° hyperextension equals 80% finger impairment (Figure 16-23). Note that, for each joint, the ankylosis impairment value is at its lowest for the angle of functional position.

The actual range-of-motion measurements are recorded and applied to the various impairment pie charts. Impairment values for *motion measurements falling between those shown in a pie chart may be adjusted or interpolated proportionally* in the corresponding interval.

The techniques for clinical measurement of motion of the digital joints are described in Section 16.4a. Two methods are presented: (1) measurement of individual joints with the proximal joints stabilized in extension and (2) measurement of the total active range of motion of the digit while all three joints are flexed simultaneously. The joint measurement technique that best reflects the existing impairment is selected.

DIP Joint: Flexion and Extension

The DIP joint has a normal motion of 0° extension to 70° flexion. The functional position is 20° flexion. The relative value of this motion unit is 45% of the finger.

1. Measure the maximum flexion and extension, and record the *actual* goniometer readings (Figure 16-20).
2. Using Figure 16-21, match the measured angles (row headed V) of flexion and extension to their corresponding impairments of flexion (row headed $I_F\%$) and extension (row headed $I_E\%$). Impairment percents for positions of hyperextension are read above the 0° neutral position. Impairment values for measured angles falling between those listed in Figure 16-21 may be adjusted or interpolated proportionally in the corresponding interval.
3. *Add* $I_F\%$ and $I_E\%$ to obtain the finger impairment due to decreased motion of the DIP joint.
4. If the DIP joint is ankylosed, match the measured angle (row headed V) to the corresponding ankylosis impairment under the row headed $I_A\%$ in Figure 16-21. Interpolate impairment values for intervening angles. Ankylosis in the functional position (20° flexion) is given the lowest ankylosis impairment value (30%).

Example 16-26

Exam: A middle finger DIP joint has −10° extension lag and 50° flexion.

Analysis: $I_E\% = 2\%$, $I_F\% = 10\%$ (Figure 16-21).

Impairment Rating: 2% + 10% = 12% impairment of the middle finger, or 2% hand impairment (Table 16-1).

Example 16-27

Exam: DIP joint has +30° hyperextension and 0° flexion.

Analysis: $I_E\% = 0\%$, $I_F\% = 36\%$.

Impairment Rating: 0% + 36% = 36% finger impairment.

Example 16-28

Exam: A DIP joint has ankylosis in 35° flexion.

Impairment Rating: The interpolated $I_A\%$ of 34% finger impairment is calculated from the interval between 33% at 30° and 35% at 40°.

PIP Joint: Flexion and Extension

The PIP joint has a normal motion of 0° extension to 100° flexion. The functional position is 40° flexion. The relative value of this motion unit is 80% of the finger.

1. Measure the maximum active flexion and extension and record the *actual* goniometer readings (Figure 16-22).
2. Using Figure 16-23, match the measured angles (row headed V) of flexion and extension to their corresponding impairments of flexion (row headed $I_F\%$) and extension (row headed $I_E\%$). Impairment percents for positions of hyperextension are read above the 0° neutral position. Impairment values for measured angles falling between those listed in Figure 16-23 may be adjusted or interpolated proportionally in the corresponding interval.

Figure 16-22 Neutral Position (top) and Flexion (bottom) of Finger PIP Joint (isolated joint measurement shown)

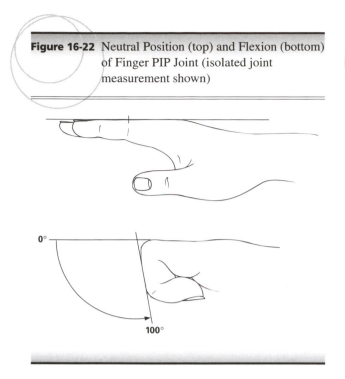

3. *Add* $I_F\%$ and $I_E\%$ to obtain the finger impairment resulting from decreased motion of the PIP joint.
4. If the PIP joint is ankylosed, match the measured angle (row headed V) to the corresponding ankylosis impairment (row headed $I_A\%$) in Figure 16-23. Interpolate impairment value for intervening angles. Ankylosis in the functional position (40° flexion) is given the lowest ankylosis impairment percent (50%).

Example 16-29

Exam: A middle finger PIP joint has −15° extension lag and 60° flexion.

Analysis: The interpolated $I_E\%$ of 5% finger impairment is calculated from the interval between 3% at −10°, and 7% at −20°. $I_E\% = 5\%$; $I_F\% = 24\%$ (Figure 16-23).

Impairment Rating: 5% + 24% = 29% impairment of the middle finger, or 6% hand impairment (Table 16-1).

Figure 16-23 Finger Impairments Due to Abnormal Motion at PIP Joint

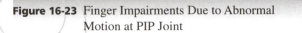

Relative value of functional unit is 80% of the finger. Ankylosis in functional position (40° flexion) receives lowest $I_A\%$ (50%).

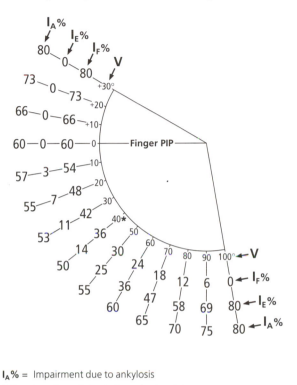

$I_A\%$ = Impairment due to ankylosis
$I_E\%$ = Impairment due to loss of extension
$I_F\%$ = Impairment due to loss of flexion
V = Measured angles of motion
* = Position of function

Adapted from Swanson AB, Hagert CG, de Groot Swanson G. Evaluation of impairment of hand function. In: Hunter JM, Schneider LH, Mackin E, Calahan A, eds. *Rehabilitation in the Hand.* St Louis, Mo: CV Mosby Co; 1978:31-69.

Example 16-30

Exam: Ankylosis of the PIP joint in 40° flexion.

Impairment Rating: $I_A\% = 50\%$ finger impairment.

Figure 16-24 Neutral Position (top) and Flexion (bottom) of Finger MP Joint (total active range-of-motion measurement shown)

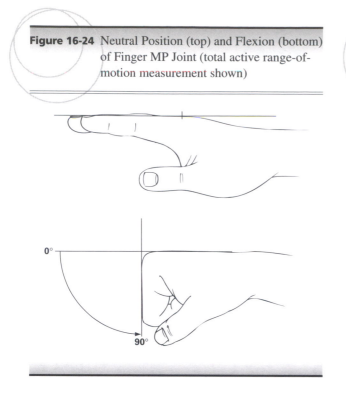

Figure 16-25 Finger Impairments Due to Abnormal Motion at the MP Joint

Relative value of functional unit is 100% of the finger. Ankylosis in functional position (30° flexion) receives lowest I_A% (45%).

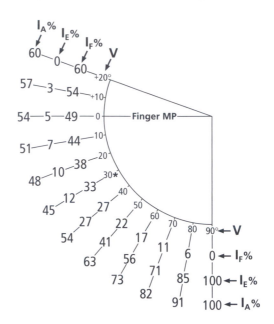

I_A% = Impairment due to ankylosis
I_E% = Impairment due to loss of extension
I_F% = Impairment due to loss of flexion
V   = Measured angles of motion
*   = Position of function

Adapted from Swanson AB, Hagert CG, de Groot Swanson G. Evaluation of impairment of hand function. In: Hunter JM, Schneider LH, Mackin E, Calahan A, eds. *Rehabilitation in the Hand.* St Louis, Mo: CV Mosby Co; 1978:31-69.

MP Joint: Flexion and Extension

The finger MP joint motion ranges from +20° hyperextension to 90° flexion. The functional position is 30° flexion. The relative value of this motion unit is 100% of the finger.

1. Measure the maximum active flexion and extension, and record the *actual* goniometer readings (Figure 16-24).
2. Using Figure 16-25, match the measured angles (row headed V) of flexion and extension to their corresponding impairments of flexion (row headed I_F%) and extension (row headed I_E%). Impairment values for positions of hyperextension are read above the 0° neutral position. Impairment values for measured angles falling between those listed in Figure 16-25 may be adjusted or interpolated proportionally in the corresponding interval.
3. *Add* I_F% and I_E% to obtain finger impairment resulting from decreased motion of the MP joint.
4. If the MP joint is ankylosed, match the measured angle (row headed V) to the corresponding ankylosis impairment (row headed I_A%) in Figure 16-25. Interpolate impairment values for intervening angles. Ankylosis in the functional position (30° flexion) is given the lowest I_A% value (45%).

Example 16-31

Exam: A middle finger MP joint has 0° extension and 50° flexion.

Analysis: I_E% = 5%; I_F% = 22% (Figure 16-25).

Impairment Rating: 5% + 22% = 27% impairment of the middle finger, or 5% hand impairment (Table 16-1).

Example 16-32

Exam: MP joint ankylosis in 55° flexion.

Impairment Rating: The interpolated I_A% of 68% finger impairment for ankylosis in 55° flexion is calculated from the interval between 63% at 50° and 73% at 60° (Figure 16-25).

Combining Abnormal Motion at More Than One Finger Joint

Method for individual joint measurements:

1. Determine the motion impairment of each joint in terms of finger impairment, as described in the preceding pages.
2. *Combine* the finger impairments derived for each joint to obtain the total finger impairment due to loss of motion (Combined Values Chart, p. 604). If all three joints are involved, *combine* the resulting impairment value from the first two joints to the value of the third joint.

Method for total active range-of-motion measurements:

1. *Combine* the $I_E\%$ of all three joints.
2. *Combine* the $I_F\%$ of all three joints.
3. *Subtract* the extension combined value from the flexion combined value to determine the finger impairment due to decreased motion.

Express the finger impairment in terms of the hand, upper extremity, and whole person impairment (Tables 16-1 through 16-3).

Example 16-33

Exam: Middle finger has a DIP joint impairment of 12%, PIP joint impairment of 31%, and MP joint impairment of 27%.

Analysis: 12% *combined* with 31% = 39% (Combined Values Chart, p. 604); 39% *combined* with 27% = 55% total middle finger motion impairment.

Impairment Rating: This is equivalent to an impairment of 11% of the hand (Table 16-1), 10% of the upper extremity (Table 16-2), and 6% of the whole person (Table 16-3).

16.4f Multiple Digit Impairments

Combining Digit Amputation, Sensory Loss, and Abnormal Motion Impairments of the Hand

1. Determine separately the digit impairments contributed by amputation, sensory loss, and abnormal motion.
2. *Combine* the digit impairment percents using the Combined Values Chart (p. 604) to obtain the total digit impairment.

3. Use Tables 16-1 through 16-3 to relate the digit impairment in succession to impairment of the hand, the upper extremity, and the whole person. If more than one digit is involved, the impairment values contributed by each digit are *added* to obtain the total hand impairment before making the conversion to upper extremity impairment.

Example 16-34

Exam: A middle finger amputation impairment of 20%, a sensory impairment of 10%, and an abnormal motion impairment of 10%.

Analysis: 20% *combined* with 10% = 28%; 28% *combined* with 10% = 35% middle finger impairment (Combined Values Chart, p. 604).

Impairment Rating: This corresponds to 7% impairment of the hand (Table 16-1), 6% impairment of the upper extremity (Table 16-2), and 4% impairment of the whole person (Table 16-3).

Example 16-35

Exam: Thumb has 30% amputation impairment, 10% sensory impairment, and 10% abnormal motion impairment.

Analysis: 30% *combined* with 10% = 37%; 37% *combined* with 10% = 43% thumb impairment (Combined Values Chart, p. 604).

Impairment Rating: This corresponds to 17% impairment of the hand, 15% impairment of the upper extremity, and 9% impairment of the whole person (Tables 16-1, 16-2, and 16-3).

Determining Hand Impairment From Two or More Digits

1. If two or more digits are involved, calculate separately the total digit impairment for each.
2. Using Table 16-1, convert each digit impairment to a hand impairment value.
3. *Add* the hand impairment values contributed by each digit to obtain the total hand impairment.
4. In a hand presenting an upper extremity impairment from amputation of the thumb proximal to the MP joint, the hand impairment resulting from involvement of the other digits is converted to upper extremity impairment (Table 16-2) and then *added* directly to the upper extremity impairment value resulting from amputation of the thumb ray (Table 16-4).
5. Using Tables 16-2 and 16-3, the hand impairment is related to that of the upper extremity and the whole person.

Example 16-36

Exam: A 10% impairment of the thumb, 20% impairment of the index finger, 30% impairment of the middle finger, 40% impairment of the ring finger, and 50% impairment of the little finger.

Analysis: Digit impairments are converted to hand impairments (Table 16-2) and *added* to obtain the total impairment.

% Impairment of Digit	% Impairment of Hand
10, thumb	4
20, index finger	4
30, middle finger	6
40, ring finger	4
50, little finger	5
Total hand impairment	23

Impairment Rating: Tables 16-2 and 16-3 show that 23% hand impairment is equivalent to 21% impairment of the upper extremity and 13% impairment of the whole person.

16.4g Wrist Motion Impairment

The wrist functional unit represents 60% of the upper extremity function. The wrist has two units of motion (see Figure 16-26), each contributing a relative value to its function. The units-of-motion impairments are converted to upper extremity impairments by multiplying their respective values by 60% as follows:

1. Flexion and extension unit: 70% of wrist function; 70% × 60% = 42% of upper extremity function.
2. Radial and ulnar deviation unit: 30% of wrist function; 30% × 60% = 18% of upper extremity function.

For each wrist functional unit of motion, impairment curves were derived according to the basic formula, A = E + F and expressed on a 100% motion unit scale (Figures 16-27 and 16-30). These impairment curves were converted to pie charts of upper extremity impairment by applying their relative upper extremity functional value as a conversion factor (Figures 16-28 and 16-31).

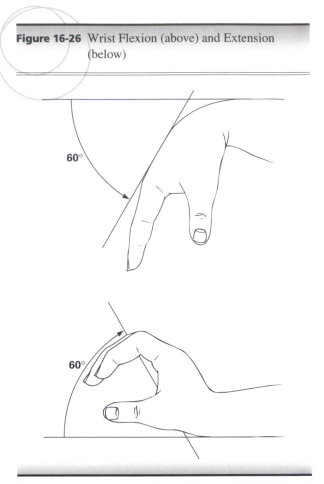

Figure 16-26 Wrist Flexion (above) and Extension (below)

60°

60°

Redrawn with permission from Swanson AB, Hagert CG, de Groot Swanson G. Evaluation of impairment of hand function. In: Hunter JM, Schneider LH, Mackin E, Calahan A, eds. *Rehabilitation in the Hand.* St Louis, Mo: CV Mosby Co; 1978:31-69.

The upper extremity impairment due to abnormal wrist motion is calculated from the pie charts by *adding* directly together the upper extremity impairment contributed by each motion unit.

The actual range-of-motion measurements are recorded and applied to the various impairment pie charts. *Impairment values for motion measurements falling between those shown in the pie chart may be adjusted or interpolated proportionally in the corresponding interval.*

Figure 16-27 Motion Unit Impairment Curves for Ankylosis ($I_A\%$), Loss of Flexion ($I_F\%$), and Loss of Extension ($I_E\%$) of Wrist Joint

Ankyloses in functional positions (10° extension to 10° flexion) are given the lowest $I_A\%$ value (50%).

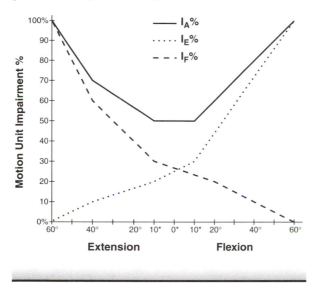

Extension   Flexion

Redrawn with permission from Swanson AB, Hagert CG, de Groot Swanson G. Evaluation of impairment of hand function. In: Hunter JM, Schneider LH, Mackin E, Calahan A, eds. *Rehabilitation in the Hand.* St Louis, Mo: CV Mosby Co; 1978:31-69.

Figure 16-28 Pie Chart of Upper Extremity Motion Impairments Due to Lack of Flexion and Extension of Wrist Joint

Relative value of this functional unit to upper extremity impairment is 42%.

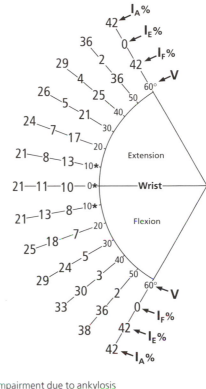

$I_A\%$ = Impairment due to ankylosis
$I_E\%$ = Impairment due to loss of extension
$I_F\%$ = Impairment due to loss of flexion
V = Measured angles of motion
★ = Positions of function

Redrawn with permission from Swanson AB, Hagert CG, de Groot Swanson G. Evaluation of impairment of hand function. In: Hunter JM, Schneider LH, Mackin E, Calahan A, eds. *Rehabilitation in the Hand.* St Louis, Mo: CV Mosby Co; 1978:31-69.

Flexion and Extension

The normal range of wrist motion is from 60° extension to 60° flexion. The position of function is from 10° extension to 10° flexion. The relative value of this motion unit is 42% of the upper extremity function.

1. Measure maximum active wrist flexion and extension, and record the *actual* goniometer readings (Figure 16-26).
2. In Figure 16-28, match the measured flexion and extension angles (row headed V) to their corresponding impairments of flexion (row headed $I_F\%$) and extension (row headed $I_E\%$). Impairment values for angles falling between those listed in Figure 16-28 may be adjusted or interpolated proportionally in the corresponding interval.
3. *Add* $I_F\%$ and $I_E\%$ to obtain the percent of upper extremity impairment contributed by decreased wrist flexion and extension.
4. If the wrist is ankylosed, match the measured angle (row headed V) to its corresponding ankylosis impairment (row headed $I_A\%$) in Figure 16-28. Interpolate impairment values for intervening angles.

Ankyloses in functional positions (10° extension to 10° flexion) are given the lowest $I_A\%$, or 50% of this motion unit value (Figure 16-27). This corresponds to 21% impairment of the upper extremity (Figure 16-28). Wrist ankylosis in 60° flexion or 60° extension represents 100% loss of wrist extension and flexion function (Figure 16-27). This is equivalent to 70% impairment of wrist function, or 42% impairment ($70\% \times 60\%$) of the upper extremity resulting from loss of this wrist motion unit (Figure 16-28).

Example 16-37

Exam: Wrist extension of 10°and flexion of 10° (Figure 16-28).

Analysis: $I_E\% = 8\%$ impairment of the upper extremity; $I_F\% = 8\%$ impairment of the upper extremity.

Impairment Rating: *Add* 8% + 8% = 16% impairment of the upper extremity resulting from decreased wrist flexion and extension.

Example 16-38

Exam: Wrist ankylosis in 35° flexion.

Impairment Rating: The interpolated value for $I_A\%$ in 35° flexion = 31% impairment of the upper extremity.

Radial and Ulnar Deviation

The normal range of wrist motion is from 20° radial deviation to 30° ulnar deviation. The position of function is from neutral to 10° ulnar deviation. The relative value of this motion unit is 18% of upper extremity function.

1. Measure the maximum active wrist radial and ulnar deviation, and record the *actual* goniometer readings (Figure 16-29).
2. Using Figure 16-31, match the measured ulnar and radial deviation angles (row headed V) to the corresponding impairments of radial deviation (row headed $I_{RD}\%$) and ulnar deviation (row headed $I_{UD}\%$). Impairment values for angles falling between those listed in Figure 16-31 may be adjusted or interpolated proportionally in the corresponding interval.
3. *Add* $I_{RD}\% + I_{UD}\%$ to obtain the upper extremity impairment value contributed by decreased wrist lateral deviation.
4. If the wrist is ankylosed, match the measured angle (row headed V) to its corresponding ankylosis impairment value (row headed $I_A\%$) in Figure 16-31. Interpolate impairment values for intervening angles.

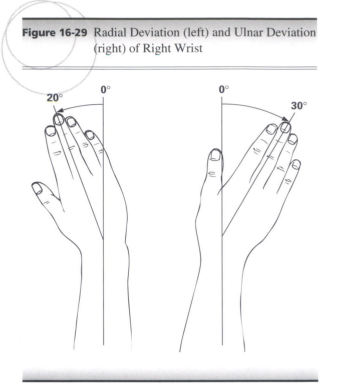

Figure 16-29 Radial Deviation (left) and Ulnar Deviation (right) of Right Wrist

Redrawn with permission from Swanson AB, Hagert CG, de Groot Swanson G. Evaluation of impairment of hand function. In: Hunter JM, Schneider LH, Mackin E, Calahan A, eds. *Rehabilitation in the Hand.* St Louis, Mo: CV Mosby Co; 1978:31-69.

Ankyloses in functional positions (0° to 10° ulnar deviation) receive the lowest $I_A\%$, or 50% of this motion unit value (Figure 16-30). This corresponds to 9% impairment of the upper extremity (Figure 16-31). Wrist ankylosis in either 30° ulnar deviation or 20° radial deviation represents 100% loss of wrist lateral deviation function (Figure 16-30). This is equivalent to 30% impairment of wrist function and 18% impairment (60% × 30%) of the upper extremity (Figure 16-31).

Figure 16-30 Motion Unit Impairment Curves for Ankylosis (I_A%), Loss of Radial Deviation (I_{RD}%), and Loss of Ulnar Deviation (I_{UD}%) of Wrist Joint

Ankyloses in functional positions (0° to 10° ulnar deviation) are given the lowest ankylosis impairment (50%).

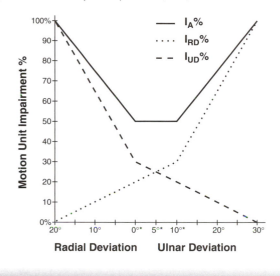

Redrawn with permission from Swanson AB, Hagert CG, de Groot Swanson G. Evaluation of impairment of hand function. In: Hunter JM, Schneider LH, Mackin E, Calahan A, eds. *Rehabilitation in the Hand.* St Louis, Mo: CV Mosby Co; 1978:31-69.

Figure 16-31 Pie Chart of Upper Extremity Motion Impairments Due to Abnormal Radial and Ulnar Deviations of Wrist Joint

Relative value of this functional unit to upper extremity impairment is 18%.

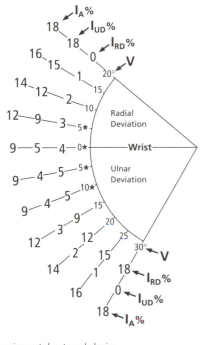

I_A% = Impairment due to ankylosis
I_{RD}% = Impairment due to loss of radial deviation
I_{UD}% = Impairment due to loss of ulnar deviation
V   = Measured angles of motion
*   = Positions of function

Redrawn with permission from Swanson AB, Hagert CG, de Groot Swanson G. Evaluation of impairment of hand function. In: Hunter JM, Schneider LH, Mackin E, Calahan A, eds. *Rehabilitation in the Hand.* St Louis, Mo: CV Mosby Co; 1978:31-69.

Example 16-39

Exam: Wrist ulnar deviation 0° and radial deviation 10° (Figure 16-31).

Analysis: I_{UD}% = 5% impairment of the upper extremity. I_{RD}% = 2% impairment of the upper extremity.

Impairment Rating: *Add* 5% + 2% = 7% impairment of the upper extremity resulting from decreased wrist lateral deviation.

Example 16-40

Exam: Wrist ankylosis in 15° radial deviation.

Impairment Rating: I_A% = 16% impairment of the upper extremity resulting from loss of wrist lateral deviation.

Determining Impairment Due to Abnormal Wrist Motion

1. Using Figures 16-28 and 16-31, determine the impairment of the upper extremity contributed by each wrist unit of motion (flexion and extension, radial and ulnar deviation) by *adding* $I_F\% + I_E\%$ and $I_{RD}\% + I_{UD}\%$.
2. Because the relative upper extremity value of each wrist functional unit has been taken into consideration in the impairment pie charts, the impairments contributed by each unit of motion are *added* directly to determine the impairment of the upper extremity due to abnormal wrist motion, or it equals $(I_F\% + I_E\%) + (I_{RD}\% + I_{UD}\%)$.
3. If the wrist joint is ankylosed, *add* the ankylosis impairment contributed by each unit of motion to determine the upper extremity impairment due to loss of wrist motion.
4. Use Table 16-3 to relate the impairment of the upper extremity to impairment of the whole person.

Example 16-41

Exam: 16% upper extremity impairment due to loss of wrist flexion and extension and 7% impairment resulting from loss of wrist radial and ulnar deviation.

Analysis: *Add* 16% + 7% = 23% impairment of the upper extremity.

Impairment Rating: 14% impairment of the whole person (Table 16-3).

Example 16-42

Exam: Wrist ankylosis in 0° flexion and 0° lateral deviation (functional position range) (Figures 16-28 and 16-31).

Analysis: Flexion $I_A\% = 21\%$; lateral deviation $I_A\% = 9\%$.

Impairment Rating: *Add* 21% + 9% = 30% impairment of the upper extremity, or 18% impairment of the whole person (Table 16-3).

16.4h Elbow Motion Impairment

The elbow functional unit represents 70% of upper extremity function. The elbow joint has two functional units of motion, each contributing a relative value to its function. The unit-of-motion impairments are converted to upper extremity impairments by multiplying their respective values by 70% as follows:

1. Flexion and extension: 60% of elbow function; 60% × 70% = 42% of upper extremity function.
2. Pronation and supination: 40% of elbow function; 40% × 70% = 28% of upper extremity function.

For each elbow functional unit of motion, impairment curves were derived according to the basic formula, A = E + F and expressed on a 100% motion unit scale (Figures 16-33 and 16-36). These impairment curves were converted to pie charts of upper extremity impairment by applying the upper extremity functional value of each motion unit as a conversion factor (Figures 16-34 and 16-37).

The upper extremity impairment due to abnormal elbow motion is calculated from the pie charts by *adding* directly the upper extremity impairment values contributed by each motion unit.

The actual range-of-motion measurements are recorded and applied to the various impairment pie charts. *Impairment values for motion measurements falling between those shown in the pie chart may be adjusted or interpolated proportionally in the corresponding interval.*

Flexion and Extension

The normal range of motion is considered to be from 140° flexion to 0° extension. The position of function is 80° flexion. The relative value of this motion unit is 42% of the upper extremity function.

1. Measure the maximum active elbow flexion and extension, and record the *actual* goniometer readings (Figure 16-32).
2. In Figure 16-34, match the measured flexion and extension angles (row headed V) to their corresponding impairments of flexion (row headed $I_F\%$) and extension (row headed $I_E\%$). Impairment values for angles falling between those listed in Figure 16-34 may be adjusted or interpolated proportionally in the corresponding interval.
3. *Add* $I_F\%$ and $I_E\%$ to obtain the upper extremity impairment percent contributed by decreased elbow flexion and extension.
4. If the elbow is ankylosed, match the measured angle (row headed V) to its corresponding ankylosis impairment (row headed $I_A\%$) in Figure 16-34. Interpolate impairment values for intervening angles.

Ankylosis in the functional position (80° flexion) is given the lowest $I_A\%$, or 50% of this motion unit value (Figure 16-33). This corresponds to 21% impairment of the upper extremity (Figure 16-34). Ankylosis in either 0° extension or 140° flexion represents a 100% loss of elbow flexion and extension function (Figure 16-33). This is equivalent to 60% impairment of elbow function and 42% impairment (60% × 70%) of the upper extremity due to loss of this elbow motion unit (Figure 16-34).

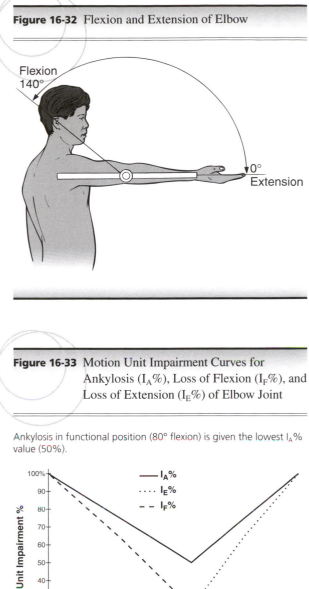

Figure 16-32 Flexion and Extension of Elbow

Figure 16-33 Motion Unit Impairment Curves for Ankylosis ($I_A\%$), Loss of Flexion ($I_F\%$), and Loss of Extension ($I_E\%$) of Elbow Joint

Ankylosis in functional position (80° flexion) is given the lowest $I_A\%$ value (50%).

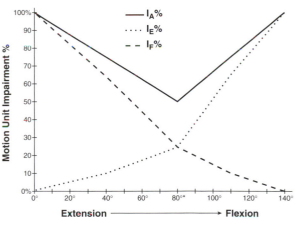

Redrawn with permission from Swanson AB, Hagert CG, de Groot Swanson G. Evaluation of impairment of hand function. In: Hunter JM, Schneider LH, Mackin E, Calahan A, eds. *Rehabilitation in the Hand.* St Louis, Mo: CV Mosby Co; 1978:31-69.

Figure 16-34 Pie Chart of Upper Extremity Motion Impairments Due to Lack of Flexion and Extension of Elbow Joint

Relative value of this functional unit to upper extremity impairment is 42%.

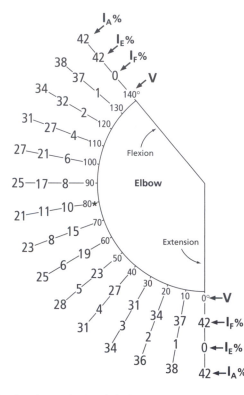

I_A% = Impairment due to ankylosis
I_E% = Impairment due to loss of extension
I_F% = Impairment due to loss of flexion
V   = Measured angles of motion
*   = Position of function

Redrawn with permission from Swanson AB, Hagert CG, de Groot Swanson G. Evaluation of impairment of hand function. In: Hunter JM, Schneider LH, Mackin E, Calahan A, eds. *Rehabilitation in the Hand.* St Louis, Mo: CV Mosby Co; 1978:31-69.

Example 16-43

Exam: Elbow extension lag of −40° and flexion to 65° (Figure 16-34).

Analysis: I_E% = 4% impairment of the upper extremity; the interpolated value for I_F% at 65° = 17% impairment of the upper extremity.

Impairment Rating: *Add* 4% + 17% = 21% impairment of the upper extremity due to decreased elbow flexion and extension.

Example 16-44

Exam: Elbow ankylosis in 80° flexion.

Impairment Rating: I_A% = 21% impairment of the upper extremity resulting from loss of flexion and extension.

Pronation and Supination

The normal range of motion is from 80° supination to 80° pronation. The position of function is 20° pronation. The relative value of this motion unit is 28% of the upper extremity function.

Impairments of pronation and supination are ascribed to the elbow because the major muscles for this function are inserted about the elbow. This applies even if the loss of forearm rotation results primarily from wrist involvement in the presence of an intact elbow.

1. Measure the maximum active elbow pronation and supination, and record the *actual* goniometer readings (Figure 16-35).
2. In Figure 16-37, match the measured supination and pronation angles (row headed V) to their corresponding impairments of pronation (row headed I_P%) and supination (row headed I_S%). Impairment values for angles falling between those listed in Figure 16-37 may be adjusted or interpolated proportionally in the corresponding interval.
3. *Add* I_P% and I_S% to obtain the upper extremity impairment percent contributed by decreased forearm rotation.
4. If the elbow is ankylosed, match the measured angle (row headed V) to its corresponding ankylosis impairment (row headed I_A%) in Figure 16-37. Interpolate impairment values for intervening angles.

Ankylosis in the functional position (20° pronation) is given the lowest I_A%, or 30% of this motion unit value (Figure 16-36). This is equivalent to 8% impairment of the upper extremity (Figure 16-37). Ankylosis in 80° of pronation or supination represents 100% impairment of the forearm rotation unit (Figure 16-36). This is equivalent to 40% impairment of elbow function and 28% impairment (40% × 70%) of the upper extremity due to loss of forearm rotation (Figure 16-37).

Figure 16-35 Pronation and Supination of Forearm

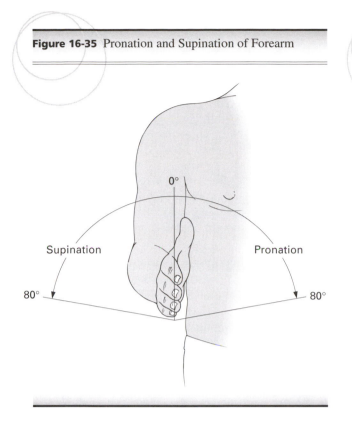

Figure 16-36 Motion Unit Impairment Curves for Ankylosis ($I_A\%$), Loss of Supination ($I_S\%$), and Loss of Pronation ($I_P\%$) of Elbow Joint

Ankylosis in functional position (20° pronation) is given the lowest $I_A\%$ value (30%).

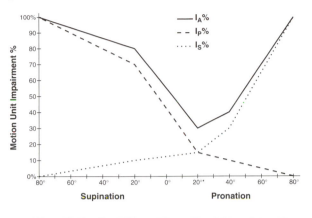

Redrawn with permission from Swanson AB, Hagert CG, de Groot Swanson G. Evaluation of impairment of hand function. In: Hunter JM, Schneider LH, Mackin E, Calahan A, eds. *Rehabilitation in the Hand.* St Louis, Mo: CV Mosby Co; 1978:31-69.

Example 16-45

Exam: Pronation of the forearm to 30° and supination to 10° (Figure 16-37).

Analysis: $I_P\% = 3\%$ impairment of the upper extremity. $I_S\% = 3\%$ impairment of the upper extremity.

Impairment Rating: *Add* 3% + 3% = 6% upper extremity impairment due to decreased forearm rotation.

Example 16-46

Exam: Elbow ankylosis in 30° supination.

Impairment Rating: $I_A\% = 23\%$ impairment of the upper extremity due to loss of forearm rotation.

Determining Impairment Due to Abnormal Elbow Motion

1. Using Figures 16-34 and 16-37, determine the impairment of the upper extremity contributed by each elbow unit of motion (flexion and extension, pronation and supination), as described in preceding parts, by *adding* $I_F\% + I_E\%$ and $I_P\% + I_S\%$.

2. Because the relative upper extremity value of each elbow functional unit has been taken into consideration in the impairment pie charts, the impairment values contributed by each unit of motion are *added* directly to determine the impairment of the upper extremity due to abnormal elbow motion, or it equals $(I_F\% + I_E\%) + (I_P\% + I_S\%)$.

3. If the elbow joint is ankylosed, *add* the ankylosis impairments contributed by each unit of motion to determine the upper extremity impairment resulting from loss of elbow motion.

4. Use Table 16-3 to relate the impairment of the upper extremity to impairment of the whole person.

Example 16-47

Analysis: 19% upper extremity impairment due to loss of elbow flexion and extension and 6% impairment due to loss of pronation and supination (Figures 16-34 and 16-37).

Add 19% + 6% = 25% impairment of the upper extremity.

Impairment Rating: 15% impairment of the whole person (Table 16-3).

Figure 16-37 Pie Chart of Upper Extremity Motion Impairments Due to Lack of Pronation and Supination

Relative value of this functional unit to upper extremity impairment is 28%.

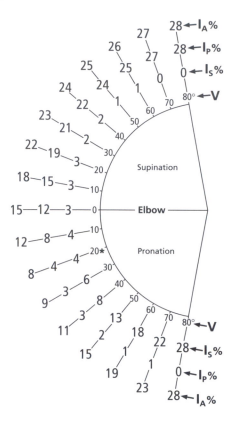

I_A% = Impairment due to ankylosis

I_P% = Impairment due to loss of pronation

I_S% = Impairment due to loss of supination

V   = Measured angles of motion

*   = Position of function

Redrawn with permission from Swanson AB, Hagert CG, de Groot Swanson G. Evaluation of impairment of hand function. In: Hunter JM, Schneider LH, Mackin E, Calahan A, eds. *Rehabilitation in the Hand.* St Louis, Mo: CV Mosby Co; 1978:31-69.

Example 16-48

Exam: Elbow ankylosis in 80° flexion and 30° supination.

Analysis: Flexion I_A% = 21%; supination I_A% = 23%. *Add* 21% + 23% = 44% impairment of the upper extremity.

Impairment Rating: 26% impairment of the whole person (Table 16-3).

16.4i Shoulder Motion Impairment

The shoulder functional unit represents 60% of the upper extremity function. The shoulder has three functional units of motion, each contributing a relative value to its function. The unit-of-motion impairments are converted to upper extremity impairments by multiplying their respective values by 60% as follows:

1. Flexion: 40% of shoulder function.
   Extension: 10% of shoulder function.
   Flexion and extension unit: 50% of shoulder function, or 50% × 60% = 30% of upper extremity function.
2. Abduction: 20% of shoulder function.
   Adduction: 10% of shoulder function.
   Abduction and adduction unit: 30% of shoulder function, or 30% × 60% = 18% of upper extremity function.
3. Internal rotation: 10% of shoulder function.
   External rotation: 10% of shoulder function.
   Internal and external rotation unit: 20% of shoulder function, or 20% × 60% = 12% of upper extremity function.

For each shoulder functional unit of motion, impairment curves were derived according to the basic formula, A = E + F, and expressed on a 100% motion unit scale (Figures 16-39, 16-42, and 16-45). These impairment curves were converted to pie charts of upper extremity impairments by applying the upper extremity functional value of each motion unit as a conversion factor (Figures 16-40, 16-43, and 16-46).

The upper extremity impairment resulting from abnormal shoulder motion is calculated from the pie charts by *adding* directly the upper extremity impairment values contributed by each motion unit.

The actual range-of-motion measurements are recorded and applied to the various impairment pie charts. *Impairment values for motion measurements falling between those shown in the pie chart may be adjusted or interpolated proportionally in the corresponding interval.*

Flexion and Extension

The normal range of motion is considered to be from 180° flexion to 50° extension. The positions of function range from 40° flexion to 20° flexion. The relative value of this motion unit is 30% of the upper extremity function.

1. Measure the maximum active shoulder flexion and extension, and record the goniometer readings (Figure 16-38).
2. In Figure 16-40, match the measured flexion and extension angles (row headed V) to their corresponding impairments of flexion (row headed $I_F\%$) and extension (row headed $I_E\%$). Impairment values for measured angles falling between those listed in Figure 16-40 may be adjusted or interpolated proportionally in the corresponding interval.
3. *Add* $I_F\% + I_E\%$ to obtain the percent of upper extremity impairment contributed by decreased shoulder flexion and extension.
4. If the shoulder is ankylosed, match the measured angle (row headed V) to its corresponding ankylosis impairment (row headed $I_A\%$) in Figure 16-40. Interpolate impairment values for intervening angles.

Ankyloses in functional positions (40° flexion to 20° flexion) are given the lowest $I_A\%$, or 50% of this motion unit value (Figure 16-39). This corresponds to 15% impairment of the upper extremity (Figure 16-40). Ankylosis in 50° extension or 180° flexion represents 100% loss of this shoulder motion unit (Figure 16-39). This is equivalent to 50% impairment of shoulder function, or 30% impairment (50% × 60%) of the upper extremity resulting from loss of this shoulder unit of motion (Figure 16-40).

Figure 16-38 Shoulder Flexion and Extension

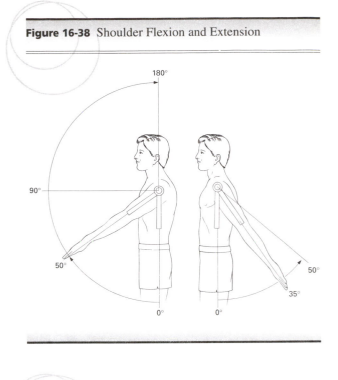

Figure 16-39 Motion Unit Impairment Curves for Ankylosis ($I_A\%$), Loss of Flexion ($I_F\%$), and Loss of Extension ($I_E\%$) of Shoulder

Ankyloses in functional positions (40° to 20° flexion) are given the lowest $I_A\%$ value (50%).

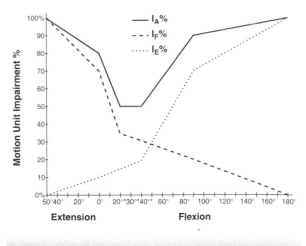

Redrawn with permission from Swanson AB, Hagert CG, de Groot Swanson G. Evaluation of impairment of hand function. In: Hunter JM, Schneider LH, Mackin E, Calahan A, eds. *Rehabilitation in the Hand.* St Louis, Mo: CV Mosby Co; 1978:31-69.

Figure 16-40 Pie Chart of Upper Extremity Motion Impairments Due to Lack of Flexion and Extension of Shoulder

Relative value of this functional unit to upper extremity impairment is 30%.

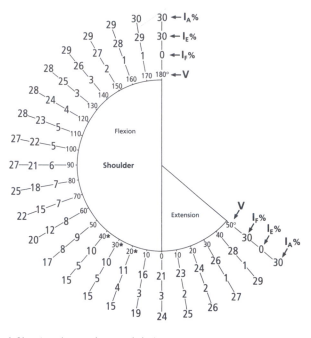

$I_A\%$ = Impairment due to ankylosis

$I_E\%$ = Impairment due to loss of extension

$I_F\%$ = Impairment due to loss of flexion

V   = Measured angles of motion

*   = Positions of function

Redrawn with permission from Swanson AB, Hagert CG, de Groot Swanson G. Evaluation of impairment of hand function. In: Hunter JM, Schneider LH, Mackin E, Calahan A, eds. *Rehabilitation in the Hand.* St Louis, Mo: CV Mosby Co; 1978:31-69.

Example 16-49

Exam: Shoulder flexion of 90° and extension of 0° (Figure 16-39).

Analysis: $I_F\% = 6\%$ impairment of the upper extremity. $I_E\% = 3\%$ impairment of the upper extremity.

Impairment Rating: *Add* 6% + 3% = 9% impairment of the upper extremity due to decreased shoulder flexion and extension.

Example 16-50

Exam: Shoulder ankylosis in 30° flexion.

Impairment Rating: $I_A\% = 15\%$ impairment of the upper extremity due to loss of this shoulder unit of motion.

Abduction and Adduction

The normal range of motion is considered to be from 180° abduction to 50° adduction. The positions of function range from 50° abduction to 20° abduction. The relative value of this motion unit is 18% of the upper extremity function.

1. Measure the maximum active shoulder abduction and adduction, and record the *actual* goniometer readings (Figure 16-41).
2. In Figure 16-43, match the measured abduction and adduction angles (row headed V) to their corresponding impairments of abduction (row headed $I_{ABD}\%$) and adduction (row headed $I_{ADD}\%$). Impairment values for motion measurements falling between those listed in Figure 16-43 may be adjusted or interpolated proportionally in the corresponding interval.
3. *Add* $I_{ABD}\% + I_{ADD}\%$ to obtain the upper extremity impairment contributed by decreased shoulder abduction and adduction.
4. If the shoulder is ankylosed, match the measured angle (row headed V) to its corresponding ankylosis impairment (row headed $I_A\%$) in Figure 16-43. Interpolate impairment values for intervening angles.
5. Ankyloses in functional positions (50° abduction to 20° abduction) are given the lowest impairment percent, or 50% of this motion unit value (Figure 16-42). This corresponds to 9% impairment of the upper extremity (Figure 16-43). Ankylosis in either 50° adduction or 180° abduction represents 100% loss of this shoulder unit of motion (Figure 16-42). This is equivalent to 30% impairment of shoulder function, or 18% impairment (30% × 60%) of the upper extremity resulting from loss of this shoulder motion unit (Figure 16-43).

Figure 16-41 Shoulder Abduction and Adduction

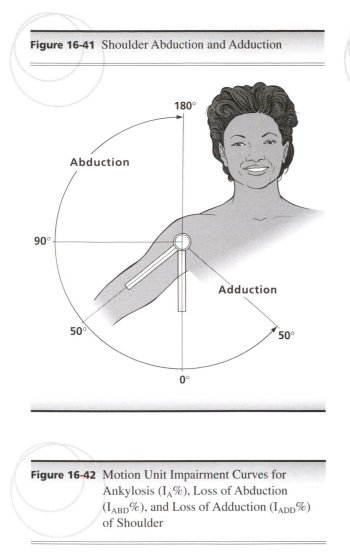

Figure 16-42 Motion Unit Impairment Curves for Ankylosis (I$_A$%), Loss of Abduction (I$_{ABD}$%), and Loss of Adduction (I$_{ADD}$%) of Shoulder

Ankyloses in functional positions (50° to 20° abduction) are given the lowest I$_A$% (50%).

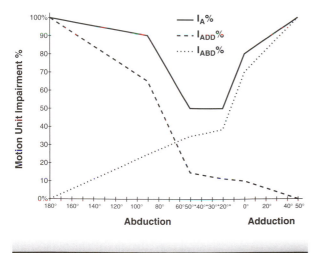

Redrawn with permission from Swanson AB, Hagert CG, de Groot Swanson G. Evaluation of impairment of hand function. In: Hunter JM, Schneider LH, Mackin E, Calahan A, eds. *Rehabilitation in the Hand.* St Louis, Mo: CV Mosby Co; 1978:31-69.

Figure 16-43 Pie Chart of Upper Extremity Motion Impairments Due to Lack of Abduction and Adduction of Shoulder

Relative value of this functional unit to upper extremity impairment is 18%.

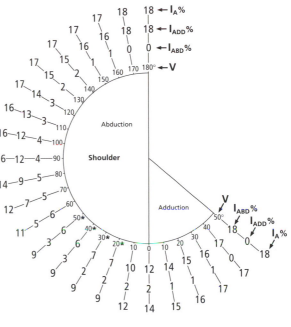

I$_A$% = Impairment due to ankylosis
I$_{ABD}$% = Impairment due to loss of abduction
I$_{ADD}$% = Impairment due to loss of adduction
V = Measured angles of motion
* = Positions of function

Redrawn with permission from Swanson AB, Hagert CG, de Groot Swanson G. Evaluation of impairment of hand function. In: Hunter JM, Schneider LH, Mackin E, Calahan A, eds. *Rehabilitation in the Hand.* St Louis, Mo: CV Mosby Co; 1978:31-69.

Example 16-51

Exam: Shoulder abduction to 100° and adduction to 0° (Figure 16-43).

Analysis: I$_{ABD}$% = 4% impairment of the upper extremity. I$_{ADD}$% = 2% impairment of the upper extremity.

Impairment Rating: *Add* 4% +2% = 6% impairment of the upper extremity resulting from decreased shoulder abduction and adduction.

Example 16-52

Exam: Shoulder ankylosis in 40° abduction.

Impairment Rating: 9% impairment of the upper extremity due to loss of this shoulder motion unit.

Internal and External Rotation

The normal range of motion is from 90° internal rotation to 90° external rotation. The positions of function range from 30° internal rotation to 50° internal rotation. The relative functional value of this motion unit is 12% of the upper extremity function.

1. Measure the maximum active shoulder internal and external rotation, and record the *actual* goniometer readings (Figure 16-44).
2. From Figure 16-46, match the measured internal and external rotation angles (row headed V) to their corresponding impairments of internal rotation (row headed $I_{IR}\%$) and external rotation (row headed $I_{ER}\%$). Impairment values for angles falling between those listed in Figure 16-46 may be adjusted or interpolated proportionally in the corresponding interval.
3. *Add* $I_{IR}\% + I_{ER}\%$ to obtain the value for upper extremity impairment contributed by decreased shoulder rotation.
4. If the shoulder is ankylosed, match the measured angle (row headed V) to its corresponding ankylosis impairment (row headed $I_A\%$) in Figure 16-46. Interpolate impairment values for intervening angles.

Ankyloses in functional positions (30° to 50° internal rotation) are given the lowest $I_A\%$, or 50% of this motion unit value (Figure 16-45). This corresponds to 6% impairment of the upper extremity (Figure 16-46). Ankylosis in either 90° internal or external rotation represents 100% loss of shoulder rotation function (Figure 16-45). This is equivalent to 20% impairment of shoulder function, or 12% impairment (20% × 60%) of the upper extremity resulting from loss of shoulder rotation (Figure 16-46).

Figure 16-44 Shoulder External Rotation and Internal Rotation

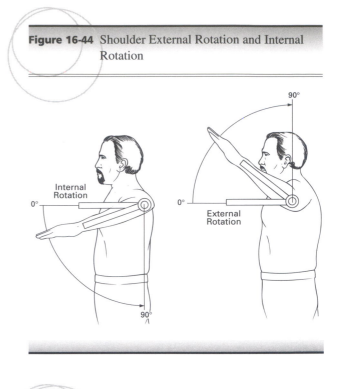

Figure 16-45 Motion Unit Impairment Curves for Ankylosis ($I_A\%$), Loss of Internal Rotation ($I_{IR}\%$), and Loss of External Rotation ($I_{ER}\%$) of Shoulder

Ankyloses in functional positions (30° internal rotation to 50° internal rotation) are given the lowest $I_A\%$ (50%).

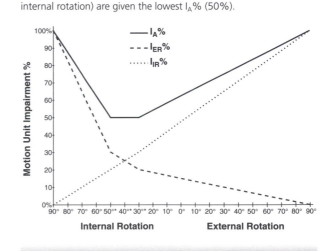

Figure 16-46 Pie Chart of Upper Extremity Impairments Due to Lack of Internal and External Rotation of Shoulder

Relative value of this functional unit to upper extremity impairment is 12%.

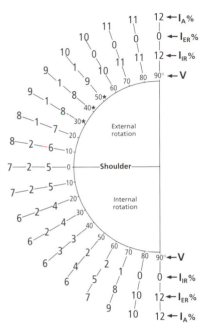

I_A% = Impairment due to ankylosis

I_{IR}% = Impairment due to loss of internal rotation

I_{ER}% = Impairment due to loss of external rotation

V = Measured angles of motion

* = Positions of function

Redrawn with permission from Swanson AB, Hagert CG, de Groot Swanson G. Evaluation of impairment of hand function. In: Hunter JM, Schneider LH, Mackin E, Calahan A, eds. *Rehabilitation in the Hand.* St Louis, Mo: CV Mosby Co; 1978:31-69.

Example 16-53

Exam: Shoulder internal rotation of 40° and external rotation of 50° (Figure 16-46).

Analysis: I_{IR}% = 3% impairment of upper extremity. I_{ER}% = 1% impairment of upper extremity.

Impairment Rating: *Add* 3% + 1% = 4% impairment of upper extremity resulting from decreased shoulder rotation.

Example 16-54

Exam: Shoulder ankylosis in 10° external rotation.

Impairment Rating: I_A% = 8% impairment of the upper extremity resulting from loss of shoulder rotation.

Determining Impairment Due to Abnormal Shoulder Motion

1. Using Figures 16-40, 16-43, and 16-46, determine the impairment of the upper extremity contributed by each shoulder unit of motion (flexion and extension, abduction and adduction, internal and external rotation) by adding I_F% + I_E%, I_{ABD}% + I_{ADD}% and I_{IR}% + I_{ER}%, as described in preceding sections.

2. Because the relative upper extremity value of each shoulder functional unit has been taken into consideration in the impairment pie charts, the impairment values contributed by each unit of motion are *added* to determine the impairment of the upper extremity due to abnormal shoulder motion, or it equals (I_F% + I_E%) + (I_{ABD}% + I_{ADD}%) + (I_{IR}% + I_{ER}%).

3. If the shoulder is ankylosed, *add* the ankylosis impairments contributed by each unit of motion to determine the upper extremity impairment resulting from loss of shoulder motion.

4. Use Table 16-3 to relate the impairment of the upper extremity to impairment of the whole person.

Example 16-55

Exam: Shoulder flexion and extension impairment of 9%, abduction and adduction impairment of 5%, and internal and external rotation impairment of 2% (Figures 16-40, 16-43, and 16-46).

Analysis: *Add* 9% + 5% + 2% = 16% impairment of the upper extremity.

Impairment Rating: 10% impairment of the whole person (Table 16-3).

Example 16-56

Exam: Shoulder ankylosis in 0° extension, 0° adduction, and 0° rotation.

Analysis: Extension I_A% = 24%; adduction I_A% = 14%; rotation, I_A% = 7%. *Add* 24% + 14% + 7% = 45% impairment of the upper extremity.

Impairment Rating: 27% impairment of the whole person (Table 16-3).

16.5 Impairment of the Upper Extremities Due to Peripheral Nerve Disorders

The peripheral nerves constitute an intricate system that carries neural impulses traveling in both directions between the spinal cord and other tissues of the body, and through it many important body functions are regulated. Accurate diagnosis of peripheral nerve disorders is based on a detailed history, a thorough physical examination with special emphasis on the nervous and vascular systems, and appropriate diagnostic tests, including a variety of electrical and imaging studies. Excellent knowledge of the morphologic anatomy and physiology of the nervous system is a prerequisite. Underlying causes of neuromuscular dysfunction that may mimic specific regional defects must be detected and may include diabetes mellitus, chronic alcohol abuse, systemic neurologic disorders, hypothyroidism, and other systemic diseases. A failure to recognize a preexisting alteration of sensory or motor nerve function can lead to erroneous conclusions after nerve injury.

The spinal nerves consist of 31 pairs of symmetrically arranged nerves, each leaving and entering the spinal cord via two roots: the ventral root carries motor axons originating from the ventral horn of the spinal cord and merges with the dorsal root, which contains dorsal sensory ganglion axons, to form the spinal nerve. As the spinal nerves exit the spinal column through the intervertebral foramina, they immediately divide into two primary rami. The anterior primary rami of the four lower cervical nerves (C5-8), together with a greater part of the first thoracic nerve (T1) and occasional contributions from the second thoracic nerve (T2), form the brachial plexus. The spinal nerves contain three main groups of fibers: (1) sensory (afferent) fibers that carry to the central nervous system impulses arising from various receptors in the skin, muscles, tendons, ligaments, bones, and joints; (2) motor (efferent) fibers, which include large *alpha* motor neuron fibers conducting impulses from the spinal cord to skeletal muscle fibers; small *gamma* motor neuron fibers carrying impulses to muscle spindles for feedback control; and (3) autonomic system fibers, which are efferent and are concerned with the control of smooth muscles and glands.

This section presents a method of evaluating upper extremity impairments related to disorders of the spinal nerves (C5 to C8 and T1), the brachial plexus, and major peripheral nerves of the upper extremities. It also addresses the evaluation of specific conditions, including entrapment/compression neuropathy and complex regional pain syndromes (CRPS), which include CRPS I/reflex sympathetic dystrophy (RSD) and CRPS II/causalgia.

Sensory deficits in the digits strictly due to lesions of digital nerves are evaluated according to Section 16.3. Impairments relating to the spinal cord and central nervous system are considered in Chapters 13 and 15 of the *Guides,* respectively. Impairment due to chronic pain is discussed in Chapter 18, Pain. Motivation and behavioral concerns are considered in Chapter 14, Mental and Behavioral Disorders.

16.5a Impairment Evaluation Principles

The evaluation of permanent impairment resulting from peripheral nerve disorders is based on the anatomic distribution and severity of loss of function resulting from (1) sensory deficits or pain and (2) motor deficits and loss of power. Characteristic deformities and manifestations resulting from peripheral nerve lesions, such as restricted motion, atrophy, and vasomotor, trophic, and reflex changes, have been taken into consideration in the estimated impairment values shown in this section. Therefore, when an impairment results strictly from a peripheral nerve lesion, in the absence of CRPS, the motion impairment values derived from Section 16.4 are not applied to this section to avoid duplication or unwarranted increase in the impairment estimation. For example, the claw hand deformity of MP joint hyperextension and IP joint flexion of the ring and little fingers is a classic manifestation of an ulnar nerve lesion; in absence of CRPS II/causalgia, the impairment value for motor deficit of the ulnar nerve is derived according to this section and applied without assigning additional impairment for loss of motion. However, if restricted motion cannot be attributed strictly to a peripheral nerve lesion, such as would be the case in CRPS I/RSD, the motion impairment values are evaluated separately according to Section 16.4 and then combined (Combined Values Chart, p. 604) with the peripheral nerve system impairment value derived from this section.

16.5b Impairment Evaluation Methods

The upper extremity impairment is calculated by multiplying the grade of severity of the sensory deficit (Table 16-10a) and/or of the motor deficit (Table 16-11a) by the respective maximum upper extremity impairment value resulting from sensory and/or motor deficits of each nerve structure involved, as listed in Section 16.5c, Regional Impairment Determination: spinal nerves, Table 16-13; brachial plexus, Table 16-14; and major peripheral nerves, Table 16-15. When both sensory and motor functions are involved, the impairment values derived for each are *combined* (Combined Values Chart, p. 604). The steps of the impairment determination method are detailed below.

The origins and functions of the peripheral nerves that serve the upper extremities are summarized in Table 16-12. The motor innervation of the upper extremity is shown in Figure 16-47. The cutaneous innervation and related nerves are shown in Figure 16-48, the dermatomes of the upper extremities in Figure 16-49, and a schematic diagram of the brachial plexus in Figure 16-50.

Impairment Determination Method

Use the following method to evaluate the impairment resulting from each peripheral nerve structure:

1. If sensory deficits or pain is present, localize the distribution and relate it to the nerve structure involved (Table 16-12 and Figures 16-48, 16-49, and 16-50).
2. If motor deficits or loss of power is present, identify the key muscles involved and relate the motor deficit to the nerve structure(s) involved (Table 16-12 and Figures 16-47 and 16-50).
3. *Grade the severity of sensory deficits or pain* according to Table 16-10a and/or that of the *motor deficits* according to Table 16-11a.
4. Find the values for *maximum impairment of the upper extremity* due to sensory and/or motor deficits of the nerve structure involved: individual spinal nerve (Table 16-13), brachial plexus (Table 16-14), and major peripheral nerves (Table 16-15).
5. For each nerve structure involved, *multiply* the grade of severity of the sensory and/or motor deficits (see step 3 above) by the appropriate maximum upper extremity impairment value (see step 4 above) to determine the upper extremity impairment percent for each function.

6. For a *structure with mixed motor and sensory fibers*, determine the upper extremity impairment for each function (steps 1 through 5), then *combine* the sensory and motor impairment percents (Combined Values Chart, p. 604) to obtain the total upper extremity impairment value.
7. When *more than one nerve structure* is involved, *combine* their respective upper extremity impairment values (steps 1 through 5) to obtain the total upper extremity impairment resulting from peripheral nerve disorders (Combined Values Chart).
8. When *multiple impairments of the extremity* are present because of amputation, loss of motion that is not strictly attributed to a peripheral nerve lesion, or peripheral vascular disorders, *combine* the peripheral nerve upper extremity impairment value with the other upper extremity impairment values (Combined Values Chart) to obtain the total upper extremity impairment.
9. The total upper extremity impairment is *converted* to a whole person impairment by means of Table 16-3.
10. If there is *bilateral upper extremity involvement*, determine separately the impairment values for each side, and convert them to whole person impairment. *Combine* the whole person impairment values for each side (Combined Values Chart) to obtain the total whole person impairment. Consult page 435 for further comments on bilateral upper extremity involvement.

Grading Sensory Deficits or Pain

A wide range of abnormal sensations may be associated with peripheral nerve lesions, including diminished sensation (anesthesia or hypesthesia), abnormal sensation (dysesthesia or paresthesia), and increased sensation (hyperesthesia). Another possible manifestation is pain of various types, including pain resulting from nonnoxious stimulus (allodynia), overreactive pain (hyperpathia), a state of dysesthetic pain (deafferentation), and, most significantly, the sustained, burning pain present in CRPS I (RSD) and CRPS II (causalgia). Cold intolerance may also be present.

Sensory deficits or pain associated with peripheral nerve disorders are evaluated according to the following criteria: (1) How does the sensory deficit or pain interfere with the individual's performance of daily activities? (2) To what extent does the sensory deficit or pain follow the defined anatomic pathways of the spinal nerves, brachial plexus, or peripheral nerves? (3) To what extent is the description of the sensory deficit or pain consistent with characteristics of peripheral nerve disorders? (4) To what extent does the sensory deficit or pain correspond to other disturbances (motor, trophic, vasomotor, etc) of the involved nerve structure?

The methods for clinical assessment of sensibility are detailed in Section 16.3. In individuals with nerve lacerations, the presence of two-point discrimination usually indicates significant return of function. However, in conditions such as radiculitis, causalgia, and entrapment or compression neuropathy, normal two-point discrimination does not exclude the presence of abnormal light-touch/deep-pressure thresholds and abnormal conduction studies. Conversely, the presence of a normal light-touch threshold does not necessarily indicate that two-point discrimination is normal in these cases. The use of the Semmes-Weinstein touch-pressure threshold monofilament test may be a helpful adjunct to the two-point discrimination test to help assess changes in light-touch sensibility.

Upper extremity impairments due to sensory deficits or pain resulting from peripheral nerve disorders are determined according to the grade of severity in diminution or loss of function and the relative maximum upper extremity impairment value of the nerve structure involved, as shown in the classification (a) and procedural (b) steps described in Table 16-10 and the impairment determination method detailed in Section 16.5b. Table 16-10 provides a classification for determining impairment of the upper extremity due to a sensory deficit or pain resulting from a nerve disorder. This table is to be used for pain that is due to *nerve injury* or disease that has been documented with objective physical findings or electrodiagnostic abnormalities. *It is not to be used for pain in the distribution of a nerve that has not been injured* except in diagnosed cases of complex regional pain syndromes. The examiner must use clinical judgment to estimate the appropriate percentage of sensory deficits or pain within the range of values shown for each severity grade. The maximum value for each grade is not applied automatically.

Table 16-10 Determining Impairment of the Upper Extremity Due to Sensory Deficits or Pain Resulting From Peripheral Nerve Disorders

a. Classification

Grade	Description of Sensory Deficit or Pain	% Sensory Deficit
5	No loss of sensibility, abnormal sensation, or pain	0
4	Distorted superficial tactile sensibility (diminished light touch), with or without minimal abnormal sensations or pain, that is forgotten during activity	1-25
3	Distorted superficial tactile sensibility (diminished light touch and two-point discrimination), with some abnormal sensations or slight pain, that interferes with some activities	26-60
2	Decreased superficial cutaneous pain and tactile sensibility (decreased protective sensibility), with abnormal sensations or moderate pain, that may prevent some activities	61-80
1	Deep cutaneous pain sensibility present; absent superficial pain and tactile sensibility (absent protective sensibility), with abnormal sensations or severe pain, that prevents most activity	81-99
0	Absent sensibility, abnormal sensations, or severe pain that prevents all activity	100

b. Procedure

1	Identify the area of involvement using the cutaneous innervation chart (Figure 16-48) or the dermatome chart (Figure 16-49).
2	Identify the nerve structure(s) that innervate the area(s) (Table 16-12 and Figures 16-48, 16-49, and 16-50).
3	Grade the severity of the sensory deficit or pain according to the classification given above (a). Use clinical judgment to select the appropriate percentage from the range of values shown for each severity grade.
4	Find the maximum upper extremity impairment value due to sensory deficit or pain for each nerve structure involved: spinal nerves (Table 16-13), brachial plexus (Table 16-14), and major peripheral nerves (Table 16-15).
5	*Multiply* the severity of the sensory deficit by the maximum upper extremity impairment value to obtain the upper extremity impairment for each nerve structure involved.

Adapted from Kline DG, Hudson AR. *Operative Results for Major Nerve Injuries, Entrapments, and Tumors.* Philadelphia, Pa: WB Saunders Co; 1995:89; Moberg E. Sensibility in reconstructive limb surgery. In: Fredericks S, Brody GS, eds. *Symposium on the Neurologic Aspects of Plastic Surgery.* St Louis, Mo: CV Mosby Co; 1978:30-35. Omer GE Jr, Bell-Krotoski J. Evaluation of clinical results following peripheral nerve suture. In: Omer GE Jr, Spinner M, Van Beek AL, eds. *Management of Peripheral Nerve Problems.* 2nd ed. Philadelphia, Pa: WB Saunders Co; 1998:340-349; Seddon HJ. *Surgical Disorders of the Peripheral Nerves.* 2nd ed. Edinburgh, Scotland: Churchill Livingstone; 1975; Swanson AB. Evaluation of impairment of function in the hand. *Surg Clin North Am.* 1964;44:925-940; Swanson AB, de Groot Swanson G. Evaluation of permanent impairment in the hand and upper extremity. In: Doege TC, ed. *Guides to the Evaluation of Permanent Impairment.* Fourth ed. Chicago, Ill: American Medical Association; 1993.

Table 16-10a classifies the levels of functional sensibility based on the recommendations of Seddon, Moberg, Omer and Bell-Krotoski, and Kline and Hudson for assessment of sensory recovery, and Swanson's grading of associated pain interference on activity. In interpretation of Table 16-10a, individuals in *grade 4* have diminished light touch, with fair (6-10 mm) to good two-point discrimination, localization of sensory stimuli, and good protective sensibility. Abnormal sensations or pain, if present, is minimal and forgotten during activity. Individuals in *grade 3* have diminished light touch and two-point discrimination. There is mislocalization of sensory stimuli with some abnormal or increased irritability sensations or pain that interferes with activities. Protective sensibility is normal. Individuals in *grade 2* have decreased protective sensibility, which is defined as a conscious appreciation of pain, temperature, or pressure before tissue damage results from the stimulus. They have diminished hand function. The mislocalization and overresponse (hyperesthesia or paresthesia, hyperpathia, or allodynia) to sensory stimuli result in decreased manipulative skills and gripping function and complaints of hand weakness. It is possible to have a gross appreciation of two-point discrimination (11-15 mm) at this level. Individuals in *grade 1* have no protective sensibility, have little use of the hand, cannot manipulate objects outside their line of vision, and have a tendency to injure themselves easily. However, they can feel a pinprick and have deep-pressure sensibility, and they are not totally asensory. Pain and/or overresponse can be severe. *Grade 0* represents an asensory hand with severe pain and overreactive responses and no functional usage.

Note that with the sole exception of CRPS I/RSD, Table 16-10a is exclusively used for cases presenting a documented sensory or mixed nerve involvement. In the absence of CRPS, sensory impairments strictly due to digital nerve lesions are evaluated according to Section 16.3.

Example 16-57

Exam: One year after a closed injury to the distal forearm, an individual continues to complain of vague pain and some numbness over the radial side of the dorsum of the hand, which is annoying but does not interfere with activity. The physical examination documents hypesthesia in the distribution of the superficial dorsal branch of the radial nerve and a positive percussion test over the point of nerve injury.

Analysis:
1. Nerve involved: superficial dorsal branch of the radial nerve (Table 16-12 and Figure 16-48).
2. Severity of sensory deficit: grade 4, ranging between 1% and 25% (Table 16-10a). On the basis of clinical judgment, 20% severity was selected.
3. Maximum impairment of the upper extremity due to sensory deficits or pain of the radial nerve: 5% (Table 16-15).
4. Multiply the grade of severity, 20% (step 2), by the maximum upper extremity impairment value for sensory deficit of the nerve involved, 5% (step 3), to obtain the upper extremity impairment value.

Impairment Rating: $20\% \times 5\% = 1\%$ of the upper extremity, or 1% of the whole person (Table 16-3).

Grading Motor Deficits and Loss of Power

Involvement of the peripheral nerve system structures may lead to paralysis or weakness of the muscles they supply and/or to characteristic sensory changes. Clinical examination of the upper extremity demands precise anatomic knowledge to properly select the muscle tests that correlate to the specific nerve structure(s) involved (Table 16-12). Some muscles display a dual or variable pattern of nerve supply and require special consideration.

The manual grading of muscle strength is based on the ability of a normal muscle to contract and move a bone-joint lever arm through its full active range of motion with full resistance. Palpation of the muscle-tendon unit helps evaluate muscle contractility. Other than amplitude and strength, factors in muscle function that should be considered and recorded include endurance, speed of contraction, and independence of action of individual muscles, especially those with associated function, such as the flexor digitorum superficialis and flexor digitorum profundus. Both upper extremities should be tested and the results compared.

The relaxed muscle should be palpated to identify fibrosis or painful areas that could limit excursion. Trick movements must be detected. If there is questionable motor activity based on either pain or suspected anastomotic variations, use of a local anesthetic to block either the pain point or competing innervation may assist the examiner in evaluating function. Muscle strength testing is voluntary in that it requires full individual concentration and cooperation. It remains somewhat subjective until precise methods of measuring muscle contractions become generally available. Muscle atrophy, although not rated separately, can be a more objective sign of motor dysfunction. Electromyographic studies can help confirm motor function of specific muscles or groups of muscles.

Upper extremity impairments due to motor deficits and loss of power resulting from peripheral nerve disorders are determined according to the grade of severity of loss of function and the relative maximum upper extremity impairment value of the nerve structure involved, as shown in the classification (a) and procedural (b) steps described in Table 16-11 and the impairment determination method detailed in Section 16.5b. The examiner must use clinical judgment to estimate the appropriate percentage of motor deficits and loss of power within the range of values shown for each severity grade. It is important to ascertain that weakness is due to loss of nerve function before using these tables. Weakness may be due to many causes, including pain, and Table 16-11 is not to be used for rating weakness that is not due to a diagnosed injury of a specific nerve or nerves. A diagnosis of nerve injury can usually be made by a careful physical examination done by an examiner who has sufficient knowledge of the anatomy and function of the part. If there is doubt about the presence of a nerve injury, electromyographic studies may be

Table 16-11 Determining Impairment of the Upper Extremity Due to Motor and Loss-of-Power Deficits Resulting From Peripheral Nerve Disorders Based on Individual Muscle Rating

a. Classification

Grade	Description of Muscle Function	% Motor Deficit
5	Complete active range of motion against gravity with full resistance	0
4	Complete active range of motion against gravity with some resistance	1- 25
3	Complete active range of motion against gravity only, without resistance	26- 50
2	Complete active range of motion with gravity eliminated	51- 75
1	Evidence of slight contractility; no joint movement	76- 99
0	No evidence of contractility	100

b. Procedure

1	Identify the motion involved, such as flexion, extension, etc.
2	Identify the muscle(s) performing the motion and the motor nerve(s) involved.
3	Grade the severity of motor deficit of individual muscles according to the classification given above.
4	Find the maximum impairment of the upper extremity due to motor deficit for each nerve structure involved: spinal nerves (Table 16-13), brachial plexus (Table 16-14), and major peripheral nerves (Table 16-15).
5	Multiply the severity of the motor deficit by the maximum impairment value to obtain the upper extremity impairment for each structure involved.

Adapted from Lovett RW. From Omer GE Jr, Bell-Krotoski J. Evaluation of clinical results following peripheral nerve suture. In: Omer GE Jr, Spinner M, Van Beek AL, eds. *Management of Peripheral Nerve Problems*. 2nd ed. Philadelphia, Pa: WB Saunders Co; 1998:341; Seddon HJ. *Surgical Disorders of the Peripheral Nerves*. 2nd ed. Edinburgh, Scotland: Churchill Livingstone; 1975; Swanson AB, de Groot Swanson G. Evaluation of permanent impairment in the hand and upper extremity. In: Doege TC, ed. *Guides to the Evaluation of Permanent Impairment*. Fourth ed. Chicago, Ill: American Medical Association; 1993.

necessary in order to confirm the diagnosis. Note that grade 4 covers a wide range of weakness, from minimal detectable weakness to severe weakness in which the muscles are functional through a full range with only very slight resistance. The degree of weakness should be rated from 1% to 25% depending on the degree within this grade.

Loss of strength relating to conditions not resulting from peripheral nerve disorders is discussed in Section 16.8. *The evaluator should not apply impairment values from both sections to the same condition.*

Table 16-12a Origins and Functions of the Peripheral Nerves of the Upper Extremity Emanating From the Brachial Plexus

Nerves of Plexus	Primary Branches	Secondary Branches	Function
Muscular branches Dorsal scapular (C5) Long thoracic (C5, 6, 7) Suprascapular (C5, 6) Lateral pectoral (C5, 6, 7) Medial pectoral (C8, T1) Upper subscapular (C5, 6) Lower subscapular (C5, 6) Thoracodorsal ± C6, C7, 8)	Unnamed		Motor to longus colli, scalenes, and subclavius Motor to rhomboideus major and minor, levator scapulae Motor to serratus anterior Motor to supraspinatus and infraspinatus Motor to pectoralis major and minor Motor to pectoralis major and minor Motor to subscapularis Motor to teres major and subscapularis Motor to latissimus dorsi
Medial brachial cutaneous (T1)			Sensory to anteromedial surface of arm (with intercostobrachial)
Intercostobrachial (T2)			Sensory to posteromedial surface of arm (with medial brachial cutaneous)
Medial antebrachial cutaneous (C8, T1)			Sensory to anterocentral surface of arm, anteromedial half of forearm, and posteromedial third of elbow, forearm, and wrist
Musculocutaneous (C5, 6, 7)	Unnamed		Motor to coracobrachialis, biceps brachii, brachialis
	Lateral antebrachial cutaneous		Sensory to anterolateral half and posterolateral third of forearm
Axillary (C5, C6)	Teres minor branch		Motor to teres minor
	Anterior		Motor to deltoid (middle and anterior thirds)
	Posterior	Muscular branches	Motor to deltoid (posterior third)
		Upper lateral brachial cutaneous	Sensory over lower half of deltoid
Radial (C5,6,7,8 ± T1)	Unnamed		Motor to triceps brachii, brachialis (lateral part), brachioradialis, extensor carpi radialis longus, anconeus
	Ulnar collateral		Motor to triceps brachii (medial head)
	Posterior brachial cutaneous		Sensory to distal posterocentral surface of arm as far as olecranon
	Inferior lateral brachial cutaneous		Sensory to distal posterolateral surface of arm and elbow
	Posterior antebrachial cutaneous		Sensory to posterocentral surface of forearm
	Superficial terminal	Dorsal branches	Sensory to posterolateral half of wrist and hand
		Dorsal digitals (5 branches)	Sensory to dorsum of thumb, index, middle, and ring (radial half) fingers up to middle phalanx
	Deep terminal (posterior interosseous)	Unnamed	Motor to extensor carpi radialis brevis, and supinator
		Superficial branch	Motor to extensor digitorum communis, extensor digiti minimi, extensor carpi ulnaris
		Deep branch	Motor to extensor pollicis longus, extensor pollicis brevis, abductor pollicis longus, extensor indicis proprius Sensory to wrist joint capsule

Modified from Swanson AB, de Groot Swanson G. Evaluation of permanent impairment in the hand and upper extremity. In: Engelberg AL, ed. *Guides to the Evaluation of Permanent Impairment.* Third ed. Chicago, Ill: American Medical Association; 1988.

Table 16-12b Origins and Functions of the Peripheral Nerves of the Upper Extremity Emanating From the Brachial Plexus

Nerves of Plexus	Primary Branches	Secondary Branches	Function
Median (± C5, C6, 7, 8, T1)	Unnamed	Cubital fossa and forearm branches	Motor to pronator teres, flexor carpi radialis, palmaris longus, flexor digitorum superficialis
	Anterior interosseous		Motor to radial half of flexor digitorum profundus (index and middle fingers), flexor pollicis longus, pronator quadratus
	Palmar cutaneous		Sensory to central proximal surface of palm
	Thenar muscular		Motor to abductor pollicis brevis, flexor pollicis brevis (superficial head), opponens pollicis
	Common palmar radial digital	1st lumbrical branch	Motor to 1st lumbrical
		Proper palmar digitals (3 branches)	Sensory to 1st web space (palmar), palmar, and distal dorsal surfaces of thumb (both sides) and index (radial side)
	Common palmar central digital	2nd lumbrical branch	Motor to 2nd lumbrical
		Proper palmar digitals (2 branches)	Sensory to 2nd web space (palmar), palmar, and distal dorsal surfaces of contiguous sides of index and middle fingers
	Common palmar ulnar digital	Proper palmar digitals (2 branches)	Sensory to 3rd web space (palmar), palmar, and distal dorsal surfaces of contiguous sides of middle and ring fingers
Ulnar (± C7, C8, T1)	Unnamed	Forearm branches	Motor to flexor carpi ulnaris, ulnar half of flexor digitorum profundus (ring and little fingers)
	Palmar cutaneous		Sensory to ulnar surface of palm and wrist
	Dorsal cutaneous	Dorsal branches	Sensory to ulnar dorsum of wrist and hand
		Dorsal digitals (3 branches)	Sensory to dorsum of ring finger (ulnar proximal half), little finger (up to nail root), and 4th web space
	Superficial palmar	Palmaris brevis br	Motor to palmaris brevis
		Proper palmar digitals (3 branches)	Sensory to palmar and distal dorsal surface of ring (ulnar half), and little finger (both sides)
	Deep palmar		Motor to adductor pollicis, flexor pollicis brevis (deep head), abductor digiti minimi, flexor digiti minimi brevis, opponens digiti minimi, 3rd and 4th lumbricals, all interossei

Modified from Swanson AB, de Groot Swanson G. Evaluation of permanent impairment in the hand and upper extremity. In: Engelberg AL, ed. *Guides to the Evaluation of Permanent Impairment*. Third ed. Chicago, Ill: American Medical Association; 1988.

Figure 16-47 Motor Innervation of the Upper Extremity

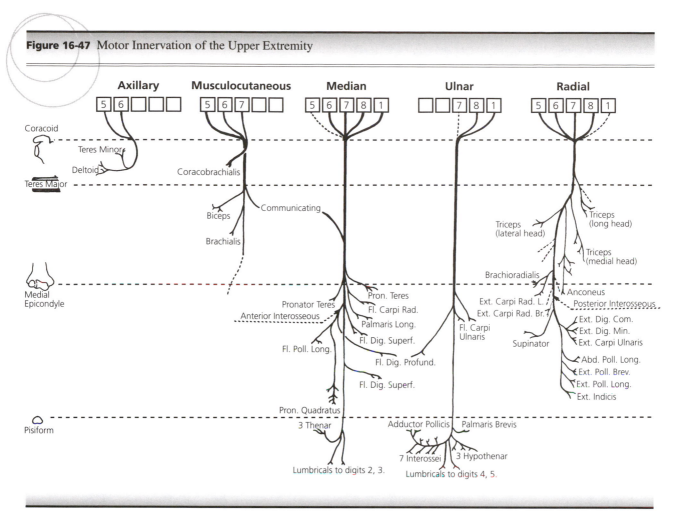

From Swanson AB, de Groot Swanson G. Evaluation of permanent impairment in the hand and upper extremity. In: Doege TC, ed. *Guides to the Evaluation of Permanent Impairment*. Fourth ed. Chicago, Ill: American Medical Association; 1993.

Example 16-58

Exam: An individual sustained a dislocation of the right shoulder, which was reduced to its anatomic position as seen on roentgenograms. However, some loss of muscle strength persisted despite an appropriate course of rehabilitation and sufficient time for maximal recovery. While in a standing position with the arm placed alongside the body and the elbow flexed, the individual could actively abduct and elevate the upper arm from 90° to 180° against gravity and slight resistance. There was some hypesthesia of the skin over the lower two thirds of the deltoid muscle that did not interfere with activity. The estimated impairment should take into consideration the motor and sensory deficits.

Analysis:

Sensory deficit calculation:

1. Cutaneous dermatome involved: lateral brachial cutaneous nerve (terminal sensory branch of the axillary nerve) (Table 16-12 and Figure 16-48).
2. Severity of sensory deficit or pain: grade 4 (1%-25%) (Table 16-10a). A severity grading of 15% was selected on clinical judgment.
3. Maximum upper extremity impairment resulting from sensory deficit of the sensory branch of the axillary nerve: 5% (Table 16-15).
4. *Multiply* the maximum upper extremity impairment for sensory deficit of the axillary nerve sensory branch (5%) by the severity of sensory deficit (15%) to obtain the impairment of the upper extremity due to sensory deficit of the axillary nerve terminal sensory branch, or 5% × 15% = 0.75%, which is rounded to 1%.

Figure 16-48 Cutaneous Innervation of the Upper Extremity and Related Peripheral Nerves and Roots

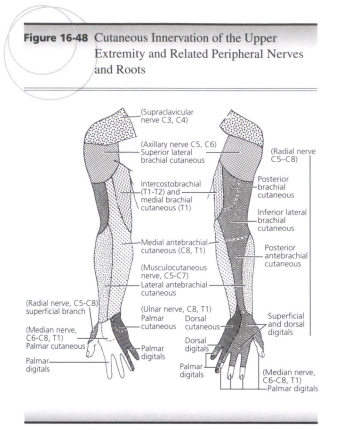

Adapted with permission from an original painting by F. H. Netter In: *The Atlas of Human Anatomy.* Summit, NJ: CIBA-GEIGY Corp; 1989.

Motor deficit calculation:

1. Muscle involved: deltoid, which is innervated by the axillary nerve (Table 16-12 and Figure 16-47).
2. Severity of motor deficit: grade 4 (1%-25%) (Table 16-11a). A severity rating of 25% was selected on clinical judgment because of the severity of the weakness.
3. Maximum upper extremity impairment due to motor deficit of the axillary nerve: 35% (Table 16-15).
4. *Multiply* the maximum upper extremity impairment for motor deficit of the axillary nerve (35%) by the severity of motor deficit (25%) to obtain the impairment of the upper extremity due to motor deficit of the axillary nerve, or $35\% \times 25\% = 9\%$.

Impairment Rating: *Combined* sensory and motor deficits: *Combine* 9% upper extremity motor deficit with 1% upper extremity sensory deficit (Combined Values Chart, p. 604) to obtain 10% upper extremity impairment resulting from axillary nerve dysfunction. This corresponds to 6% whole person impairment (Table 16-3).

16.5c Regional Impairment Determination

Impairment of the peripheral nerve system may involve the structures listed below. The impairment determination method is detailed step by step in Section 16.5b.

- Spinal nerves C5 to C8 and T1
- Brachial plexus
- Major peripheral nerves

Spinal Nerves

Evaluating impairment of the spinal nerves due to injuries or disease is based on the severity of loss of function of the peripheral nerves receiving fibers from specific spinal nerves. Because each spinal nerve transmits fibers to more than one peripheral nerve, the loss of function is greater with the involvement of two or more spinal nerves transmitting fibers to the same peripheral nerve than with the involvement of a single spinal nerve. Therefore, in multiple spinal nerve involvement, the impairment is evaluated according to the brachial plexus values (Table 16-14) rather than combining the individual spinal nerve values shown in Table 16-13.

For example, the maximum upper extremity impairment due to *combined* motor and sensory deficits resulting from a lesion of the upper trunk (C5 and C6) is 81% (Table 16-14); however, *combining* the impairment values of the individual nerves C5 (34%) and C6 (40%), as shown in Table 16-13, results in 60% upper extremity impairment (Combined Values Chart, p. 604), which does not reflect the full severity of loss of function.

Table 16-13 provides maximum upper extremity impairment values for unilateral sensory and motor deficits of the spinal nerves that are most frequently involved. A spinal nerve–related impairment is determined according to the method detailed in Section 16.5b. Impairment of a specific spinal nerve that is not mentioned in this section should be estimated by considering the percents suggested for a nerve that has fibers from the specific spinal nerve. Bilateral involvements are discussed in the Impairment Determination Method (Section 16.5b), step 10.

Table 16-13 Maximum Upper Extremity Impairment Due to Unilateral Sensory or Motor Deficits of Individual Spinal Nerves or to *Combined* 100% Deficits

Spinal Nerve	Maximum % Upper Extremity Impairment Due to:		
	Sensory Deficit or Pain*	Motor Deficit†	*Combined* Motor/Sensory Deficits
C5	5	30	34
C6	8	35	40
C7	5	35	38
C8	5	45	48
T1	5	20	24

* See Table 16-10a to grade sensory deficit or pain.

† See Table 16-11a to grade motor deficit.

From Swanson AB, de Groot Swanson G. Evaluation of permanent impairment in the hand and upper extremity. In: Doege TC, ed. *Guides to the Evaluation of Permanent Impairment*. Fourth ed. Chicago, Ill: American Medical Association; 1993.

Example 16-59

Exam: A 42-year-old man fell 30 feet and landed on his upper back. He complained of neck pain radiating down his right arm. Sixteen months later, after a maximum medical rehabilitation program and an optimal period for physiologic recovery, an examination disclosed a 20% sensory deficit in the C5 area and 50% loss of power of the muscles innervated by C5. These losses were stable and determined as permanent impairments.

Analysis:
1. Sensory deficit impairment: 20% (sensory deficit severity) × 5% (maximum upper extremity impairment for sensory deficit of C5) (Table 16-13) = 1% impairment of the upper extremity.
2. Motor deficit impairment: 50% (motor deficit severity) × 30% (maximum upper extremity impairment for motor deficit of C5) (Table 16-13) = 15% impairment of the upper extremity.

Impairment Rating: *Combine* 1% sensory deficit with 15% motor deficit (Combined Values Chart, p. 604) to obtain 16% impairment of the upper extremity, which is 10% impairment of the whole person (Table 16-3).

Brachial Plexus

The brachial plexus innervates the shoulder girdle and upper extremity and is formed by the anterior primary divisions of the fifth through eighth cervical roots and the first thoracic root. These roots anastomose to form three primary trunks: upper trunk (C5 and C6), middle trunk (C7), and lower trunk (C8 and T1) (Figure 16-50). Specific findings result from the involvement of these structures.

Total brachial plexus paralysis is manifested by flail arm, paralysis of all muscles of the hand, and no sensibility. Sudorific function is intact when the lesion is preganglionic.

In *upper trunk paralysis* (C5, C6, Erb-Duchenne), the arm hangs in adduction and internal rotation with the elbow in extension and the forearm in pronation; the biceps, deltoid, brachialis, supraspinatus, infraspinatus, and rhomboid muscles are paralyzed; the triceps, pectoralis major, and extensor carpi radialis brevis and longus muscles are weak; most finger movements are intact; biceps reflex is absent; and a sensory deficit in the C5 and C6 dermatomes is present (Figure 16-49).

Lower trunk paralysis (C8, T1, Déjerine-Klumpke) is manifested by paralysis of all intrinsic muscles of the hand; weakness of the flexor carpi ulnaris and flexor digitorum profundus of the little finger; Horner syndrome (ptosis, myosis, enophthalmos) if the T1 root is avulsed from the spinal cord; and a sensory deficit of the C8 and T1 dermatomes (Figure 16-49).

Table 16-14 provides maximum upper extremity impairment values resulting from unilateral sensory or motor deficits of the brachial plexus, or to *combined* deficits. A brachial plexus–related impairment is determined according to the method described in Section 16.5b.

Figure 16-49 Dermatomes of the Upper Limb

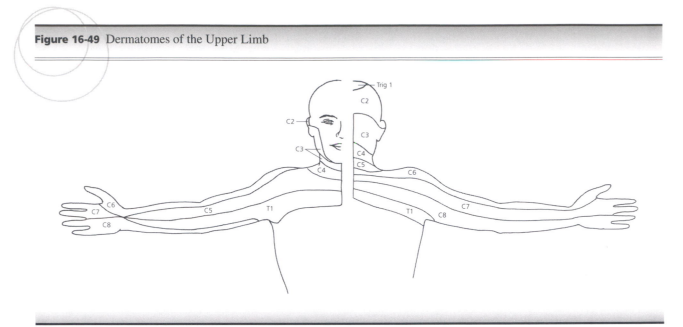

Source: Netter FH. *The Atlas of Human Anatomy.* Summit, NJ: CIBA-GEIGY Corp; 1989.

Figure 16-50 The Brachial Plexus

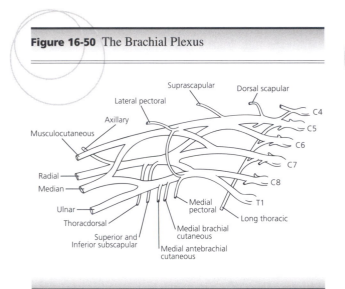

Table 16-14 Maximum Upper Extremity Impairments Due to Unilateral Sensory or Motor Deficits of Brachial Plexus or to *Combined* 100% Deficits

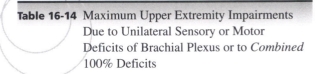

Brachial Plexus and Trunks	Maximum % Upper Extremity Impairment Due to:		
	Sensory Deficit or Pain*	Motor Deficit†	Combined Motor/Sensory Deficits
Brachial plexus (C5 through C8, T1)	100	100	100
Upper trunk (C5, C6, Erb-Duchenne)	25	75	81
Middle trunk (C7)	5	35	38
Lower trunk (C8, T1, Déjerine-Klumpke)	20	70	76

* See Table 16-10a to grade sensory deficit or pain.

† See Table 16-11a to grade motor deficit.

From Swanson AB, de Groot Swanson G. Evaluation of permanent impairment in the hand and upper extremity. In: Doege TC, ed. *Guides to the Evaluation of Permanent Impairment.* Fourth ed. Chicago, Ill: American Medical Assocation; 1993.

Example 16-60

Exam: A 22-year-old man was driving a pickup truck that flipped over during a crash. Days later the man could not move his left arm. After a period of months, he had recovered hand and forearm function but had total paralysis along the C5 and C6 root distribution. As a result of grafts from C5 and C6 to truncal divisions, he was partially recovered within 4 years.

Analysis: In the C5 and C6 distributions, the motor function of individual muscles was graded as follows: supraspinatus, 4; infraspinatus, 3; deltoid, 3; biceps brachialis, 4; brachioradialis, 3; and supinator, 3. Table 16-12 and Figure 16-47 describe the motor nerves of the upper extremity.

The whole person impairment was derived from the following:

1. Supraspinatus and infraspinatus muscles (suprascapular nerve, C5-6): a motor function grade of 4 was estimated to be 25% motor deficit (Table 16-11a). The maximum upper extremity impairment for motor deficit of the suprascapular nerve is 16% (Table 16-15). The upper extremity impairment was estimated to be 25% × 16%, or 4%.
2. Deltoid muscle (axillary nerve, C5-6): a motor function grade of 3 was estimated to be 50% motor deficit (Table 16-11a). The maximum upper extremity impairment for motor deficit of the axillary nerve is 35% (Table 16-15). The upper extremity impairment was estimated to be 50% × 35% or, rounding off, 18%.
3. Biceps brachialis muscle (musculocutaneous nerve, C5-6): a motor function grade of 4 represented 25% motor deficit (Table 16-11a). The maximum upper extremity impairment for motor deficit of the musculocutaneous nerve is 25% (Table 16-15). The upper extremity impairment was estimated to be 25% × 25%, or 6%.
4. Brachioradialis and supinator muscles (radial nerve C5-6): a motor function grade of 3 was estimated to be 40% motor deficit (Table 16-11a). The maximum upper extremity impairment for motor deficit of the radial nerve with sparing of the triceps is 35% (Table 16-15). The upper extremity impairment was estimated to be 40% × 35%, or 14%.

Impairment Rating: The upper extremity motor deficit impairments are *combined* by means of the Combined Values Chart (p. 604): 4% *combined* with 18% is 21%, 21% *combined* with 6% is 26%, and 26% *combined* with 14% is 36%. The total impairment of the upper extremity is 36%, which represents 22% whole person impairment (Table 16-3).

Major Peripheral Nerves

The sensory and motor innervation of the upper extremity is shown in Figures 16-47 through 16-50 and in Table 16-12. Table 16-15 shows the maximum upper extremity impairment resulting from sensory and/or motor deficits of the major peripheral nerves most frequently involved.

Impairment due to involvement of major peripheral nerves is derived according to the method described in Section 16.5b. An example of mixed peripheral nerve impairment is given in Example 16-58, based on the individual who sustained a shoulder dislocation followed by axillary nerve deficits.

16.5d Entrapment/Compression Neuropathy

Entrapment neuropathy is a nerve compression–type lesion that implies disproportion between the volume of the peripheral nerve and the space through which it passes. The underlying causes may be intrinsic or extrinsic, in that the nerve itself or the other contents of the passage may be enlarged or the passage space may be narrowed. The differential diagnosis of entrapment neuropathy is extensive. The local causes can relate to specific anatomic variations in the configuration of bones or soft tissue resulting from chronic irritation or an inflammatory process such as tenosynovitis; mechanical causes such as blunt trauma, fractures, or scarring; or congenital anomalies such as aberrant muscles, arteries, or a cervical rib in the thoracic outlet region. Neoplastic conditions, such as myeloma or neurofibromatosis, or space-occupying lesions, such as ganglion, lipoma, or fibroma, must be ruled out. Predisposing or associated conditions can include diabetes, arthritis, alcoholism, renal disease, hormonal changes, malnutrition, or obesity.

Table 16-15 Maximum Upper Extremity Impairment Due to Unilateral Sensory or Motor Deficits or to *Combined* 100% Deficits of the Major Peripheral Nerves

Nerve	Maximum % Upper Extremity Impairment Due to:		
	Sensory Deficit or Pain *	Motor Deficit†	*Combined* Motor and Sensory Deficits
Pectorals (medial and lateral)	0	5	5
Axillary	5	35	38
Dorsal scapular	0	5	5
Long thoracic	0	15	15
Medial antebrachial cutaneous	5	0	5
Medial brachial cutaneous	5	0	5
Median (above midforearm)	39	44	66
Median (anterior interosseous branch)	0	15	15
Median (below midforearm)	39	10	45
Radial palmar digital of thumb	7	0	7
Ulnar palmar digital of thumb	11	0	11
Radial palmar digital of index finger	5	0	5
Ulnar palmar digital of index finger	4	0	4
Radial palmar digital of middle finger	5	0	5
Ulnar palmar digital of middle finger	4	0	4
Radial palmar digital of ring finger	3	0	3
Musculocutaneous	5	25	29
Radial (upper arm with loss of triceps)	5	42	45
Radial (elbow with sparing of triceps)	5	35	38
Subscapulars (upper and lower)	0	5	5
Suprascapular	5	16	20
Thoracodorsal	0	10	10
Ulnar (above midforearm)	7	46	50
Ulnar (below midforearm)	7	35	40
Ulnar palmar digital of ring finger	2	0	2
Radial palmar digital of little finger	2	0	2
Ulnar palmar digital of little finger	3	0	3

* See Table 16-10a to grade sensory deficits or pain.

† See Table 16-11a to grade motor deficits.

* From Swanson AB, de Groot Swanson G. Evaluation of permanent impairment in the hand and upper extremity. In: Doege TC, ed. *Guides to the Evaluation of Permanent Impairment.* Fourth ed. Chicago, Ill: American Medical Association; 1993.

Peripheral nerves can become compressed at any level from the hand to the thoracocervical region. One nerve can be trapped simultaneously at two levels, or more than one nerve can be trapped. Certain anatomic constraints make particular nerves at specific sites more vulnerable, leading to well-defined patterns or syndromes. Generally, each nerve lesion can be described clinically as a high or a low lesion, that is, a high or a low median, radial, or ulnar lesion. The most frequently encountered entrapment is of the median nerve at the wrist, leading to the carpal tunnel syndrome, followed by the ulnar nerve at the elbow. The recurrent motor branch of the median nerve can be involved singly or in combination with the median nerve at the wrist. Knowledge

of normal and variant anatomy, both gross and microscopic, is essential for accurate diagnosis and precise localization of the lesion.

Diagnosis of Entrapment/Compression Neuropathy

The diagnosis of entrapment/compression neuropathy is based on (1) the history and symptoms; (2) objective clinical signs and findings on detailed examination; and (3) documentation by electroneuromyographic studies. Standard roentgenograms and more involved imaging studies are also useful.

The history should include a listing of occupation(s), activities of daily living, factors that alleviate or aggravate the symptoms, medical conditions, and past surgical procedures or trauma. The entrapment of a major peripheral nerve or one of its branches is reflected by a disturbance of a specific motor, sensory, or autonomic function. Functionally, the symptoms may vary from slight paresthesia, motor weakness, or both to complete sensibility loss, muscle paralysis, or both. The severity of the nerve damage and symptoms depends on the duration, magnitude, and type of compression as well as on the microanatomy of the nerve involved.

The physical examination evaluates sensibility alterations, muscle power, range of motion, grip strength, and tendon reflexes. Increased pressure over an entrapped nerve, or its irritation by tapping or stretching, is reflected by paresthesia (sensation of electrical shock) in its autonomous zone and possibly by limitation of motion because of pain. Individuals with compression neuropathies show different patterns of loss and recovery than individuals with lacerations. They may have normal two-point discrimination but abnormal light-touch/deep-pressure recognition. Semmes-Weinstein monofilament testing can be indicated in these cases. Provocative tests are helpful to induce clinical symptoms; these include, for example, the tourniquet, Phalen's or reverse Phalen's, elbow flexion, and Adson's tests. Nerve percussion tests are performed distal to proximal and then directly over the area of a sensitive cutaneous or major mixed nerve. Testing of Tinel's sign should be reserved for regenerating nerves to document the progress and speed of axon regeneration after repair of a lacerated nerve or decompression of a severely compressed nerve.

The electroneurodiagnostic examination includes electromyographic (needle and cutaneous) examinations, which evaluate only motor unit potentials, and motor and sensory nerve conduction studies. These procedures assess only the largest, most heavily myelinated axons; the lightly myelinated and unmyelinated axons that transmit pain are not directly evaluated. A fundamental point is that, regardless of the cause of nerve damage, the electrodiagnostic studies essentially can detect only two types of pathophysiology of the peripheral nerve system fibers: (1) axon loss (axonotmetic lesion), which is manifested as conduction failure, and (2) focal demyelination (neuropraxic lesion), which can cause either conduction slowing or conduction block, depending on the severity of the process. *The severity of conduction slowing has no correlation with the severity of clinical symptoms,* such as weakness or static large-fiber sensory loss. If these are present, substantial amounts of either conduction block, axon loss, or a combination of both must be present.

Impairment Rating of Entrapment/Compression Neuropathies

Only individuals with an *objectively verifiable diagnosis* should qualify for a permanent impairment rating. The diagnosis is made not only on believable symptoms but, more important, on the presence of *positive clinical findings and loss of function.* The diagnosis should be documented by electromyography as well as sensory and motor nerve conduction studies. However, it is critical to understand that there is *no correlation* between the severity of conduction delay on nerve conduction velocity testing and the severity of either symptoms or, more important, impairment rating. The surgical findings of evidence of nerve compression and reactive hyperemia upon nerve release help confirm the diagnosis.

Postoperatively, a sufficient amount of time for optimal physiologic recovery and rehabilitation should elapse before an individual qualifies for permanent impairment rating should there be residual symptoms or clinical findings. Factors affecting nerve recovery in compression lesions include nerve fiber pathology, level of injury, duration of injury, and status of the end organs. Age is not a prognostic factor. Sensory function usually returns before motor function. High axonotmetic lesions may take 1 to 2 years for maximal recovery, whereas even lesions at the wrist may take 6 to 9 months for maximal recovery of nerve function. During the recovery time, individuals can experience some of the preoperative symptoms. An advancing Tinel's sign can be monitored and is a good prognostic sign.

The sensory deficits or pain, and/or the motor deficits and loss of power, are evaluated according to the impairment determination method described in Section 16.5b. Sensory impairments strictly due to lesions of digital nerves are evaluated according to Section 16.3. In compression neuropathies, additional impairment values are not given for decreased grip strength. In the absence of CRPS, additional impairment values are not given for decreased motion. In the presence of associated CRPS II (causalgia), the compression neuropathy is evaluated according to the principles of CRPS II described in Section 16.5e.

Example 16-61

History: A 30-year-old forest ranger fell in the woods and sustained a severe laceration on the medial side of the left elbow. Medical care was not immediately accessible. Surgical exploration 20 hours after injury showed wound contamination with foreign material and an exposed but not visibly damaged ulnar nerve. Despite appropriate antibiotic therapy, the man developed a wound infection that required operative debridements, followed ultimately by delayed primary closure. Symptoms of ulnar nerve dysfunction first appeared during the time of active infection and progressively increased over 3 weeks. Despite considerable difficulties, he refused surgical intervention.

Current Symptoms: One year later, back at work as a forest ranger, the man complains of burning pain and numbness on the medial side of the forearm radiating to the left little finger and ulnar half of the ring finger, which prevents repetitive and heavy work. He also reports hand weakness and clumsiness.

Physical Exam: Healed scar over the medial aspect of the left elbow; normal range of motion of all joints of the extremity; difficulty in crossing and snapping the fingers; loss of synchronism of MP and IP joint flexion (MP joint did not flex until all IP joint flexion was completed); atrophy of the hypothenar eminence and of the interosseous muscles; skin atrophy and decreased fingerprint pattern involving the little finger; two-point discrimination greater than 20 mm with no sharp-dull discrimination in the little finger and ulnar half of the ring finger; positive percussion test over ulnar nerve on medial side of elbow; and no muscle function in the flexor carpi ulnaris, flexor digitorum profundus to the little finger, adductor pollicis, or hypothenar eminence on manual testing.

Clinical Studies: Radiograms were negative, both initially and at follow-up. Complete loss of sensory and motor function in the ulnar nerve distal to the elbow were confirmed by electrodiagnostic studies.

Diagnosis: Ulnar nerve entrapment at the elbow secondary to scarring.

Analysis:
   Sensory deficit calculation:
   1. Severity of sensory deficit or pain: 100% (grade 0) (Table 16-10a).
   2. Maximum upper extremity impairment due to sensory deficit of the ulnar nerve (above mid-forearm): 7% (Table 16-15).
   3. *Multiply* the maximum upper extremity impairment for sensory deficit of the ulnar nerve (7%) by the severity of sensory deficit (100%) to obtain impairment of the upper extremity due to sensory deficit of the ulnar nerve, or 7%.

   Motor deficit calculation:
   1. Severity of motor deficit: 100% (grade 0) (Table 16-11a).
   2. Maximum upper extremity impairment due to motor deficit of the ulnar nerve (above mid-forearm): 46% (Table 16-15).
   3. *Multiply* the maximum upper extremity impairment for motor deficit of the ulnar nerve (46%) by the severity of motor deficit (100%) to obtain impairment of the upper extremity due to motor deficit of the ulnar nerve, or 46%.

Impairment Rating: *Combine* 7% upper extremity sensory deficit with 46% upper extremity motor deficit (Combined Values Chart, p. 604) to obtain 50% upper extremity impairment resulting from ulnar nerve dysfunction. Note that the maximum upper extremity impairment value (50%) due to *combined complete motor and sensory deficits* of the ulnar nerve is also listed in the far right column of Table 16-15. 50% upper extremity impairment corresponds to 30% whole person impairment (Table 16-3).

Carpal Tunnel Syndrome

The carpal tunnel syndrome (CTS) is the most common of nerve compression lesions and involves the median nerve at the volar aspect of the wrist. There are many presentations of CTS. Pain and paresthesias in the median nerve distribution of the hand are the usual symptoms. Pain may radiate proximally. Nocturnal paresthesias, relieved by shaking the hand, are frequently reported and can be the only symptom in the earliest stages of nerve pathology. True sensory disturbances and muscle atrophy represent later stages, when axonotmesis with axonal degeneration is also present. The symptoms, signs, and findings may include sensory or autonomic disturbances of the radial 3½ digits, weakness or atrophy of the thenar muscles, a positive percussion sign at the wrist, presence of Phalen's sign, and motor and sensory electroneuromyographic abnormalities. Not all symptoms are necessarily present in any one case. In isolated involvement of the recurrent branch of the median nerve, there is weakness of thumb abduction and thenar atrophy without any sensory disturbance in the hand. Sensitivity to cold may be a major presenting symptom of CTS. Certain cases may be associated with reflex dystrophy (CRPS I). It has also been reported that 5% of individuals with CTS may have normal electrophysiologic studies.

If, after an *optimal recovery time* following surgical decompression, an individual continues to complain of pain, paresthesias, and/or difficulties in performing certain activities, three possible scenarios can be present:

1. Positive clinical findings of median nerve dysfunction and electrical conduction delay(s): the impairment due to residual CTS is rated according to the sensory and/or motor deficits as described earlier.
2. Normal sensibility and opposition strength with abnormal sensory and/or motor latencies or abnormal EMG testing of the thenar muscles: a residual CTS is still present, and an impairment rating not to exceed 5% of the upper extremity may be justified.
3. Normal sensibility (two-point discrimination and Semmes-Weinstein monofilament testing), opposition strength, and nerve conduction studies: there is no objective basis for an impairment rating.

16.5e Complex Regional Pain Syndromes (CRPS), Reflex Sympathetic Dystrophy (CRPS I), and Causalgia (CRPS II)

The hallmark of these syndromes is a characteristic burning pain that is present without stimulation or movement, that occurs beyond the territory of a single peripheral nerve, and that is disproportionate to the inciting event. The pain is associated with specific clinical findings, including signs of vasomotor and sudomotor dysfunction and, later, trophic changes of all tissues from skin to bone.

Sympathetic nervous system dysfunction was thought to be involved in the generation of the symptoms and signs; hence, the term *reflex sympathetic dystrophy (RSD)*. Causalgia was considered similar to RSD except, unlike RSD, it followed a lesion of a peripheral nerve, either of a major mixed nerve in the proximal extremity (major causalgia) or of a purely sensory branch more distally (minor causalgia). A recent reconsideration of these syndromes has generated new terminology and ideas concerning the underlying pathophysiology. The International Association for the Study of Pain has proposed the term *complex regional pain syndromes*, which has replaced the term *RSD* with *CRPS I* and *causalgia* with *CRPS II*. The most important difference from earlier opinions is that sympathetic dysfunction is not assumed to be the underlying basis for the symptoms and signs of CRPS. It is felt that sympathetically maintained pain is not an essential component of CRPS, as it may be present in a variety of painful conditions, including or independent of CRPS. *Contrary to previous suggestions, regional sympathetic blockade has no role in the diagnosis of CRPS.*

Since a subjective complaint of pain is the hallmark of these conditions, and many of the associated physical signs and radiologic findings can be the result of disuse, the differential diagnosis is extensive; it includes somatoform pain disorder, somatoform conversion disorder, factitious disorder, and malingering. Consequently, the approach to the diagnosis of these syndromes should be conservative and based on objective findings. The criteria listed in Table 16-16 predicate a diagnosis of CRPS upon a preponderance of objective findings that can be identified during a standard physical examination and demonstrated by radiologic techniques. At least eight of these findings must be present concurrently for a diagnosis of CRPS. Signs are objective evidence of disease perceptible to the examiner, as opposed to symptoms, which are subjective sensations of the individual.

Table 16-16 Objective Diagnostic Criteria for CRPS (RSD and causalgia)

Local clinical signs

Vasomotor changes:
- Skin color: mottled or cyanotic
- Skin temperature: cool
- Edema

Sudomotor changes:
- Skin dry or overly moist

Trophic changes:
- Skin texture: smooth, nonelastic
- Soft tissue atrophy: especially in fingertips
- Joint stiffness and decreased passive motion
- Nail changes: blemished, curved, talonlike
- Hair growth changes: fall out, longer, finer

Radiographic signs

- Radiographs: trophic bone changes, osteoporosis
- Bone scan: findings consistent with CRPS

Interpretation:

≥ 8   Probable CRPS
< 8   No CRPS

Modified from Ensalada LH. Complex regional pain syndrome. In: Brigham CR, ed. *The Guides Casebook.* Chicago, Ill: American Medical Association; 1999:14.

CRPS I (RSD) Impairment Determination

In CRPS I, neither the initiating causative factor nor the symptoms involve a specific peripheral nerve structure or territory. The impairment determination is derived as follows:

1. Rate the upper extremity impairment resulting from *loss of motion* of each individual joint involved (Section 16.4).
2. Rate the upper extremity impairment resulting from sensory *deficits and pain* according to the grade that best describes the severity of interference with activities of daily living as described in Table 16-10a. Use clinical judgment to select the appropriate severity grade and the appropriate percentage from within the range shown in each grade. The maximum value is not automatically applied. The value selected represents the upper extremity impairment. *A nerve value multiplier is not used.*
3. *Combine* the upper extremity value for loss of joint motion (step 1) and pain and sensory deficits (step 2) to determine the upper extremity impairment due to CRPS I (Combined Values Chart, p. 604).
4. *Convert* the upper extremity impairment to whole person impairment by using Table 16-3.

In contrast to CRPS II, impairment values for sensory and motor deficits of a specific nerve structure cannot be applied. No additional impairment is assigned for decreased pinch or grasp strength. The impairment rating method described for sensory deficits due to lesions of digital nerves is not applied in CRPS.

CRPS II (Causalgia) Impairment Determination

In CRPS II, a specific sensory or mixed nerve structure is involved. The impairment determination is derived as follows:

1. Rate the upper extremity impairment due to *loss of motion* of each individual joint involved (Section 16.4).
2. Rate the upper extremity impairment resulting from *sensory deficits and pain* of the injured nerves according to the determination methods described in Section 16.5b and Table 16-10a. Use clinical judgment to select the appropriate severity grade and the appropriate percentage from within the range shown in each grade.

3. Rate the upper extremity impairment resulting from *motor deficits and loss of power* of the injured nerve according to the determination method described in Section 16.5b and Table 16-11a.

4. *Combine* the upper extremity impairment percents for loss of joint motion (step 1), pain and sensory deficits (step 2), and motor deficits (step 3), if present, to determine the upper extremity impairment (Combined Values Chart, p. 604). Severe CRPS II may result in complete loss of function and in impairment of the extremity as great as 100%.

5. *Convert* the upper extremity impairment to whole person impairment by using Table 16-3.

No additional impairment is given for decreased pinch or grip strength. The impairment rating method described for sensory deficits resulting from lesions of digital nerves is not applied in CRPS.

16.6 Impairment of the Upper Extremities Due to Vascular Disorders

The criteria for evaluating Raynaud's phenomena and other extremity impairments due to peripheral vascular disorders resulting from diseases of the arteries, veins, or lymphatics is discussed in Chapter 4, The Cardiovascular System: Systemic and Pulmonary Arteries, Section 4.3.

Table 16-17 provides a similar classification of impairments due to peripheral vascular disease. Physical signs of vascular damage must be present and are the primary determinants in placing the examinee into one of these categories. Raynaud's phenomenon consists of localized blanching of one or more fingers, followed by a period of cyanosis, followed by erythema. Pain on exposure to cold or generalized paleness of the fingers on exposure to cold does not in itself indicate Raynaud's phenomenon. When amputation because of peripheral vascular disease is involved, the impairment resulting from amputation should be evaluated according to Section 16.2 and combined with the appropriate value in Table 16-17 by means of the Combined Values Chart (p. 604).

It is important to differentiate symptoms of Raynaud's phenomenon on the basis of obstructive physiology from those occurring because of vasoreactivity. Individuals with obstructive physiology will often experience symptoms more frequently and with a greater degree of severity. Establish the presence of obstructive physiology by objective testing. Arterial pressure ratios between the affected digits and the brachial pressure (finger/brachial index) are easily performed. A ratio of < 0.8 suggests obstructive physiology, even if Raynaud's symptoms are not present. Obstructive physiology can also be established by the use of cutaneous laser Doppler flowmetry. This technique is established and can reliably assess microcirculation performance and real-time changes in skin blood flow.

Impairment of 0% to 9% is indicated by documented Raynaud's phenomenon with obstructive physiology (as documented by finger-brachial indices of less than 0.8 or low digital temperatures with decreased laser Doppler signals that do not normalize with warming of affected digits) that *completely responds* to lifestyle changes and/or medical therapy.

Impairment of 10% to 39% is indicated by symptoms of Raynaud's phenomenon with obstructive physiology (as documented by finger-brachial indices of less than 0.8 or low digital temperatures with decreased laser Doppler signals that do not normalize with warming of affected digits) that *incompletely responds* to lifestyle changes and medical therapy.

Example 16-62

Exam: A 45-year-old woman had had Raynaud's phenomenon from scleroderma for 9 years. She had incomplete healing of finger ulcerations with conservative measures and prazosin hydrochloride. Physical examination showed ulcerations on the tips of the index and ring fingers of the right hand. Autoamputation of the distal half of the distal phalanges of the index and ring fingers on the left hand was noted. The finger/brachial ratio was 0.6, and laser Doppler signals were consistent with microcirculatory impairment.

—

Table 16-17 Impairment of the Upper Extremity Due to Peripheral Vascular Disease

Symptoms	Upper Extremity Impairment %				
	Class 1 (0%-9%)	Class 2 (10%-39%)	Class 3 (40%-69%)	Class 4 (70%-89%)	Class 5 (90%-100%)
Claudication	None	Intermittent with severe use	Intermittent with moderate use	Intermittent with mild use	Persistent
Pain at rest	None	None	None	Intermittent	Severe and constant
Edema	Transient	Persistent and moderate	Marked	Marked	Marked
Signs of vascular damage	Loss of pulses; minimal loss of subcutaneous tissue of fingertips; arterial calcifications on x-ray; asymptomatic dilation of veins or arteries not requiring surgery; no decreased activity	Healed painless amputation stump of one digit with persistent vascular disease or healed ulcer	Healed amputation stump of two or more digits with persistent vascular disease or superficial ulceration	Amputation of two or more digits of each extremity, or amputation at or above wrist of one extremity with persistent widespread or deep ulceration of one extremity	Amputation of all digits or amputation at or above the wrist of each extremity, with persistent vascular disease or widespread or deep ulcerations of both extremities
Raynaud's phenomenon	Raynaud's symptoms with or without obstructive physiology (as documented by finger brachial indices of < 0.8 or low digital temperatures with decreased laser Doppler signals that do not normalize with warming of affected digits) that completely responds to lifestyle changes and/or medical therapy	Raynaud's phenomena with obstructive physiology (as documented by finger/brachial indices of < 0.8 or low digital temperatures with decreased laser Doppler signals that do not normalize with warming of affected digits) that incompletely responds to lifestyle changes and/or medical therapy			
Medication control	Good	Good	Partial	Partial	Poor

Analysis:

Left upper extremity: 55% impairment of the upper extremity (middle range of class 3) due to peripheral vascular disease; 5% of the upper extremity due to finger amputations (see Section 16.2 and Figure 16-5). Combining these values yields 57% impairment of the left upper extremity, or 34% whole person impairment.

Right upper extremity: 25% of the upper extremity (middle range of class 2), or 15% whole person impairment.

Impairment Rating: *Combining* 34% with 15% gives 44% whole person impairment.

16.7 Impairment of the Upper Extremities Due to Other Disorders

Conditions not previously described that can contribute to impairments of the hand and upper extremity include bone and joint disorders (Section 16.7a), presence of resection or implant arthroplasty (Section 16.7b), musculotendinous disorders (Section 16.7c), and tendinitis (Section 16.7d), and loss of strength (Section 16.8). The severity of impairment due to these disorders is rated separately according to Tables 16-19 through 16-30 and then multiplied by the relative maximum value of the unit involved as specified in Table 16-18. Appropriate impairment percents are combined with other impairment percents by means of the Combined Values Chart (p. 604).

Table 16-18 Maximum Impairment Values for the Digits, Hand, Wrist, Elbow, and Shoulder Due to Disorders of Specific Joints or Units*

Units and Joints	Unit	Hand	Upper Extremity	Whole Person
Shoulder				
Glenohumeral	—	—	60	36
Acromioclavicular	—	—	25	15
Sternoclavicular	—	—	5	3
Elbow				
Entire elbow	—	—	70	42
Ulnohumeral	—	—	50	30
Proximal radioulnar	—	—	20	12
Wrist				
Entire wrist	—	—	60	36
Radiocarpal	—	—	40	24
Distal radioulnar	—	—	20	12
Proximal carpal row	—	—	30	18
Entire hand	—	100	90	54
Thumb				
Entire thumb	100	40	36	22
CMC	60	24	22	13
MP	15	6	5	3
IP	25	10	9	5
Index and middle				
Entire finger	100	20	18	11
MP	50	10	9	5
PIP	30	6	5	3
DIP	20	4	4	2
Ring or little				
Entire finger	100	10	9	5
MP	50	5	5	3
PIP	30	3	3	2
DIP	20	2	2	1

* Each value is related to the next larger units and the whole person

Skin disorders, including disfigurement, scars, and skin grafts, are evaluated using criteria in Chapter 8, The Skin.

Impairments from the disorders considered in this section under the category of "other disorders" are usually estimated by using other impairment evaluation criteria. *The criteria described in this section should be used only when the other criteria have not adequately encompassed the extent of the impairments.* Some of the conditions described in this section can be concurrent with each other and with decreased motion because they share overlapping pathomechanics. The evaluator must have good understanding of pathomechanics of deformities and apply proper judgment to avoid duplication of impairment ratings.

Table 16-18 shows the maximum values for the digits, hand, wrist, elbow, and shoulder resulting from the conditions described in this section and relates the percents to larger units and the whole person. Note that the relative upper extremity impairment values for the shoulder, elbow, and wrist are the same for decreased motion (Section 16.4) and "other disorders" (Table 16-18) but differ from those for amputation at similar levels (Table 16-4). The values for individual joints of both the thumb and fingers listed in Table 16-18 have been assigned on a 100% digit unit scale and differ from those listed for amputation (Table 16-4) and range of motion (Section 16.4). The hand impairment value of each digit is the same throughout this entire chapter. *If more than one joint of a specific digit is affected by impairments due to "other disorders" listed in this section, the applicable joint impairment ratings are added only when the joints involved have a full range of motion. Otherwise, the joint impairment values are combined using the Combined Values Chart.*

16.7a Bone and Joint Deformities

If the same unit presents several findings, the following rules must be followed to avoid duplication of impairments. In the digits, wrist, and elbow, manifestations of joint translocation can include lateral deviation, rotational deformity (digit), and/or subluxation or dislocation in any combination. The impairment values due to these findings cannot be combined, and only the finding with the highest impairment value is rated. Limited motion impairment is rated according to Section 16.4 and can be appropriately combined with impairments due to "other disorders" listed in this section, except with those due to joint swelling from synovial hypertrophy, persistent joint subluxation or dislocation, and musculotendinous disorders (Section 16.7c). Joint instability impairment values can be combined with other appropriate impairment values, including decreased motion, but not with arthroplasty. Joint swelling due to synovial hypertrophy is rated only when no other findings are present. Joint crepitation is not rated separately because other findings, such as those listed above, are more reliable indicators of the severity of the same arthritic process.

Table 16-19 Joint Impairment From Synovial Hypertrophy

Description of Joint Swelling	% Joint Impairment*
Mild: visibly apparent	10
Moderate: palpably apparent	20
Severe: greater than 10% increase in size	30

* Multiply by the relative value of the joint (Table 16-18) to determine the joint impairment.

Modified from Swanson AB, Mays JD, Yamauchi Y. A rheumatoid arthritis evaluation record for the upper extremity. *Surg Clin North Am.* 1968;48:1003-1013.

Table 16-20 Digit Impairment From Active Ulnar or Radial Deviation

Deviation	% Digit Impairment*
Mild: < 10°	10
Moderate: 10°-30°	20
Severe: > 30°	30

* Multiply by the relative hand value of the digit (Table 16-18) to determine the hand impairment.

Modified from Swanson AB, Mays JD, Yamauchi Y. A rheumatoid arthritis evaluation record for the upper extremity. *Surg Clin North Am.* 1968;48:1003-1013.

Joint Swelling Due to Synovial Hypertrophy

Synovial hypertrophy is a sign of an inflammatory arthritic process that can progress through varying the manifestations listed above, including decreased motion. If synovial hypertrophy is the *only finding,* the joint impairment is rated according to Table 16-19 and multiplied by the relative maximum value of the joint involved (Table 16-18). It *cannot* be combined with impairment due to decreased joint motion or other findings.

Digit Lateral Deviation

The deviation from longitudinal alignment of each of the digital joints is measured in degrees during maximum active extension. Since lateral deviation at any level affects the longitudinal arch of the digit, the deviation impairment value is applied to the entire digit. If lateral deviation is the only impairment, the severity of digit impairment (Table 16-20) is multiplied by the relative hand value of the digit (Table 16-18) to determine the hand impairment. The lateral deviation impairment percent can be *combined* with other impairments of the same digits, including motion, according to the rules outlined on page 499 (Combined Values Chart, p. 604).

Example 16-63

Exam: 35° ulnar deviation at the PIP joint of the little finger after a ligamentous injury. Range of motion at that joint is 20° extension lag through 30° flexion.

Analysis: Ulnar deviation is classified as "severe" and corresponds to 30% (Table 16-20).

Motion impairment of the little finger PIP joint: $I_E\% = 7\%$; $I_F\% = 42\%$ (Figure 16-23); 7% + 42% = 49% motion impairment.

Impairment Rating: From the Combined Values Chart (p. 604), 49% combined with 30% is 64% impairment of the little finger, which is considered to be 6% impairment of the hand and 5% impairment of the upper extremity (Tables 16-2 and 16-3).

Digit Rotational Deformity

Rotational deformity of any segment of a digit can result either from rotational *malalignment of a metacarpal or phalanx following a fracture or from imbalances of the joint* as often seen in rheumatoid arthritis (eg, pronation deformity of the index finger). Rotational deformity of the distal, middle, or proximal phalanx is measured during maximum active flexion of the digit. Malrotation of the normal axial alignment of any segment of a digit in either pronation or supination affects the function of the entire digit, and the impairment percent is applied to the entire (100%) digit value.

The digit impairment percent due to rotational deformity (Table 16-21) is multiplied by the relative hand value of the digit (Table 16-18) to obtain the hand impairment. The rotational deformity impairment can be *combined* with other impairments of the same digit, including motion, according to the rules outlined on page 499.

Table 16-21 Digit Impairment From Rotational Deformity

Digit Rotational Deformity	% Digit Impairment*
Mild: < 15°	20
Moderate: 15°-30°	40
Severe: > 30°	60

* Multiply the relative hand value of the digit (Table 16-18) to determine the hand impairment percent.

Adapted from Swanson AB, Mays JD, Yamauchi Y. A rheumatoid arthritis evaluation record for the upper extremity. *Surg Clin North Am.* 1968;48:1003-1013.

Table 16-22 Joint Impairment From Persistent Subluxation or Dislocation

Severity of Joint Subluxation or Dislocation	% Joint Impairment*
Mild: can be completely reduced manually	20
Moderate: cannot be completely reduced manually	40
Severe: cannot be reduced	60

* Multiply by the relative value of the joint (Table 16-18) to determine the joint impairment.

Modified from Swanson AB, Mays JD, Yamauchi Y. A rheumatoid arthritis evaluation record for the upper extremity. *Surg Clin North* Am. 1968;48:1003-1013.

Example 16-64

Exam: A 20° pronation deformity of the index finger is present after a healed fracture of the second metacarpal.

Analysis: According to Table 16-21, this is a "moderate" deformity and corresponds to 40% digit impairment. Relative value of the entire index finger to the hand is 20% (Table 16-18).

Impairment Rating: Hand impairment is 40% × 20% = 8%; this is equivalent to 7% impairment of the upper extremity (Table 16-2).

Persistent Joint Subluxation or Dislocation

Persistent joint subluxation or dislocation usually results in restricted motion. If there is no restricted motion, the values shown in Table 16-22 are multiplied by the relative value of the joint (Table 16-18) to determine the joint impairment. If the same joint presents other findings, the rules outlined on page 499 must be followed to avoid duplication of impairments.

Instability and translocation of the wrist and shoulder joints are evaluated according to methods described on pages 502 and 503.

Joint Passive Mediolateral Instability

Mediolateral laxity or instability is tested by passive manipulation in various positions of flexion and extension, and the maximum medial or lateral joint angulation is measured in degrees. The severity of mediolateral joint instability is rated according to the excess number of angulation degrees compared to the opposite, "normal" side (Table 16-23). If both sides are involved, a comparison to accepted normal average values is made. The percentage of impairment is then multiplied by the relative value of the joint (Table 16-18) to determine the joint impairment. Carpal and shoulder instabilities are discussed on pages 502 and 503.

If the same joint presents other findings, the rules outlined on page 499 must be followed to avoid duplication of impairments.

Table 16-23 Joint Impairment Due to Excessive Passive Mediolateral Instability

Severity of Excessive Passive Mediolateral Joint Deviation Degrees Compared to Normal Control	% Joint Impairment*
Mild: < 10°	20
Moderate: 10°-20°	40
Severe: > 20°	60

* Multiply by the relative value of the joint (Table 16-18) to determine the joint impairment.

Modified from Swanson AB, Mays JD, Yamauchi Y. A rheumatoid arthritis evaluation recorded for the upper extremity. *Surg Clin North Am.* 1968;48:1003-1013.

Table 16-24 Wrist and Elbow Joint Impairment From Excessive Active Mediolateral Deviation

Severity of Excessive Active Mediolateral Deviation	% Joint Impairment*
Mild: < 20°	10
Moderate: 20°-30°	20
Severe: > 30°	30

* Multiply by the relative value of the joint (Table 16-18) to determine the upper extremity impairment.

Modified from Swanson AB, Mays JD, Yamauchi Y. A rheumatoid arthritis evaluation record for the upper extremity. *Surg Clin North Am.* 1968;48:1003-1013.

Example 16-65

Physical Exam: Passive radial deviation of the MP joint of the thumb of 60°, compared to 30° on the normal side.

Analysis: The difference in angulation of 30° is graded as severe and represents a 60% joint impairment (Table 16-23). The MP joint represents 15% of the thumb ray unit (Table 16-18).

Impairment Rating: The thumb impairment is 16% × 15% = 9%; this is equivalent to 4% hand impairment (Table 16-1) and 4% upper extremity impairment (Table 16-2).

Wrist Elbow Joint Active Radial and Ulnar Deviations

Active radial or ulnar deviation of the wrist or elbow is measured in maximum active extension of the joint. The severity of lateral deviation is rated according to the excess number of angulation degrees compared to the normal opposite side (Table 16-24). The percentage of impairment is multiplied by the relative value of the joint (Table 16-18) to obtain the upper extremity impairment.

If the same joint presents other findings, the rules outlined on page 499 must be followed to avoid duplication of impairments.

Example 16-66

Exam: A displaced supracondylar fracture of the humerus healed in a 10° cubitus varus deformity. The elbow range of motion was normal. The opposite, normal elbow measured 15° cubitus valgus. The radiograms showed good bone healing, with incomplete angular reduction.

Analysis: Excessive medial angulation on full active elbow extension is 10° (varus) + 15° (valgus angle lost) = 25°. A 25° excessive ulnar angulation represents a "moderate," or 20% joint impairment (Table 16-24). The elbow joint's relative functional value is 70% of the upper extremity (Table 16-18).

Impairment Rating: Impairment of the upper extremity is 20% × 70%, or 14%.

Carpal Instability

Carpal instability patterns are classified as mild, moderate, or severe. The classification is usually based on the roentgenographic findings listed in Table 16-25. A mild carpal instability exists also when a ligament tear has been diagnosed by arthrogram, arthroscopy, or MRI, even though the static roentgenographic findings may be normal. Certain individuals may have wrist pain and loss of strength related to a dynamic or nondissociative carpal instability that cannot be measured by changes of angles on static roentgenograms. Symptoms of nondissociative wrist instability are painful clicking and clunking with activities of daily living. The radiocarpal joint represents 40% of the upper extremity (Table 16-18). Therefore, the grades of mild (20%), moderate (40%), and severe (60%) impairment represent upper extremity impairments of 8%, 16%, and 24%, respectively. Only one category of severity of carpal instability impairment is selected, based on the greatest severity of the

Table 16-25 Upper Extremity Impairment Due to Carpal Instability Patterns

Roentgenographic Findings*	% of Upper Extremity Impairment		
	Mild (8%)	Moderate (16%)	Severe (24%)
Radiolunate angle†	11°-20°	21°-30°	>30°
Scapholunate angle	61°-70°	71°-80°	>80°
Scapholunate gap	>3 mm	>5 mm	>8 mm
Triquetrolunate stepoff	>1 mm	>2 mm	>3 mm
Ulnar translation‡	Mild	Moderate	Severe

* Clenched fist neutral PA views.

† A positive angle (lunate extension) represents a DISI deformity A negative angle (lunate flexion) represents a VISI deformity

‡ See text for description.

Adapted from Lichtman DM, Alexander AH, eds. *The Wrist and Its Disorders*. 2nd ed. Philadelphia, Pa: WB Saunders; 1997:chaps 7, 12, 35.

Figure 16-51 Techniques for Measuring the Scaphoid (S), Lunate Axis (L), and Long Axis of the Radius (R) and Corresponding Angles

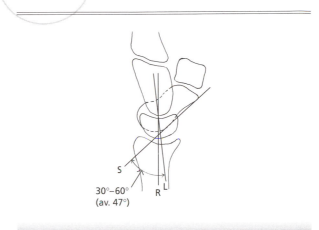

Source: David M. Lichtman, Fort Worth, Texas.

roentgenographic findings. The severity categories *cannot* be added or combined. The selected upper extremity impairment value may be *combined only with limited wrist motion*. Pain and decreased strength are not rated separately.

The *scapholunate* and *radiolunate angles* are measured on a lateral radiograph taken with the fist forcefully clenched (stressed view) and the wrist in neutral flexion/extension and lateral deviation. Lines are drawn on the film parallel to the long axis of the radius, through the long axis of the scaphoid (palmar surface), and a line representing the long axis of the lunate (a line perpendicular to the line connecting the two distal poles [Figure 16-51]). The angles between these lines are measured. The normal radiolunate relationship should be less than 10° of either volar or dorsal lunate angulation. The scapholunate angle ranges from 30° to 60° (average of 47°). The *triquetrolunate stepoff* is measured on the neutral posteroanterior (PA) view and represents proximal or ulnar translation of the triquetrum. The *scapholunate gap* is best profiled on a neutral PA view with the ulnar aspect of the hand elevated 10° to 15° or on a neutral anteroposterior (AP) view.

Ulnar translation may occur secondary to injury or arthritis. It is measured on the neutral PA view with the fist forcefully clenched. Normally, greater than 50% of the lunate overlies the ulnar border of the distal radius. As ulnar translation becomes more severe, progressively less of the lunate overlies the radius. The grades of severity of upper extremity impairment are classified as *mild* (8%), wherein less than 50% of the lunate overlies the distal radius ulnar

border; *moderate* (16%), wherein less than 25% of the lunate overlies the distal radius ulnar border; and *severe* (24%), wherein the lunate is displaced ulnarly off the radius (Table 16-25).

Example 16-67

Exam: Roentgenographic evidence of a scapholunate angle of 65°, a radiolunate angle of 5°, and a scapholunate gap of 6 mm.

Analysis: The greatest impairment is "moderate" (16%) for the scapholunate gap (Table 16-25).

Impairment Rating: Impairment for carpal instability is 16% of the upper extremity.

Shoulder Instability

Shoulder instability, recurrent joint subluxation, or dislocation usually occurs when the integrity of either the glenoid labrum and/or of the surrounding capsuloligamentous and musculotendinous structures becomes compromised following either one or more acute traumatic dislocations, repetitive microtrauma, or arthritic conditions. Predisposing factors can include abnormal contour or alignment of the joint itself from either congenital or posttraumatic origins; congenital laxity of the capsuloligamentous structures (eg, Ehlers-Danlos syndrome); or musculotendinous imbalances. Shoulder instability can be classified by direction (anterior, posterior, or inferior), etiology (traumatic or atraumatic), or volition (voluntary or involuntary).

Shoulder instability, recurrent subluxation, or dislocation *must be adequately documented* through a complete medical history, physical examination, and radiographic findings. Magnetic resonance imaging (MRI), arthroscopy, and examination under anesthesia may be useful components of the evaluation. An individual's complaint of feeling or fearing that a joint is "popping" or "going out of place" without adequate clinical findings is not a basis for permanent impairment rating.

True shoulder instability must be differentiated from hyperlaxity. *Laxity* refers to the normal sliding of the humeral head in the glenoid socket. *Instability* is the inability to maintain a normal relationship between the head and the socket and can be manifested by pain and muscular defense induced by provocative movements in the direction of the instability. If a provocative test shows increased humeral head motion without reproducing the individual's symptoms, hyperlaxity instead of instability is considered to be present and no permanent impairment rating is assigned. The impingement-type shoulder pain must be differentiated from neck pain or radiating pain. The "dead arm" syndrome caused by stretching of the brachial plexus can be transiently experienced by certain athletes (eg, pitchers during the act of throwing) due to humeral head subluxation, but in itself it is not diagnostic of shoulder instability.

The shoulder examination includes range-of-motion measurements and laxity and provocative tests. The tests can be difficult to interpret if the individual is not fully relaxed, as muscular contraction can temporarily stabilize a pathologically unstable shoulder. Since a certain amount of shoulder laxity is normal, it is critical for the examiner to determine whether the *physical findings reproduce the individual's symptoms.* Comparison to the healthy side is also helpful.

The *sulcus sign* is elicited by applying downward traction on the humerus and tests the inferior translation of the humeral head. A positive sign may merely be an indication of hyperlaxity and should not be given too much significance unless the maneuver clearly reproduces the individual's discomfort or sense of instability.

The *loading posterior/anterior drawer test* is performed with the individual supine and the shoulder in neutral rotation, 60° abduction, and 30° flexion. One hand stabilizes the extremity in neutral rotation, and the other applies a posteriorly directed force to subluxate the shoulder posteriorly. The position of the examiner's hands is reversed to reproduce the maneuver applying an anteriorly directed force. Note that in a clinical setting, the examiner can usually evaluate the severity of instability without inducing a shoulder dislocation.

The posterior/anterior glenohumeral translation has been classified as follows:
   Trace: Small movement of the humeral head.
   Class I: Humeral head rides up the glenoid but not over the rim.
   Class II: Humeral head subluxes over the glenoid rim but reduces spontaneously in position when the axial load is withdrawn.
   Class III: Humeral head frankly dislocates over the glenoid rim and remains dislocated with removal of force.

The apprehension and relocation tests are best carried out with the individual in a supine position. The *anterior apprehension test* is performed by applying external rotation as the shoulder is held in 90° abduction. If the test is positive, the individual fears that the humeral head will slide out, causing pain. Muscular defense against the motion is usually present. However, presence of pain alone is not necessarily diagnostic of instability. The *anterior relocation test* (Jobe's) is performed by applying a posteriorly directed force to the proximal humerus while the shoulder is in 90° abduction and external rotation with the individual supine. This posterior stabilizing force should reduce the humeral head and relieve any apprehension of anterior instability.

Shoulder instability patterns are based on the parameters listed in Table 16-26 and can be classified as occult instability, instability with a subluxating humeral head, and instability with a dislocating humeral head. The shoulder representing 60% of the upper extremity (Table 16-18), the patterns of occult (10%), subluxating (20%), and dislocating (40%) instabilities represent upper extremity impairments of 6%, 12%, and 24%, respectively. *This value may be combined only with impairments due to decreased motion (Section 16.4). Pain and decreased muscle strength are not rated separately.*

Table 16-26 Upper Extremity Impairment Due to Symptomatic Shoulder Instability Patterns

Parameters	% Upper Extremity Impairment Due to Symptomatic Shoulder Instability Patterns		
	Occult (6%)	With Subluxating Humeral Head (12%)	With Dislocating Humeral Head (24%)
Confirmed history of acute trauma	No	Yes	Yes
Consistent relationship of symptoms with specific activities/motion ranges	Yes	Yes	Yes
Clinical symptoms reproducible on shoulder stability testing	Yes/No	Yes	Yes
Glenohumeral translation class	I + II	II	III
Demonstrable etiological anatomic lesion	No	Yes	Yes

Compiled by EG McFarland, MD, Baltimore, Maryland.

Example 16-68

History: A 30-year-old athletic male sustained a third episode of anterior shoulder subluxation while delivering an overhead serve during a tennis match. He reported that he had sustained two previous episodes of shoulder subluxation while playing tennis at ages 18 and 25.

Current Symptoms: One year later he reports decreased ability to abduct and externally rotate his shoulder due to pain and a feeling that it is going to "pop" out.

Exam: The shoulder active range of motion is 50° adduction, 130° abduction, 80° internal rotation, and 80° external rotation with normal flexion and extension. The tests for anterior instability, anterior apprehension, and anterior relocation (Jobe's) all are positive. The axial load test showed that the humeral head could be subluxated anteriorly over the glenoid rim, but reduced spontaneously in place when the force-load was withdrawn (class II glenohumeral translation). This maneuver reproduced the clinical symptoms. The shoulder radiogram was normal, but an MRI confirmed an anterior glenoid labrum tear. The man refuses surgery for personal reasons.

Analysis: According to Table 16-26, a class II humeral translation (subluxating head) with a history of previous trauma, consistent relationship of symptoms with specific motions, reproducible symptoms on clinical testing, and positive radiographic findings corresponds to 12% upper extremity impairment.

The upper extremity impairment due to decreased shoulder motion is found in Section 16.4: $I_{ADD}\% = 0\%$ and $I_{ABD}\% = 2\%$ (Figure 16-43); $I_{IR}\% = 0\%$ and $I_{ER}\% = 0\%$ (Figure 16-46). The upper extremity motion impairment is 2%.

Impairment Rating: The upper extremity impairments due to shoulder instability (12%) and decreased motion (2%) are *combined* (Combined Values Chart, p. 604) and equal 14% of the upper extremity, or 8% of the whole person (Table 16-3).

16.7b Arthroplasty

Resection arthroplasty of a joint may be carried out with or without implant replacement. Impairment ratings for the upper extremity following arthroplasty of specific joints are listed in Table 16-27 and reflect upgraded information.

In the presence of *decreased motion,* motion impairments are derived separately (Section 16.4) and *combined* with the arthroplasty impairment (Combined Values Chart, p. 604). If the same joint presents other findings, the rules outlined on page 499 must be followed to avoid duplication of impairments. However, impairment due to arthroplasty *cannot be combined* with impairments due to instability, subluxation, or dislocation.

After *arthrodesis* procedures, the impairment is based on the *ankylosis impairment* ($I_A\%$) for the corresponding angle of fusion (V) according to the guidelines in Section 16.4.

A severe symptomatic failure of an implant arthroplasty procedure (eg, symptomatic breakage or subluxation of the device) is given 100% of the joint value as listed in Table 16-18.

Impairments involving the resection of malignant tumors with reconstructive surgery including arthroplasty should receive individual consideration.

Table 16-27 Impairment of the Upper Extremity After Arthroplasty of Specific Bones or Joints

Level of Arthroplasty	% Impairment of Upper Extremity	
	Implant Arthroplasty	Resection Arthroplasty
Total shoulder	24	30
Distal clavicle (isolated)	—	10
Proximal clavicle (isolated)	—	3
Total elbow	28	35
Radial head (isolated)	8	10
Total wrist	24	—
Radiocarpal	16	—
Ulnar head (isolated)	8	10
Proximal row carpectomy	—	12
Carpal bone (isolated)	8	10
Radial styloid (isolated)	—	5
Thumb		
CMC	9	11
MP	2	3
IP	4	5
Index or middle finger		
MP	4	5
PIP	2	3
DIP	1	2
Ring or little finger		
MP	2	2
PIP	1	1
DIP	1	1

CMC: thumb carpometacarpal; IP: thumb interphalangeal; MP: metacarpophalangeal; PIP: proximal interphalangeal; DIP: distal interphalangeal.

Modified from Swanson AB, de Groot Swanson G. Principles and methods of impairment evaluation in the hand and upper extremity. In: Engelberg AE, ed. *Guides to the Evaluation of Permanent Impairment.* Third ed. Chicago, Ill: American Medical Association; 1989:47; prepared with the assistance of DM Lichtman, Fort Worth, Texas, and EG McFarland, Baltimore, Maryland.

Example 16-69

Exam: An individual with a total wrist (radiocarpal and distal radioulnar joints) replacement has 30° flexion and 20° extension, 0° radial deviation, and 30° ulnar deviation.

Analysis: Wrist implant arthroplasty = 24% impairment of the upper extremity (Table 16-27). The impairments of the upper extremity due to restricted motion are found in Figures 16-28 and 16-31:

$I_F\% = 5\%$; $I_E\% = 7\%$
$I_{RD}\% = 4\%$; $I_{UD}\% = 0\%$
$5\% + 7\% + 4\% = 16\%$

Impairment Rating: 24% *combined* with 16% = 36% upper extremity impairment (Combined Values Chart, p. 604).

Table 16-28 Digit Impairment Due to Intrinsic Tightness

Intrinsic Tightness Severity (Passive Flexion of PIP Joint With MP Joint Hyperextended)	% Digit Impairment*
Mild: PIP flexion 80°-60°	20
Moderate: PIP flexion 59°-20°	40
Severe: PIP flexion ≤ 20°	60

* Multiply by the relative hand value of the digit (Table 16-18) to determine the hand impairment.

Modified from Swanson AB, Mays JD, Yamauchi Y. A rheumatoid arthritis evaluation record for the upper extremity. *Surg Clin North* Am. 1968;48:1003-1013.

16.7c Musculotendinous Impairments
Intrinsic Tightness
Intrinsic tightness in the hand may be demonstrated by a test described by Bunnell. Hyperextension of the metacarpophalangeal (MP) joint in a normal hand still allows passive flexion of the proximal interphalangeal (PIP) joint. If the intrinsic muscles are tight or contracted, the available stretch of these muscles is taken up by the hyperextended position of the MP joint, and passive flexion of the PIP joint will be difficult. The digit impairment due to intrinsic tightness is rated according to Table 16-28 and multiplied by the relative hand value of the digit (Table 16-18) to derive the hand impairment value.

The impairment due to intrinsic tightness can be *combined* with other impairments of the same digit, *providing they do not share the same pathomechanics,* eg, in extensor tendon subluxation over the MP joint (Table 16-30). Intrinsic tightness impairment *cannot be combined* with that due to decreased motion at the MP or PIP joints.

Constrictive Tenosynovitis
The impairment percent due to constrictive tenosynovitis (Table 16-29) is multiplied by the relative hand value of the digit (Table 16-18) to derive its hand impairment. This impairment *may be combined* with other impairments of the digit (Combined Values Chart, p. 604) but *not* with decreased motion.

Table 16-29 Digit Impairment Due to Constrictive Tenosynovitis

Constrictive Tenosynovitis Severity	% Digit Impairment*
Mild: inconstant triggering during active range of motion	20
Moderate: constant triggering during active range of motion	40
Severe: constant triggering during passive range of motion	60

* Multiply by the relative hand value of the digit (Table 16-18) to determine the hand impairment.

Modified from Swanson AB, Mays JD, Yamauchi Y. A rheumatoid arthritis evaluation record for the upper extremity. *Surg Clin North Am.* 1968;48:1003-1013.

Table 16-30 Digit Impairment Due to Extensor Tendon Subluxation Over the MP Joint

Severity of Extensor Tendon Subluxation in Intermetacarpal Groove	% Digit Impairment*
Mild: tendon subluxation on MP joint flexion only	10
Moderate: reducible tendon subluxation	20
Severe: nonreducible tendon subluxation	30

* Multiply by the relative hand value of the digit (Table 16-18) to determine the hand impairment.

Modified from Swanson AB, Mays JD, Yamauchi Y. A rheumatoid arthritis evaluation record for the upper extremity. *Surg Clin North Am.* 1968;48:1003-1013.

Extensor Tendon Subluxation at the MP Joint of the Fingers

The digit impairment due to extensor tendon subluxation at the metacarpophalangeal (MP) joint (Table 16-30) is multiplied by the relative hand value of the digit (Table 16-18) to obtain its hand impairment value. It *cannot be combined* with impairment due to restricted motion at the MP joint or to other related manifestations of the same pathomechanical disturbance.

16.7d Tendinitis

Several syndromes involving the upper extremity are variously attributed to tendinitis, fasciitis, or epicondylitis. The most common of these are the stubborn conditions of the origins of the flexor and extensor muscles of the forearm where they attach to the medial and lateral epicondyles of the humerus. Although these conditions may be persistent for some time, they are not given a permanent impairment rating unless there is some other factor that must be considered.

If an individual has had tendon rupture or has undergone surgical release of the flexor or extensor origins or medial or lateral epicondylitis, or has had excision of the epicondyle, there may be some permanent weakness of grip as a result of the tendon rupture or the surgery. In this case, impairment can be given on the basis of weakness of grip strength according to Section 16.8b. Although there is no good data on the time required to regain maximum strength after surgery, the data on strength loss after carpal tunnel release suggests that impairment rating according to Section 16.8b should not be determined less than 1 year after surgery.

16.8 Strength Evaluation

Because strength measurements are functional tests influenced by subjective factors that are difficult to control and the *Guides* for the most part is based on anatomic impairment, the *Guides* does not assign a large role to such measurements. Those who have contributed to the *Guides* believe that further research is needed before loss of grip and pinch strength is given a larger role in impairment evaluation.

Strength measures the power with which musculotendinous units act across a bone-joint lever-arm system to actively generate motion, or passively resist movement against gravity and variable resistance. The effectiveness and magnitude of muscle contraction depends on the integrity of the dynamic and passive elements of a complex lever system, including its muscles and tendons, normal passive motion in the joints across which the muscles act, and the quality of innervation of the muscles. Many subjective or nonmeasurable factors, including fatigue, handedness, time of day, age, nutritional state, pain, and the individual's cooperation, further influence strength measurements. Voluntary muscle strength testing remains somewhat subjective until a precise way of measuring muscle contraction is generally available. It should also be noted that the correlation of strength with performance of activities of daily living is poor and that increased strength does not necessarily equate with increased function.

16.8a Principles

In a rare case, if the examiner believes the individual's loss of strength represents an impairing factor that has not been considered adequately by other methods in the *Guides*, the loss of strength may be rated separately. An example of this situation would be loss of strength due to a severe muscle tear that healed leaving a palpable muscle defect. If the examiner judges that loss of strength should be rated separately in an extremity that presents other impairments, the impairment due to loss of strength *could be combined* with the other impairments, *only* if based on unrelated etiologic or pathomechanical causes. *Otherwise, the impairment ratings based on objective anatomic findings take precedence.* Decreased strength *cannot* be rated in the presence of decreased motion, painful conditions, deformities, or absence of parts (eg, thumb amputation) that prevent effective application of maximal force in the region being evaluated.

Motor weakness associated with disorders of the peripheral nerve system and various degenerative neuromuscular conditions are evaluated according to guidelines described in Section 16.5 and the Chapter 13, The Central and Peripheral Nervous System. It should be understood that weakness or loss of strength can occur without muscle atrophy.

When evaluating strength, the examiner must have good reason to believe the individual has reached maximal medical improvement and that the condition is a "permanent" one as defined in Chapter 1 and the Glossary. Maximum strength is usually not regained for at least a year after an injury or surgical procedure. Because impairment is evaluated when the individual has reached MMI, strength can only be applied as a measure when a year or more has passed since the time of injury or surgery. This determination is best made with measurements taken over a period of time. Two methods are used to determine loss of strength in the upper extremity. Measurements of grip and pinch strength are used to evaluate power weaknesses relating to the structures in the hand, wrist, or forearm. Manual muscle testing of major groups is used for testing strength about the elbow and shoulder.

16.8b Grip and Pinch Strength

Tests repeated at intervals during an examination are considered to be reliable if there is less than 20% variation in the readings. If there is more than 20% variation in the readings, one may assume the individual is not exerting full effort. The test is usually repeated three times with each hand at different times during the examination, and the values are recorded and later compared.

Grip strength measurements must be performed in a standard manner because altering wrist, forearm, and/or elbow position will change the results. The generally accepted position for measurements is for the individual to be seated with back against the chair and feet flat on the floor. The arm should be relaxed beside the lateral torso, the elbow flexed at 90°, and the forearm and wrist in neutral position. *Grip strength* measurements may be taken with a Jamar dynamometer. The second (4 cm) or third (6 cm) position, according to the size of the hand, usually allows the individual to apply maximal force comfortably.

Two techniques have been reported to help detect individuals who exert less than maximal effort on grip strength testing. Stokes pointed out that the plotting of grip strength measurements from each of the five handle settings of the Jamar dynamometer would produce a bell-shaped curve. Those individuals not exerting maximal effort will produce results yielding a straight line or a flat curve.

An alternate method is the rapid exchange grip technique. The grip strength first is determined by standard techniques. The individual then is instructed to grip the dynamometer with maximal effort, first with one hand, then quickly with the other hand, for at least five exchanges. Individuals who did not exert maximal effort with the standard technique will record significantly higher strength readings. If they become aware of this, the strength of both hands will drop dramatically.

Pinch strength measurements are done with a pinch gauge and may include chuck or three-digit pinch, key or lateral pinch, and tip pinch with separate digits. Key pinch measurements usually are sufficient. Measurements are repeated three times. The three readings each for grip and pinch strength are averaged and compared to those of the opposite extremity, which usually is normal. If both extremities are involved, the strength measurements are compared to the average normal strengths listed in Tables 16-31 through 16-33.

Table 16-31 Average Strength of Unsupported Grip by Occupation in 100 Subjects

| | Grip Strength (kg) | | | |
| | Males | | Females | |
Occupation	Major Hand	Minor Hand	Major Hand	Minor Hand
Skilled	47.0	45.4	26.8	24.4
Sedentary	47.2	44.1	23.1	21.1
Manual	48.5	44.6	24.2	22.0
Average	47.6	45.0	24.6	22.4

Adapted with permission from Swanson AB, Matev IB, de Groot Swanson. The strength of the hand. *Bull Prosthet Res.* Fall 1970:145-153.

Table 16-33 Average Strength of Lateral Pinch by Occupation in 100 Subjects

| | Lateral Pinch (kg) | | | |
| | Males | | Females | |
Occupation	Major Hand	Minor Hand	Major Hand	Minor Hand
Skilled	6.6	6.4	4.4	4.3
Sedentary	6.3	6.1	4.1	3.9
Manual	8.5	7.7	6.0	5.5
Average	7.5	7.1	4.9	4.7

Adapted with permission from Swanson, AB, Matev IB, de Groot Swanson. The strength of the hand. *Bull Prosthet Res.* Fall 1970:145-153.

Table 16-32 Average Strength of Grip by Age in 100 Subjects

| | Grip Strength (kg) | | | |
| | Males | | Females | |
Age Group (yrs)	Major Hand	Minor Hand	Major Hand	Minor Hand
< 20	45.2	42.6	23.8	22.8
20-29	48.5	46.2	24.6	22.7
30-39	49.2	44.5	30.8	28.0
40-49	49.0	47.3	23.4	21.5
50-59	45.9	43.5	22.3	18.2

Adapted with permission from Swanson AB, Matev IB, de Groot Swanson. The strength of the hand. *Bull Prosthet Res.* Fall 1970:145-153.

Table 16-34 Upper Extremity Joint Impairment Due to Loss of Grip or Pinch Strength

% Strength Loss Index	% Upper Extremity Impairment
10- 30	10
31- 60	20
61-100	30

If there is evidence that the individual is exerting less than maximal effort, the grip strength measurements are invalid for estimating impairment. It is acknowledged that wide variations exist in strength, even among persons doing the same kind of work. Little evidence exists of a significant difference in grip strength between the dominant and nondominant hand. If the evaluator believes that a significant difference in grip strength was lost in the dominant hand and that it impacts the ability to perform activities of daily living, this should be addressed in the evaluation report (see Section 16.1b).

An index of loss of strength uses the following formula:

$$\frac{\text{Normal strength} - \text{Limited strength}}{\text{Normal strength}} = \frac{\text{Strength loss}}{\text{index \%}}$$

Impairments of the upper extremity due to loss of pinch and grip strength are based on the values of the strength loss index shown in Table 16-34.

Rate the function that measures the greatest loss of strength. Both measurements are not applied.

16.8c Manual Muscle Testing

Manual muscle testing assesses an individual's ability to move a joint through a full range of motion against gravity, or move it against additional resistance applied by the examiner, and/or hold the joint position against resistance. Manual muscle testing is subject to the individual's conscious or unconscious control. Individuals whose performance is inhibited by pain or fear of pain may not be good candidates for this testing. Results of strength testing should be reproducible on different occasions or by two or more trained observers.

Table 16-35 Impairment of the Upper Extremity Due to Strength Deficit From Musculoskeletal Disorders Based on Manual Muscle Testing of Individual Units of Motion of the Shoulder and Elbow

Joint Relative Value	Unit of Motion Relative Value	% Upper Extremity Impairment	
		Strength Deficit*	
		5%-25%†	30%-50%‡
Shoulder (60%)			
Flexion	24	1-6	7-12
Extension	6	0-2	2- 3
Abduction	12	1-3	4- 6
Adduction	6	0-2	2- 3
Internal rotation	6	0-2	2- 3
External rotation	6	0-2	2- 3
Elbow (70%)			
Flexion	21	1-5	6- 11
Extension	21	1-5	6- 11
Pronation	14	1-4	4- 7
Supination	14	1-4	4- 7

* Use clinical judgment to select the appropriate percentage from the range of values shown for each severity grade.

† Complete range of motion against gravity only without resistance.

‡ Complete range of motion against gravity with some resistance.

Derived from Section 16.4 and Table 16-11 by G. de Groot Swanson, Grand Rapids, Michigan.

Upper extremity impairment ratings for strength deficits about the elbow and shoulder (Table 16-35) were derived by multiplying the maximum relative value of each unit of motion by the percentage of severity of strength deficit found on manual muscle testing. The relative functional value of each unit of motion is the same as in Section 16.4, Evaluating Abnormal Motion. The severity of strength deficits is classified and rated on the same principles used for evaluation of the peripheral nerves (Table 16-11). The numeric grades are sometimes also named 5, normal; 4, good; 3, fair; 2, poor; 1, trace; and 0, no muscle contraction. In the absence of peripheral nerve involvement, most weaknesses usually fall in the grade 4 category: "complete active range of motion against gravity with some resistance." Few injuries result in a more profound weakness, such as a grade 3 category: "complete active range of motion against gravity only, without resistance." Muscle strength graded 3 or lower is usually accompanied by other clinical findings such as atrophy. *Because the functional units of motion of each joint were assigned on a 100% scale, the upper extremity impairment values derived for weakness of each unit of motion are added directly together.*

Example 16-70

History: Healed Bennett's fracture.

Physical Exam: Individual complained of pain and weakness when he applied and removed strong alligator clamps. Full active range of motion of the thumb ray. Positive "grind" test at the carpometacarpal (CMC) joint. Lateral (key) pinch was 6 kg on the injured side and 10 kg on the normal side.

Clinical Studies: Radiographs: irregularities of the CMC joint surfaces with arthritic changes.

Analysis: $\dfrac{10\% - 6\%}{10\%} = 40\%$ strength loss index %

This corresponds to a 20% joint impairment (Table 16-34). The maximum impairment value of the CMC joint is 22% of the upper extremity (Table 16-18).

Impairment Rating: $20\% \times 22\% = 4\%$ impairment of the upper extremity due to symptomatic post-traumatic arthritis at the CMC joint.

Example 16-71

History: A worker sustained an open injury to the lateral side of the elbow with proximal damage to the extensor carpi radialis longus and brevis, and pronator teres, and loss of a portion of the lateral epicondyle of the humerus.

Physical Exam: Normal neurologic examination. Full active range of elbow extension and supination against gravity with full resistance. Full active range of flexion and pronation against gravity with some resistance: grade 4 (Table 16-35).

Analysis: Flexion weakness: 5% impairment of the upper extremity. Pronation weakness: 4% impairment of the upper extremity.

Impairment Rating: 5% + 4% = 9% impairment of the upper extremity due to strength deficit about the elbow.

Example 16-72

History: An individual "pulled" his shoulder while sorting some lumber. A full-thickness tear of the rotator cuff was diagnosed on MRI. He failed to respond to conservative management and underwent open surgical repair.

Current Symptoms: Currently works with restrictions due to shoulder weakness, easy fatiguability, and some pain with overhead movement.

Clinical Studies: After optimal healing time and therapy, the MRI showed a healed rotator cuff with some scarring.

Physical Exam: Full active range of shoulder rotation, extension, and adduction. Full active range of shoulder flexion and abduction against gravity with some resistance: grade 4 (Table 16-35).

Analysis: Flexion weakness: 6% upper extremity impairment. Abduction weakness: 3% upper extremity impairment.

Impairment Rating: 6% + 3% = 9% impairment of the upper extremity due to weakness about the shoulder.

16.9 Summary of Steps for Evaluating Impairments of the Upper Extremity

I. Determine the upper extremity impairment derived for the hand region.
Determine and record each of the following on the Upper Extremity Evaluation Record, Part 1 (Figure 16-1).

Hand Region

1. Individual digit impairment due to *amputation* (Sections 16.2c and 16.2d).
   Note: Thumb amputations proximal to the MP joint are rated in terms of upper extremity impairment (Table 16-4 and page 440) and *added* to the upper extremity impairment value obtained from step 8 below.

2. Individual digit impairment due to *sensory* loss from digital nerve lesions (Section 16.3; Figures 16-6 and 16-7; and Tables 16-6 and 16-7).
   Note: Impairment related to neuromas of digital nerves is discussed in Section 16.3c.

3. Individual joint impairment due to *abnormal motion* (Section 16.4: thumb IP, p. 454; MP, p. 456; CMC, p. 458; finger DIP, p. 462; PIP, p. 462; MP, p. 464).
   Note: The motion impairments at the DIP, PIP, and MP joints of the fingers are *combined* (p. 465 and Combined Values Chart, p. 604) to determine the digit impairment. The thumb motion impairments at the IP, MP, and CMC joints are *added* (p. 460).

4. Individual digit impairments due to *other disorders* (Section 16.7).

5. **Total individual digit impairment**: *combine* impairments due to amputation (step 1), sensory loss (step 2), abnormal motion (step 3), and other disorders (step 4)(Combined Values Chart, p. 604).

6. *Convert individual digit impairments to hand impairments* (Table 16-1).

7. **Total hand impairment**: *add* the hand impairment values contributed by each digit.

8. Convert the total hand impairment to **impairment of the upper extremity** (Table 16-2).

9. If applicable, *add* the upper extremity impairment due to *thumb amputation proximal to the MP joint* (Table 16-4) to the upper extremity impairment derived from the hand region (step 8).

10. If applicable, determine the upper extremity impairment due to *loss of strength* and *combine* with the upper extremity impairment derived from the hand region (step 8).

11. If no other upper extremity impairment exists, **convert the upper extremity impairment related to the hand region to an impairment of the whole person** (Table 16-3).

12. If other impairments of the upper extremity are present, enter the upper extremity impairment value due to the Hand Region on Line II of Part 2 of the Evaluation Record.

II. Determine the upper extremity impairment derived from the Wrist, Elbow, and Shoulder Regions and enter on the appropriate space or line of Upper Extremity Evaluation Record, Part 2 (Figure 16-1).

1. **Wrist Region**
Determine upper extremity impairments due to *loss of motion* (Section 16.4g) and *other disorders* (Section 16.7), and *combine* the values to determine the upper extremity impairment related to the wrist region. Enter on line II.

2. **Elbow Region**
Determine upper extremity impairments due to *loss of motion* (Section 16.4h) and *other disorders* (Section 16.7), and *combine* the values to determine the upper extremity impairment related to the elbow region. Enter on line II.

3. **Shoulder Region**
Determine upper extremity impairments due to *loss of motion* (Section 16.4i) and *other disorders* (Section 16.7), and *combine* the values to determine the upper extremity impairment involving the shoulder region. Enter on line II.

III. Determine the upper extremity impairment due to *amputation through the arm or forearm* (Section 16.2b) and enter on line I of the Evaluation Record, Part 2.

IV. Determine the upper extremity impairment due to *peripheral nerve disorders* (Section 16.5) and enter on line III of the Evaluation Record, Part 2.

V. Determine the upper extremity impairment due to *peripheral vascular disorders* (Section 16.6) and enter on line IV of the Evaluation Record, Part 2.

VI. Determine the upper extremity impairments due *to other disorders not included in regional impairment* (Section 16.7) and enter on line V of the Evaluation Record, Part 2.

VII. Determine the total upper extremity impairment and enter on the bottom of Part 2 of the Record.
Combine the upper extremity impairments due to *amputation* (other than hand) (Line I of Part 2), *regional disorders* (hand, wrist, elbow, shoulder) (Line II of Part 2), *peripheral vascular disorders* (Line III of Part 2*), peripheral nerve disorders* (Line IV of Part 2*),* and *other disorders not included in regional impairment* (Line V of Part 2) (Combined Values Chart, p. 604).

VIII. Convert the upper extremity impairment to a *whole person impairment* (Table 16-3).

IX. When *both upper extremities* are involved, derive the whole person impairment percent for each and then *combine* both values using the Combined Values Chart (p. 604).

16.10 Clincal Examples

Example 16-73

History: Table saw injury. Maximum medical rehabilitation reached.

Findings: Index finger: Amputation at DIP joint with painful neuroma on radial side that prevents use of the digit for most activities. Thumb: Amputation through CMC joint.

Analysis:

Index finger:
DIP joint amputation = 45% digit impairment (Table 16-5), or 9% hand impairment (Table 16-1) and 8% upper extremity impairment (Table 16-2).

Radial nerve neuroma: Grade 1 pain or sensory deficit = 95% deficit (Table 16-10a); maximum impairment of the upper extremity for deficit of radial palmar digital nerve of index finger = 5% (Table 16-15). 95% × 5% = 5% (rounded) impairment of the upper extremity.

8% (amputation) *combined* with 5% (neuroma) equals 13% impairment of the upper extremity due to the index finger (See Section 16.4f and Combined Values Chart, p. 604).

Thumb:
Amputation at the CMC joint = 38% impairment of the upper extremity (Table 16-4).

Impairment Rating: 13% (index) + 38% (thumb) = 51% impairment of the upper extremity, or 31% impairment of the whole person (Table 16-3). See the rating method for thumb amputation proximal to the MP joint.

Example 16-74

History: A 36-year-old man who sustained a crush injury of the left hand is now at maximum medical improvement.

Physical Exam: Decreased motion of all digits. Ring finger amputation through the PIP joint. Impaired sensibility on both sides of ring finger stump and little finger.

Analysis: Rate decreased motion of thumb (Figures 16-12 and 16-15, and Tables 16-8a, 16-8b, and 16-9) and fingers (Figures 16-21, 16-23, and 16-25).

Rate sensory loss of digits (Figures 16-6 and 16-7, and Tables 16-6 and 16-7).

Impairment Rating: Specific findings and impairments ratings are given in Figure 16-52.

Example 16-75

History: A 35-year-old man sustained a deep laceration of the right middle finger, volar aspect, at the level of the PIP joint without joint involvement, but with complete laceration of the flexor digitorum profundus (FDP) and flexor digitorum superficialis (FDS) tendons, and of the radial digital nerve. A primary flexor tenorrhaphy of the FDP and FDS tendons and a microneurorrhaphy of the radial digital nerve were done, followed by a 3-month hand rehabilitation program.

Current Symptoms: Numbness on radial side of the middle finger, pain on flexion, and weakness of the right hand.

Findings and Analysis:

Sensory impairment:
9 mm of two-point discrimination on the radial side of the distal and middle phalanges of the middle finger.

Partial longitudinal sensory loss on radial side of middle finger over an 80% length (Figure 16-7) corresponds to a 12% impairment of the finger (Table 16-7).

Motion impairment:
$$I_E\% + I_F\% = \text{finger impairment \%}.$$
DIP: 0° to 50°   0% + 10% = 10% (Figure 16-21).
PIP: –0° to 60°   7% + 24% = 31% (Figure 16-23).
MP: +20° to 90° 0% +   0% =   0% (Figure 16-25).
10% *combined* with 31% = 38% finger impairment (see Section 16.4f).

Impairment Rating: The total finger impairment is obtained by *combining* the sensory impairment (12%) with the motion impairment (38%) by means of the Combined Values Chart (see Section 16.4f). This equals 45% finger impairment, or 9% hand impairment (Table 16-1), 8% upper extremity impairment (Table 16-2), and 5% impairment of the whole person (Table 16-3). Additional estimates are not given for pain and loss of strength.

Example 16-76

History: A 45-year-old firefighter sustained a severe thermal burn to the left hand. Multiple skin grafting procedures and joint releases were performed.

Physical Exam: Decreased motion of digits and wrist (See Figure 16-53a and 16-53b). Static two-point discrimination measured between 7 and 12 mm in all digits.

Analysis: Decreased motion of thumb (Figures 16-12 and 16-15, and Tables 16-8a, 16-8b, and 16-9), fingers (Figures 16-21, 16-23, and 16-25), wrist (Figures 16-28 and 16-31), and elbow (Figure 16-37). Partial transverse sensory loss of digits (Figures 16-6 and 16-7; Tables 16-6 and 16-7).

Impairment Rating: A completed Upper Extremity Impairment Evaluation Record (Figures 16-53a and 16-53b) summarizes the clinical findings and impairment ratings.

Example 16-77

History: A 28-year-old operator had multiple amputations of the right hand from a punch press injury.

Physical Exam: Stumps with good skin coverage. No evidence of neuroma formation.

Impairment Rating: The examination results and impairment calculations are shown in the Upper Extremity Impairment Evaluation Record (Figure 16-54).

Example 16-78

History: A 45-year-old woman fell in a parking lot and sustained a Colles' fracture of the right distal radius.

Physical Exam: Full range of motion at the finger joints, some limitation of wrist motion, some deformity of the wrist, moderate pain with heavy activity, and 40% grip strength loss index.

Impairment Rating: The factors to be rated are the loss of motion of the wrist and forearm rotation. Strength loss should not be rated because it shares the same pathomechanics as decreased motion (See Section 16.8). No impairment estimate for deformity or pain is given. Based on the anatomic examination, the impairment evaluation is determined as follows.

Wrist motion impairment:

Wrist Motion	Degrees	% Upper Extremity Impairment
Extension (Figure 16-28)	30°	$I_E\% = 5\%$
Flexion	40°	$I_F\% = 3\%$
Radial deviation (Figure 16-31)	20°	$I_{RD}\% = 0\%$
Ulnar deviation	10°	$I_{UD}\% = 4\%$

Add the upper extremity impairments contributed by the wrist units of motion: 5% + 3% + 4% = 12% impairment of the upper extremity.

Elbow motion impairment:
Forearm rotation is discussed in Section 16.4h (Figure 16-36).

Elbow Motion	Degrees	% Upper Extremity Impairment
Pronation	40°	$I_P\% = 3\%$
Supination	30°	$I_S\% = 2\%$

Add the upper extremity impairments contributed by the elbow units of motion: 3% + 2% + 5% impairment.

Impairment Rating: *Combine* the upper extremity regional impairments: 12% (wrist) and 5% (elbow) = 16% impairment of the upper extremity (Combined Values Chart, p. 604), or 10% impairment of the whole person (Table 16-3).

Example 16-79

Findings: An individual sustained multiple injuries of the upper extremity and had the following regional impairments: 50% of the thumb, 10% of the index finger, 5% of the upper extremity due to the wrist, and 2% of the upper extremity due to the elbow.

Analysis: Hand region:
50% thumb impairment corresponds to 20% hand impairment (Table 16-1). 10% index finger impairment corresponds to 2% hand impairment. 20% + 2% = 22% impairment of the hand, or 20% impairment of the upper extremity (Table 16-2).

Wrist region:
5% upper extremity impairment.

Elbow region:
2% upper extremity impairment.

Impairment Rating: The regional impairments of the upper extremity are *combined*: 20% *combined* with 5% is 24%; 24% *combined* with 2% is 26% impairment of the upper extremity, or 16% whole person impairment (Table 16-3).

Figure 16-52 Upper Extremity Impairment Evaluation Record–**Part 1 (Hand)**   Side ☐R ☒L

Name __A.B. Example 16-74__   Age __36__   Sex ☒M ☐F   Dominant hand ☐R ☒L   Date _____

Occupation __Construction Worker__   Diagnosis __Crush Injury__

		Abnormal Motion				Amputation	Sensory Loss	Other Disorders	Hand Impairment%
		Record motion or ankylosis angles and digit impairment %				Mark level & impairment %	Mark type, level, & impairment %	List type & impairment %	●Combine digit imp % ★Convert to hand imp %

Thumb

			Flexion	Extension	Ankylosis	Imp %
IP	Angle°	30	-10		6
	Imp %	4	2		
MP	Angle°	30	-15		4
	Imp %	3	1		

			Motion	Ankylosis	Imp %
CMC	Radial abduction	Angle°	30		3
		Imp %	3		
	Adduction	Cm	4		4
		Imp %	4		
	Opposition	Cm	4		9
		Imp %	9		

Add digit impairment %   CMC + MP + IP = 26 [1]

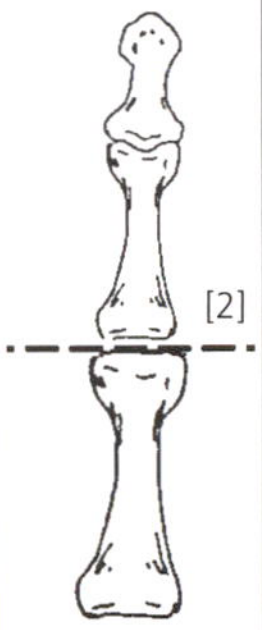

[2] ‡UE IMP % = [5]

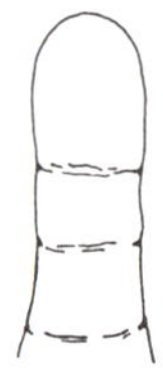

Digit [2] IMP % =   Digit [3] IMP % =   Digit [4] IMP % =

Abnormal motion [1]	26
Amputation [2]	
Sensory loss [3]	
Other disorders [4]	
Total digit imp % ●Combine 1, 2, 3, 4	26
Hand impairment % ★Convert above	10

Index

		Flexion	Extension	Ankylosis	Imp %
DIP	Angle°	30	-10		23
	Imp %	21	2		
PIP	Angle°	70	-10		21
	Imp %	18	3		
MP	Angle°	50	-10		29
	Imp %	22	7		

●Combine digit impairment % MP, PIP, DIP = 56 [1]

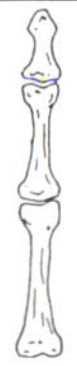

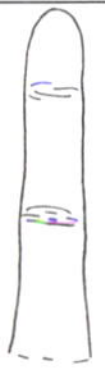

Digit [2] IMP % =   Digit [3] IMP % =   Digit [4] IMP % =

Abnormal motion [1]	56
Amputation [2]	
Sensory loss [3]	
Other disorders [4]	
Total digit imp % ●Combine 1, 2, 3, 4	56
Hand impairment % ★Convert above	11

Middle

		Flexion	Extension	Ankylosis	Imp %
DIP	Angle°	30	-10		23
	Imp %	21	2		
PIP	Angle°	70	-10		21
	Imp %	18	3		
MP	Angle°	50	-10		29
	Imp %	22	7		

●Combine digit impairment %   MP, PIP, DIP = 56 [1]

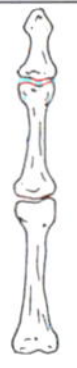

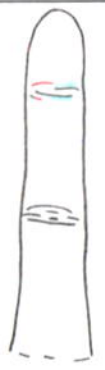

Digit [2] IMP % =   Digit [3] IMP % =   Digit [4] IMP % =

Abnormal motion [1]	56
Amputation [2]	
Sensory loss [3]	
Other disorders [4]	
Total digit imp % ●Combine 1, 2, 3, 4	56
Hand impairment % ★Convert above	11

Ring

		Flexion	Extension	Ankylosis	Imp %
DIP	Angle°				
	Imp %				
PIP	Angle°				
	Imp %				
MP	Angle°	50	-20		32
	Imp %	22	10		

●Combine digit impairment %   MP, PIP, DIP = 32 [1]

Digit [2] IMP % = 80   Digit [3] IMP % = 40   Digit [4] IMP % =

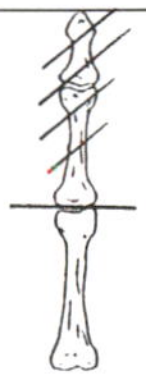

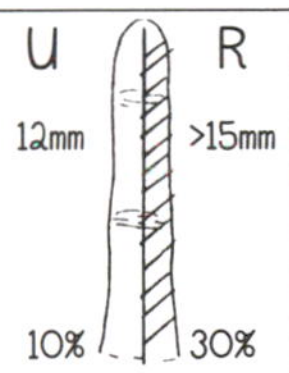

U   R   12mm >15mm   10% 30%

Abnormal motion [1]	32
Amputation [2]	80
Sensory loss [3]	40
Other disorders [4]	
Total digit imp % ●Combine 1, 2, 3, 4	92
Hand impairment % ★Convert above	9

Little

		Flexion	Extension	Ankylosis	Imp %
DIP	Angle°		10		33
	Imp %		33		
PIP	Angle°		60		60
	Imp %		60		
MP	Angle°	50	-20		32
	Imp %	22	10		

●Combine digit impairment %   MP, PIP, DIP = 84 [1]

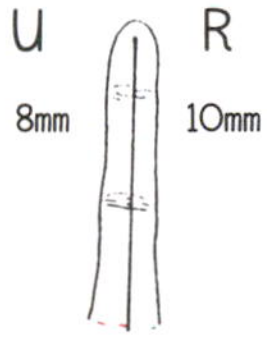

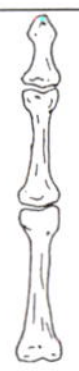

Digit [2] IMP % =   Digit [3] IMP % = 25   Digit [4] IMP % =

U   R   8mm 10mm

Abnormal motion [1]	84
Amputation [2]	
Sensory loss [3]	25
Other disorders [4]	
Total digit imp % ●Combine 1, 2, 3, 4	88
Hand impairment % ★Convert above	9

Total hand impairment: Add hand impairment % for thumb + index + middle + ring + little finger =	50	%
Convert total hand impairment to upper extremity impairment† (if thumb metacarpal intact, enter on Part 2, line II) =	45	%
‡Add thumb ray upper extremity amputation imp [5] ____ % + hand upper extremity imp ____ % =		%
If hand region impairment is only impairment, convert upper extremity impairment to whole person impairment§ =	27	%

● Combined Values Chart (p. 604).   *Use Table 16-1 (digits to hand).   †Use Table 16-2 (hand to upper extremity).   §Use Table 16-3.
Courtesy of G. de Groot Swanson, MD, Grand Rapids, Michigan.

Figure 16-53a Upper Extremity Impairment Evaluation Record–**Part 1 (Hand)** Side ☐R ☒L

Name C.D. Example 16-76 Age 40 Sex ☒M ☐F Dominant hand ☒R ☐L Date ______

Occupation Fire Fighter Diagnosis Thermal Burn

Abnormal Motion	Amputation	Sensory Loss	Other Disorders	Hand Impairment%
Record motion or ankylosis angles and digit impairment %	Mark level & impairment %	Mark type, level, & impairment %	List type & impairment %	•Combine digit imp % *Convert to hand imp %

Thumb

			Flexion	Extension	Ankylosis	Imp %
IP	Angle°		40	-20		6
	Imp %		3	3		
MP	Angle°				10	6
	Imp %				6	
				Motion	Ankylosis	Imp %
CMC	Radial abduction	Angle°		10		9
		Imp %		9		
	Adduction	Cm		6		8
		Imp %		8		
	Opposition	Cm		3		13
		Imp %		13		

[1] Add digit impairment % CMC + MP + IP = 42

Amputation: 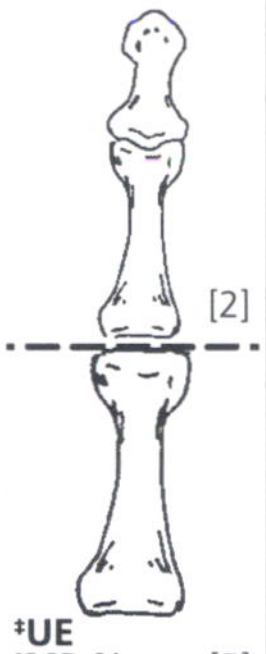 [2] ‡UE IMP % = [5]

Sensory Loss: 8mm 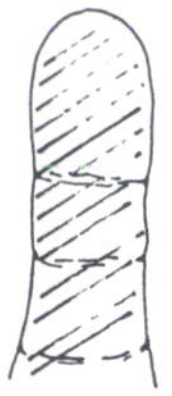

Hand Impairment%		
Abnormal motion	[1]	42
Amputation	[2]	
Sensory loss	[3]	25
Other disorders	[4]	
Total digit imp % •Combine 1, 2, 3, 4		57

Digit IMP % = [2]	Digit IMP % = 25 [3]	Digit IMP % = [4]	Hand impairment % *Convert above	23

Index

		Flexion	Extension	Ankylosis	Imp %
DIP	Angle°			10	33
	Imp %			33	
PIP	Angle°	60	-40		38
	Imp %	24	14		
MP	Angle°			0	54
	Imp %			54	

[1] •Combine digit impairment % MP, PIP, DIP = 81

Amputation:

Sensory Loss: 8 mm 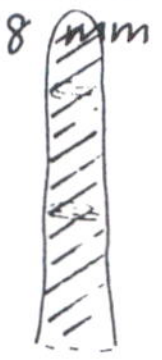

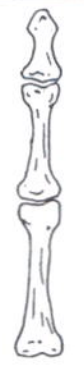

Hand Impairment%		
Abnormal motion	[1]	81
Amputation	[2]	
Sensory loss	[3]	25
Other disorders	[4]	
Total digit imp % •Combine 1, 2, 3, 4		86

Digit IMP % = [2]	Digit IMP % = 25 [3]	Digit IMP % = [4]	Hand impairment % *Convert above	17

Middle

		Flexion	Extension	Ankylosis	Imp %
DIP	Angle°			10	33
	Imp %			33	
PIP	Angle°	60	-40		38
	Imp %	24	14		
MP	Angle°			0	54
	Imp %			54	

[1] •Combine digit impairment % MP, PIP, DIP = 81

Amputation:

Sensory Loss: 8 mm 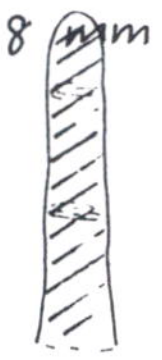

Hand Impairment%		
Abnormal motion	[1]	81
Amputation	[2]	
Sensory loss	[3]	25
Other disorders	[4]	
Total digit imp % •Combine 1, 2, 3, 4		86

Digit IMP % = [2]	Digit IMP % = 25 [3]	Digit IMP % = [4]	Hand impairment % *Convert above	17

Ring

		Flexion	Extension	Ankylosis	Imp %
DIP	Angle°			10	33
	Imp %			33	
PIP	Angle°	60	-40		38
	Imp %	24	14		
MP	Angle°			0	54
	Imp %			54	

[1] •Combine digit impairment % MP, PIP, DIP = 81

Amputation:

Sensory Loss: 8 mm 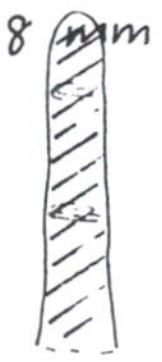

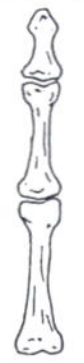

Hand Impairment%		
Abnormal motion	[1]	81
Amputation	[2]	
Sensory loss	[3]	25
Other disorders	[4]	
Total digit imp % •Combine 1, 2, 3, 4		86

Digit IMP % = [2]	Digit IMP % = 25 [3]	Digit IMP % = [4]	Hand impairment % *Convert above	9

Little

		Flexion	Extension	Ankylosis	Imp %
DIP	Angle°			10	33
	Imp %			33	
PIP	Angle°	70	-50		43
	Imp %	18	25		
MP	Angle°			0	54
	Imp %			54	

[1] •Combine digit impairment % MP, PIP, DIP = 83

Amputation:

Sensory Loss: 8 mm 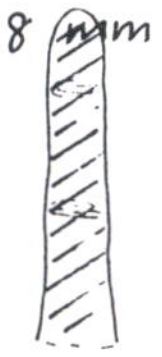

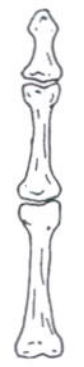

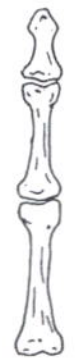

Hand Impairment%		
Abnormal motion	[1]	83
Amputation	[2]	
Sensory loss	[3]	25
Other disorders	[4]	
Total digit imp % •Combine 1, 2, 3, 4		87

Digit IMP % = [2]	Digit IMP % = 25 [3]	Digit IMP % = [4]	Hand impairment % *Convert above	9

Total hand impairment: Add hand impairment % for thumb + index + middle + ring + little finger =	75 %
Convert total hand impairment to upper extremity impairment† (if thumb metacarpal intact, enter on Part 2, line II) =	68 %
‡Add thumb ray upper extremity amputation imp [5] ___% + hand upper extremity imp ___% =	%
If hand region impairment is only impairment, convert upper extremity impairment to whole person impairment§ =	%

• Combined Values Chart (p. 604). *Use Table 16-1 (digits to hand). †Use Table 16-2 (hand to upper extremity). §Use Table 16-3.

Courtesy of G. de Groot Swanson, MD, Grand Rapids, Michigan.

Figure 16-53b Upper Extremity Impairment Evaluation Record–**Part 2 (Wrist, elbow, and shoulder)** Side ☐R ☒L

Name C.D. Example 16-76   Age 40   Sex ☒M ☐F   Dominant hand ☒R ☐L   Date _____

Occupation Fire Fighter   Diagnosis Thermal Burn

	Abnormal Motion					Other Disorders	Regional Impairment %	Amputation
	Record motion or ankylosis angles and impairment %					List type & impairment %	•Combine [1] + [2]	Mark level & impairment %
Wrist		Flexion	Extension	Ankylosis	Imp %			
	Angle°	40	20		10			
	Imp %	3	7					
		RD	UD	Ankylosis	Imp %			
	Angle°	5	10		7			
	Imp %	3	4					
	Add Imp % Flex/Ext + RD/UD = 17				[1]	Imp % = [2]	17	
Elbow		Flexion	Extension	Ankylosis	Imp %			
	Angle°							
	Imp %							
		Pronation	Supination	Ankylosis	Imp %			
	Angle°	50	40		4			
	Imp %	2	2					
	Add Imp % Flex/Ext + Pro/Sup = 4				[1]	Imp % = [2]	4	
Shoulder		Flexion	Extension	Ankylosis	Imp %			
	Angle°							
	Imp %							
		Adduction	Abduction	Ankylosis	Imp %			
	Angle°							
	Imp %							
		Int Rot	Ext Rot	Ankylosis	Imp %			
	Angle°							
	Imp %							
	Add Imp % Flex/Ext + Add/Abd + Int Rot/Ext Rot =				[1]	Imp % = [2]		Imp % =

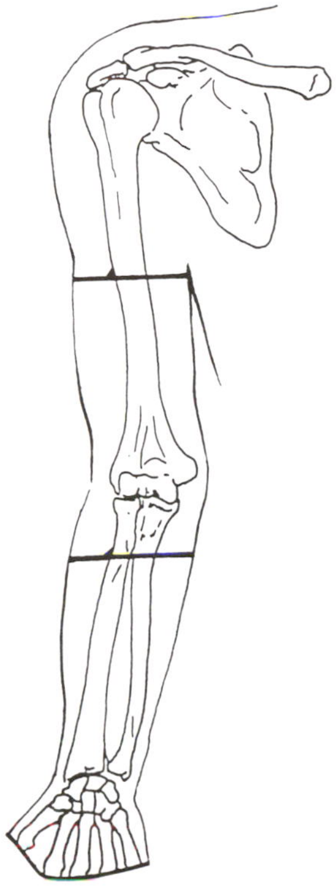

I. Amputation impairment (other than digits)   =   %

II. Regional impairment of upper extremity
   •(Combine hand 68 % + wrist 17 % + elbow 4 % + shoulder _____%)   = 74   %

III. Peripheral nerve system impairment   =   %

IV. Peripheral vascular system impairment   =   %

V. Other disorders (not included in regional impairment)   =   %

Total upper extremity impairment (•Combine I, II, III, IV, and V)   = 74   %

Impairment of the whole person (Use Table 16-3)   = 44   %

• Combined Values Chart (p. 604).

If both limbs are involved, calculate the whole person impairment for each on a separate chart and *combine* the percents (Combined Values Chart).

Figure 16-54 Upper Extremity Impairment Evaluation Record–**Part 1 (Hand)**   Side ☒ R ☐ L

Name: E.F. Example 16-77   Age 40   Sex ☒ M ☐ F   Dominant hand ☐ R ☒ L   Date _____
Occupation: Punch Press Operator   Diagnosis: Multiple Amputations

Abnormal Motion					Amputation	Sensory Loss	Other Disorders	Hand Impairment%
Record motion or ankylosis angles and digit impairment %					Mark level & impairment %	Mark type, level, & impairment %	List type & impairment %	●Combine digit imp % ★Convert to hand imp %

Thumb

		Flexion	Extension	Ankylosis	Imp %
IP	Angle° / Imp %				5
MP	Angle° / Imp %				4

		Motion	Ankylosis	Imp %
CMC	Radial abduction — Angle° / Imp %			
	Adduction — Cm / Imp %			
	Opposition — Cm / Imp %			

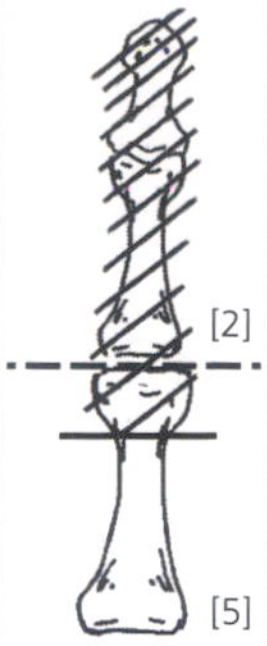

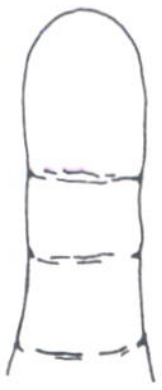

[2] ... [5]

‡UE IMP % = 37

Add digit impairment % CMC + MP + IP = [1]

Amputation	Sensory Loss	Other Disorders	Hand Impairment %
Abnormal motion [1]			
Amputation [2]			
Sensory loss [3]			
Other disorders [4]			
Total digit imp % ●Combine 1, 2, 3, 4			
Digit [2] IMP % =	Digit [3] IMP % =	Digit [4] IMP % =	Hand impairment % ★Convert above

Index

		Flexion	Extension	Ankylosis	Imp %
DIP	Angle° / Imp %				
PIP	Angle° / Imp %				
MP	Angle° / Imp %	60 / 17	+20 / 0		17

●Combine digit impairment % MP, PIP, DIP = 17   [1]

Hand Impairment %
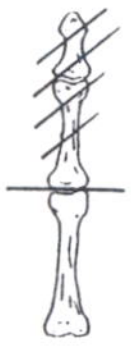 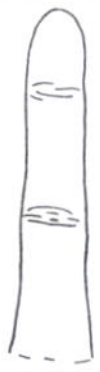 Abnormal motion [1] 17
Amputation [2] 80
Sensory loss [3]
Other disorders [4]
Total digit imp % ●Combine 1, 2, 3, 4 83
Digit [2] IMP % = 80	Digit [3] IMP % =	Digit [4] IMP % =	Hand impairment % ★Convert above 17

Middle

		Flexion	Extension	Ankylosis	Imp %
DIP	Angle° / Imp %				
PIP	Angle° / Imp %	30 / 42	0 / 0		42
MP	Angle° / Imp %	70 / 11	+20 / 0		11

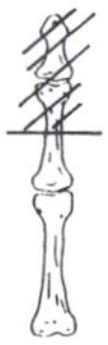

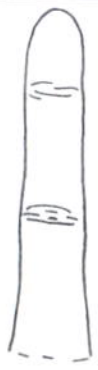

●Combine digit impairment % MP, PIP, DIP = 48   [1]

Hand Impairment %
Abnormal motion [1] 48
Amputation [2] 60
Sensory loss [3]
Other disorders [4]
Total digit imp % ●Combine 1, 2, 3, 4 79
Digit [2] IMP % = 60	Digit [3] IMP % =	Digit [4] IMP % =	Hand impairment % ★Convert above 16

Ring

		Flexion	Extension	Ankylosis	Imp %
DIP	Angle° / Imp %	30 / 21	-10 / 2		23
PIP	Angle° / Imp %	70 / 18	0 / 0		18
MP	Angle° / Imp %	80 / 6	+20 / 0		6

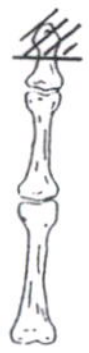

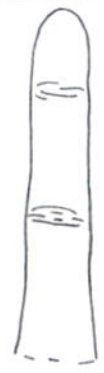

●Combine digit impairment % MP, PIP, DIP = 41   [1]

Hand Impairment %
Abnormal motion [1] 41
Amputation [2] 25
Sensory loss [3]
Other disorders [4]
Total digit imp % ●Combine 1, 2, 3, 4 56
Digit [2] IMP % = 25	Digit [3] IMP % =	Digit [4] IMP % =	Hand impairment % ★Convert above 6

Little

		Flexion	Extension	Ankylosis	Imp %
DIP	Angle° / Imp %	30 / 21	0 / 0		21
PIP	Angle° / Imp %	90 / 6	0 / 0		6
MP	Angle° / Imp %	90 / 0	+20 / 0		0

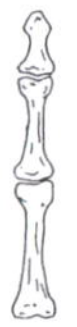

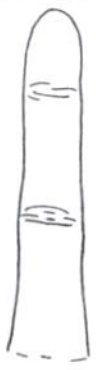

●Combine digit impairment % MP, PIP, DIP = 26   [1]

Hand Impairment %
Abnormal motion [1] 26
Amputation [2]
Sensory loss [3]
Other disorders [4]
Total digit imp % ●Combine 1, 2, 3, 4 26
Digit [2] IMP % =	Digit [3] IMP % =	Digit [4] IMP % =	Hand impairment % ★Convert above 3

Total hand impairment: Add hand impairment % for thumb + index + middle + ring + little finger =	42 %
Convert total hand impairment to upper extremity impairment† (if thumb metacarpal intact, enter on Part 2, line II) =	38 %
‡Add thumb ray upper extremity amputation imp [5] 37 % + hand upper extremity imp 38 % =	75 %
If hand region impairment is only impairment, convert upper extremity impairment to whole person impairment§ =	45 %

● Combined Values Chart (p. 604).   *Use Table 16-1 (digits to hand).   †Use Table 16-2 (hand to upper extremity).   §Use Table 16-3.
Courtesy of G. de Groot Swanson, MD, Grand Rapids, Michigan.

Chapter 16

Bibliography

Amadio PC. The Mayo Clinic and carpal tunnel syndrome. *Mayo Clin Proc.* 1992;67:42.

American Academy of Orthopaedic Surgeons. *Joint Motion: Method of Measuring and Recording.* Chicago, Ill: American Academy of Orthopaedic Surgeons; 1965.

American Board of Electrodiagnostic Medicine; American Association of Electrodiagnostic Medicine; 21 Second St SW, Rochester, MN 55902.

American Society of Hand Therapists. *Clinical Assessment Recommendations.* 2nd ed. Chicago, Ill: American Society of Hand Therapists; 1992.

American Society for Surgery of the Hand. *The Hand: Examination and Diagnosis.* 2nd ed. New York, NY: Churchill Livingstone; 1983.

Aulicino PL. Clinical examination of the hand. In: Hunter J, Mackin E, Callahan AD, eds. *Rehabilitation of the Hand.* 5th ed. Philadelphia, Pa: CV Mosby Co; 1995:53-75.

Bechtol CO. Grip test, the use of a dynamometer with adjustable handle spacings. *J Bone Joint Surg Am.* 1954;36:820-824.

Bell JA. Sensibility evaluation. In: Hunter J, Schneider L, Mackin E, eds. *Rehabilitation of the Hand.* Philadelphia, Pa: CV Mosby Co; 1978:278-279.

Bell-Krotoski J, Tomanick E. The repeatability of testing with Semmes-Weinstein monofilaments. *J Hand Surg Am.* 1987;12:155-161.

Bell-Krotoski JA. Sensibility testing: current concepts. In: Hunter J, Mackin E, Callahan AD, eds. *Rehabilitation of the Hand.* 5th ed. Philadelphia, Pa: CV Mosby Co; 1995:109-128.

Boyes JH, ed. *Bunnell's Surgery of the Hand.* 5th ed. Philadelphia, Pa: JB Lippincott Co; 1970.

Brand PW, Hollister A. *Clinical Mechanics of the Hand.* 3rd ed. St Louis, Mo: CV Mosby Co; 1999.

Braun RM, Davidson K, Doehr S. Provocative testing in the diagnosis of dynamic carpal tunnel syndrome. *J Hand Surg Am.* 1989;14:195-197.

Braun RM, Doehr S, Leonard N. Quantitative management of hand function: application to medical decision-making and return to the work place after cumulative nerve trauma. In: Omer GE Jr, Spinner M, Van Beek AL, eds. *Management of Peripheral Nerve Problems.* 2nd ed. Philadelphia, Pa: WB Saunders Co; 1998:543-549.

Brigham CR. *The Guides Casebook: Cases to Accompany Guides to Evaluation of Permanent Impairment, Fourth Edition.* Chicago, Ill: American Medical Association; 1999.

Callahan AD. Sensibility assessment: prerequisites and techniques for nerve lesions in continuity and nerve lacerations. In: Hunter J, Mackin E, Callahan AD, eds. *Rehabilitation of the Hand.* 5th ed. Philadelphia, Pa: CV Mosby Co; 1995:129-152.

Cambridge-Kelling CA. Range-of-motion measurement of the hand. In: Hunter J, Mackin E, Callahan AD, eds. *Rehabilitation of the Hand.* 5th ed. Philadelphia, Pa: CV Mosby Co; 1995:93-107.

Cohen MS. Instability of the wrist. In: Brigham CR, Talmage JB, eds. *The Guides Newsletter.* Chicago, Ill: American Medical Association; March-April 1998:1-3.

Culver J. Personal written and oral communication. The Cleveland Clinic, Cleveland, Ohio, 1990-1992.

Dellon AL, Kallman CH. Evaluation of functional sensation in the hand. *J Hand Surg Am.* 1983;8:865-870.

Demeter SL, Andersson GBJ, Smith GM, eds. *Disability Evaluation.* St Louis, Mo: CV Mosby Co; 1996.

De Palma A. *Surgery of the Shoulder.* 2nd ed. Philadelphia, Pa: JB Lippincott Co; 1973.

Fess E. Documentation: essential elements of an upper extremity assessment battery. In: Hunter J, Mackin E, Callahan AD, eds. *Rehabilitation of the Hand.* 5th ed. Philadelphia, Pa: CV Mosby Co; 1995:185-214.

Fess E. The need for reliability and validity in hand assessment instruments. *J Hand Surg Am.* 1986;11:621-623.

Green DP. Carpal dislocations and instabilities. In: Green DP. *Operative Hand Surgery.* 3rd ed. New York, NY: Churchill Livingstone; 1993:861-928.

Hawkins RJ, Bokor DJ. Clinical evaluation of shoulder problems. In: Rockwood CA, Matsen III FA, eds. *The Shoulder.* Philadelphia, Pa: WB Saunders Co; 1990:149-177.

Katz J. Symptoms, functional status, and neuromuscular impairment following carpal tunnel release. *J Hand Surg Am.* 1995;20:549-555.

Kline DG. Caution in the evaluation of results of peripheral nerve surgery. In Samiit M, ed. *Peripheral Nerve Lesions.* Berlin, Germany: Springer-Verlag; 1990.

Kline DG, Hudson AR. *Operative Results for Major Nerve Injuries, Entrapments, and Tumors.* Philadelphia, Pa: WB Saunders Co; 1995:89.

Kendall H, Kendall F, et al. *Muscle Testing and Function.* 4th ed. Baltimore, Md: Williams & Wilkins; 1993.

Lankford LL. Reflex sympathetic dystrophy. In: Omer GE Jr, Spinner M, eds. *Management of Peripheral Nerve Problems.* Philadelphia, Pa: WB Saunders Co; 1980:chap 12.

Lichtman DM. Introduction to the carpal instabilities. In: Lichtman DM, Alexander AH, eds. *The Wrist and Its Disorders.* 2nd ed. Philadelphia, Pa: WB Saunders Co; 1988:181-188.

Linscheid RL, Dobyns JH, Bebout JW. Traumatic instability of the wrist: diagnosis, classification, and pathomechanics. *J Bone Joint Surg Am.* 1972;54:1612-1632.

Louis DS. The carpal tunnel syndrome in the work place. In: Millender LH, Louis DS, Simmons BP, eds. *Occupational Disorders of the Upper Extremity.* New York, NY: Churchill Livingstone; 1992:145-153.

Luck JV Jr, Florence DW. A brief history and comparative analysis of disability systems and impairment rating guides. *Orthop Clin North Am.* 1988;19:839-844.

Lundborg G, Dahlin L. Pathophysiology of peripheral nerve trauma. In: Omer GE Jr, Spinner M, Van Beek AL, eds. *Management of Peripheral Nerve Problems.* 2nd ed. Philadelphia, Pa: WB Saunders Co; 1998:353-363.

Mann FA, Gilula LA. Post-traumatic wrist pain and instability: a radiographic approach to diagnosis. In: Lichtman DM, Alexander AH, eds. *The Wrist and Its Disorders.* 2nd ed. Philadelphia, Pa: WB Saunders Co; 1988:91-108.

McBride ED. *Disability Evaluation.* 6th ed. Philadelphia, Pa: JB Lippincott Co; 1963.

McFarland EG, Torpey B, Curl LA. Evaluation of shoulder laxity. *Sports Med.* 1996;22:264-272.

McFarland EG, Campbell G, McDowell J. Posterior shoulder laxity in asymptomatic athletes. *Sports Med.* 1996;24:468-471.

Medical Research Council. *Aids to the Examination of the Peripheral Nervous System.* London, England: Her Majesty's Stationery Office; 1976. Memorandum No. 45.

Moberg E. Objective methods for determining the functional value of sensibility in the hand. *J Bone Joint Surg Br.* 1958;40:454-476.

Moberg E. Sensibility in reconstructive limb surgery. In: Fredericks S, Brody GS, eds. *Symposium on the Neurologic Aspects of Plastic Surgery.* St Louis, Mo: CV Mosby Co; 1978:30-35.

Moberg E. Two-point discrimination test. *Scand J Rehabil Med.* 1990;22:127-134.

Ochoa JL. Nerve fiber pathology in acute and chronic compression. In: Omer GE Jr, Spinner M, Van Beek AL, eds. *Management of Peripheral Nerve Problems.* 2nd ed. Philadelphia, Pa: WB Saunders Co; 1998:475-483.

Omer GE Jr. Sensation and sensibility in the upper extremity. *Clin Orthop.* 1974;104:30-36.

Omer GE Jr. Methods of assessment of injury and recovery of peripheral nerves. *Surg Clin North Am.* 1981;61:303-319.

Omer GE Jr. Report of the committee for evaluation of the clinical result in peripheral nerve injury. *J Hand Surg Am.* 1983;8(part 2):754-758.

Omer GE Jr. Nerve compression syndromes. *Hand Clin.* 1992;8:317-324.

Omer GE Jr, Bell-Krotoski J. Sensibility testing. In: Omer GE Jr, Spinner M, Van Beek AL, eds. *Management of Peripheral Nerve Problems.* 2nd ed. Philadelphia, Pa: WB Saunders Co; 1998:11-28.

Omer GE Jr, Bell-Krotoski J. The evaluation of clinical results following peripheral nerve suture. In: Omer GE Jr, Spinner M, Van Beek AL, eds. *Management of Peripheral Nerve Problems.* 2nd ed. Philadelphia, Pa: WB Saunders Co; 1998:340-349.

Phalen GS. The carpal tunnel syndrome. Seventeen years experience in diagnosis and treatment of six-hundred forty-four hands. *J Bone Joint Surg Am.* 1966;48:211.

Pirela-Cruz MA. Surgical exposures of the peripheral nerves in the extremities. In: Omer GE Jr, Spinner M, Van Beek AL, eds. *Management of Peripheral Nerve Problems.* 2nd ed. Philadelphia, Pa: WB Saunders Co; 1998:175-209.

Prendergast Lauckhardt KH. Decision pathways for the therapist's management of peripheral nerve injury. In: Omer GE Jr, Spinner M, Van Beek AL, eds. *Management of Peripheral Nerve Problems.* 2nd ed. Philadelphia, Pa: WB Saunders Co; 1998:94-104.

Rayan GM, Asal NR, Bohr PC. Epidemiology and economic impact of compression neuropathy. In: Omer GE Jr, Spinner M, Van Beek AL, eds. *Management of Peripheral Nerve Problems.* 2nd ed. Philadelphia, Pa: WB Saunders Co; 1998:484-493.

Richards LG. Posture effects on grip strength. *Arch Phys Med Rehabil.* 1997;78:1154-1156.

Russell RC, Hussmann J, Burns M. Clinical motor function testing—upper extremity. In: Omer GE Jr, Spinner M, Van Beek AL, eds. *Management of Peripheral Nerve Problems.* 2nd Philadelphia, Pa: WB Saunders Co; 1998:39-55.

Seddon HJ. *Surgical Disorders of the Peripheral Nerves.* 2nd ed. Edinburgh, Scotland: Churchill Livingstone; 1975:32-56.

Slocum DB, Pratt DR. Disability evaluation for the hand. *J Bone Joint Surg.* 1946;28:491-450.

Spinner M, Spinner RJ. Management of nerve compression lesions of the upper extremity. In: Omer GE Jr, Spinner M, Van Beek AL, eds. *Management of Peripheral Nerve Problems.* 2nd ed. Philadelphia, Pa: WB Saunders Co; 1998:501-533.

Stokes HM. The seriously injured hand: weakness of grip. *J Occup Med.* 1983;25:683-684.

Swanson AB. Evaluation of impairment of function in the hand. *Surg Clin North Am.* 1964;44:925-940.

Swanson AB, Mays JD, Yamauchi Y. A rheumatoid arthritis evaluation record for the upper extremity. *Surg Clin North Am.* 1968;48:1003-1013.

Swanson AB, Matev IB, de Groot Swanson G. The strength of the hand. *Bull Prosthet Res.* Fall 1970:145-153.

Swanson AB. Evaluation of disabilities and recordkeeping. In: Swanson AB. *Flexible Implant Resection Arthroplasty in the Hand and Extremities.* St Louis, Mo: CV Mosby Co; 1973:chap 5.

Swanson AB, Hagert CG, de Groot Swanson G. Evaluation of impairment of hand function. *J Hand Surg Am.* 1983;8(part 2):709-722.

Swanson AB, de Groot Swanson G. Implant arthroplasty in the carpal and radiocarpal joints. In: Lichtman DM, Alexander AH, eds. *The Wrist and Its Disorders.* 2nd ed. Philiadelphia, Pa: WB Saunders Co; 1988:616-641.

Swanson AB, de Groot Swanson G, Blair SJ. Evaluation of impairment of hand and upper extremity function. In: Barr JS Jr, ed. *Instructional Course Lectures, American Academy of Orthopaedic Surgery.* St Louis, Mo: CV Mosby Co; 1989;38(part B):77-102.

Swanson AB, de Groot Swanson G. Principles and methods of impairment evaluation in the hand and upper extremity. In: Doege TC, Houston TP, eds. *Guides to the Evaluation of Permanent Impairment.* Fourth ed. Chicago, Ill: American Medical Association; 1993:13-74.

Swanson AB. Pathomechanics of deformities in hand and wrist. In: Hunter J, Mackin E, Callahan AD, eds. *Rehabilitation of the Hand.* 5th ed. Philadelphia, Pa: CV Mosby Co; 1995:1315-1328.

Swanson AB, de Groot Swanson G, Hagert CG. Evaluation of impairment of hand function. In: Hunter J, Mackin E, Callahan AD, eds. *Rehabilitation of the Hand.* 5th ed. Philadelphia, Pa: CV Mosby Co; 1995:1839-1896.

Swanson AB, de Groot Swanson G. Impairment evaluation of the peripheral nerve system of the upper extremity. In: Omer GE Jr, Spinner M, Van Beek AL, eds. *Management of Peripheral Nerve Problems.* 2nd ed. Philadelphia, Pa: WB Saunders Co; 1998:767-779.

Szabo R, Gelberman R, Dimick M. Sensibility testing in patients with carpal tunnel syndrome. *J Bone Joint Surg Am.* 1984;66:61-64.

Tubiana R, Valentin P. Opposition of the thumb. *Surg Clin North Am.* 1968;48:967-977.

Tubiana R, Thomine JM, Mackin E. *Examination of the Hand and Upper Limb.* Philadelphia, Pa: WB Saunders Co; 1984.

Van't Hof A, Heiple KG. Flexor-tendon injuries of the fingers and thumb: a comparative study: a report on sixty primary tendon repairs by the authors, to which reports of other series have been added to furnish statistics on 310 cases. *J Bone Joint Surg Am.* 1958;40:256-262.

Wilbourn AJ, Shields RW Jr. Generalized polyneuropathies and other nonsurgical peripheral nervous system disorders. In: Omer GE Jr, Spinner M, Van Beek AL, eds. *Management of Peripheral Nerve Problems.* 2nd ed. Philadelphia, Pa: WB Saunders Co; 1998:648-660.

Chapter 17

The Lower Extremities

17.1 Principles of Assessment

17.2 Methods of Assessment

**17.3 Lower Extremity Impairment Evaluation
Procedure Summary and Examples**

Introduction

This chapter provides criteria for evaluating permanent impairment of the lower extremities, including impairment ratings that reflect an individual's ability to perform the activities of daily living (ADL). For evaluation purposes, the lower extremities are divided into six sections: the feet, the hindfeet, the ankles, the legs, the knees, the hips, and the pelvis. In addition to the skeletal framework, assessment of the lower extremities also requires an assessment of its joints and the associated soft tissues, vascular system, and nervous system. The lower extremities are evaluated on the basis of anatomic changes, diagnostic categories, and functional changes. Impairment evaluations pertain to conditions that have reached maximum medical improvement (MMI), as defined in Chapter 1 and the Glossary.

The following revisions have been made for the fifth edition: (1) The principles of assessment have been expanded to clarify when the different evaluation methods should be used; (2) a new table, Guide to the Appropriate Combination of Evaluation Methods (Table 17-2), has been added to indicate which methods are appropriate to use in combination;

(3) the evaluation of causalgia and complex regional pain syndrome now follows the same principles used to evaluate central nervous system lesions; (4) additional case examples are provided; and (5) a lower extremity worksheet is provided as a template to simplify making the assessment and recording the evaluation.

17.1 Principles of Assessment

Before using the information in this chapter, the *Guides* user should become familiar with Chapters 1 and 2 and the Glossary. Chapters 1 and 2 discuss the *Guides'* purpose, applications, and methods for performing and reporting impairment evaluations. The Glossary provides definitions of common terms used by many specialties in impairment evaluation.

The evaluation should include a comprehensive, accurate medical history; a review of all pertinent records; a comprehensive description of the individual's current symptoms and their relationship to daily activities; a careful and thorough physical examination; and all findings of relevant laboratory, radiologic (imaging), and ancillary tests. It is also essential that the rater include in the report a description of how the impairment was calculated. Because many ratings are reviewed by other physicians and third-party administrators, the explanation of the calculation will lead to a better understanding of the method used and the report will be considered more reliable.

17.1a Interpretation of Symptoms and Signs

History
The case history should be based mainly on the individual's own statements rather than on secondhand information. The evaluator should consider information from other sources, including medical records. The physician should use this information cautiously, especially if it is subjective. It is not appropriate to question the individual's integrity. If information from the individual is inconsistent with what is known about the medical condition, the circumstances, or the written record, this should be reported and comment should be included about the inconsistencies.

The medical history must describe the chief complaint. Discuss the quality, frequency, duration, and anatomic location of pain, numbness, paresthesias, and weakness in detail. Further, report how the condition interferes with daily activities. The physician should elicit the facts about when and how the condition started and the relationship to any related problems elsewhere in the lower extremity or in other areas of the musculoskeletal system, such as the spine. The report should describe any precipitating events or factors.

Ideally, include the individual's description as to how the symptoms developed and the assumed cause. In addition, discuss the results of special studies and treatment. The physician should review available x-rays and other imaging studies personally or report the findings as being those of another reviewer (based on reports). A review of organ systems and of the general medical history can provide potentially helpful information, including complicating medical problems that can affect the diagnosis and care plan.

Examination
Physical examination of nonmusculoskeletal areas (eg, the nervous system) is discussed in other parts of the *Guides*. A targeted neurologic assessment is needed for individuals with lower extremity problems. Guided by the history and physical examination, the physician records lower extremity–related physical findings, such as range of motion, limb length discrepancy, deformity, reflexes, muscle strength and atrophy, ligamentous laxity, motor and sensory deficits, and specific diagnoses such as fractures and bursitis.

Neurologic examination of the lower extremities includes measurement of knee and ankle reflexes and motor and sensory functions. It is important to ensure that lower extremity impairment discussed in this chapter is not due to underlying spine pathology. If lower extremity impairment is due to an underlying spine disorder, the lower extremity impairment would, in most cases, be accounted for in the spine impairment rating.

17.1b Description of Clinical Studies

Specific Lower Extremity Techniques

The physician needs to review and record findings from diagnostic studies, including laboratory tests, electromyographic, vascular, and roentgenographic studies, CT scans, and MRI studies with or without contrast. A summary of the studies should be included as a separate paragraph or section. While imaging and other studies may assist physicians in making a diagnosis and help determine the method for assessment, they are not the sole determinants.

17.2 Methods of Assessment

Thirteen methods can be used to assess the lower extremities, as listed in Table 17-2. Table 17-1 classifies the 13 methods into three non–mutually exclusive categories to reflect their primary mode of assessment: (1) anatomic, (2) functional, or (3) diagnosis based. Detailed discussions of each method are provided in the sections noted.

Table 17-1 Methods Used to Evaluate Impairments of the Lower Extremities

Assessment Type	Method	Section Number
Anatomic (1-9)	1. Limb length discrepancy	17.2b
	2. Muscle atrophy	17.2d
	3. Ankylosis	17.2g
	4. Amputation	17.2i
	5. Arthritis of joints	17.2h
	6. Skin loss	17.2k
	7. Peripheral nerve injury	17.2l
	8. Vascular	17.2n
	9. Causalgia/reflex sympathetic dystrophy (CRPS)	17.2m
Functional (10-12)	10. Range of motion	17.2f
	11. Gait derangement	17.2c
	12. Muscle strength (manual muscle testing)	17.2e
Diagnosis based (13)	Fractures	17.2j
	Ligament injuries	17.2j
	Meniscectomies	17.2j
	Foot deformities	17.2j
	Hip and pelvic bursitis	17.2j
	Lower extremity joint replacements	17.2j

Anatomic changes, including range of motion (ROM), any limb length discrepancy, arthritis, skin changes, amputation, muscle atrophy, nerve impairment, and vascular derangement are assessed in the physical examination and supported with clinical studies. Arthritis has its own diagnostic category, which applies to individuals with documented arthritis who are impaired by pain, weakness, or stiffness, but who have maintained functional ranges of motion. Arthritis is evaluated based on narrowing of the joint space as measured from x-rays. Causalgia and complex regional pain syndrome (reflex sympathetic dystrophy) are evaluated using a combination of ROM and peripheral neurologic evaluation techniques.

Diagnosis-based estimates are used to evaluate impairments caused by specific fractures and deformities, as well as ligamentous instability, bursitis, and various surgical procedures, including joint replacements and meniscectomies. In certain situations, diagnosis-based estimates are combined with other methods of assessment.

Functional impairments are chosen for conditions when anatomic changes are difficult to categorize or when functional implications have been documented. Functional impairments are assessed last.

The evaluator should read this chapter in its entirety and understand and follow the evaluation methods using the worksheet given in Figure 17-10 at the end of the chapter or a similar, comprehensive checklist. The evaluator's first step is to establish the diagnosis(es) and whether or not the individual has reached MMI. The next step is to identify each part of the lower extremity that might possibly warrant an impairment rating (pelvis, hip, thigh, etc, down to the toes). Figure 17-10 lists potential methods for each lower extremity part. The evaluator determines whether ROM impairment or other regional impairments are present for each relevant part and records the impairment values in the appropriate locations on the worksheet. The selection of the most specific method(s) and the appropriate combination are later considerations.

After all potentially impairing conditions have been identified and the correct ratings recorded, the evaluator should select the clinically most appropriate (ie, most specific) method(s) and record the estimated impairment for each. The **cross-usage chart** (Table 17-2) indicates which methods and resulting impairment ratings may be combined. It is the responsibility of the evaluating physician to explain in writing why a particular method(s) to assign the impairment rating was chosen. When uncertain about which method to choose, the evaluator should calculate the impairment using different alternatives and choose the method or combination of methods that gives the most clinically accurate impairment rating.

Table 17-2 Guide to the Appropriate Combination of Evaluation Methods

Open boxes indicate impairment ratings derived from these methods can be combined.

	Limb Length Discrepancy	Gait Derangement	Muscle Atrophy	Muscle Strength	ROM Ankylosis	Arthritis (DJD)	Amputation	Diagnosis-Based Estimates (DBE)	Skin Loss	Peripheral Nerve Injury	Complex Regional Pain Syndrome (CRPS)	Vascular
Limb Length Discrepancy		X					X					
Gait Derangement	X		X	X	X	X	X	X	X	X	X	X
Muscle Atrophy		X		X	X	X	X	X		X	X	
Muscle Strength		X	X		X	X		X		X	0	
ROM Ankylosis		X	X	X		X		X			0	
Arthritis (DJD)		X	X	X	X							
Amputation	X	X	X	X								
Diagnosis-Based Estimates (DBE)		X	X	X	X							
Skin Loss		X										
Peripheral Nerve Injury		X	X	X							X	
Complex Regional Pain Syndrome (CRPS)		X	X	0	0					X		X
Vascular		X									X	

X = Do not use these methods together for evaluating a single impairment.

0 = See specific instructions for CRPS of the lower extremity.

Typically, one method will adequately characterize the impairment and its impact on the ability to perform ADL. In some cases, however, more than one method needs to be used to accurately assess all features of the impairment. When more than one rating method is used, the individual impairment ratings are combined using the Combined Values Chart (p. 604).

Avoid combining methods that rate the same condition. Selecting the optimal approach or combining several methods requires judgment and experience. A careful examination and review of supporting material is essential to produce accurate and consistent results. If more than one method can be used, the method that provides the higher rating should be adopted.

17.2a Converting From Lower Extremity to Whole Person Impairment

To make this chapter easier to use, the tables in this chapter show the impairment percentages of the whole person, the lower extremity, and the specific lower extremity part together. The whole person impairments are not in parentheses; the lower limb impairment percents are in parentheses ( ); and, when applicable, the specific part impairments are in brackets [ ]. To calculate the lower extremity impairment percent from a specific part impairment percent (eg, foot), multiply by 0.7. To calculate whole person impairment from a lower extremity impairment, multiply by 0.4. These values are shown in Table 17-3.

Table 17-3 Whole Person Impairment Values Calculated From Lower Extremity Impairment

% Impairment of		% Impairment of		% Impairment of	
Lower Extremity	Whole Person	Lower Extremity	Whole Person	Lower Extremity	Whole Person
0 =	0	34 =	14	68 =	27
1 =	0	35 =	14	69 =	28
2 =	1	36 =	14	70 =	28
3 =	1	37 =	15	71 =	28
4 =	2	38 =	15	72 =	29
5 =	2	39 =	16	73 =	29
6 =	2	40 =	16	74 =	30
7 =	3	41 =	16	75 =	30
8 =	3	42 =	17	76 =	30
9 =	4	43 =	17	77 =	31
10 =	4	44 =	18	78 =	31
11 =	4	45 =	18	79 =	32
12 =	5	46 =	18	80 =	32
13 =	5	47 =	19	81 =	32
14 =	6	48 =	19	82 =	33
15 =	6	49 =	20	83 =	33
16 =	6	50 =	20	84 =	34
17 =	7	51 =	20	85 =	34
18 =	7	52 =	21	86 =	34
19 =	8	53 =	21	87 =	35
20 =	8	54 =	22	88 =	35
21 =	8	55 =	22	89 =	36
22 =	9	56 =	22	90 =	36
23 =	9	57 =	23	91 =	36
24 =	10	58 =	23	92 =	37
25 =	10	59 =	24	93 =	37
26 =	10	60 =	24	94 =	38
27 =	11	61 =	24	95 =	38
28 =	11	62 =	25	96 =	38
29 =	12	63 =	25	97 =	39
30 =	12	64 =	26	98 =	39
31 =	12	65 =	26	99 =	40
32 =	13	66 =	26	100 =	40
33 =	13	67 =	27		

Some individuals may have several impairments involving different parts of the same lower extremity; others may have several impairments of the same lower extremity part. If there are several impairments involving different regions of the lower extremity (eg, the thigh and the foot), evaluate each impairment separately, convert these regional impairments to whole person impairments, and combine the whole person impairment rating using the Combined Values Chart (p. 604). If there are multiple impairments within a region (eg, the toes and the ankle), combine these regional, lower extremity impairments of the foot and convert the combined foot impairment to a whole person impairment. Similarly, when using separate methods on the same region, combine the regional impairments before converting to a whole person impairment rating.

The 13 assessment methods listed in Table 17-1 are discussed separately below.

17.2b Limb Length Discrepancy

To determine limb length discrepancy, place the individual supine on the examination table with the legs in the same position, measure the distance between the anterior superior iliac spine and the medial malleolus on the involved side, and compare it with the opposite side. To identify where on the leg the discrepancy is, the knee is flexed to 90° while the feet are kept flat on the table. If one knee is higher than the other, the tibia is longer on that leg. Another method sometimes used is to evaluate the level of the iliac crest when the individual is standing. This is not recommended because differences in iliac crest levels may be due to pelvic obliquity, flexion, or adduction deformity of the hip. When these reasons exist for the obliquity, it is referred to as apparent leg length discrepancy.

Both clinical methods have at least a 0.5- to 1.0-cm variance, and both measurements are difficult to perform in a person with pelvic angulation, knee flexion contracture, or significant ankle edema. For this reason, **teleroentgenography** is recommended. If surface measurements with a tape measure from the anterior superior iliac spine to medial malleolus are used, they should be repeated three times and averaged to reduce measurement error. Impairments from limb length discrepancy depend on the magnitude of the leg length difference and are provided in Table 17-4. When applicable, the leg length discrepancy impairment is combined with other impairments.

Table 17-4 Impairment Due to Limb Length Discrepancy

Discrepancy (cm)	Whole Person (Lower Extremity) Impairment (%)
0-1.9	0
2-2.9	2-3 (5- 9)
3-3.9	4-5 (10-14)
4-4.9	6-7 (15-19)
5+	8 (20)

In case of shortening due to overriding or malalignment or fracture deformities, but not to include flexion or extension deformities, combine the following values with other functional sequelae, using the Combined Values Chart:

0-1.25 cm (0-½ in) = 5% of lower extremity
1.25-2.5 cm (½-1 in) = 10% of lower extremity
2.5-3.75 cm (1-1½ in) = 15% of lower extremity
3.75-5.0 cm (1½-2 in) = 20% of lower extremity

Example 17-1
2% Impairment Due to Limb Length Discrepancy

Subject: 35-year-old man.

History: A 108-kg (240-lb), 172.5-cm (5 ft 8 in), unbelted passenger sustained an open, comminuted fracture of the right femur in an automobile accident. He was treated with an unlocked nail. The fracture healed with shortening.

Current Symptoms: Walks with a decided limp. No pain or weakness.

Physical Exam: Full, pain-free range of motion of the hip and knee. No apparent atrophy of the thigh or calf; no loss of strength. The left leg measures 94 cm (37 in) from the iliac crest to the tip of the medial malleolus. The right leg measures 96.5 cm (38 in).

Clinical Studies: Teleroentgenography: left leg measures 81.5 cm (32.1 in), and the right leg measures 83.5 cm (33 in).

Diagnosis: Healed femur fracture with shortening.

Impairment Rating: 2% impairment of the whole person.

Comment: Although the individual has a limp (gait abnormality), gait derangement should be used only when no other method is available to rate the person. Limb length discrepancy is a more specific method. According to Table 17-4, the 2 cm of shortening results in an impairment of 5% of the leg, or 2% impairment of the whole person. Because the teleroentgenography is more accurate than tape measurements, especially in an obese individual (as this person was), it is the preferred method of determining leg length. Limb shortening may be combined with other methods (eg, diagnosis of femur fracture, as listed in Table 17-2).

17.2c Gait Derangement

Gait derangement is present with many different types of lower extremity impairments and is always secondary to another condition. An impairment rating due to a gait derangement should be supported by pathologic findings, such as x-rays. Except as otherwise noted, the percentages given in Table 17-5 are for full-time gait derangements of persons who are dependent on **assistive devices.**

Table 17-5 Lower Limb Impairment Due to Gait Derangement

Severity	Individual's Signs	Whole Person Impairment
Mild	a. Antalgic limp with shortened stance phase and documented moderate to advanced arthritic changes of hip, knee, or ankle	7%
	b. Positive Trendelenburg sign and moderate to advanced osteoarthritis of hip	10%
	c. Same as category a or b above, but individual requires part-time use of cane or crutch for distance walking but not usually at home or in the workplace	15%
	d. Requires routine use of short leg brace (ankle-foot orthosis [AFO])	15%
Moderate	e. Requires routine use of cane, crutch, or long leg brace (knee-ankle-foot orthosis [KAFO])	20%
	f. Requires routine use of cane or crutch and a short leg brace (AFO)	30%
	g. Requires routine use of two canes or two crutches	40%
Severe	h. Requires routine use of two canes or two crutches and a short leg brace (AFO)	50%
	i. Requires routine use of two canes or two crutches and a long leg brace (KAFO)	60%
	j. Requires routine use of two canes or two crutches and two lower-extremity braces (either AFOs or KAFOs)	70%
	k. Wheelchair dependent	80%

Whenever possible, the evaluator should use a more specific method. When the gait method is used, a written rationale should be included in the report. The lower limb impairment percents shown in Table 17-5 stand alone and are not combined with any other impairment evaluation method.

Section 17.2c does not apply to abnormalities based only on subjective factors, such as pain or sudden giving-way, as with, for example, an individual with low-back discomfort who chooses to use a cane to assist in walking.

Example 17-2
20% Impairment Due to Gait Derangement From Hip Pain

Subject: 61-year-old woman.

History: Fell on snow-covered steps and landed on her right knee. Developed severe pain in the right groin and later in the hip. No previous problems with her hip. She was last year's club tennis champion in the over-60 age bracket.

Current Symptoms: Difficulty walking for more than 5 blocks; continued pain; needs a cane when walking outside her home; can no longer play tennis or run.

Physical Exam: Walks with a Trendelenburg gait; full range of motion of the hip and knee. Complains of pain with full internal rotation of the hip. Neurovascular status intact.

Clinical Studies: Original x-rays: normal. Bone scan and MRI: did not reveal specific abnormalities. Follow-up x-rays 12 months later: slight narrowing of the hip joint space, which is measured at 3 mm, compared to 4 mm on the left.

Diagnosis: Hip pain with difficulty walking.

Impairment Rating: 20% impairment of the whole person.

Comment: Mild narrowing of the hip joint space on x-ray and pain at the extreme of internal rotation indicate early osteoarthritis is a possibility. The narrowing would result in an impairment of 3% of the whole person according to Table 17-3. However, the gait derangement results in a higher rating according to Table 17-5, and the higher rating should be used when it seems to more accurately represent the clinical situation. The two methods should not be combined because a gait evaluation is never combined with any other method. A rationale for its use should be provided by the evaluator.

17.2d Muscle Atrophy (Unilateral)

In evaluating muscle atrophy, the leg circumference should be measured and compared to the opposite leg at equal distances from either the joint line or another palpable anatomic structure. For example, a thigh atrophy may involve measuring the thigh circumference with a tape measure 10 cm above the patella and comparing it to a similar measure on the other leg. Calf circumference is compared at the maximum level bilaterally. Neither limb should have swelling or varicosities that would invalidate the measurements. Diminished muscle function can be estimated using four different methods. Only one should be used; that is, use only one method for assessing muscle function. Atrophy ratings should not be combined with any of the other three possible ratings of diminished muscle function (gait derangement, muscle weakness, and peripheral nerve injury). When muscle dysfunction is present, assess the condition with all four methods. Use the method that most accurately and objectively reflects the individual's impairment. Atrophy at both the thigh and calf is evaluated separately and the whole person impairment combined. Impairment ratings from atrophy are provided in Table 17-6.

Table 17-6 Impairment Due to Unilateral Leg Muscle Atrophy

Difference in Circumference (cm)	Impairment Degree	Whole Person (Lower Extremity) Impairment (%)
a. Thigh: The circumference is measured 10 cm above the patella with the knee fully extended and the muscles relaxed.		
0-0.9	None	0
1-1.9	Mild	1-2 (3-8)
2-2.9	Moderate	3-4 (8-13)
3+	Severe	5 (13)
b. Calf: The maximum circumference on the normal side is compared with the circumference at the same level on the affected side.		
0-0.9	None	0
1-1.9	Mild	1-2 (3-8)
2-2.9	Moderate	3-4 (8-13)
3+	Severe	5 (13)

Example 17-3

1% Impairment Due to Unilateral Muscle Atrophy From a Fracture

Subject: 78-year-old woman.

History: Sustained a closed fracture of her left tibia in a fall at the grocery store. The fracture was undisplaced and treated with a short leg cast for 3 months.

Current Symptoms: Healed fracture; no pain; leg weakness despite extensive physical therapy. Limited walking.

Physical Exam: Normal gait without support. No malalignment of the leg; neurovascular status is intact. The left calf measures 1.3 cm less than the right at the lower extremity's greatest circumference. The thigh circumferences 10 cm above the patella are within 1 cm. No discernible weakness by manual muscle testing.

Clinical Studies: X-rays of the tibia: complete healing of the fracture in good alignment.

Diagnosis: Healed tibia fracture.

Impairment Rating: 1% impairment of the whole person.

Comment: Fractures can lead to atrophy of an extremity when the limb immobilization is protracted. Especially in older people, it is difficult to regain full girth, despite adequate physical therapy. If no other abnormalities are present, these individuals can be rated by measuring the amount of atrophy. Other measures of muscle function, such as muscle strength or gait derangement, should not be combined with this method.

Example 17-4

4% Impairment Due to Unilateral Leg Muscle Atrophy From a Fracture

Subject: 49-year-old man.

History: Fractured the right tibia in a fall while mountain climbing. Completed rehabilitation and is at MMI 12 months later.

Current Symptoms: Pain-free walking with a mild limp. Symptoms of fatigue when walking or running. Minimal impact on ADL.

Physical Exam: 2 cm of thigh muscle atrophy and 1 cm of calf muscle atrophy. Manual muscle testing shows normal strength.

Clinical Studies: X-rays: undisplaced, healed tibial fracture.

Diagnosis: Healed tibia fracture.

Impairment Rating: 4% impairment of the whole person.

Comment: The healing times of fractured tibias are highly variable. Some individuals require prolonged immobilization and inactivity, which may result in significant atrophy. Younger individuals are more likely to be able to rebuild leg muscle mass and function compared with older individuals. Although manual muscle tests were normal, the injured extremity may fatigue more rapidly than usual. Evaluating the impairment in terms of atrophy gives an impairment estimate that more closely matches the person's capabilities when results of manual muscle testing are normal but atrophy exists. Combine 8% lower extremity thigh impairment (3% whole person impairment) and 3% lower extremity calf impairment (1% whole person impairment) (Table 17-6) to give an estimated 4% whole person impairment (Combined Values Chart, p. 604).

17.2e Manual Muscle Testing

Manual muscle testing, which typically involves groups of muscles, depends on the examinee's cooperation and is subject to his or her conscious and unconscious control. To be valid, the results should be concordant with other observable pathologic signs and medical evidence. In general, this method is best used for pathology that does not have a primary neurologic basis, eg, a compartment syndrome or direct muscle trauma. Weakness caused by an identifiable motor deficit of a specific peripheral nerve should be assessed according to Section 17.2l, Peripheral Nerve Injuries.

Measurements can be made by one or two observers. If the measurements are made by one examiner, they should be consistent on different occasions. If made by two, they should be consistent between examiners. Even in a fully cooperative individual, strength may vary from one examination to another, but not by more than one grade. If they vary by more than one grade between observers, or by the same examiner on separate occasions, the measurement should be considered invalid. In those individuals, impairment estimates should not be made using this section. Individuals whose performance is inhibited by pain or the fear of pain are not good candidates for manual muscle testing, and other evaluation methods should be considered for them. Table 17-7 shows the criteria on which estimates and grades of the lower extremity's strength are based, and Table 17-8 lists the actual ratings based on lower extremity weakness.

Table 17-7 Criteria for Grades of Muscle Function of the Lower Extremity

Grade	Description of Muscle Function
5	Active movement against gravity with full resistance
4	Active movement against gravity with some resistance
3	Active movement against gravity only, without resistance
2	Active movement with gravity eliminated
1	Slight contraction and no movement
0	No contraction

Table 17-8 Impairment Due to Lower Extremity Muscle Weakness

Muscle Group		Whole Person (Lower Extremity) [Foot] Impairment (%)												
		Grade 0			Grade 1			Grade 2			Grade 3			Grade 4	
Hip	Flexion	6	(15)		6	(15)		6	(15)		4	(10)		2	(5)	
	Extension	15	(37)		15	(37)		15	(37)		15	(37)		7	(17)	
	Abduction*	25	(62)		25	(62)		25	(62)		15	(27)		10	(25)	
Knee	Flexion	10	(25)		10	(25)		10	(25)		7	(17)		5	(12)	
	Extension	10	(25)		10	(25)		10	(25)		7	(17)		5	(12)	
Ankle	Flexion (plantar flexion)	15	(37)	[53]	15	(37)	[53]	15	(37)	[53]	10	(25)	[35]	7	(17)	[24]
	Extension (dorsiflexion)	10	(25)	[35]	10	(25)	[35]	10	(25)	[35]	10	(25)	[35]	5	(12)	[17]
	Inversion	5	(12)	[17]	5	(12)	[17]	5	(12)	[17]	5	(12)	[17]	2	(5)	[7]
	Eversion	5	(12)	[17]	5	(12)	[17]	5	(12)	[17]	5	(12)	[17]	2	(5)	[7]
Great toe	Extension	3	(7)	[10]	3	(7)	[10]	3	(7)	[10]	3	(7)	[10]	1	(2)	[3]
	Flexion			[17]			[12]	[17]	5	(12)	[17]	5	(12)	[17]	2	(5)	[7]

* Hip adduction weakness is evaluated as an obturator nerve impairment (see Table 17-37).

Example 17-5

10% Impairment Due to Muscle Weakness From a Patella Fracture

Subject: 55-year-old man.

History: Sustained a displaced fracture of the patella with multiple deep abrasions. The fracture required open reduction and internal fixation, but because of the deep, dirty abrasions and superficial infection, the surgery had to be delayed for 5 weeks, during which time he ambulated on crutches. Postoperatively, he was placed in a long leg cast for 6 weeks, followed by physical therapy for 8 weeks with a home exercise program.

Current Symptoms: Occasional discomfort about the knee, inability to walk fast or run, pain after long periods of sitting with the knee flexed, and a general weakness of the leg.

Physical Exam: Healed abrasions; surgical scar. Full range of motion of the knee and no instability. A 1-cm atrophy of the thigh. Manual muscle testing demonstrates weakness of both the quadriceps and the hamstring muscles; both are grade 4. Can flex and extend the knee against some resistance.

Clinical Studies: X-rays: healed patella fracture; no joint space narrowing.

Diagnosis: Residual muscle weakness and surgical scar following a patella fracture.

Impairment Rating: 10% impairment of the whole person.

Comment: Manual muscle testing is difficult to perform, but sometimes it is the best method available. Gait is less specific; the atrophy is minor and does not fully reflect the amount of weakness. There is no peripheral nerve injury. Use Table 17-7 to determine the grade of the muscle deficit, in this case grade 4. Referring to Table 17-8, extension of the knee with muscular function of grade 4 results in a lower extremity impairment of 12% (5% whole person impairment). Similarly, flexion of the knee at grade 4 results in a lower extremity impairment of 12% (5% whole person impairment). Converting to whole person and combining the two impairments results in a total whole person impairment of 10%.

Example 17-6
12% Impairment Due to Muscle Weakness From a Tibia Fracture With Compartment Syndrome

Subject: 30-year-old man.

History: Fell, sustaining a tibia fracture. Postoperatively, developed an anterior compartment syndrome, which was treated surgically.

Current Symptoms: Walks with an ankle-foot orthosis (AFO). When walking without this, he limps and walks with a drop foot. No pain.

Physical Exam: Ankle extension strength is grade 3; thus, he requires an AFO. Also has grade 3 weakness of the extensor hallucis longus. There is calf atrophy of 2 cm, consistent with the weakness observed on manual muscle testing.

Clinical Studies: Radiograph: healed tibia fracture.

Diagnosis: Tibia fracture with compartment syndrome.

Impairment Rating: 12% impairment of the whole person.

Comment: The 10% whole person impairment due to ankle weakness (25% lower extremity impairment) (Table 17-8) is combined with 3% whole person impairment (7% lower extremity impairment) for the loss of great toe extension using the Combined Values Chart (p. 604), giving 12% whole person impairment. A muscle strength deficit should not be combined with any other measure of muscle function, such as atrophy.

17.2f Range of Motion

Lower extremity impairment can be evaluated by assessing the range of motion of its joints, recognizing that pain and motivation may affect the measurements. If it is clear to the evaluator that a restricted range of motion has an organic basis, three measurements should be obtained and the greatest range measured should be used. If multiple evaluations exist, and there is inconsistency of a rating class between the findings of two observers, or in the findings on separate occasions by the same observer, the results are considered invalid. Figures 17-1 to 17-6 illustrate one method of measuring range of motion in the lower extremity. The ranges listed in Tables 17-9 through 17-14 are examples of mild, moderate, and severe impairments and are to be used as guides. Range-of-motion restrictions in multiple directions do increase the *impairment. Add* range-of-motion impairments for a single joint to determine the total joint range-of-motion impairments. For example, hip motion is evaluated and any impairment *added* in each of the six principal directions of motion.

Figure 17-1 Using a Goniometer to Measure Flexion of the Right Hip*

(a) Goniometer is placed at the right hip, and the pelvis is locked in the neutral position by flexing the left hip until the lumbar spine is flat.

(b) Examinee flexes the right hip until the anterior superior iliac spine begins to move, when the angle is recorded.

(c) To measure loss of extension of the right hip, the left hip is flexed until the lumbar spine is flat on the examining table, as determined by the examiner's hand, which is placed between the lumbar spine and table surface. The right thigh should rest flat on the table; any right hip flexion is recorded as a flexion contracture.

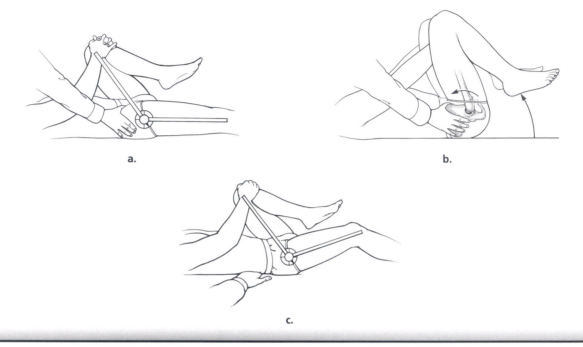

a.

b.

c.

* Accurate measurements of the lower extremity can also be obtained using a proper inclinometer (see Appendix).

Figure 17-2 Neutral Position (a), Abduction (b), and Adduction (c) of Right Hip

The examinee is supine on a flat surface. To improve consistency, flex the knee to stabilize the pelvis.

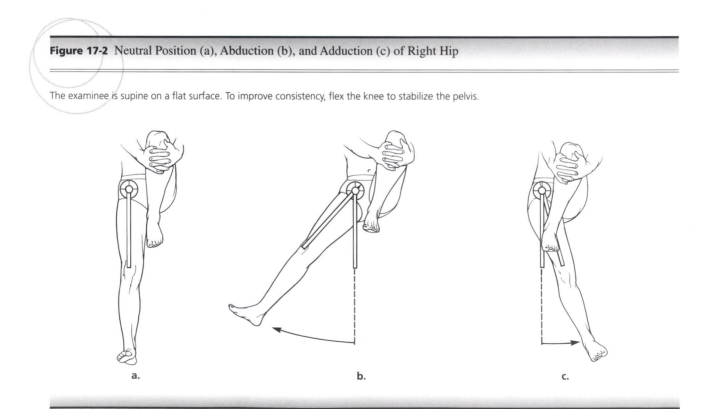

a.

b.

c.

Figure 17-3 Measuring Internal and External Hip Rotation*

The examinee is prone on a flat surface, and the knee is flexed 90°. One part of the goniometer is parallel to the flat surface, and the other is along the tibia. While testing, the examiner should place the hand on the knee to determine whether there is significant laxity of the knee joint. Keep the pelvis flat on the table.

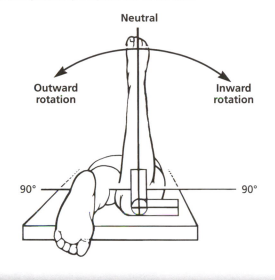

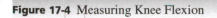

* Adapted from American Orthopaedic Association. *Manual of Orthopedic Surgery.* Rosemont, Ill: American Orthopaedic Association; 1966.

Figure 17-5 Measuring Foot Dorsiflexion and Plantar Flexion

The goniometer's pivot is centered over the ankle, and one arm parallels the tibia. The examiner reads the angles subtending the maximum arcs of motion for dorsiflexion and plantar flexion. The test is repeated with the knee flexed to 45°. The averages of the maximum angles represent dorsiflexion and plantar flexion ranges of motion.

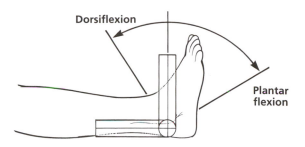

Figure 17-4 Measuring Knee Flexion

(a) The examinee is supine and the goniometer is next to the knee joint; one goniometer arm is parallel to the lower leg, and the other is parallel to the femur. Any deviation from 0° is recorded.

(b) The examinee exerts maximum effort to flex the knee. The flexion angle is obtained from the goniometer.

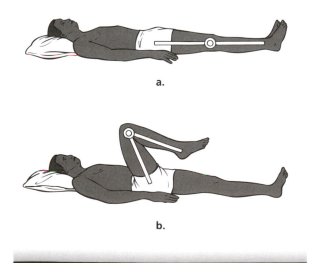

Figure 17-6 Evaluating the Range of Motion of a Toe: the Metatarsophalangeal (MTP) Joint of the Great Toe

(a) The examinee is seated in the position for evaluation of the toes. The knee is flexed to 45°, and the foot and MTP joint are in the neutral position.

(b) Extension: The goniometer is under the MTP joint, and its angle is read as a baseline. The examinee extends (dorsiflexes) the toe maximally, and the angle subtending the maximum arc of motion is read; the baseline angle is subtracted.

(c) Flexion: The goniometer is placed over the MTP joint. The baseline angle is read. The examinee plantar flexes the MTP joint maximally. The angle subtending the maximum arc of motion is read, and the baseline angle is subtracted.

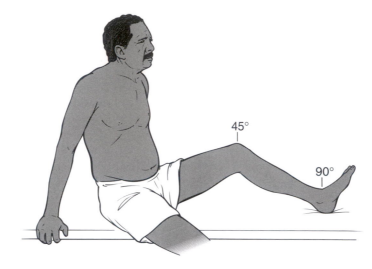

a.

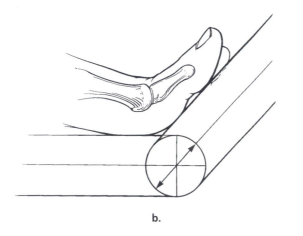

b.

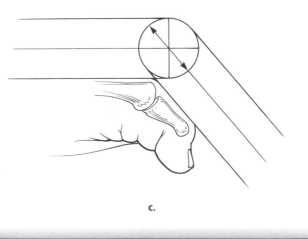

c.

Range-of-motion impairment values for the lower extremity are listed in Tables 17-9 to 17-14.

Table 17-9   Hip Motion Impairment

Motion	Whole Person (Lower Extremity) Impairment (%)		
	Mild 2% (5%)	Moderate 4% (10%)	Severe 8% (20%)
Flexion	Less than 100°	Less than 80°	Less than 50°
Extension	10°-19° flexion contracture	20°-29° flexion contracture	30° flexion contracture
Internal rotation	10°-20°	0°- 9°	—
External rotation	20°-30°	0°-19°	—
Abduction	15°-25°	5°-14°	Less than 5°
Adduction	0°- 15°	—	—
Abduction contracture*	0°- 5°	6°-10°	11°-20°

* An abduction contracture of greater than 20° = 15% whole person impairment.

Table 17-10   Knee Impairment

Motion	Whole Person (Lower Extremity) Impairment (%)		
	Mild 4% (10%)	Moderate 8% (20%)	Severe 14% (35%)
Flexion	Less than 110°	Less than 80°	Less than 60° + 1% (2%) per 10° less than 60°
Flexion contracture	5°-9°	10°-19°	20°+
Deformity measured by femoral-tibial angle; 3° to 10° valgus is considered normal			
Varus	2° valgus-0° (neutral)	1°-7° varus	8°-12° varus; add 1% (2%) per 2° over 12°
Valgus	10°-12°	13°-15°	16°-20°; add 1% (2%) per 2° over 20°

Table 17-11   Ankle Motion Impairment Estimates

Motion	Whole Person (Lower Extremity) [Foot] Impairment		
	Mild 3% (7%) [10%]	Moderate 6% (15%) [21%]	Severe 12% (30%) [43%]
Plantar flexion capability	11°-20°	1°-10°	None
Flexion contracture	—	10°	20°
Extension	10°-0° (neutral)	—	—

Table 17-12   Hindfoot Impairment Estimates

Motion	Whole Person (Lower Extremity) [Foot] Impairment	
	Mild 1% (2%) [3%]	Moderate and Severe 2% (5%) [7%]
Inversion	10°-20°	0°-9°
Eversion	0°-10°	—

Table 17-13   Ankle or Hindfoot Deformity Impairments

Position	Whole Person (Lower Extremity) [Foot] Impairment		
	Mild 5% (12%) [17%]	Moderate 10% (25%) [35%]	Severe 20% (50%) [72%]
Varus	10°-14°	15°-24°	25°+
Valgus	10°-20°	—	—

Table 17-14   Toe Impairments

Type of Impairment	Whole Person (Lower Extremity) [Foot] Impairment	
	Mild 1% (2%) [3%]	Moderate and Severe 2% (5%) [7%]

Great toe
  Metatarsophalangeal, extension
  Interphalangeal, flexion
	15°-30°
	
	Less than 20°
		Less than 15°
		
		—

Lesser toes* Metatarsophalangeal, extension	Less than 10°	—

* The maximum whole person impairment percent for impairment of two or more lesser toes of one foot is 2%.

Example 17-7
8% Impairment Due to Decreased Range of Motion From a Tibia Fracture

Subject: 45-year-old woman.

History: Sustained a tibia fracture in a motor vehicle accident.

Current Symptoms: No pain; stiffness about the ankle and foot, with some swelling of the foot and ankle toward evening. Cannot stand for long periods and cannot use shoes with elevated heels.

Physical Exam: Ankle flexion is 6°; ankle extension is 5°. Toe extension is less than 10° for all toes. 1-cm atrophy of the left calf. It is difficult to determine the strength of the ankle and toe extensors, but a mild weakness is noted.

Clinical Studies: X-rays: healed tibia fracture with no malalignment.

Diagnosis: Healed tibia frature.

Impairment Rating: 11% impairment of the whole person.

Comment: Moderate (6%) loss of ankle flexion (Table 17-11); mild (3%) loss of ankle extension; severe (2%) loss of toe motion (Table 17-14). Ankle flexion and extension losses are added (6% + 3% = 9%). Combine these with loss of toe motion by means of the Combined Values Chart (p. 604). The whole person impairment is 11%. The range-of-motion (ROM) method is preferable to the atrophy or muscle testing methods. Comparing impairment values from Tables 17-11 and 17-14 (ROM) with those from Table 17-6 (atrophy), the impairment from a ROM assessment is greater than one for atrophy and more accurately characterizes the individual's impairment. Manual muscle testing is difficult to perform when close to normal because of the lower leg muscles' limited excursion about the ankle and toes when motion is severely restricted.

17.2g Joint Ankylosis

An immobile joint is an impairment even when the position of ankylosis is optimal. Malposition in angulation or rotation of an arthrodesed or fused joint increases the magnitude of the impairment. Surgical correction usually is preferable to accepting a significant malposition, but it is not always possible or practical. Impairment estimates for malposition are therefore included for the infrequently encountered individual who is not a candidate for surgical correction.

The following text and Tables 17-15 through 17-30 indicate the optimal neutral positions for ankyloses of the lower extremity joints and provide the impairment percents for ankyloses in those optimal positions. Any variation from the optimal neutral position of an ankylosed joint increases the baseline impairment percent as indicated in the tables. The values listed are for the maximum end of the deformity range. Specific deformities should be rated using interpolation of the ranges in the tables as illustrated by examples in this section. Multiple malposition deformities of the same joint, ie, angulation and malrotation, are *added,* whereas deformities of different joints are *combined* using the Combined Values Chart (p. 604). The baseline rating for ankylosis in the neutral position is used only once for each joint. As noted elsewhere, added or combined impairment ratings can never exceed 100% of the lower extremity.

Hip

The optimal position of ankylosis is 25° to 40° flexion and neutral rotation, adduction, and abduction. This position represents a 20% whole person impairment and a 50% lower extremity impairment.

Tables 17-15 through 17-19 provide impairment estimates for hip ankyloses in various positions. See Figures 17-1 through 17-3 for illustration of the measurement of hip motion and ankylosis. Impairment estimates for rotation, abduction, and adduction deformities are added. The maximum hip impairment or lower limb impairment is 100%, which is a 40% whole person impairment.

Table 17-15 Impairment Due to Ankylosis in Hip Flexion

Ankylosis in Flexion (°)	Whole Person (Lower Extremity) Impairment (%)
0- 9	15 (37)
10-19	10 (25)
20-24	5 (12)
25-39	0 (0)
40-49	5 (12)
50-59	10 (25)
60-69	15 (37)
70+	20 (50)

* The appropriate ankylosis impairment percent is added to the impairment percent for ankylosis in the neutral position given in the text.

Table 17-16 Impairment Due to Ankylosis in Hip
Internal Rotation*

Ankylosis in Internal Rotation (°)	Whole Person (Lower Extremity) Impairment (%)
5- 9	5 (12)
10-19	10 (25)
20-29	15 (37)
30+	20 (50)

* The appropriate ankylosis impairment percent is added to the impairment percent for
ankylosis in the neutral position given in the text.

Table 17-17 Impairment Due to Ankylosis in Hip
External Rotation*

Ankylosis in External Rotation (°)	Whole Person (Lower Extremity) Impairment (%)
10-19	5 (12)
20-29	10 (25)
30-39	15 (37)
40+	20 (50)

* The appropriate ankylosis impairment percent is added to the impairment percent for
ankylosis in the neutral position given in the text.

Table 17-18 Impairment Due to Ankylosis in Hip
Abduction*

Ankylosis in Abduction (°)	Whole Person (Lower Extremity) Impairment (%)
5-14	10 (25)
15-24	15 (37)
25+	20 (50)

* The appropriate ankylosis impairment percent is added to the impairment percent for
ankylosis in the neutral position given in the text.

Table 17-19 Impairment Due to Ankylosis in Hip
Adduction*

Ankylosis in Adduction (°)	Whole Person (Lower Extremity) Impairment (%)
5- 9	10 (25)
10-14	15 (37)
15+	20 (50)

* The appropriate ankylosis impairment percent is added to the impairment percent for
ankylosis in the neutral position given in the text.

Example 17-8
40% Impairment Due to Hip Ankylosis After a Fracture Dislocation of the Hip

Subject: 64-year-old man.

History: Sustained an injury to the right hip in an industrial accident involving a fall from a moving forklift. Landed on the right hip with a central fracture dislocation of the hip joint. An open reduction was performed with less than satisfactory reduction. In the postoperative period, sustained a myocardial infarction, preempting further surgery. The fractures healed, but the hip was ankylosed. With rehabilitation completed, he is at MMI 16 months after injury.

Current Symptoms: No pain in the hip, but difficulty walking, particularly up and down stairs. Can sit comfortably, but has difficulty getting up from a chair and getting in and out of a car.

Physical Exam: Walks with the aid of one crutch. No motion in the right hip, which is ankylosed in 55° of flexion, 12° of external rotation, and 10° of abduction. Neurovascular status is intact.

Clinical Studies: Radiograph: healed right hip fracture-dislocation fused in flexion; external rotation and abduction deformity.

Diagnosis: Fracture dislocation of right hip with malunion.

Impairment Rating: 40% impairment of the whole person.

Comment: The impairment rating for a hip that is ankylosed in the optimal position is 50% of the lower extremity. Add additional impairment percentages when the position is less than optimal. In this case, the flexion position of 55° results in 25% additional lower extremity impairment, external rotation of 12° results in another 12% lower extremity impairment, and abduction of 10° results in a 25% lower extremity impairment. Adding 50% + 25% + 12% + 25% = 112%. Since no impairment can be greater than that for an amputation, the impairment of the lower extremity is 100%, which is equivalent to a 40% whole person impairment.

Knee

The optimal position is 10° to 15° of flexion with neutral alignment. Figure 17-4 shows how the goniometer is used to measure knee flexion. Ankylosis in the optimal position is a 67% lower extremity impairment or 27% whole person impairment.

Impairments beyond those of the optimal position are evaluated according to Tables 17-20 through 17-23. Malpositions of the knee include varus, valgus, and malrotation deformities, which can increase the impairment up to 100% impairment of the lower extremity.

Table 17-20 Impairment Due to Knee Ankylosis in Varus*

Ankylosis in Varus (°)	Whole Person (Lower Extremity) Impairment (%)
0- 9	5 (12)
10-19	10 (25)
20+	13 (33)

* The appropriate ankylosis impairment percent is added to the impairment percent for ankylosis in the neutral position given in the text.

Table 17-21 Impairment Due to Knee Ankylosis in Valgus*

Ankylosis in Valgus (°)	Whole Person (Lower Extremity) Impairment (%)
10-19	5 (12)
20-29	10 (25)
30+	13 (33)

* The appropriate ankylosis impairment percent is added to the impairment percent for ankylosis in the neutral position given in the text.

Table 17-22 Impairment Due to Knee Ankylosis in Flexion*

Ankylosis in Flexion (°)	Whole Person (Lower Extremity) Impairment (%)
20-29	5 (12)
30-39	10 (25)
40+	13 (33)

* The appropriate ankylosis impairment percent is added to the impairment percent for ankylosis in the neutral position given in the text.

Table 17-23 Impairment Due to Knee Ankylosis in Internal or External Malrotation*

Ankylosis in Internal or External Malrotation (°)	Whole Person (Lower Extremity) Impairment (%)
10-19	5 (12)
20-29	10 (25)
30+	13 (33)

* The appropriate ankylosis impairment percent is added to the impairment percent for ankylosis in the neutral position given in the text.

Example 17-9
32% Impairment Due to Ankylosis of the Knee

Subject: 41-year-old man.

History: Sustained a comminuted open distal right femur and proximal tibia fracture in a car accident; became infected and healed with ankylosis.

Current Symptoms: No pain. Has difficulty walking, sitting, and driving. Some swelling of the lower leg by the end of the day.

Physical Exam: Several well-healed scars about the knee. There is ankylosis in 20° of flexion with 7° valgus and normal rotation compared to the left leg.

Clinical Studies: X-rays: well-healed tibia and femur fractures.

Diagnosis: Tibia and femur fractures with ankylosis of the knee joint.

Impairment Rating: 32% impairment of the whole person.

Comment: Ankylosis in the optimal position results in a 27% whole person impairment (67% lower extremity impairment). This man has a 20° flexion deformity, rather than a 10° to 15° position, which would be optimal. Adding 5% whole person impairment from Table 17-22 to the 27% yields a total whole person impairment rating of 32%.

Ankle

The optimal ankylosis position is the neutral position without flexion, extension, varus, or valgus. Ankylosis of the ankle in the neutral position is a 4% whole person impairment, a 10% lower extremity impairment, and a 14% foot impairment. A variation from the neutral position should be evaluated according to Tables 17-24 through 17-28. The maximum impairments are 25% whole person impairment, 62% lower extremity impairment, and 88% ankle impairment. Figure 17-5 illustrates a measurement of dorsiflexion and plantar flexion.

Table 17-24 Ankle Impairment Due to Ankylosis in Plantar Flexion or Dorsiflexion*

Position	Whole Person (Lower Extremity) [Foot] Impairment (%)
20°+ dorsiflexion	15 (37) [53]
10°-19° dorsiflexion	7 (17) [24]
10°-19° plantar flexion	7 (17) [24]
20°-29° plantar flexion	15 (37) [53]
30°+ plantar flexion	21 (52) [74]

* The appropriate ankylosis impairment percent is added to the impairment percent for ankylosis in the neutral position given in the text.

Table 17-25 Ankle Impairment Due to Ankylosis in Varus Position*

Varus Position (°)	Whole Person (Lower Extremity) [Foot] Impairment (%)
5- 9	10 (25) [35]
10-19	15 (37) [53]
20-29	18 (43) [61]
30+	21 (52) [74]

* The appropriate ankylosis impairment percent is added to the impairment percent for ankylosis in the neutral position given in the text.

Table 17-26 Ankle Impairment Due to Ankylosis in Valgus Position*

Valgus Position (°)	Whole Person (Lower Extremity) [Foot] Impairment (%)
10-19	10 (25) [35]
20-30	15 (37) [53]
30+	21 (52) [74]

* The appropriate ankylosis impairment percent is added to the impairment percent for ankylosis in the neutral position given in the text.

Table 17-27 Ankle Impairment Due to Ankylosis in Internal Malrotation*

Internal Malrotation (°)	Whole Person (Lower Extremity) [Foot] Impairment (%)
0- 9	5 (12) [17]
10-19	10 (25) [35]
20-29	15 (37) [53]
30+	21 (52) [74]

* The appropriate ankylosis impairment percent is added to the impairment percent for ankylosis in the neutral position given in the text.

Table 17-28 Ankle Impairment Due to Ankylosis in External Malrotation

External Malrotation (°)	Whole Person (Lower Extremity) [Foot] Impairment (%)
15-19	5 (12) [17]
20-29	10 (25) [35]
30-39	15 (37) [53]
40+	21 (52) [74]

* The appropriate ankylosis impairment percent is added to the impairment percent for ankylosis in the neutral position given in the text.

Example 17-10
11% Impairment Due to Ankle Fracture

Subject: 55-year-old man.

History: Sustained a severe distal tibial and intra-articular ankle fracture in a fall from a height. The fracture was treated with external fixation and healed with bony ankylosis of the ankle. History of insulin-dependent diabetes mellitus.

Current Symptoms: No pain; walks slowly; difficulty walking on uneven surfaces.

Physical Exam: The ankle is ankylosed in 15° dorsiflexion and 7° varus.

Clinical Studies: X-rays: healed distal tibial and intra-articular ankle fracture. Fusion across the ankle joint.

Diagnosis: Ankle fracture with ankylosis.

Impairment Rating: 20% impairment of the whole person.

Comment: 11% whole person impairment related to ankle flexion (Table 17-24) and 10% whole person impairment related to the varus deformity (Table 17-25). These ankle impairments are combined, giving a 20% whole person impairment (Combined Values Chart, p. 604). Because of the diabetic condition and marginal circulation to the ankle region, corrective surgery is not recommended. The impairment method for malpositioning and ankylosis is more appropriate than using the method for an intra-articular ankle fracture (see Table 17-33). An impairment percent related to diabetes, if appropriate, should be combined with the lower extremity impairment.

Foot (Hindfoot, Midfoot, Forefoot)

For the subtalar part of the foot, the optimal ankylosis position is neutral, or 0°, without varus or valgus. The ankylosis impairment in the neutral position is 4% for the whole person, 10% for the lower extremity, and 14% for the foot. Malpositioning may increase the whole person impairment up to 25%. Varus or valgus malpositioning is estimated in the same way as for the ankle (Tables 17-25 and 17-26).

Ankylosis impairment for loss of the tibia–os calcis angle is estimated according to Table 17-29. The tibia–os calcis angle is made by the longitudinal axis of the os calcis and the longitudinal axis of the tibia with the ankle in neutral position (Figure 17-7).

Table 17-29 Impairments for Loss of the Tibia–Os Calcis Angle*

Angle (°)	Whole Person (Lower Extremity) [Foot] Impairment (%)
110-100	10 (25) [35]
99- 90	15 (37) [53]
Less than 90	21 (52) [74]

* The tibia–os calcis angle is shown in Figure 17-7.

Figure 17-7 Tibia–Os Calcis Angle*

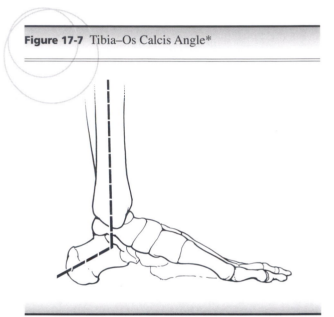

* The tibia–os calcis angle is the angle between the longitudinal axis of the os calcis and the vertical tibia, as shown by this drawing based on a lateral x-ray of the foot and ankle in the *neutral* position.

For pantalar ankylosis, the optimal position is neutral; the impairment estimates for that position are 10% for the whole person, 25% for the lower extremity, and 35% for the foot. Further flexion, varus, and valgus impairments are estimated as shown in Tables 17-25 to 17-29.

Example 17-11
14% Impairment Due to Ankle Ankylosis and Calcaneus Fracture

Subject: 41-year-old woman.

History: Fractured her ankle and calcaneal tuberosity in a fall from a height. Treated with a cast and healed with a bony fusion.

Current Symptoms: Walks without support but with special shoes. Difficulty walking on uneven ground and has swelling when she sits for long periods of time.

Physical Exam: Considerable swelling about the heel with widening; no tenderness; no motion at the ankle.

Clinical Studies: X-rays: fused ankle with fractured calcaneus and a 5° flexion angle at ankle joint. The tibia–os calcis angle is 100°.

Diagnosis: Ankle ankylosis with a healed fracture of the distal tibia and calcaneus.

Impairment Rating: 14% impairment of the whole person.

Comment: The optimal ankle position is neutral; 5° of flexion is a small deformity and does not add to the impairment. The ankle rating for ankylosis is 4% whole person impairment. The normal tibia–os calcis angle is >120°; 100° indicates an additional 10% whole person impairment. Both impairments are added, resulting in a 14% whole person impairment.

Toes

Figure 17-6 illustrates the use of a goniometer to measure a toe's range of motion. Table 17-30 provides impairment estimates related to ankylosis of one or several toes.

Example 17-12
3% Impairment Due to Crush Injury of the Toes

Subject: 52-year-old man.

History: A metal object weighing over 68 kg (150 lb) fell on his toes at work. He sustained a crush injury to the right forefoot involving the soft tissues as well as multiple fractures to the toes. Treatment was nonoperative, and the soft tissue and fractures healed.

Current Symptoms: Difficulty walking fast or long distances; inability to run; stiffness of all toes.

Physical Exam: The forefoot is mildly swollen and has several healed scars. Range of motion of the metatarsophalangeal joint of the great toe is 15° of extension and 15° of flexion. There is no motion of the other toe joints. The toes are in a normal position of function. Walks with a mild limp; unable to push off normally.

Clinical Studies: X-rays: healed toe fractures.

Table 17-30 Impairment of the Foot Due to Ankylosis of Toes

| Digit(s) Involved | Whole Person (Lower Extremity) [Foot] Impairment (%) | | |
| | Ankylosed in | | |
	Full Extension	Position of Function	Full Flexion
Great	4 (10) [14]	4 (9) [13]	5 (13) [18]
Great, second	5 (12) [17]	4 (11) [15]	6 (15) [21]
Great, second, third	6 (14) [20]	5 (12) [17]	7 (17) [24]
Great, second, fourth	6 (14) [20]	5 (12) [17]	7 (17) [24]
Great, second, fifth	6 (14) [20]	5 (12) [17]	7 (17) [24]
Great, second, third, fourth	6 (16) [23]	5 (13) [19]	8 (19) [27]
Great, second, third, fifth	6 (16) [23]	5 (13) [19]	8 (19) [27]
Great, second, fourth, fifth	6 (16) [23]	5 (13) [19]	8 (19) [27]
Great, second, third, fourth, fifth	7 (18) [26]	6 (15) [21]	8 (21) [30]
Great, third	5 (12) [17]	4 (11) [15]	6 (15) [21]
Great, third, fourth	6 (14) [20]	5 (12) [17]	7 (17) [24]
Great, third, fifth	6 (14) [20]	5 (12) [17]	7 (17) [24]
Great, third, fourth, fifth	6 (16) [23]	5 (13) [19]	8 (19) [27]
Great, fourth	5 (12) [17]	4 (11) [15]	6 (15) [21]
Great, fourth, fifth	6 (14) [20]	5 (12) [17]	7 (17) [24]
Great, fifth	5 (12) [17]	4 (11) [15]	6 (15) [21]
Second	1 (2) [3]	0 (1) [2]	1 (2) [3]
Second, third	2 (4) [6]	1 (3) [4]	2 (4) [6]
Second, third, fourth	2 (6) [9]	1 (3) [4]	2 (6) [9]
Second, third, fifth	2 (6) [9]	2 (4) [6]	2 (6) [9]
Second, third, fourth, fifth	3 (8) [12]	2 (6) [8]	3 (8) [12]
Second, fourth	2 (4) [6]	1 (3) [4]	2 (4) [6]
Second, fourth, fifth	2 (6) [9]	2 (4) [6]	3 (8) [12]
Second, fifth	2 (4) [6]	1 (3) [4]	2 (4) [6]
Third	1 (2) [3]	0 (1) [2]	1 (2) [3]
Third, fourth	2 (4) [6]	1 (3) [4]	2 (4) [6]
Third, fourth, fifth	2 (6) [9]	2 (4) [6]	2 (6) [9]
Third, fifth	2 (4) [6]	1 (3) [4]	2 (4) [6]
Fourth	1 (2) [3]	0 (1) [2]	1 (2) [3]
Fourth, fifth	2 (4) [6]	1 (3) [4]	2 (4) [6]
Fifth	1 (2) [3]	0 (1) [2]	1 (2) [3]

Diagnosis: Crush injury to the forefoot with multiple fractures.

Impairment Rating: 3% impairment of the whole person.

Comment: Mild loss of motion of the great toe corresponds to a 1% whole person impairment (Table 17-14). Add this to the 2% whole person impairment due to ankylosis of toes 2 through 5 in a functional position (Table 17-30).

17.2h Arthritis

Roentgenographic grading systems for inflammatory and degenerative arthritis are well established and widely used for treatment decisions and scientific investigation. For most individuals, roentgenographic grading is a more objective and valid method for assigning impairment estimates than physical findings, such as the range of motion or joint crepitation. While there are some individuals with arthritis for whom loss of motion is the principal impairment, most people are impaired more by pain and sometimes weakness, but they still can maintain functional ranges of motion, at least in the early stages of the process. Range-of-motion techniques are therefore of limited value for estimating impairment secondary to arthritis in many individuals. Crepitation is an inconstant finding that depends on such factors as forces on joint surfaces and synovial fluid viscosity.

Certain roentgenographic findings that are of diagnostic importance, such as osteophytes and reactive sclerosis, have no direct bearing on impairment. The best roentgenographic indicator of disease stage and impairment for a person with arthritis is the cartilage interval or joint space. The hallmark of all types of arthritis is thinning of the articular cartilage; this correlates well with disease progression.

The need for joint replacement or major reconstruction usually corresponds with complete loss of the articular surface (joint space). The impairment estimates in a person with arthritis (Table 17-31) are based on standard x-rays taken with the individual standing, if possible. The ideal film-to-camera distance is 90 cm (36 in), and the beam should be at the level of and parallel to the joint surface. The estimate for the patellofemoral joint is based on a "sunrise view" taken at 40° flexion or on a true lateral view.

In the case of the knee, the joint must be in neutral flexion-extension position (0°) to evaluate the x-rays. Impairments of individuals with knee flexion contractures should not be estimated using x-rays because measurements are unreliable. In these individuals, the range-of-motion method should be used. X-rays of the hip joint are taken in the neutral position. The cartilage interval (joint space) of the hip is relatively constant in the various positions; therefore, positioning is not as critical as for the knee x-rays. The ankle x-ray must be taken in a mortise view, which is 10° internal rotation: 10° flexion or extension is permissible. Evaluation of the foot joints requires a lateral view for the hindfoot and an anteroposterior view for the midfoot and forefoot. If there is doubt or controversy about the suitability of the

Table 17-31 Arthritis Impairments Based on Roentgenographically Determined Cartilage Intervals

Joint	Whole Person (Lower Extremity) [Foot] Impairment (%)			
	Cartilage Interval			
	3 mm	2 mm	1 mm	0 mm
Sacroiliac (3 mm)*	—	1 (2)	3 (7)	3 (7)
Hip (4 mm)	3 (7)	8 (20)	10 (25)	20 (50)
Knee (4 mm)	3 (7)	8 (20)	10 (25)	20 (50)
Patellofemoral†	—	4 (10)	6 (15)	8 (20)
Ankle (4 mm)	2 (5) [7]	6 (15) [21]	8 (20) [28]	12 (30) [43]
Subtalar (3 mm)	—	2 (5) [7]	6 (15) [21]	10 (25) [35]
Talonavicular (2-3 mm)	—	—	4 (10) [14]	8 (20) [28]
Calcaneocuboid	—	—	4 (10) [14]	8 (20) [28]
First metatarsophalangeal	—	—	2 (5) [7]	5 (12) [17]
Other metatarsophalangeal	—	—	1 (2) [3]	3 (7) [10]

* Normal cartilage intervals are given in parentheses.

† In an individual with a history of direct trauma, a complaint of patellofemoral pain, and crepitation on physical examination. but without joint space narrowing on x-rays, a 2% whole person or 5% lower extremity impairment is given.

radiographic method in a specific individual, range-of-motion techniques may be used instead.

A person who has an intra-articular fracture and subsequent rapid onset of arthritis should be evaluated using the arthritis section combined with Section 17.2j on diagnosis-based estimates.

Example 17-13
15% Impairment Due to Arthritis and Malalignment From a Tibia Fracture

Subject: 48-year-old man.

History: Fell from a loading dock 23 years ago, sustaining a right tibia fracture.

Current Symptoms: Resumed work. Over the last several years, had right knee pain toward the end of the day. Occasional mild swelling of the knee joint.

Physical Exam: The fracture healed with a 10° varus deformity of the right tibia. He has almost full range of motion of the injured knee, 0° through 125°, and mild crepitation.

Clinical Studies: Standing x-rays: cartilage interval is 2 mm on the medial side of the right knee.

Diagnosis: Moderate degenerative arthritis of the right knee.

Impairment Rating: 15% impairment of the whole person.

Comment: Symptoms worsen after a day's work. The cause of pain and impairment is the development of osteoarthritis in the knee joint. Accurate x-rays are an objective way to estimate this impairment. Based on the x-rays, this individual has an 8% whole person impairment and 20% impairment of the lower extremity due to arthritis (Table 17-31). The 8% whole person impairment related to knee arthritis should be combined with an 8% whole person impairment due to the tibia fracture malalignment, 10° varus of the tibia (see Table 17-33). Combining two 8% whole person impairments yields a 15% whole person impairment (Combined Values Chart, p. 604).

17.2i Amputations
Impairments of the lower extremity due to amputations are estimated according to Table 17-32.

Example 17-14
28% Impairment Due to Amputation From a Crush Injury

Subject: 35-year-old man.

History: Sustained a crush injury to the left leg in a motor vehicle accident. Below-knee amputation.

Current Symptoms: Ambulates with a below-knee prosthesis, without the need for a cane or support. Has no pain in the stump and no phantom pain.

Physical Exam: The left knee is stable, has no sign of arthritis, and has full motion.

Clinical Studies: X-rays: 13 cm (5 in) of retained proximal tibia in the stump. The stump is well healed, and he has not had any trouble with stump breakdown.

Diagnosis: Below-knee left leg amputation.

Impairment Rating: 28% impairment of the whole person.

Comment: Table 17-32 shows that this condition receives a 28% whole person impairment rating. In this case, there was no concomitant knee injury. If there is an injury to the knee, or more proximal to the leg, that may also need to be rated.

Table 17-32 Impairment Estimates for Amputations

Amputation	Whole Person (Lower Extremity) [Foot] Impairment (%)
Hemipelvectomy	50
Hip disarticulation	40 (100)

Above knee
  Proximal
  Midthigh
  Distal
	
	40 (100)
	36 (90)
	32 (80)

Knee disarticulation	32 (80)

Below knee
  Less than 3"
  3" or more
	
	32 (80)
	28 (70)

Syme (hindfoot)	25 (62) [100]
Midfoot	18 (45) [64]
Transmetatarsal	16 (40) [57]
First metatarsal	8 (20) [28]
Other metatarsals	2 (5) [7]
All toes at metatarsophalangeal (MTP) joint	9 (22) [31]
Great toe at MTP joint	5 (12) [17]
Great toe at interphalangeal joint	2 (5) [7]
Lesser toes at MTP joint	1 (2) [3] each

17.2j Diagnosis-Based Estimates
Some impairment estimates are assigned more appropriately on the basis of a diagnosis than on the basis of findings on physical examination. A good example is that of an individual impaired because of a successful replacement of a hip. This person may function well but require prophylactic restrictions of activities of daily living to prevent a further impairment, such as premature failure of the prosthesis. Table 17-33 provides impairment estimates for certain lower extremity impairments. For most diagnosis-based estimates, the ranges of impairment are broad, and the estimate will depend on the clinical manifestations and their impact on the ability to perform activities of daily living. Hip replacements should first be rated using Table 17-34 and knee replacements using Table 17-35. The points obtained from the assessment are then applied to Table 17-33 for the diagnosis impairment rating. If limb length discrepancy also exists, that impairment rating should be combined with the impairment from the joint replacement using the Combined Values Chart (p. 604).

Chapter 17

Table 17-33 Impairment Estimates for Certain Lower Extremity Impairments

Region and Condition	Whole Person (Lower Extremity) [Foot] Impairment (%)
Pelvis*	
Pelvic fracture Undisplaced, nonarticular, healed, without neurologic deficit or other sign	0
Displaced nonarticular fracture: estimate by evaluating shortening and weakness	—
Acetabular fracture: estimate according to range of motion and joint changes	—
Sacroiliac joint fracture: consider displacement	1-3 (2-7)
Ischial bursitis (weaver's bottom) requiring frequent unweighting and limiting of sitting time	3 (7)
Hip	
Total hip replacement; includes endoprosthesis, unipolar or bipolar Good results, 85-100 points†	15 (37)
Fair results, 50-84 points†	20 (50)
Poor results, less than 50 points†	30 (75)
Femoral neck fracture, healed in Good position	Evaluate according to examination findings
Malunion	12 (30) plus range-of-motion criteria
Nonunion	15 (37) plus range-of-motion criteria
Girdlestone arthroplasty Or estimate according to examination findings; use the greater estimate	20 (50)
Trochanteric bursitis (chronic) with abnormal gait	3 (7)
Femoral shaft fracture	
Healed with 10°-14° angulation or malrotation 15°-19°	10 (25) 18 (45)
20°	+1 (2) per degree up to 25 (62)

Region and Condition	Whole Person (Lower Extremity) [Foot] Impairment (%)
Knee	
Patellar subluxation or dislocation with residual instability	3 (7)
Patellar fracture Undisplaced, healed	3 (7)
Articular surface displaced more than 3 mm	5 (12)
Displaced with nonunion	7 (17)
Patellectomy Partial	3 (7)
Total	9 (22)
Meniscectomy, medial *or* lateral Partial	1 (2)
Total	3 (7)
Meniscectomy, medial *and* lateral Partial	4 (10)
Total	9 (22)
Cruciate *or* collateral ligament laxity Mild	3 (7)
Moderate	7 (17)
Severe	10 (25)
Cruciate *and* collateral ligament laxity Moderate	10 (25)
Severe	15 (37)
Plateau fracture Undisplaced	2 (5)
Displaced 5°-9° angulation	5 (12)
10°-19° angulation	10 (25)
20°+ angulation	+1 (2) per degree up to 20 (50)
Supracondylar or intercondylar fracture Undisplaced fracture	2 (5)
Displaced fracture 5°-9° angulation	5 (12)
10°-19° angulation	10 (25)
20°+ angulation	+1 (2) per degree up to 20 (50)

* Refer also to Section 15.14 on the pelvis.

† See Table 17-34 or Table 17-35 for point rating system.

‡ A stress x-ray is an anterior-posterior view taken with a varus or valgus stress applied by a knowledgeable physician.

§ The tibia–os calcis angle is measured as shown in Figure 17-7.

Region and Condition	Whole Person (Lower Extremity) [Foot] Impairment (%)
Total knee replacement including unicondylar replacement	
Good result, 85-100 points†	15 (37)
Fair results, 50-84 points†	20 (50)
Poor results, less than 50 points†	30 (75)
Proximal tibial osteotomy	
Good result	10 (25)
Poor result	Estimate impairment according to examination and arthritic degeneration
Tibial shaft fracture, malalignment of	
10°-14°	8 (20)
15°-19°	12 (30)
20°+	+1 (2) per degree up to 20 (50)
Ankle	
Ligamentous instability (based on stress x-rays‡)	
Mild (2-3 mm excess opening)	2 (5) [7]
Moderate (4-6 mm)	4 (10) [14]
Severe (> 6 mm)	6 (15) [21]
Fracture	
Extra-articular with angulation	
10°-14°	6 (15) [21]
15°-19°	10 (25) [35]
20°+	+1 (2) [3] per degree up to 15 (37) [53]
Intra-articular with displacement	8 (20) [28]
Hindfoot	
Fracture	
Extra-articular (calcaneal)	
With varus angulation 10°-19°	5 (12) [17]
With varus angulation 20°+	0.5 (1) [1] per degree up to 10 (25)
With valgus angulation 10°-19°	3 (7) [11]
With valgus angulation 20°+	0.5 (2) [1] per degree up to 10 (25) [35]

Region and Condition	Whole Person (Lower Extremity) [Foot] Impairment (%)
Loss of tibia–os calcis angle§	
Angle is 120°-110°	5 (12) [17]
Angle is 100°-90°	8 (20) [28]
Angle is less than 90°	+1 (2) [3] per degree up to 15 (37) [54]
Intra-articular fracture with displacement	
Subtalar bone	6 (15) [21]
Talonavicular bone	3 (7) [10]
Calcaneocuboid bone	3 (7) [10]
Midfoot deformity	
Cavus	
Mild	1 (2) [3]
Moderate	3 (7) [10]
"Rocker bottom"	
Mild	2 (5) [7]
Moderate	4 (10) [14]
Severe	8 (20) [28]
Avascular necrosis of the talus	
Without collapse	3 (7) [10]
With collapse	6 (15) [21]
Forefoot deformity	
Metatarsal fracture with loss of weight transfer	
1st metatarsal	4 (10) [14]
5th metatarsal	2 (5) [7]
Other metatarsal	1 (2) [3]
Metatarsal fracture with plantar angulation and metatarsalgia	
1st metatarsal	4 (10) [14]
5th metatarsal	2 (5) [7]
Other metatarsal	1 (2) [3]

The evaluating physician must determine whether diagnostic or examination criteria best describe the impairment of a specific individual. The evaluator should, in general, use only one approach for each anatomic part. There are, however, a few instances in which elements from both diagnostic and examination approaches will apply to a specific situation (see Figure 17-2). An individual with an acetabular fracture and a sciatic nerve palsy should have estimates made for both the hip joint impairment and the nerve palsy. The estimates for the fracture and the nerve condition are then combined using the Combined Values Chart (p. 604) to provide the final impairment estimate. The final lower extremity impairment cannot exceed the impairment estimate for amputation of the extremity (100%), or 40% whole person impairment.

Table 17-34 Rating Hip Replacement Results*

	Number of Points			Number of Points
a. Pain			**d. Deformity**	
None	44		Fixed adduction	
Slight	40		< 10°	1
Moderate, occasional	30		≥ 10°	0
Moderate	20			
Marked	10		Fixed internal rotation	
			< 10°	1
b. Function			≥ 10°	0
Limp				
None	11		Fixed external rotation	
Slight	8		< 10°	1
Moderate	5		≥ 10°	0
Severe	0			
			Flexion contracture	
Supportive device			< 15°	1
None	11		≥ 15°	0
Cane for long walks	7			
Cane	5		Leg length discrepancy	
One crutch	3		< 1.5 cm	1
Two canes	2		≥ 1.5 cm	0
Two crutches	0			
			e. Range of Motion	
Distance walked			Flexion	
Unlimited	11		> 90°	1
Six blocks	8		≤ 90°	0
Three blocks	5			
Indoors	2		Abduction	
In bed or chair	0		> 15°	1
			≤ 15°	0
c. Activities				
Stairs climbing			Adduction	
Normal	4		> 15°	1
Using railing	2		≤ 15°	0
Cannot climb readily	1			
Unable to climb	0		External rotation	
			> 30°	1
Putting on shoes and socks			≤ 30°	0
With ease	4			
With difficulty	2		Internal rotation	
Unable to do	0		> 15°	1
			≤ 15°	0
Sitting				
Any chair, 1 hour	4			
High chair	2			
Unable to sit comfortably	0			
Public transportation				
Able to use	1			
Unable to use	0			

* Add the points from categories a, b, c, d, and e to determine the total and characterize the result of replacement. Source: modified from Gross AE, McDermott AGP, Lavoie MV, et al. The use of allograft bone in revision hip arthroplasty. In: Brand R, ed. *Proceeding of the Fourteenth Open Scientific Meeting of the Hip Society.* St Louis, Mo: CV Mosby Co; 1987:49; and Harris AH. Traumatic arthritis of the hip after dislocation and acetabular fractures: treatment by mold arthroplasty. *J Bone Joint Surg Am.* 1969;51A:741-742.

Table 17-35 Rating Knee Replacement Results*

	Number of Points
a. Pain	
None	50
Mild or occasional	45
Stairs only	40
Walking and stairs	30
Moderate	
Occasional	20
Continual	10
Severe	0
b. Range of Motion	
Add 1 point per 5°	25
c. Stability	
(maximum movement in any position)	
Anteroposterior	
< 5 mm	10
5-9 mm	5
> 9 mm	0
Mediolateral	
5°	15
6°-9°	10
10°-14°	5
≥ 15°	0
Subtotal	
Deductions (minus) d, e, f	
d. Flexion contracture	
5°-9°	2
10°-15°	5
16°-20°	10
> 20°	20
e. Extension lag	
< 10°	5
10°-20°	10
> 20°	15
f. Alignment	
0°- 4°	0
5°-10°	3 points per degree
11°-15°	3 points per degree
> 15°	20
Deductions subtotal	—

* The point total for estimating knee replacement results is the sum of the points in categories a, b, and c minus the sum of the points in categories d, e, and f. Modified from Insall JN, Dorr LD, Scott RD. Rationale of the Knee Society clinical rating system. *Clin Orthop.* 1989;248:14.

Fractures in and about joints with degenerative changes should be rated either by using this section and combining the rating with that for arthritis (Table 17-31 and Combined Values Chart, p. 604) or by using the loss of range-of-motion method. It is recommended that the method providing the greater of the two impairment estimates be used. A diagnosis of isolated full-thickness articular cartilage defects and ununited osteochondral fractures requires arthroscopic or surgical confirmation.

Example 17-15
11% Impairment Due to a Tibia Fracture

Subject: 40-year-old woman.

History: Sustained a comminuted midshaft tibial fracture in a skiing accident. The fracture healed with shortening and angulation. She was advised of the risks of midshaft tibial osteotomy and lengthening, and she declined surgery.

Current Symptoms: Mild pain about the right knee and ankle, particularly when walking on uneven surfaces. Mild swelling of the lower leg; difficulty walking more than 5 blocks without a rest period.

Physical Exam: There is a right leg shortening of 2.5 cm. The lower leg fracture has healed with a 10° varus angle. Ranges of motion of the knee and ankle are normal.

Clinical Studies: Radiograph: healed tibia fracture with varus angulation and 2.5 cm of shortening.

Diagnosis: Healed tibia fracture with varus angulation.

Impairment Rating: 11% impairment of the whole person.

Comment: The lower extremity impairment estimate for a tibia fracture that heals with a 10° varus angulation is 20% (Table 17-33), or 8% whole person impairment; the lower extremity impairment estimate for 2.5 cm of shortening, using interpolation, is 7%, or 3% whole person impairment (Table 17-4). The 8% and 3% whole person impairments are combined using the Combined Values Chart (p. 604). The whole person impairment is 11%. Impairment due to malunion of a fracture should be estimated according to the diagnosis. Any associated muscle weakness or atrophy is included in the diagnosis-related estimates, but shortening is a separate impairment. (See cross-usage Table 17-2.) If there were an associated nerve palsy, the fracture and nerve palsy impairment percents would be combined (Combined Values Chart).

17.2k Skin Loss

Full-thickness skin loss about certain areas in the lower extremity results in significant impairment, as shown in Table 17-36, even when the areas are successfully covered with an appropriate type of skin graft. Chronic osteomyelitis is also evaluated using this method.

Table 17-36 Impairments for Skin Loss

Description	Whole Person (Lower Extremity) [Foot] Impairment (%)
Ischial covering that requires frequent unweighting and limits sitting time	5 (12)
Tibial tuberosity covering that limits kneeling	2 (5)
Heel covering that limits standing and walking time	10 (25) [35]
Plantar surface, metatarsal head covering that limits standing and walking time	
First metatarsal	5 (12) [17]
Fifth metatarsal	5 (12) [17]
Chronic osteomyelitis with active drainage	
Of femur	3 (7) [10]
Of tibia	3 (7) [10]
Of foot, requiring periodic redressing and limiting time using footwear	10 (25) [35]

Example 17-16
10% Impairment Due to Skin Loss

Subject: 56-year-old man.

History: Insulin-dependent diabetic who stepped on a nail at work and developed *Pseudomonas* cellulitis of the heel. The heel pad became necrotic and required debridement. A subsequent full-thickness skin graft was successfully applied to the plantar aspect of the heel.

Current Symptoms: 1 year later, standing tolerance is limited to 45 minutes and walking tolerance is limited to 1 mile. Occasional minor breakdown of the full-thickness graft. Never developed osteomyelitis or recurring infections.

Physical Exam: Normal motion in the ankle and subtalar joints. Graft site well healed.

Clinical Studies: None.

Diagnosis: Puncture wound with 2° infection of right heel. Status post–split thickness skin graft.

Impairment Rating: 10% impairment of the whole person.

Comment: Table 17-36 indicates a 10% whole person impairment since his condition limits daily activities, as well as standing and walking time. Any subsequent impairment from the diabetes should be combined with the musculoskeletal impairment.

17.2l Peripheral Nerve Injuries

Peripheral nerve injuries are divided into two components: motor deficits and sensory deficits. Figures 17-8 and 17-9 show the sensory and motor nerves of the lower extremity. All estimates listed in Table 17-37 are for complete motor or sensory loss for the named peripheral nerves. Partial sensory and motor deficits should be rated as in the upper extremity (Tables 16-10 and 16-11). First identify the injured nerve and find the maximum impairment of the lower extremity due to motor deficit in Table 17-37. Grade the severity of motor deficit of the individual muscle groups innervated by that nerve according to the classification given in Table 16-11. Assign a motor deficit concordant with that grade and multiply the maximum impairment value of the nerve for motor loss by the percent motor deficit to obtain the lower extremity impairment for this partial loss. Sensory deficits follow a similar method, as described in Table 16-10. Motor and sensory estimates should be combined, but impairments from multiple peripheral nerve injuries should not exceed the whole person impairment from complete loss of a lower extremity (40%).

Figure 17-8 Sensory Nerves of the Lower Extremity, Their Areas of Innervation and Roots of Origin

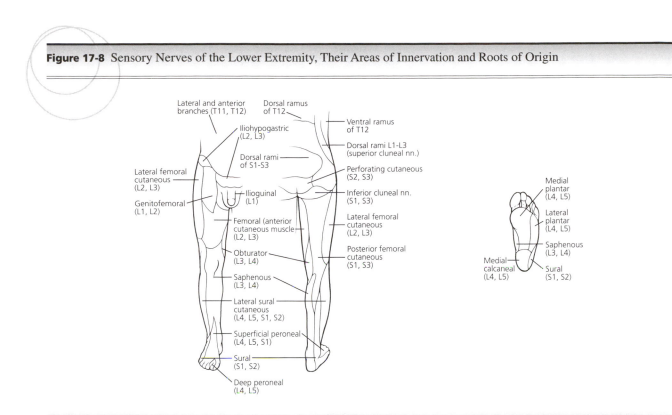

Figure 17-9 Motor Nerves of the Lower Extremity, Their Muscle Innervations and Roots of Origin

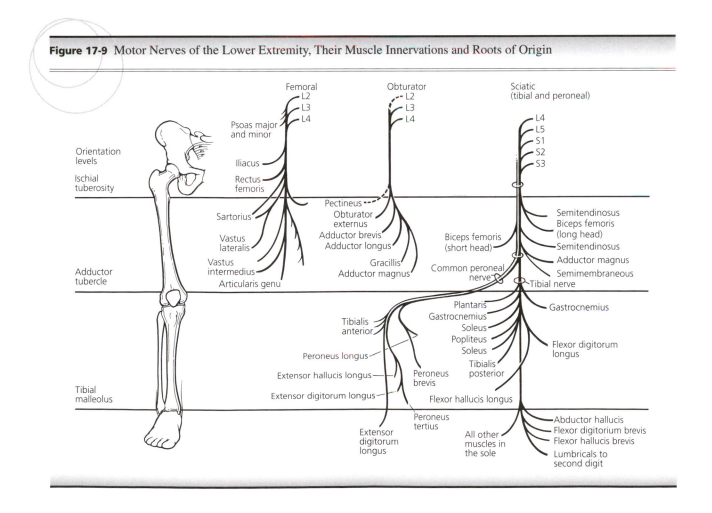

Table 17-37 Impairments Due to Nerve Deficits

Nerve	Whole Person (Lower Extremity) [Foot] Impairment (%)		
	Motor	Sensory	Dysesthesia
Femoral	15 (37)	1 (2)	3 (7)
Obturator	3 (7)	0	0
Superior gluteal	25 (62)	0	0
Inferior gluteal	15 (37)	0	0
Lateral femoral cutaneous	0	1 (2)	3 (7)
Sciatic	30 (75)	7 (17)	5 (12)
Common peroneal	15 (42)	2 (5)	2 (5)
Superficial peroneal	0	2 (5)	2 (5)
Sural	0	1 (2)	2 (5)
Medial plantar	2 (5) [7]	2 (5) [7]	2 (5) [7]
Lateral plantar	2 (5) [7]	2 (5) [7]	2 (5) [7]

Sensory deficits, including dysesthesias, are subjective and must be carefully evaluated. Ideally, two examiners should agree. Estimates for peripheral nerve impairments may be combined with those for other types of lower extremity impairments, except those for muscle weakness, atrophy, and gait derangement, using the Combined Values Chart (p. 604). See cross-usage Table 17-2.

Example 17-17
4% Impairment Due to Peripheral Nerve Injury

Subject: 22-year-old man.

History: Sustained a shrapnel-type injury at work when a part in his lathe broke and a sharp metal fragment struck him near the groin. The wound was surgically explored, and he was found to have a totally transected femoral nerve. The femoral vessels were not injured. The nerve was repaired, with return of significant function.

Current Symptoms: 2 years postinjury, walks without a cane or brace but with an abnormal gait, hyperextending his knee by using his hip extensors, just prior to weight-bearing.

Physical Exam: Decreased light touch perception in the leg in the distribution of the saphenous nerve (the distal sensory branch of the femoral nerve). This area of skin on the medial leg has retained sharp dull perception. Blisters on the medial

malleolus from his shoe rubbing on an area where the skin has decreased sensation. Quadriceps strength is judged as grade 4; moderate resistance by the examiner prevents full knee extension.

Clinical Studies: None.

Diagnosis: Partial femoral nerve palsy.

Impairment Rating: 4% impairment of the whole person.

Comment: The operation report documents that the femoral nerve was injured. Examination confirms that the sensory deficit is in the saphenous nerve distribution, and the motor weakness affects the quadriceps muscle (knee extension). This is consistent with a femoral nerve injury with incomplete recovery.

Sensory impairment can be rated using Tables 17-37 and 16-10. According to Table 17-37, the maximum value for a totally destroyed and nonfunctioning femoral nerve due to sensory loss and pain is 9% lower extremity impairment. The sensory deficit and pain are forgotten with activity, so a severity multiplier of grade 4 may be chosen from Table 16-10; grade 4 includes a range of multipliers from 1% to 25%. If a multiplier of 20% is chosen, 20% of the 9% maximum value of the nerve is 2% lower extremity impairment for loss of sensation and pain.

The motor weakness impairment can be calculated in a similar manner. Table 17-37 indicates that the maximal impairment for total loss of femoral nerve motor function is 37% lower extremity impairment. The exam shows that the man can move the leg through a full range of motion against gravity, but with only minimal added resistance. This is grade 4 weakness according to manual muscle testing criteria. Table 16-11 indicates that grade 4 weakness can qualify for a severity multiplier of anywhere from 1% to 25%. If a multiplier of 25% is chosen since the weakness is very significant, 25% multiplied by the 37% maximal value of the nerve for weakness yields a total of 9% lower extremity impairment.

Using the Combined Values Chart (p. 604) to combine the 9% lower extremity impairment for motor weakness with the 2% lower extremity impairment for loss of sensation and pain yields a rating of 11% lower extremity impairment. The 11% lower extremity impairment is equivalent to 4% whole person impairment ($11\% \times 0.4 = 4\%$).

17.2m Causalgia and Complex Regional Pain Syndrome (Reflex Sympathetic Dystrophy)

Causalgia is a burning pain resulting from injury of a peripheral nerve. As a term, **complex regional pain syndrome (CRPS)** is preferred to **reflex sympathetic dystrophy (RSD)** because the relationship to the sympathetic nervous system is uncertain. CRPS is characterized by pain, swelling, stiffness, discoloration, and skeletal demineralization, and it may follow a sprain, fracture or nerve or vascular injury. CRPS is further described in Section 13.8. When causalgia or CRPS occurs in an extremity, the evaluator should use the method described in Chapter 13, The Central and Peripheral Nervous System.

Example 17-18
39% Impairment Due to Causalgia

Subject: 32-year-old woman.

History: Fell and struck the anterior aspect of her knee; sustained a bruise with ecchymosis but no fractures when she jumped 4.5 feet from a truck dock to the ground below. She was much worse 1 month later, with "terrible pain," swelling (edema), and a red, warm leg that sweated when no other part of her was sweating.

Current Symptoms: 2 years later, ambulating with two crutches and not bearing weight on the right leg. Constant severe pain in the leg, despite treatment that included all known modalities for causalgia.

Physical Exam: Leg remains swollen and pale, with skin atrophy and atrophy of the toes equivalent to "fingerprints." On active range-of-motion testing, she does not cooperate due to pain, with very little active motion in any joint in the leg. Does not cooperate with manual muscle testing, as the testing provokes pain. On sensory exam, there is no loss of sensation; rather, any touching of the leg provokes severe pain (allodynia).

Clinical Studies: Bone scan postinjury: diffuse periarticular increased uptake at the knee, ankle, and foot on the "third phase" or 3- to 4-hour delayed images. Current x-rays of the leg: only extensive osteoporosis.

Diagnosis: Causalgia, right leg.

Impairment Rating: 39% impairment of the whole person.

Comment: This case is typical of severe, type 1 CRPS, or causalgia. The leg is very difficult to examine, as traditional physical examination maneuvers such as manual muscle testing, reflex testing, sensory examination, and active range of motion all provoke complaints of severe pain and limited or no cooperation. This makes an impairment evaluation based on the traditional physical examination impossible. In this individual, no single peripheral nerve has been injured, and the pain involves the entire limb. Thus, trying to rate this as a peripheral nerve injury is inappropriate. No specific method described in the lower extremity or upper extremity chapters adequately covers this unique circumstance.

The pathology in CRPS is currently believed to occur in the central nervous system, so the evaluator should use the station and gait impairment criteria in Table 13-15 to rate lower extremity impairments due to lesions in the central nervous system (brain and/or spinal cord). Table 13-15 rates this individual's impairment at 20% to 39% impairment of the whole person. Since her pain is severe and functional ADL are compromised, a 39% impairment rating is appropriate.

Comparing this woman's status with the guidelines for gait derangement indicated in Table 17-5 suggests that since she requires routine use of two canes or two crutches, she could be rated at 39% whole person impairment. The leg is totally nonfunctional; thus, she is similar to an amputee and should be rated at 39% whole person impairment. The rating of at 39% whole person impairment is thus supportable by several lines of reasoning.

17.2n Vascular Disorders

Table 17-38 classifies and provides criteria for impairments due to peripheral vascular disease of the lower extremity. When amputation due to peripheral vascular disease is involved, the impairment due to amputation should be evaluated according to the criteria in section 17.2i, and the impairment percent should be combined (Combined Values Chart, p. 604) with an appropriate percent based on Table 17-38 for the remaining vascular disease.

Table 17-38 Lower Extremity Impairment Due to Peripheral Vascular Disease

Class 1 0%-9% Impairment	Class 2 10%-39% Impairment	Class 3 40%-69% Impairment	Class 4 70%-89% Impairment	Class 5 90%-100% Impairment
Neither claudication nor pain at rest *and* only transient edema *and* on physical examination, not more than the following findings are present: loss of pulses; minimal loss of subcutaneous tissue; calcification of arteries as detected by x-ray examination; asymptomatic dilation of arteries or of veins, not requiring surgery and not resulting in curtailment of activity	Intermittent claudication on walking at least 100 yards at an average pace *or* persistent edema of a moderate degree, incompletely controlled by elastic supports *or* vascular damage as evidenced by a sign such as a healed, painless stump of an amputated digit showing evidence of persistent vascular disease or healed ulcer	Intermittent claudication on walking as few as 25 yards and no more than 100 yards at average pace *or* marked edema that is only partially controlled by elastic supports *or* vascular damage as evidenced by a sign such as healed amputation of two or more digits of one extremity, with evidence of persisting vascular disease or superficial ulceration	Intermittent claudication on walking less than 25 yards or intermittent pain at rest *or* marked edema that cannot be controlled by elastic supports *or* vascular damage as evidenced by signs such as an amputation at or above an ankle, or amputation of two or more digits of two extremities with evidence of persistent vascular disease, or persistent widespread or deep ulceration involving one extremity	Severe and constant pain at rest *or* vascular damage as evidenced by such signs as amputations at or above the ankles of two extremities, or amputation of all digits of two or more extremities, with evidence of persistent vascular disease or of persistent, widespread, or deep ulceration involving two or more extremities

Example 17-19
8% Impairment Caused by Vascular Disease Due to a Deep Venous Thrombosis (DVT)

Subject: 45-year-old man.

History: Sustained a closed but displaced tibial fracture at work. Treated with cast immobilization until the fracture healed. Postoperative course was complicated by a DVT in the injured left leg.

Current Symptoms: At MMI, 1 year postinjury, standing tolerance is described as 1 hour and walking tolerance is described as almost 1 mile. Only medication is aspirin. He has not had recurrent venous thrombosis. Able to do most ADL.

Physical Exam: No weakness on manual muscle testing. Knee, ankle, and subtalar joints all have full motion. Chronic venous insufficiency of the left leg as a result of the DVT. The right lower extremity is normal, with no edema or varices. The left leg has 2+ pitting edema when examined in the morning, despite the use of Jobst compression hose 16 hours every day. Intermittent stasis dermatitis about the ankle, but no permanent skin changes other than discoloration.

Clinical Studies: Healed fracture with no angulation, displacement, or shortening.

Diagnosis: Peripheral vascular disease, post-DVT, and healed tibia fracture.

Impairment Rating: 8% impairment of the whole person.

Comment: Table 17-38 shows that the impairment for peripheral vascular (venous) disease can be estimated as a class 2 impairment, which ranges from 10% to 39% lower extremity impairment. He has the criterion of persistent edema of a moderate degree, incompletely controlled by elastic supports. The impairment can be estimated at midway between the lower and the higher impairment for class 2, or at 20% lower extremity impairment (20% × 0.4 = 8% whole person impairment).

17.3 Lower Extremity Impairment Evaluation Procedure Summary and Examples

When evaluating an individual with lower extremity impairment, first obtain the person's detailed history and perform a thorough and careful physical examination, then follow the steps suggested below.

1. Establish the diagnosis.
2. Determine whether the individual has reached maximal medical improvement (MMI).
3. Identify each anatomic region of the lower extremity(ies) with abnormalities related to the illness/injury being evaluated. List potential methods. Use the worksheet shown in Figure 17-10.
4. Calculate the impairment according to the text and tables for each applicable method (Table 17-1).
5. Identify and calculate impairment related to the peripheral nervous system.
6. Identify and calculate impairment related to the peripheral vascular system.
7. Identify and calculate any impairment that is related to a complex regional pain syndrome.
8. If no other methods are available, use the gait derangement method if clinically applicable; document its validity.

9. Select the most appropriate method(s) based on the history and physical examination. Use the cross-usage table (Table 17-2) to ensure only the proper methods are combined. Although diminished muscle function can be evaluated by means of four methods (peripheral nervous system impairment, atrophy, manual muscle testing, or gait), use only the method that has the greatest specificity (eg, a peripheral nerve injury, if present). Anatomically based, specific methods are used to evaluate skin loss and osteomyelitis (Section 17.2k), peripheral nerve injuries (Section 17.2l), and vascular disorders (Section 17.2n). If a vascular impairment results in an amputation, any remaining vascular and amputation impairments are combined. Neurologic and vascular impairments are recorded separately since they are not limited to one region of the lower extremity. Gait derangements should be used only infrequently, when other, more specific measures are not appropriate.
10. If there are several alternatives, use the grouping that provides the greatest impairment percent. Convert a lower extremity impairment rating to whole person impairment using the appropriate tables. Combine whole person impairments for each injury/illness for the same extremity using the Combined Values Chart (p. 604).
11. If more than one leg is involved, each lower extremity is rated separately and converted to whole person; then both whole person ratings (right and left leg) are combined using the Combined Values Chart.

Example 17-20

7% Impairment Due to Peripheral Nervous System Injury

Subject: 22-year-old man.

History: Fell approximately 20 feet from a ladder, injuring his right knee and left toe. Sustained an anterior cruciate ligament rupture to the right knee and a lateral meniscus tear, treated with an anterior cruciate ligament reconstruction and partial lateral meniscectomy. Sustained a common peroneal nerve neuropraxia that was treated with observation and a temporary ankle/foot orthosis. Had a fracture/dislocation of the left great toe at the interphalangeal (IP) joint that required closed reduction only.

Current Symptoms: Postrehabilitation, has residual soreness in the right knee after vigorous activities and constant stiffness in the left great toe.

Physical Examination: *Right lower extremity:* Walks normally without support. Uses an occasional sport brace for vigorous activities, but does not require this for most ADL. The scars around the right knee are well healed. No incisional tenderness. There is no effusion or tenderness along the joint lines. There is 1-cm atrophy of the right thigh compared to the left, as well as 1-cm calf atrophy compared to the left. Manual muscle testing is normal except for right foot evertor strength, which is 4/5. Range of motion of the right knee is from 0° to 130° of flexion, as compared to 0° to 138° on the left. Stability testing reveals 1+ Lachman and anterior drawer and a negative pivot shift exam. Sensation is decreased to light touch in the superficial peroneal distribution on the dorsum of the foot and is forgotten with activity. No obvious deep peroneal deficit. *Left lower extremity:* The only gross abnormality identified is great toe IP flexion, which is limited to 10°.

Clinical Studies: Based on the operative report, the individual had an anterior cruciate ligament reconstruction with a mid–one third patellar tendon graft using interference screw fixation. The report suggested that approximately one half of the posterior portion of the lateral meniscus had been removed. X-rays of the right knee: prior anterior cruciate ligament reconstruction, but no degenerative changes seen. X-rays of the great toe: healed, nondisplaced fracture of the proximal phalanx. The joints appear normal.

Diagnosis: Residual, partial common peroneal nerve neuropraxia, status post-lateral meniscectomy. Healed left great toe fracture

Impairment Rating: 7% impairment of the whole person.

Comment: See Box 17-1 for a step-by-step explanation of how this impairment rating was calculated.

Example 17-21

8% Impairment Due to Decreased Range of Motion From Hip Dislocation and Fixation

Subject: 35-year-old woman.

History: Sustained a dislocation of the right hip with severe comminution of the posterior acetabulum. Underwent open reduction and internal fixation of the posterior acetabular wall. Because of the comminution and inability to obtain a stable fracture fixation, the surgeon elected to keep her in skeletal traction for 4 weeks. She healed, but with some loss of joint space and significant loss of range of motion.

Current Symptoms: Aching pain in the right groin toward the end of the day, after household activities and caring for her children.

Physical Exam: Walks with a slight antalgic gait on the right. Range-of-motion measurements of the hip are as follows: flexion = 50°; extension = 15°; flexion contracture, internal rotation = 20°, external rotation = 15°; abduction = 20°; adduction = 5°. There is 3 cm of atrophy of the thigh and 2 cm of atrophy of the calf.

Clinical Studies: Repeat x-rays of the pelvis: only 1 mm of joint space in the right hip.

Diagnosis: Right hip dislocation with internal fixation; secondary osteoarthritis.

Impairment Rating: 8% impairment of the whole person.

Comment: Range of motion, atrophy, and arthritis are the three possible methods of rating this individual's impairment. According to Table 17-2, range-of-motion parameters should not be combined with either arthritis or atrophy. Use the range-of-motion method because it is more specific and best characterizes the impairment. Flexion of 50° qualifies for severe impairment according to Table 17-9. The other measurements qualify as less than severe, but since one of the measurements qualifies for severe, it should be used as the basis; the impairment is therefore 20% of the lower extremity. This converts to a whole person impairment of 8% (20% × 0.4 = 8%).

Example 17-22
10% Impairment Due to Limb Length Discrepancy, Malalignment of the Tibial Shaft Fracture, and Atrophy

Subject: 45-year-old man.

History: Fell from a scaffold and sustained an undisplaced tibial plateau fracture of the right leg and an open fracture of the left tibia and fibula. The open tibia/fibula fracture was treated by irrigation and debridement and internal fixation with an intramedullary Rush pin. The tibial plateau fracture was treated with a Bledsoe brace, locked in extension for 3 weeks, and then treated with progressive mobilization.

Current Symptoms: Unable to do some activities of daily living because of pain in both legs when lifting or standing.

Physical Exam: Full range of motion of both knees. There is a 12° valgus deformity of the left leg. Both knees are stable. There is 2 cm of atrophy of the left calf compared to the right. Neurovascular status of both legs is intact. No muscle weakness.

Clinical Studies: X-rays: healing of all fractures; the right knee fracture has healed without displacement, but the left tibial fracture has healed with 12° of valgus angulation. Teleroentgenograms: 1.5 cm of shortening.

Diagnosis: Healed right tibia plateau fracture; healed left tibia fracture with malalignment.

Impairment Rating: 10% impairment of the whole person.

Comment: The undisplaced right tibia plateau fracture has a 5% lower extremity impairment rating, and the valgus angulation of the left tibial fracture has 20% impairment of the lower extremity according to Table 17-33. There is no further impairment rating for leg shortening since it is less than 2 cm. The individual does not receive an impairment rating for left calf atrophy according to Table 17-6 since diagnosis-based estimates are used. The left lower extremity rating of 20% converts to 8% whole person impairment (20% × 0.4). The right lower extremity impairment of 5% equates to 2% whole person impairment (5% × 0.4). Combining the 8% whole person impairment from the left leg and the 2% whole person impairment from the right leg equals a 10% whole person impairment for the injuries. The pain is accounted for in the impairment ratings.

Example 17-23
10% Impairment Due to Undisplaced Tibial Plateau Fracture and Peroneal Neuropathy

Subject: 55-year-old man.

History: Sustained a lateral tibial plateau and proximal fibula fracture when a metal lathe threw a piece of scrap metal against his leg. Also had a complete peroneal nerve laceration. Treated with open reduction and internal fixation of the fracture and repair of the peroneal nerve. Postoperatively, he was placed in a locked Bledsoe brace for 3 weeks and then was progressively mobilized. The fracture healed without deformity, but there was only partial return of nerve function.

Current Symptoms: Aching along the lateral side of the leg. Walks without a brace but has a slight steppage gait, and when walking long distances, prefers to use an AFO.

Physical Exam: 2° limitation in the extension of the knee; flexes to 100°. No malalignment. There is 2.5 cm of atrophy of the calf. Knee ligaments are stable. Numbness on the lateral side of the lower leg and foot that is judged to be grade 2 according to Table 16-12. He has weakness of the peroneal innervated muscles that is judged to be grade 3 according to Table 16-11.

Clinical Studies: Radiograph: healed tibial and fibula fracture.

Diagnosis: Undisplaced tibial plateau fracture; peroneal neuropathy.

Impairment Rating: 10% impairment of the whole person.

Comment: According to Table 17-33, this individual receives a 5% lower extremity impairment for the undisplaced tibial plateau fracture. According to Table 17-2, the rater should not use atrophy in conjunction with a diagnosis-based estimate. The neurologic deficit requires a separate rating. Table 16-10 states that a grade 4 sensory lesion results in a 1% to 25% sensory deficit. Since this man has considerable numbness, he is rated at 25%. Multiplying the 25% by the 5% assigned from Table 17-37 for a complete common peroneal sensory deficit equals 1.25%, rounded down to a 1% sensory deficit. Table 16-11 states that a grade 3 motor lesion equates to a 26% to 50% deficit. Since the man must wear a brace part-time, 50% is appropriate. Multiplying that 50% by the 42% from Table 17-37 for a complete common peroneal motor deficit equals 21%. Combining the 1% lower extremity impairment for the sensory deficit with the 21% lower extremity impairment for the motor deficit results in 22% lower extremity impairment for the nerve injury. Combining the 5% lower extremity impairment for the fracture and the 22% impairment for the nerve injury results in a 26% lower extremity impairment, or a 10% whole person impairment ($26\% \times 0.4 = 10.4\%$, or 10%).

Example 17-24
15% Impairment Due to Hip Replacement

Subject: 35-year-old woman (same individual as in Example 17-21).

History: The individual described in Example 17-21 developed progressive arthritis of the hip and underwent total hip arthroplasty. She is now 2 years postoperative and is seen for repeat impairment evaluation.

Current Symptoms: Slight pain, and walks with a slight limp. Climbs stairs normally, puts on socks and shoes with difficulty because of persistent limitation of flexion and limited external rotation, sits unlimited amounts of time, and does not use public transportation, although she thinks she could. Never uses a cane and can walk six blocks without stopping. Has difficulty doing activities with her family.

Physical Exam: Continued atrophy of the thigh and calf. A flexion contracture of 15°. No other contractures, and her leg lengths are equalized. Flexion is 90°, abduction is 20°, adduction is 10°, external rotation is 20°, and internal rotation is 20°.

Clinical Studies: Hip replacement well positioned.

Diagnosis: Hip replacement.

Impairment Rating: 15% impairment of the whole person.

Comment: According to Table 17-2, atrophy should not be considered if the diagnosis method is used (Table 17-34). The individual is assigned 40 points for pain, 8 points for a slight limp, 11 points for not using a cane, and 8 points for being able to walk six blocks. She is also assigned 4 points for stair climbing, 2 points for difficulty putting on socks, 4 points for unlimited sitting ability, and 1 point for the ability to use public transportation. She has a fixed flexion contracture without leg length discrepancy, so she receives an additional 3 points for deformity. For range of motion, she receives no points for flexion motion but receives 1 each for the other four motions (given the flexion contracture). That totals 85 points. According to Table 17-33, the impairment is 37% lower extremity or 15% whole person.

Example 17-25
25% Impairment Due to Transmetatarsal Amputation

Subject: 60-year-old man.

History: Caught his right foot in a construction ditch with a machine operating and sustained a mangled foot. Treated with debridement and internal fixation of multiple fractures of the metatarsals, os calcus, and ankle. The forefoot became infected and required a transmetatarsal amputation. He finally healed, but he had significant residual stiffness of the foot. Was unable to do heavy work.

Current Symptoms: Stiffness in the foot and ankle. Able to walk in lace-up shoes with a shoe insert. Limps and has atrophy of the calf. Unable to stand for sustained periods of time without pain.

Physical Exam: Multiple scars, all healed. Ankle flexion contracture of 10° and can plantar flex to 25°. Fixed valgus deformity of the os calcus measuring 15°. No further inversion from 15°.

Clinical Studies: Radiographs: healed foot and ankle fractures with valgus deformity.

Diagnosis: Healed transmetatarsal amputation.

Impairment Rating: 25% impairment of the whole person.

Comment: The amputation results in an impairment of 57% of the foot or 40% of the lower extremity according to Table 17-32. Impairments other than the amputation need to be considered. According to Table 17-13, the heel deformity results in a lower extremity impairment of 25%. Since this is a deformity, subtalar motion is not considered. Loss of ankle dorsiflexion, according to Table 17-11, results in a lower extremity impairment of 15% (moderate). Combining the 40%, the 25%, and the 15% results in a lower extremity impairment of 62%. By multiplying the lower extremity impairment by 0.4, a whole person impairment of 24.8%, or 25%, is obtained.

Notice that to calculate the lower extremity impairment, all the impairment ratings must be calculated for the lower extremity. Thus, the lower extremity amputation impairment rating must be used, not the foot impairment rating. Calculating the whole person impairment by combining the lower extremity impairments and multiplying by 0.4 should be the same as converting each lower extremity impairment to whole person impairment and then combining the whole person impairments. In cases where they are not equal, the evaluator should use the higher rating.

Figure 17-10 Lower Extremity Impairment Evaluation Record and Worksheet

Name _____ Age _____ Sex _____ Side □R □L Date _____

Diagnosis _____

Potential Impairments							Final Impairment Utilized	
Region	**Abnormal Motion**	**Regional Impairments**	**Table #**	**Percent**	**Amputation** Location	Percent	**Methodology**	**Percent**
Pelvis		DBE DJD Skin Leg Length Amp	17-33 17-31 17-36 17-4 17-32	% % % % %			DBE DJD Skin Leg Length Amputation	% % % % %
Hip	Tables 17-9 and 17-15 to 17-19 Angle Impairment: Flexion / Extension / Ankylosis / Impairment % Angle Impairment: Abduction / Adduction / Ankylosis / Impairment % Angle Impairment: Internal Rot / External Rot / Ankylosis / Impairment % Add impairment % ROM or use largest ankylosis = ____ %	DBE DJD Skin Leg Length Weakness Amp	17-33/34 17-31 17-36 17-4 17-8 17-32	% % % % % %			DBE DJD Skin Leg Length Weakness ROM Amputation	% % % % % % %
Thigh	(Consider related pathology at hip and knee)	Atrophy DJD Skin Leg Length Amp	17-6 17-31 17-36 17-4 17-32	% % % % %			Atrophy DJD Skin Leg Length Amputation	% % % % %
Knee	Tables 17-10 and 17-20 to 17-23 Angle Impairment: Flexion / Extension / Ankylosis / Impairment % Add impairment % ROM or use largest ankylosis = ____ %	DBE DJD Skin Weakness Amp	17-33/35 17-31 17-36 17-8 17-32	% % % % %			DBE DJD Skin Weakness Amputation	% % % % %
Calf	(Consider related pathology at knee and ankle)	Atrophy DBE Skin Leg Length Amp	17-6 17-33 17-36 17-4 17-32	% % % % %			Atrophy DBE Skin Leg Length Amputation	% % % % %
Ankle/ Foot	Tables 17-11 to 17-13 and 17-24 to 17-28 Angle Impairment: Dorsiflex / Plantarflex / Ankylosis / Impairment % Angle Impairment: Inversion / Eversion / Ankylosis / Impairment % Add impairment % ROM or use largest ankylosis = ____ %	DBE DJD Skin Weakness Amp	17-29/33 17-31 17-36 17-8/9 17-32	% % % % %			DBE DJD Skin Weakness ROM Amputation	% % % % % %
Toe	Tables 17-14 and 17-30 Great Toe Angle Impairment: MP Dorsiflex / IP Plantarflex / Ankylosis / Impairment % Lesser Toes Angle Impairment: MP Dorsiflex / Ankylosis / Impairment % Add impairment % ROM or use largest ankylosis = ____ %	DBE DJD Skin Weakness Amp	17-33 17-31 17-36 17-8/14 17-32	% % % % %			DBE DJD Skin Weakness ROM Amputation	% % % % % %

Peripheral Nervous System Impairment	Grade %	Nerve %	Total %	Nerve	Maximum Motor %	Maximum Sensory %	Maximum Dysesthesia %	
Motor Grade (Table 16-14)	_____	_____ ×	_____ =	_____	_____			
Sensory Grade (Table 16-15)	_____	_____ ×	_____ =	_____	_____			
Dysesthesia Grade	_____	_____ ×	_____ =	_____	_____	Combine all neurologic components	%	

Peripheral Vascular System Impairment (Table 17-38)

Grade _____   Total vascular system impairment ____ %

Gait Derangement (This is a *stand-alone* impairment and may *not* be combined) (Table 17-5)   ____ %

Final Combined Impairment (An explanation should be provided if more than one methodology is used, justifying the rationale for each methodology used)   ____ %

DBE = diagnosis-based estimates; DJD = degenerative joint disease (arthritis).

Box 17-1 Choosing a Lower Extremity Impairment Rating

1. Establish the diagnosis.

   Right Lower Extremity
   Anterior cruciate ligament tear; lateral meniscus tear; common peroneal nerve neuropraxia.

   Left Lower Extremity
   Fracture/dislocation, left great toe IP joint.

2. Determine whether MMI has been reached.

   Right Lower Extremity
   Right lower extremity injuries meet definitional requirements and MMI.

   Left Lower Extremity
   Left lower extremity injuries meet definitional requirements and MMI.

3. Identify each lower extremity anatomic region with abnormalities that are related to illness/injury in question. List potential methods.

   Right Lower Extremity
   Thigh—Atrophy
   Knee—Diagnosis-based estimate
   Calf—Atrophy

   Left Lower Extremity
   Great toe—Range of motion

4. Calculate impairment according to text and tables for each applicable method.

   Right Lower Extremity
   Thigh atrophy—3% impairment of the lower extremity (1% whole person impairment); see Table 17-6.

   Partial lateral meniscectomy—2% impairment of the lower extremity (1% whole person impairment); see Table 17-33.

   Calf atrophy—3% impairment of the lower extremity (1% whole person impairment); see Table 17-6.

   Anterior cruciate laxity, mild—7% impairment of the lower extremity (3% whole person impairment); total diagnosis-based estimate combines 7% (ACL laxity) with 2% (for partial meniscectomy) for a lower extremity diagnosis estimate of 9%.

   Left Lower Extremity
   Great toe range of motion—2% impairment of the lower extremity (1% whole person impairment); see Table 17-14.

5. Identify and calculate illness/injury related to peripheral nervous system impairment.

   Right Lower Extremity
   Partial common peroneal nerve injury with some motor and sensory residuals.

   Motor: According to Table 16-11, 4/5 evertor strength would allow for 25% of the motor value of the involved nerve (25% of 15% lower extremity impairment [see Table 17-37]) or approximately 4% of the lower extremity.

   Sensory deficits: Partial; able to do all activities of daily living. Using Table 16-10 from The Upper Extremities as a guide, take the sensory deficit in the 25% sensory deficit category. This would be 25% of the total value of superficial peroneal nerve (7% is total value), which results in an impairment of approximately 2% of the lower extremity for partial sensory loss. Combine motor and sensory losses for total peripheral nerve impairment, which would be 4% of the lower extremity for motor losses *and* 2% for partial sensory losses, for a total rating of 6% of the lower extremity.

   Left Lower Extremity
   None.

6. Identify and calculate all illness/injury related to the peripheral vascular system.

   Right Lower Extremity
   None.

   Left Lower Extremity
   None.

7. Identify and calculate all injury impairment related to CRPS.

   Right Lower Extremity
   None.

   Left Lower Extremity
   None.

8. If no other method is available, then determine impairment due to gait derangement if clinically applicable.

Right Lower Extremity
Not applicable.

Left Lower Extremity
Not applicable.

9. Consult lower extremity cross-usage table (Table 17-2) to determine possible method groupings.

Right Lower Extremity
Methods used: Atrophy; diagnosis-based estimate; peripheral nervous system.

Possible groupings: Atrophy alone; diagnosis-based estimate and peripheral nervous system.

Left Lower Extremity
Range of motion only method available; no specific grouping used since single parameter present.

10. Consider all medical data available and select the largest and most clinically appropriate methods for each illness/injury; combine each parameter within each individual grouping in order to determine impairment for each leg. Numeric figures should be in whole person units.

Right Lower Extremity
Use diagnosis-based estimate combined with peripheral nervous system injury. That is, combine 9% impairment of the lower extremity with 6% impairment of the lower extremity, which results in an impairment rating of 14% of the right lower extremity for this illness/injury.

Left Lower Extremity
Range of motion is the only parameter available; for that reason, the rating is 2% impairment of the left lower extremity.

11. Use the Combined Values Chart (p. 604) to combine whole person impairments from each regional impairment calculated in step 10 of the same limb. This allows the examiner to determine the lower extremity rating for that particular extremity. The lower extremity impairment rating for each limb is then converted to whole person impairment using Table 17-3. If both lower extremities are involved, the impairment rating for each extremity is first converted to a whole person impairment before being combined with the whole person impairment for the contralateral extremity.

Right Lower Extremity
Final impairment is 14% of the lower extremity as the only condition being rated due to the injuries to the knee and common peroneal nerve. Therefore, the 14% lower extremity impairment is converted to 6% whole person impairment.

Left Lower Extremity
The IP fracture/dislocation was the only illness/injury rated in the left lower extremity. Therefore, the 2% lower extremity impairment rating does not need to be combined with any other illnesses/injuries in the left lower extremity. The final rating is 2% of the lower extremity or 1% whole person impairment.

Now that the lower extremity impairment rating for each limb has been converted to a whole person impairment rating, the two whole person ratings for each limb are then combined to give the final whole person impairment for this particular individual. The 6% whole person impairment for the right lower extremity is combined with 1% whole person impairment for the left lower extremity, resulting in a total whole person impairment rating of 7%.

References

1. American Orthopaedic Association (AOA). *Manual of Orthopaedic Surgery.* Rosemont, Ill: American Orthopaedic Association; 1966.

2. Anderson G. Hip assessment: a comparison of nine different methods. *J Bone Joint Surg Br.* 1972;54B: 621-625.

3. Callaghan JJ, Dysart SH, Savory CF, Hopkinson WJ. Assessing the results of hip replacement: a comparison of five different rating systems. *J Bone Joint Surg Br.* 1990;72B:1008-1009.

4. Feagin JA. The ACL-deficient knee. In: Feagin JA, Applewhite LB, eds. *The Crucial Ligaments: Diagnosis and Treatment of Ligamentous Injuries About the Knee.* 2nd ed. New York, NY: Churchill Livingstone; 1994:4-6.

5. Feagin JA. Principles of diagnosis and treatment. In: Feagin JA, Applewhite LB, eds. *The Crucial Ligaments: Diagnosis and Treatment of Ligamentous Injuries About the Knee.* 2nd ed. New York, NY: Churchill Livingstone; 1994:9-26.

6. Gerhardt JJ. *Documentation of Joint Motion.* 4th ed. Portland, Ore: ISOMED, Inc; 1994.

7. Gross AE, McDermott AGP, Lavoie MV, et al. The use of allograft bone in revision hip arthroplasty. In: Brand R, ed. *Proceeding of the Fourteenth Open Scientific Meeting of the Hip Society.* St Louis, Mo: CV Mosby Co; 1987:49.

8. Harris AH. Traumatic arthritis of the hip after dislocation and acetabular fractures: treatment by mold arthroplasty. *J Bone Joint Surg Am.* 1969;51A:741-742.

9. Insall JN, Dorr LD, Scott RD. Rationale of the Knee Society clinical rating system. *Clin Orthop.* 1989;248:14.

10. Kelly MA, Insall JN. Clinical examination. In: Insall JN, Windsor RE, Scott WN, et al, eds. *Surgery of the Knee.* 2nd ed. New York, NY: Churchill Livingstone; 1993: 63-82.

11. Larson RL. Clinical evaluation. In: Larson RL, Grana WA, eds. *The Knee: Form, Function, Pathology, and Treatment.* Philadelphia, Pa: WB Saunders Co; 1993:73-102.

12. Lea RD, Gerhardt JJ. Current concepts review: range-of-motion measurements. *J Bone Joint Surg.* 1995;77A: 784-798.

13. Luck JV, Beardmore TD, Kaufman R. Disability evaluation in arthritis. *Clin Orthop.* 1987;221:59-67.

14. Luck JV, Florence DW. Brief history and comparative analysis of disability systems and impairment rating guides. *Orthop Clin North Am.* 1988;19:839-844.

15. Luck JV. Joint systems: knee and hip. In: Demeter SL, Andersson GBJ, Smith GM, eds. *Disability Evaluation.* St Louis, Mo: Mosby-Year Book, Inc, and American Medical Association; 1996:238-253.

16. Lysholm J, Gillquist J. Evaluation of knee ligament surgery results with special emphasis on use of a scoring scale. *Am J Sports Med.* 1982;10:150-154.

17. Marshall JL, Fetto JF, Botero PM. Knee ligament injuries: a standardized evaluation method. *Clin Orthop.* 1977;123:115-129.

18. Ranawat C, Shine JJ. Duo-condylar total knee arthroplasty. *Clin Orthop.* 1973;94:188-189.

19. Tegner Y, Lysholm J. Rating systems in the evaluation of knee ligament injuries. *Clin Orthop.* 1985;198:43-49.

Chapter 18

Pain

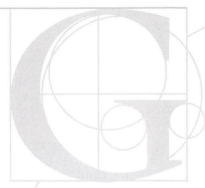

Introduction

This chapter provides information that will enable physicians to understand pain and develop a method to distinguish pain that accompanies illnesses and injuries from pain that has become an autonomous process, and provide physicians with a qualitative method for evaluating permanent impairment due to chronic pain.

This chapter has been completely revised from the fourth edition. Its new features include (1) an overview of pain; (2) a discussion of the complexity of assessing impairment due to pain; (3) a review of situations in which pain is a major cause of suffering, dysfunction, or medical intervention rather than a part of injuries and illnesses of specific organ systems as covered in other chapters of the *Guides*; (4) a qualitative method for evaluating impairment due to chronic pain; and (5) a description of when to use the methods described in this chapter and how they can be integrated with the impairment rating methods used in other chapters of the *Guides*.

Physicians need to use their clinical judgment as to what constitutes normal or expected pain in conditions that produce widely variable amounts of pain; a herniated lumbar disk, for example, may be completely painless or incapacitatingly painful. This chapter focuses on those situations in which the pain itself is a major cause of suffering, dysfunction, or medical intervention. Pain as considered in this chapter is persistent, which is not to say that it is refractory to all treatment, but that it is likely to be permanent and stationary.

18.1 Principles of Assessment

Before using the information in this chapter, the *Guides* user should become familiar with Chapters 1 and 2 and the Glossary. Chapters 1 and 2 discuss the *Guides'* purpose, applications, and methods for performing and reporting impairment evaluations. The Glossary provides definitions of common terms used by many specialties in impairment evaluation.

It is considerably more difficult to provide a method for assessing chronic, persistent pain than acute pain. In chronic pain states, there is often no demonstrable active disease or unhealed injury, and the autonomic changes that accompany acute pain, even in the anesthetized individual, are typically absent. Historically, it was assumed that pain derived from underlying peripheral tissue pathology and that its severity should correlate highly with the identified pathology. Current research, however, shows that pain perception is less a moment-to-moment analysis of afferent input than a dynamic process influenced by the effects of past experiences. Sensory stimuli act on neural systems that have been modified by earlier inputs, and the output of these systems is significantly influenced by the "memory" of these prior events.

18.2 Overview of Pain

18.2a Definitions
Pain is defined by the International Association for the Study of Pain[1] as "an unpleasant sensory and emotional experience associated with actual or potential tissue damage or described in terms of such damage."

Pain is a plural concept with biological, psychological, and social components. Its perception is influenced by cognitive, behavioral, environmental, and cultural factors. At first glance, it seems at odds with scientific medicine because of the difficulty accounting for it with obvious pathophysiologic changes.

Pain is subjective. Its presence cannot be readily validated or objectively measured. Physicians are confronted with ambiguity as they attempt to assess the severity and significance of chronic pain in their patients. In large part, this stems from the fundamental divide between a person who suffers from pain and an observer who attempts to understand that suffering. Observers tend to view pain complaints with suspicion and disbelief, akin to complaints of dizziness, fatigue, and malaise. As Scarry remarked, "To have great pain is to have certainty, to hear that another person has pain is to have doubt."[2]

The concept of chronic pain as an extension of acute nociceptive pain is not valid. **Chronic pain** is an evolving process in which injury may produce one pathogenic mechanism, which in turn produces others, so that the cause(s) of pain change over time. Support for this concept includes evidence that primary afferent discharge actually has the ability to injure or kill spinal inhibitory neurons (excitotoxicity), leading to hyperexcitability due to disinhibition. Peripheral nerve injury can initiate evolving abnormalities in spinal cord neurons, which in turn generate abnormal responsiveness of thalamic neurons, which in turn generate cortical dysfunction. In time, these higher-level abnormalities may become independent of the abnormalities that produced them.[3]

Even in situations that might be expected to provide clear correlations between perceived pain and identified peripheral pathology, there are perplexing observations. For example, in up to 85% of individuals who report back pain, no pain-producing pathology can be identified[4]; conversely, some 30% of asymptomatic people have significant pathology on magnetic resonance imaging (MRI)[5] and computed tomographic (CT) scans[6] that might be expected to cause pain. Headache is another common disabling condition in which impairment must be assessed primarily on the basis of individuals' reports of pain rather than on tissue pathology or anatomic abnormality. The reason is straightforward: in the majority of cases there is no demonstrable tissue pathology. Thus, pain can exist without tissue damage, and tissue damage can exist without pain. In summary, there is no "pain thermometer," that is, no biological measure that correlates highly with individuals' complaints of pain.

18.2b Impact of Pain on Population Health and Disability

Pain is among the most common reasons for seeking medical attention, accounting for more than 70 million office visits to physicians each year.[7] It is also the most common cause of disability, with chronic low back pain alone accounting for more disability than any other condition, resulting in nearly 150 million lost work days in 1988.[8] Disability related to back pain has increased dramatically, although there is no reason to suspect that back problems by themselves have increased.[9,10] Headache disorders are also a major cause of work loss.[11] Despite advances in physiologic understanding, surgical interventions, and pharmacologic therapies, the prevalence of chronic pain shows no signs of abating and continues to be of epidemic proportions. Notwithstanding this fact, the importance of pain is often discounted. Morris has averred that pain reported by somebody else falls into the category we reserve for whatever is invisible, subjective, immaterial, and therefore unreal.[12] A 1987 report of the Social Security Administration opined that it is impossible to understand the pain that another person is suffering.[13]

Pain is an essential determinant of the incapacitation of many individuals who undergo impairment evaluation. As observed by the Institute of Medicine Committee on Pain and Disability and Chronic Illness Behavior,[14] "The notion that all impairments should be verifiable by objective evidence is administratively necessary for an entitlement program. Yet this notion is fundamentally at odds with a realistic understanding of how disease and injury operate to incapacitate people. Except for a very few conditions, such as the loss of a limb, blindness, deafness, paralysis, or coma, most diseases and injuries do not prevent people from working by mechanical failure. Rather, people are incapacitated by a variety of unbearable sensations when they try to work."

When pain persists, it has the capacity to dominate a person's existence, contributing to significant impairment, reduction in the quality of life, functional limitations, and disability. The ravages of chronic pain often extend beyond the person who has it, as the lives of family members are often dominated by the pain of a loved one. Indeed, the children of individuals with chronic pain are at risk for suffering a similar fate.[15] In addition to the human costs, chronic pain is extremely costly to society. Medical expenditures for pain-related assessment and treatment, indemnity costs, loss of productivity, and loss of tax revenues are estimated to be $125 billion each year in the United States.[16]

18.2c Medical Advances in Understanding and Managing Pain
Behavioral/Psychological

Several major currents of thought and investigation in the last three decades have profoundly altered medical understanding of pain and its associated behaviors. The first was the behavioral hypothesis that much of the behavior associated with chronic pain was not intrinsic to a disease or injury but, rather, reflected environmental contingencies.[17] This development led to the introduction of powerful clinical interventions, but it had the unfortunate effect of increasing skepticism about the validity of the suffering in those with persistent pain.

The considerable role of cognitive factors and coping skills in augmenting and mitigating the suffering and dysfunction of chronic pain has been compellingly demonstrated. These insights have provided the foundation of efficacious treatments.[18]

Associated with these developments has been the introduction of the term *chronic pain syndrome (CPS)* into common parlance. Although not official nomenclature, it is frequently used to describe an individual who is markedly impaired by chronic pain with substantial psychological overlay.[19] CPS is largely a behavioral syndrome that affects a minority of those with chronic pain. It may best be understood as a form of **abnormal illness behavior** that consists mainly of excessive adoption of the sick role. The term is useful in that it properly directs therapy toward the reversal of regression and away from an exclusive focus on elimination of nociception. It does not, however, substitute for a careful diagnosis of the physiologic, psychological, and conditioning components that comprise the syndrome. The term *CPS* must be used with caution, as grouping pain problems together under a generic disorder may mask and leave untreated important physiologic differences.

Neurophysiologic

A second major current has derived from explosive growth in our understanding of the pathophysiology of pain, which has rendered many older concepts untenable. Processes of peripheral and central sensitization have been clarified, along with such phenomena as the development of adrenergic sensitivity in injured nociceptive fibers and the accumulation of ion channels at sites of nerve injury, all of which may produce severe pain in response to trivial stimulation. Processes have been identified by which unilateral inflammation, trauma, or illness can lead to pain and sensitivity in uninvolved, often contralateral, structures. Physiologic processes underlying such symptoms, which were often dismissed as "not real," have been found at the level of the dorsal horn, thalamus, and sensory cortex. Intense stimulation and peripheral nerve damage have been found to induce persistent changes in the spinal cord that, over time, alter the receptive field mapping and the phenotype of neurons rostral to them, which in turn may induce changes at the cortical level. These findings are of major import. They demonstrate that pain need not be symptomatic of a disease or injury but, in fact, can become a disease unto itself.

A major implication of recent research on sensitization is that the failure of medical and surgical investigation to account for a given pain may result not from looking in the wrong place, but from looking at the wrong time. That is, the investigations may be directed toward the organ or body part that was historically responsible for the individual's pain, but they may be unrevealing because the pain, having been initiated by an injury or illness in the past, is now relatively independent.

Although sensitization of the peripheral and central nervous system has been demonstrated repeatedly in basic neuroscience research, there are currently no widely accepted methods for determining whether the symptoms of an individual with chronic pain can be ascribed to sensitization. Thus, while the concept of sensitization is extremely important to a conceptual understanding of chronic pain, there is currently no systematic way to incorporate it into impairment ratings.

Implications

The scientific advances described above have important implications for the assessment of pain-related impairment. The AMA *Guides* as a whole embodies the premise that injuries and illnesses cause deficits in the functioning of organs or body parts, and these deficits can be quantitatively assessed during an impairment evaluation. In the simplest situations, an individual experiences a definite biological insult that creates a clear-cut abnormality in his or her biological functioning. This abnormality, in turn, leads directly to deficits in activities of daily living (ADL) that can be quantified during the course of an impairment evaluation. An example is an individual who sustains a below-elbow amputation in a sawmill accident.

The behavioral concept of CPS and the neurophysiologic concept of peripheral or central nervous system sensitization imply that pain and pain-related activity restrictions may be dissociated from the biological insult to which a person was exposed and from any measurable biological dysfunction in that person's organs or body parts. Both concepts thus challenge the assumed linkages among biological insult, organ or body part dysfunction, and ADL deficits that are fundamental to the AMA rating system.

Physicians differ sharply in the way in which they conceptualize the relations among biological insult, measurable organ or body part dysfunction, and self-reported activity limitations in individuals with chronic pain. Some physicians have a low threshold for using diagnoses like "chronic pain syndrome" or "psychogenic pain" to describe these people. The diagnoses highlight the lack of association between the complaints of the individuals and any well-defined biological abnormality.

Other physicians attempt to link the complaints of pain patients to a biological abnormality. In general, they do this by employing one of two strategies. The first is to view the person as having an atypical presentation of a well-accepted syndrome. For example, thoracic outlet syndrome is a well-recognized condition that can be caused by measurable abnormalities in arterial, venous, or neural structures in the thoracic outlet. Some physicians view people with chronic pain and paresthesias in an upper extremity as having a variant of thoracic outlet syndrome, even though vascular studies and electrodiagnostic studies are either normal or equivocal.[20] The other strategy is to construct diagnoses based on the person's symptoms and on subjective physical examination findings. The assumption of physicians employing this strategy is that a biological underpinning for the symptoms exists, but that medical science has not yet identified it. For example, the diagnosis of fibromyalgia is based on individuals' reports of widespread pain and their reports of tenderness during physical examination. Despite extensive research, no specific underlying biological abnormality has been discovered to explain the reports of these people.

Acrimonious debates have occurred between physicians who favor biological explanations for controversial pain syndromes and those who construe the syndromes as dissociated from any definable biological abnormality. The interpretation has significant practical implications because many of the administrative agencies that provide benefits for people with impairments emphasize the importance of (1) objective findings of biological dysfunction and (2) a clear causal link between an index injury and an individual's present symptoms and findings. If a painful condition is construed as a CPS or a psychogenic pain syndrome, both of these criteria are violated.

The distinction between well-accepted conditions and those that are ambiguous or controversial is itself ambiguous. Sometimes disagreements arise about individuals with atypical presentations of well-recognized painful syndromes. The example of thoracic outlet syndrome was given above. Another example is a person with chronic low back pain, vague symptoms in one lower extremity, and an MRI with questionable compromise of a lumbar nerve root. The person might be described as having an atypical presentation of a lumbar radiculopathy; an alternative assessment is that the individual has a nonspecific chronic pain syndrome involving the low back. In other instances, disagreements center around the validity of the diagnostic procedures used to diagnose conditions. For example, a practitioner of manual medicine might ascribe an individual's back pain to a lumbar subluxation or torsion of the ilium, whereas physicians not practiced in manual medicine might discount these diagnoses because they do not accept the validity of the physical examination maneuvers underlying them. Finally, as in the case of fibromyalgia, reliable diagnostic criteria exist, but physicians disagree about whether the condition diagnosed by use of these criteria has a specific, definable biologic basis.

The controversies described above cannot be resolved in this chapter of the *Guides* for the simple reason that the medical community has not achieved consensus about how to construe such conditions as myofascial pain syndrome, fibromyalgia, and "disputed neurogenic" thoracic outlet syndrome.[20] A practical approach for performing impairment ratings on individuals with ambiguous or controversial syndromes is given below.

18.3 Integrating Pain-Related Impairment Into the Conventional Impairment Rating System

There are several difficulties associated with integrating pain-related impairment into an impairment rating system such as the *Guides*. A basic challenge for a system of rating pain-related impairment is to incorporate the subjectivity associated with pain into an impairment rating system whose fundamental premise is that impairment assessment should be based on objective findings. The inherent subjectivity of pain is incongruent with the *Guides'* attempts to assess impairment on the basis of objective measures of organ dysfunction, as it requires that determinations of pain intensity and the restrictions imposed by it must be largely based on patients' reports.

A second issue is that an individual's pain behaviors are influenced by his or her social environment. Impairment ratings are usually performed not to establish academic facts or to make treatment decisions but, rather, to establish the financial obligations of payers to individuals or, conversely, the entitlements of individuals to monetary rewards. Thus, the social context surrounding impairment ratings might provide an incentive for individuals to exaggerate their reports of pain so as to maximize awards. Conversely, since insurance companies and government agencies often hire the professionals who perform impairment ratings, evaluators may have an incentive to doubt the complaints of individuals. An ideal rating system would validate the genuine suffering of individuals and resist influence by those who exaggerate their incapacitation for secondary gain. In the absence of objective criteria for assessing the severity and functional significance of pain, it has proved exceedingly difficult to achieve this goal.

Third, this chapter assesses pain qualitatively. Because percentages for pain-related impairment have not been used and tested on a widespread basis, as have other impairment ratings used in the *Guides,* it was decided that impairment ratings for pain disorders would not be expressed as percentages of whole person impairment. Future scientific evidence may emerge that will enable a more quantifiable approach to be adopted. Nevertheless, the value of a qualitative assessment is that any identification of a significant pain component warrants additional consideration when interpreting impairment ratings used for allocation of medical resources, work placement, or financial compensation.

Finally, at a practical level, a chapter of the *Guides* devoted to pain-related impairment should not be redundant of or inconsistent with principles of impairment rating described in other chapters. The *Guides'* impairment ratings currently include allowances for the pain that individuals typically experience when they suffer from various injuries or diseases, as articulated in Chapter 1 of the *Guides*: "Physicians recognize the local and distant pain that commonly accompanies many disorders. Impairment ratings in the *Guides* already have accounted for pain. For example, when a cervical spine disorder produces radiating pain down the arm, the arm pain, which is commonly seen, has been accounted for in the cervical spine impairment rating" (p. 10). Thus, if an examining physician determines that an individual has pain-related impairment, he or she will have the additional task of deciding whether or not that impairment has already been adequately incorporated into the rating the person has received on the basis of other chapters of the *Guides*.

18.3a When This Chapter Should Be Used to Evaluate Pain-Related Impairment

Organ and body system ratings of impairment should be used whenever they adequately capture the actual ADL deficits that individuals experience. However, the organ and body system impairment rating does not adequately address impairment in several situations, discussed below.

When There Is Excess Pain in the Context of Verifiable Medical Conditions That Cause Pain

Individuals in this group have pain associated with medical conditions that are verifiable by objective means. An example is an individual with a persistent lumbar radiculopathy following a lumbar diskectomy. Such an individual will usually have objective findings, including atrophy of the affected leg, muscle weakness, and MRI evidence of epidural scarring. An individual with these findings would receive an impairment rating of 10% on the basis of the DRE spine impairment rating system described in Chapter 15. Although the DRE rating is usually appropriate, some individuals with persistent lumbar radiculopathies report "excess" pain. That is, they report that their pain causes severe ADL deficits, suggesting a level of impairment greater than 10%. Procedures in this chapter can be used to assess this additional impairment and to classify it as mild, moderate, moderately severe, or severe.

When There Are Well-Established Pain Syndromes Without Significant, Identifiable Organ Dysfunction to Explain the Pain

Individuals in this group have pain syndromes that are widely accepted by physicians based on the individuals' clinical presentation but that are not associated with definable tissue pathology. These syndromes are not ratable under the conventional rating system and also they do not fit any of the other chapters in the *Guides* since there is no measurable organ dysfunction. Individuals with these well-established pain syndromes can be evaluated on the basis of concepts elaborated in this chapter. These individuals must have symptoms and signs that can plausibly be attributed to a well-defined medical condition. Some of the most common of these syndromes are listed in Table 18-1. The list is not comprehensive and may change as the body of medical information about various pain syndromes grows. If an examiner determines that an individual has a diagnosis that is not on the list, he or she may rate the individual's pain-related impairment if he or she is convinced that the diagnosed condition is well recognized and that the pain-related impairment is a consequence of the condition. An explanation should be provided in writing.

Table 18-1	Illustrative List of Well-Established Pain Syndromes Without Significant, Identifiable Organ Dysfunction to Explain the Pain

Headache (most)

Postherpetic neuralgia

Tic douloureux

Erythromelalgia

Complex regional pain syndrome, type 1 (reflex sympathetic dystrophy)

Any injury to the nervous system

Table 18-2	Illustrative List of Associated Pain Syndromes

Postparaplegic pain

Syringomyelia pain

Thalamic syndrome

Brachial plexus avulsion pain

Nerve entrapment syndromes

Peripheral neuropathy

Complex regional pain syndrome, type 2 (causalgia)

When There Are Other Associated Pain Syndromes

Use this chapter to evaluate pain-related impairment when dealing with syndromes with the following characteristics: (*a*) They are associated with identifiable organ dysfunction that is ratable according to other chapters in the *Guides*; (*b*) they *may be* associated with well-established pain syndromes, but the occurrence or nonoccurrence of the pain syndromes is not predictable; so that (*c*) the impairment ratings provided in other chapters of the *Guides* do not capture the added burden of illness borne by individuals who have the associated pain syndromes.

Examples of syndromes in this category are given in Table 18-2. Again, the list is not comprehensive, so an examiner must use his or her judgment to decide whether an individual with an unlisted condition should be placed in this category.

18.3b When This Chapter Should Not Be Used to Rate Pain-Related Impairment

When Conditions Are Adequately Rated in Other Chapters of the Guides

Examiners should not use this chapter to rate pain-related impairment for any condition that can be adequately rated on the basis of the body and organ impairment rating systems given in other chapters of the *Guides*.

When Rating Individuals With Low Credibility

Since the assessment of pain-related impairment depends heavily on the verbal reports of individuals, examiners must be careful to provide ratings only for those who provide information that appears to be reasonable and accurate. The reports of individuals may lack credibility for a variety of reasons. Some people appear unable or unwilling to provide information that is sufficiently detailed for an examiner to assess pain-related impairment. The reasons for this are multiple, including psychosis, severe depression, memory deficits secondary to brain injury, and a lack of cooperation. Other individuals provide detailed information, but the validity of the information is questionable.

When There Are Ambiguous or Controversial Pain Syndromes

As noted above, physicians disagree sharply about whether individuals with chronic pain should be construed as having conditions with definite, albeit obscure, biologic underpinnings. The alternative is to describe these people as having CPS, psychogenic pain syndromes, or some other term implying that their pain cannot be associated with a well-accepted biologic abnormality. For purposes of this chapter, the pain of individuals with ambiguous or controversial pain syndromes is considered *unratable*.

As noted earlier, the distinctions between well-recognized conditions and ambiguous or controversial ones is subtle, so that no definitive list of ambiguous or controversial conditions can be given. The examining physician can, however, identify ambiguous or controversial syndromes by asking the following questions:

1. Do the individual's symptoms and/or physical findings match any known medical condition?
2. Is the individual's presentation typical of the diagnosed condition?
3. Is the diagnosed condition one that is widely accepted by physicians as having a well-defined pathophysiologic basis?

If the answer to all three of the above questions is yes, the examiner should consider the individual's pain-related impairment to be ratable and should proceed according to the rating protocol described in Section 18.3d. If the answer to any of the above three questions is no, the examiner should consider the individual's pain-related impairment to be *unratable* on the basis of concepts in this chapter. In that instance, he or she should still use the assessment protocol described in Section 18.3d to determine the severity and impact of the individual's pain and report the results. That is, even if the examiner considers the person to have unratable pain, he or she needs to characterize the apparent pain-related impairment.

The fact that pain-related impairment may be unratable either on the basis of the organ and body rating system or on the basis of this chapter highlights the limits that exist in the science and practice of impairment evaluation. The judgment that pain-related impairment is unratable does not mean that the evaluating physician considers the pain to be "unreal" or fabricated. In fact, individuals with ambiguous or controversial pain syndromes may suffer from severe pain and report significant restrictions in ADL. These reports are often corroborated by information provided by family members and treating physicians. Thus, when a physician judges pain-related impairment to be unratable, he or she is simply asserting an inability to determine how the activity restrictions reported by an individual are linked to a disease or injury. The decision regarding how to construe these reports must therefore be administrative, not medical.

Advances in diagnostic technology and clinical experience may eventually make pain-related impairment rating feasible for individuals with ambiguous or controversial pain syndromes. At the present time, however, the best option available to an examiner is to report that the individual has apparent impairment that is unratable on the basis of current medical knowledge. Insurance companies and administrative agencies that dispense benefits for impairments will need to make the final decision about how to use this information.

18.3c Administrative Issues Associated With Pain-Related Impairment

In essence, this chapter divides apparent impairment into three categories: (1) impairment ratable on the basis of the conventional rating system used throughout *Guides* Chapters 3 through 17; (2) pain-related impairment ratable according to concepts outlined in this chapter; and (3) pain-related impairment that is unratable according to the concepts outlined in this chapter.

There are two major reasons why these distinctions are crucial. First, agencies that provide benefits for individuals with impairments function under different legal mandates with respect to pain-related impairment. For example, workers' compensation laws in some states mandate that pain-related impairment be considered in disability awards for injured workers.[21] In other states pain-related impairment is not considered.[22]

The system described here distinguishes between an impairment rating using the organ system approach and impairment awarded on the basis of pain. This distinction permits administrative agencies to count "conventional" impairment ratings and pain-related impairment ratings on an equal footing, to discount pain-related impairment ratings, or to disregard them entirely. Similarly, the present system identifies individuals with unratable pain-related impairment so that administrative agencies can make informed decisions about whether or not to compensate these individuals.

Second, the distinction between ratable and unratable pain-related impairment embodies a key premise of this chapter: physicians do not currently possess reliable, valid techniques for assessing impairment associated with pain in all clinical settings. It is then more appropriate for the examining physician to describe the individual's pain-related impairment as unratable than to give a rating that cannot be supported by either scientific evidence or consensus.

18.3d How to Rate Pain-Related Impairment: Overview

The system described in this chapter relies largely on self-reports by individuals. Thus, it differs significantly from the conventional rating system, which relies primarily on objective indices of organ dysfunction or failure. The present system assesses pain intensity, emotional distress related to pain, and ADL deficits secondary to pain. ADL deficits are given the greatest weight. An individual's pain-related impairment is considered unratable if (*a*) his or her behavior during the evaluation raises significant issues of credibility, (*b*) he or she has clinical findings atypical of a well-accepted medical condition, or (*c*) he or she is diagnosed with a condition that is vague or controversial.

A detailed protocol for assessing pain-related impairment is described below and outlined in Figure 18-1.

A. Evaluate the individual according to the body or organ rating system, and determine an impairment percentage. During the evaluation, the examiner should informally assess pain-related impairment.

B. If the body system impairment rating appears to adequately encompass the pain experienced by the individual due to his or her medical condition, his or her impairment rating is as indicated by the body system impairment rating.

C. If the individual appears to have pain-related impairment that has increased the burden of his or her condition *slightly,* the examiner may increase the percentage found in A by up to 3%.

D. The examiner should perform a formal pain-related impairment assessment if any of the following conditions are met:

1) The individual appears to have pain-related impairment that is *substantially* in excess of the impairment determined in step A

   or

2) The individual has a well-recognized medical condition that is characterized by pain in the absence of measurable dysfunction of an organ or body part (see Table 18-1 for examples)

   or

3) The individual has a syndrome with the following characteristics: (*a*) it is associated with identifiable organ dysfunction that is ratable according to other chapters in the *Guides*; (*b*) it *may be* associated with a well-established pain syndrome, but the occurrence or nonoccurrence of the pain syndrome is not predictable; so that (*c*) the impairment ratings provided in step A do not capture the added burden of illness borne by the individual because of his or her associated pain syndrome (see Table 18-2 for examples).

E. If the examiner performs a formal pain-related impairment rating, he or she may increase the percentage found in step A by up to 3%, *and* he or she should classify the individual's pain-related impairment into one of four categories: mild, moderate, moderately severe, or severe. In addition, the examiner should determine whether the pain-related impairment is *ratable* or *unratable.*

Chapter 18

Figure 18-1 Algorithm for Rating Pain-Related Impairment in Conditions Associated With Conventionally Ratable Impairment

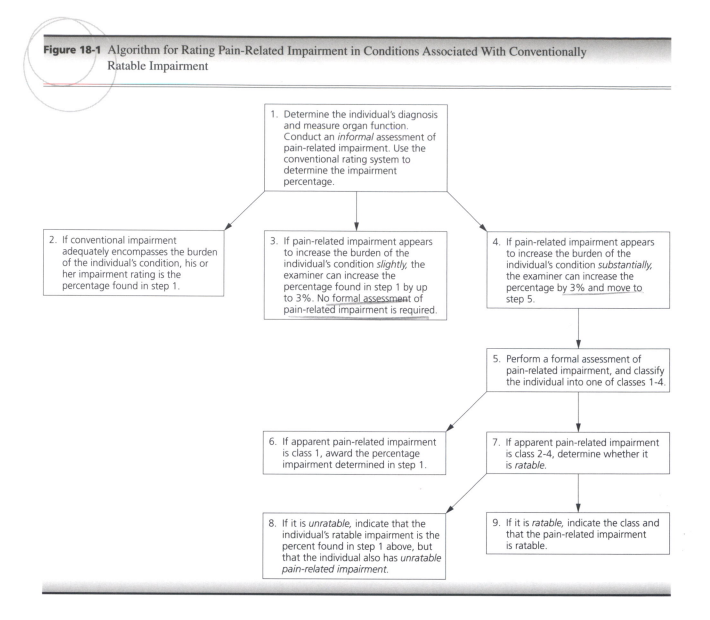

1. Determine the individual's diagnosis and measure organ function. Conduct an *informal* assessment of pain-related impairment. Use the conventional rating system to determine the impairment percentage.

2. If conventional impairment adequately encompasses the burden of the individual's condition, his or her impairment rating is the percentage found in step 1.

3. If pain-related impairment appears to increase the burden of the individual's condition *slightly*, the examiner can increase the percentage found in step 1 by up to 3%. No formal assessment of pain-related impairment is required.

4. If pain-related impairment appears to increase the burden of the individual's condition *substantially*, the examiner can increase the percentage by 3% and move to step 5.

5. Perform a formal assessment of pain-related impairment, and classify the individual into one of classes 1-4.

6. If apparent pain-related impairment is class 1, award the percentage impairment determined in step 1.

7. If apparent pain-related impairment is class 2-4, determine whether it is *ratable*.

8. If it is *unratable*, indicate that the individual's ratable impairment is the percent found in step 1 above, but that the individual also has *unratable pain-related impairment*.

9. If it is *ratable*, indicate the class and that the pain-related impairment is ratable.

Table 18-3 Impairment Classification Due to Pain Disorders

Class 1 Mild	Class 2 Moderate	Class 3 Moderately Severe	Class 4 Severe
Pain severity, based on a combination of intensity and frequency, is mild	Pain severity, based on a combination of intensity and frequency, is moderate	Pain is present most of the time and may reach an intensity of 9-10/10	Pain is essentially continuous, with intensity reaching 9-10/10 at its worst
Individual's pain is mildly aggravated by performing ADL; is able to perform them with few modifications	Individual has moderate difficulty managing ADL; must make significant modifications in order to perform them (eg, move to a ground floor apartment, buy a car with automatic transmission)	Individual can perform ADL only with substantial modifications; unable to perform many routine activities (eg, driving a car)	Individual must either get help from others for many ADL (eg, preparing food, dressing), modify them drastically (eg, stop bathing), or spend an inordinate amount of time accomplishing them (eg, 2 hours to get out of bed and dressed)
Individual demonstrates no or only minimal emotional distress in response to his or her pain	Individual demonstrates mild to moderate affective distress in relation to his or her pain	Individual demonstrates moderate to severe affective distress in relation to his or her pain	Individual demonstrates severe affective distress in relation to his or her pain and communicates the perception that the pain is completely out of control
Individual is not receiving treatment for pain on a regular basis	Individual requires ongoing medical monitoring and is taking medication much of the time	Individual receives medication to control pain on a maintenance basis	Individual is receiving maximal pharmacologic support for his or her pain on an ongoing basis
Pain-related limitations during physical examination are mild and appear appropriate; few pain behaviors (overt expressions of pain, distress, and suffering, such as moaning, limping, moving in a guarded fashion, facial grimacing) are observed during examination	Individual demonstrates significant pain-related limitations on physical examination; relatively few pain behaviors appear during the examination, and they are of indeterminate appropriateness	On physical examination, individual demonstrates severe pain-related limitations that may make the examination difficult to perform and results difficult to interpret A number of pain behaviors are observed during the examination, and they appear to be congruent with organ dysfunction	Physical examination is virtually impossible to perform because individual is intolerant of many examination maneuvers (eg, refuses to ambulate or to allow examiner to palpate symptomatic area); a significant number of pain behaviors are observed during the examination, and they appear to be congruent with organ dysfunction

18.3e Classes of Pain-Related Impairment

There are four general classes of impairment due to pain: class 1, mild; class 2, moderate; class 3, moderately severe; and class 4, severe (see Table 18-3).

18.3f How to Rate Pain-Related Impairment: Practical Steps

There are six steps in the pain-related impairment evaluation process, each discussed below. Several alternative methods are available to evaluate the severity of pain, activity restrictions, emotional distress, and pain behaviors, some of which are discussed subsequently. One such methodology is provided in Table 18-4. The first three parts of the protocol included in Table 18-4 rely on the individual's self-report. The questions may be provided to the individual to complete on his or her own, or they can be presented in interview format. If the individual is asked to complete the questionnaire on his or her own, someone should be available to answer questions and to review the completed form to make sure the individual has responded to all the items. If the individual has a question about completion of any of the items in Sections I to III, he or she should be instructed to make the best estimate possible. Although Table 18-4 provides a numerical score, this should not be misunderstood to represent a quantitative impairment rating, but rather is used to classify individuals into the four qualitative classes. To that purpose, alternative methods may be used so long as they are valid and appropriately referred to in the report.

Table 18-4 Ratings Determining Impairment Associated With Pain

Name:_____ Date:_____

I. Pain (Self-report of Severity)

A. Rate how severe your pain is **right now, at this moment** (circle a number):

0   1   2   3   4   5   6   7   8   9   10

No pain   Most severe pain can imagine

B. Rate how severe your pain is **at its worst** (circle a number):

0   1   2   3   4   5   6   7   8   9   10

None   Excruciating

C. Rate how severe your pain is **on the average** (circle a number):

0   1   2   3   4   5   6   7   8   9   10

None   Excruciating

D. Rate how much your pain is **aggravated by activity** (circle a number):

0   1   2   3   4   5   6   7   8   9   10

Activity does not   Excruciating following
aggravate pain   any activity

Sum score of Section I: A–D = Total pain severity/4 = _____

E. Rate how **frequently** you experience pain (circle a number):

0   1   2   3   4   5   6   7   8   9   10

Rarely   All of the time

Add total pain severity score
(items A–D/4) to score for item E = _____

Total pain severity score (range from 0 to 20) = _____

II. Activity Limitation or Interference

A. How much does your pain interfere with your ability to **walk 1 block**? (circle a number):

0   1   2   3   4   5   6   7   8   9   10

Does not restrict   Pain makes it impossible
ability to walk   for me to walk

B. How much does your pain prevent you from **lifting 10 pounds** (a bag of groceries)? (circle a number):

0   1   2   3   4   5   6   7   8   9   10

Does not prevent from   Impossible to lift
lifting 10 pounds   10 pounds

C. How much does your pain interfere with your ability to **sit for 1/2 hour**? (circle a number):

0   1   2   3   4   5   6   7   8   9   10

Does not restrict ability   Impossible to sit
to sit for 1/2 hour   for 1/2 hour

D. How much does your pain interfere with your ability to **stand for 1/2 hour**? (circle a number):

0   1   2   3   4   5   6   7   8   9   10

Pain does not interfere   Unable to
with ability to stand at all   stand at all

E. How much does your pain interfere with your ability to **get enough sleep**? (circle a number):

0   1   2   3   4   5   6   7   8   9   10

Does not prevent me   Impossible
from sleeping   to sleep

F. How much does your pain interfere with your ability to **participate in social activities**? (circle a number):

0   1   2   3   4   5   6   7   8   9   10

Does not interfere   Completely interferes
with social activities   with social activities

G. How much does your pain interfere with your ability to **travel up to 1 hour by car**? (circle a number):

0   1   2   3   4   5   6   7   8   9   10

Does not interfere with ability   Completely unable to
to travel 1 hour by car   travel 1 hour by car

H. In general, how much does your pain interfere with your **daily activities**? (circle a number):

0   1   2   3   4   5   6   7   8   9   10

Does not interfere   Completely interferes
with my daily activities   with my daily activities

I. How much do you **limit your activities to prevent your pain from getting worse**? (circle a number):

0   1   2   3   4   5   6   7   8   9   10

Does not limit   Completely limits
activities   activities

J. How much does your pain interfere with your **relationship with your family/partner/significant others?** (circle a number):

0   1   2   3   4   5   6   7   8   9   10

Does not interfere   Completely interferes
with relationships   with relationships

K. How much does your pain interfere with your ability to do **jobs around your home**? (circle a number):

0   1   2   3   4   5   6   7   8   9   10

Does not interfere   Completely unable to
                                                  do any job around home

L. How much does your pain interfere with your ability to **shower or bathe without help from someone else?** (circle a number):

0   1   2   3   4   5   6   7   8   9   10

Does not interfere   My pain makes it impossible to
at all   shower or bathe without help

M. How much does your pain interfere with your ability to **write or type?** (circle a number):

0   1   2   3   4   5   6   7   8   9   10

Does not interfere   My pain makes it
at all   impossible to write or type

N. How much does your pain interfere with your ability to **dress yourself**? (circle a number):

0   1   2   3   4   5   6   7   8   9   10

Does not interfere   My pain makes it
at all   impossible to dress myself

O. How much does your pain interfere with your ability to **engage in sexual activities**? (circle a number):

0   1   2   3   4   5   6   7   8   9   10

Does not interfere   My pain makes it almost
at all   impossible to engage in
                                       any sexual activity

P. How much does your pain interfere with your ability to **concentrate**? (circle a number):

0   1   2   3   4   5   6   7   8   9   10

Never   All the time

Sum score of Section II:
A-P = Total score for activity limitation/16 =
Mean activity limitation = _____

III. Individual's Report of Effect of Pain on Mood

A. Rate your **overall mood** during the past week. (circle a number):

0   1   2   3   4   5   6   7   8   9   10

Extremely high/good   Extremely low/bad

B. During the past week, how **anxious or worried** have you been because of your pain? (circle a number):

0   1   2   3   4   5   6   7   8   9   10

Not at all anxious/worried   Extremely anxious/worried

C. During the past week, how **depressed** have you been because of your pain? (circle a number):

0   1   2   3   4   5   6   7   8   9   10

Not at all depressed   Extremely depressed

D. During the past week, how **irritable** have you been because of your pain? (circle a number):

0   1   2   3   4   5   6   7   8   9   10

Not at all irritable   Extremely irritable

E. In general, how anxious/worried are you about performing activities because they **might make your pain/symptoms worse**?

0   1   2   3   4   5   6   7   8   9   10

Not at all anxious/worried   Extremely anxious/worried

Sum score of Section III:
A-E = Total pain impairment attributed to mood state/5 =
Mean score = _____

Assess Whether the Individual Is at MMI

This concept is particularly important in the assessment of pain-related impairment. A person should not be judged medically stable, and therefore ratable, unless he or she has undergone a thorough evaluation for the entire range of factors that can affect pain and has undergone a vigorous trial of rehabilitative treatment.

For example, there may be no further orthopedic interventions available for a lumbar pseudarthrosis. Spinal arachnoiditis may be refractory to any intervention. Yet in both cases, appropriate pain management may reduce all the components of impairment, with reduced pain severity, functional restoration, and mood normalization. Consultation with a specialist in pain medicine may be required to determine whether the impairment is fixed or potentially useful treatments are available.

Determine the Severity of the Pain

Although absolute quantification of pain is not possible, severity may be estimated using, for example, a visual analog scale, a numeric, or a box-rating scale. A horizontal or vertical line of known length is anchored by "no pain at all" at one end and "worst pain ever" at the other. A line of consecutive boxes also anchored with these end points, with a number in each one and in which the individual is asked to place an "X" in the box, may be of particular use because some people have difficulty understanding how to use a VAS scale.[23] It is useful to obtain least, worst, and current levels, as well as the usual level. Exacerbating and mitigating factors should be sought. The character or quality of pain may assist with diagnosis and help establish that the pain is compatible with a known medical syndrome.

Chapter 18

The McGill Pain Questionnaire is widely used in pain medicine. It contains lists of words chosen to reflect the sensory (eg, dull, cramping), affective (eg, agonizing, terrifying), and evaluative (eg, annoying, unbearable) components of the pain experience.[24] There are also descriptors of the temporal qualities of the pain (momentary, steady, intermittent). Line drawings of the body permit the individual to shade in the location of the pain. Numeric descriptors of the overall present pain intensity are provided (1 = mild, 2 = discomforting, 3 = distressing, 4 = horrible, 5 = excruciating).

Determine Activity Restrictions

The reported severity of pain may not correlate well with its functional impact. Indeed, some individuals report well-preserved function despite pain of 9/10 in severity, while others portray a vegetative existence with a pain level of 4/10. It is essential to know the extent to which the following functions are impeded by *pain*: ADL, socialization, recreation, work, sleep, sexuality, and cognition.

A quasi-quantification of functional status can be derived by scoring the extent to which pain interferes with each (applicable) activity. The individual should be queried as to how often he or she leaves the home (with documentation if housebound), gets out only for medical appointments, and the like. "Down time," the total number of hours a day the person is reclining, is a useful measure.

It is useful to provide quantification of functional limitations via accepted, standardized instruments that permit interrater comparisons. The Pain Disability Index provides 0 to 10 scales on which individuals rate pain-related interference in seven domains, including family/home responsibilities, recreation, social activity, occupation, sexual behavior, self-care, and life support activities (eating, sleeping, breathing).[25] The SF-36 is widely used to determine the degree of functional impairment and changes in overall wellness following treatment of those with pain as well as of other populations.[26] The Oswestry[27] and Roland-Morris[28] are brief questionnaires that provide an economical office assessment of function in individuals with back pain. A large number of other instruments exist, as reported in the literature. It is also possible to correlate estimates of function to actual impairment using questionnaires and scales.

The ADL listed in Table 1-2 are commonly classified within one of eight different areas: physical activity, nonspecialized hand activities, sleep, travel, self-care and personal hygiene, sexual function, communication, and sensory function.[29] The first six of these are most relevant for impairment due to pain, as it is extremely rare for pain to create major restrictions in communication and sensory functioning. A number of measures have been developed to assess ADL, some of which are general and others of which are designed for use with specific diseases and injuries.[30,31] Physicians may choose to select from among the available ADL scales if they wish a more detailed assessment. Although individuals may have difficulty separating the effect of specific diseases or injuries from the pain on their activities, some estimate is necessary to help in determining the extent of impairment due to pain that exceeds activity restriction due to the disease or injury. For example, an individual with a below-the-knee amputation may have some activity limitations in ambulation; he or she may have additional limitations due to severe stump pain.

Several well-established general measures have been standardized on chronic pain sufferers and have been used in numerous published studies that may be of particular use as they assess several important domains relevant to the assessment of impairment. For example, the Sickness Impact Profile (SIP) is a widely used health status measure that has been shown to reliably assess the impact of health problems on function and quality of life.[32] The West Haven–Yale Multidimensional Pain Inventory (MPI)[33] is another reliable and valid health status measure that has been used extensively.

Determine the Presence of Emotional Distress

An important component of chronic pain-related impairment is its associated affective distress, which often includes sadness, anger or irritability, and anxiety.[34] In some cohorts, the depression seems to be primarily a function of life interference and cognitive changes, while in others it seems to be primarily a function of the pain itself.[35] In either case, it is unnecessary that an individual meet diagnostic criteria for a mood, anxiety, or other psychiatric disorder for there to be substantial suffering related to such issues as pain, loss of meaningful and pleasurable life activities, and a bleak future.

It may be appropriate to use rating scales to provide some quantification of affective changes. Brief self-administered screens for depression, such as the Beck Depression Inventory,[36] the Zung Depression Index,[37] and rater-administered screens such as the Hamilton Self-rating Scale for Depression,[38] may alert the physician to the presence of a mood disorder that requires treatment, as well as to the possibility of suicide. Similar instruments are available for anxiety and include the Beck Anxiety Scale and Hamilton Rating Scale for Anxiety. The Profile of Mood States (POMS),[39] which has also been useful in providing quantification of various mood states in individuals with chronic pain, has scales reflecting impaired concentration, anxiety, depression, fatigue, and others.

As with pain reports, these instruments all are subject to minimization or exaggeration on the part of the individual. People are seen who score four times the cutoff for depression on the Beck Depression Inventory, yet who are animated and playful in the gym. When such discrepancies occur, the weighting given the instrument should be minimal. Moreover, caution must be taken in interpreting responses on these measures, as they were not standardized on samples of individuals with medical disorders, and using the usual cutoff scores may lead to an excessively large number of false positives.

It is important to obtain information from the individual regarding the impact of pain on his or her mood state. As noted in the discussion of activity restrictions, it may be difficult for the individual to separate the effect of specific diseases or injuries from the pain on activities; however, the items are designed to obtain a rough estimate of the individual's beliefs.

Determine if Pain Behaviors Are Present

Pain behaviors are the ways that individuals communicate about their pain. These behaviors may be verbal or nonverbal. The individual may be unaware of them, as they may be emitted and maintained due to responses that have been received from significant others, including health care professionals. In other instances, individuals may exaggerate their behaviors to signal pain and distress with the intent to achieve some desired response from those who observe the behaviors. Thus, both the antecedents and consequences of the behaviors are important.

Some individuals appear stoic as they go through evaluations, and the pain behaviors they do demonstrate are concordant with other medical information regarding their condition. In this instance, the pain behaviors provide valuable clues regarding a person's diagnosis and tend to validate the fact that he or she is suffering because of the diagnosed condition. For example, consider an individual with suspected degenerative joint disease of the hip who walks with a characteristic limp. The limp provides a clue to the diagnosis and tends to support the individual's reports that he or she has significant pain when walking.

At the opposite extreme, an individual may demonstrate pain behaviors that appear exaggerated and discordant with his or her presumed medical condition. These pain behaviors may appear to be driven by a variety of factors, such as overwhelming somatic anxiety or the person's desire to convince an examiner that he or she is suffering greatly. The common denominator underlying them is that they do not appear to be direct, inevitable consequences of a definable medical condition. Exaggerated, discordant pain behaviors tend to cast doubt on the validity of the information that people provide regarding their condition.

Thus, an examiner has a twofold task regarding pain behaviors demonstrated by a person undergoing an impairment rating: to identify the pain behaviors, and to interpret their significance, that is, to decide whether they tend to authenticate the validity of the individual's suffering or to raise questions about his or her communication style.

It is hard to specify a generic list of pain behaviors. The behaviors to look for depend on the individual's medical condition, examination maneuvers that are performed, previous responses obtained, and intent. Physicians probably differ significantly in what they view as exaggerated pain behaviors. Sources of variation include different concepts of what represents "legitimate disease" and thresholds for calling a behavior abnormal.

Despite the limitations noted, pain behaviors provide useful information regarding both the impact of pain on observable behavior and the individual's style of communicating (eg, demonstrative, stoic) about their pain. The physician should observe the individual's pain behaviors as he or she enters the examination room, during the interview, and during the history taking. This will eliminate the increase in pain behaviors that might be directly associated with the physical examination.

The examiner should give a score between +10 and −10 to indicate his or her global evaluation of an individual's pain behavior during the interview and physical examination. A positive score is given when the individual demonstrates pain behaviors that are concordant with the overall clinical findings and, in the opinion of the examiner, tend to authenticate his or her suffering. A negative score is given when an individual demonstrates grossly "nonorganic" or "exaggerated" pain behaviors. A score close to 0 should be given when the examiner is uncertain about how to interpret the individual's pain behaviors.

The specific behaviors an examiner considers vary according to the individual's medical condition and the examination maneuvers performed. Potentially significant behaviors that commonly occur during evaluations are listed in Table 18-5. Note that the significance of pain behavior cannot be determined unless related to a particular individual and context. Thus, a pain behavior that would be considered concordant in one clinical context would be considered discordant in a different one. Also, note that pain behaviors that tend to validate an individual's pain are generally specific to that person's medical condition. In contrast, exaggerated pain behaviors—such as emotional displays and pain-limited weakness—tend to occur in conjunction with a wide variety of medical conditions.

The physician can record the pain behaviors observed using the behaviors listed in Table 18-5.[40] These behaviors may be viewed as indicating symptom magnification, especially when several are present and they grossly exceed what might be expected from individuals with a similar diagnosis. These systematic observations should be used as the basis for determining a global rating regarding the presence and congruence of pain behaviors given the individual's diagnosis and organ dysfunction.

Table 18-5 Assessment of Pain Behavior

Observable Pain Behaviors

Note the presence of any of the following behaviors during the interview and examination:

1. Facial grimacing
2. Holding or supporting affected body part or area
3. Limping or distorted gait
4. Frequent shifting of posture or position
5. Extremely slow movements
6. Sitting with a rigid posture
7. Moving in a guarded or protective fashion
8. Moaning
9. Using a cane, cervical collar, or other device
10. Stooping while walking
11. Other: _____

Based on the behaviors above and knowledge of the individual's diagnosis and organ dysfunction, rate the pain behaviors by giving them a score between +10 and −10. You may give any score between +10 and −10.

−10	0	+10
Pain behaviors are exaggerated, nonphysiologic	Pain behaviors are mixed or ambiguous	Pain behaviors are appropriate and tend to confirm other clinical findings

Global pain behavior score = _____

Credibility of the Individual

Physicians routinely assess the credibility of individuals in the course of their clinical work. This kind of assessment is particularly important in the context of rating pain-related impairment because the ratings depend on verbal and nonverbal behaviors of people that are at least partly under voluntary control. Although there are no definite rules for assessing credibility, Section 18.4, Behavioral Confounders, discusses several issues that a physician should consider when making a judgment about a person's credibility.

The key question the examiner should ask is, Do the limitations that an individual describes and demonstrates accurately reflect the burden of illness he or she bears during everyday activity?

18.4 Behavioral Confounders

An extensive literature demonstrates what common sense suggests: pain behaviors and perception of pain are strongly influenced by beliefs, expectations, rewards, attention, and training. In the absence of a direct measure of pain, such behaviors function as markers by which pain is judged. However, voluminous literature demonstrates that these markers reflect social and environmental factors as much as they reflect pain. It has been shown, for example, that individual ratings of pain severity diminish when "well talk" is reinforced. With repeated identical pain stimuli, intensity reports vary with feedback. Verbal reinforcement increases performance in individuals with back pain. Studies consistently show that spouse solicitousness is correlated with pain behavior.[41]

Prospective studies consistently show that onset of disabling pain is highly associated with such factors as job dissatisfaction, lack of support at work, stress, and perceived inadequacy of income.[42-45] Once initiated, the progression of pain to chronicity is contingent on similar factors.[46,47] Financial compensation, receipt of work-related sickness payments, and compensation-related litigation are also associated with chronicity, as are such social and economic factors as poor education, language problems, and low income. Chronicity is also favored by individual tendencies to be preoccupied with one's body and symptoms.[48,49] Even in individuals with clear-cut radicular pain from disk prolapse/protrusion, application for retirement at 6 months was best predicted by depression and daily hassles at work.[50,51] In the case of injured workers, performance on functional capacity evaluation is reduced if the worker is informed that the test results will be used to determine work classification.[52] Industrial injuries and compensation situations appear to provide a disproportionate number of individuals with such issues.[53,54]

Although the suffering induced by a miserable vocational situation may equal or exceed that from disease or injury, it is the intent of the *Guides* to assign impairment based on disease and injury, not on such environmental situations as an individual's fear of returning to a hostile work environment. Similarly, the physician charged with assigning an impairment rating expects to discharge the obligation by assessing the state of the person as an organism, and he or she rightly considers such external factors as the state of the economy, the market for particular skills, and the local tolerance for language barriers to be distracters that lower the "signal-to-noise" ratio in the assessment.

Thus, examiners face a dilemma. They know that a variety of nonbiological factors strongly influence the disability status and ADL deficits of individuals they rate, but they are charged with the task of rating impairment on the basis of measurable dysfunctions of organ or body parts.

18.4a Assessing Behavioral Reliability

A primary step in radiographic interpretation is evaluation of the quality of the image. Incorrect exposure, motion artifact, and other technical deficiencies may weaken the conclusions that may be drawn from the image. The principal gauge of pain is its associated behaviors, which include reports. Thus, it is critical that this measure of pain be assessed for reliability. Inappropriate pain behavior, embellishment, and symptom magnification are common, particularly in medicolegal circumstances and entitlement programs. The following is a guide to their assessment.

Congruence With Established Conditions

In cases of phantom pain, the individual describes pain in an absent extremity. While this might be expected to evoke incredulity, it does not because this condition has been well described for decades, long before its pathophysiology was understood. Similarly, the person with complex regional pain syndrome (previously called reflex sympathetic dystrophy, or RSD) may describe exquisite pain on light touch of a healthy-appearing extremity following a trivial injury. A constellation of associated signs and symptoms, such as cold sensitivity, autonomic changes, trophic changes, dystonic phenomena, and others help to confirm that the pain complaint is consistent with a known clinical syndrome. Intolerance of light touch over a region of the lower back in individuals with mechanical low back pain is inconsistent with a defined disease process and thus fails to meet this criterion.

Most known conditions have such expected concomitants. Typically, an individual would not watch television or read while waiting for a migraine to abate, and there would be an expected response to ergots, triptans, or other antimigraine preparations. An individual with neuropathic pain will likely, but not always, show some response to certain antiepileptic drugs (eg, gabapentin, carbamazepine) or antidepressants (eg, tricyclics). A person with persistent pain of pancreatitis would be unlikely to gain weight.

Consistency Over Time and Situation

There is risk in placing unwarranted confidence in the validity of assessments that are numeric and therefore often considered "objective" and "scientific." Such confidence is challenged by such observations as a person who can tolerate only 10° forward flexion while standing, yet can sit with legs outstretched and touch his or her toes. Similarly, a person may demonstrate collapsing with pain on manual testing of plantar flexion, yet be able to tiptoe. Others may limp on one leg walking forward, the other walking backward, but neither on a treadmill. Grip strength may be measured repeatedly and coefficients of variation calculated, although these methods have been criticized.[55] Rapid exchange grip strength testing may provide similar information.[56] Isokinetic strength testing may discriminate between maximal and submaximal effort.[57] Complaints and dysfunction should be relatively independent of the observers present and should generally persist, despite distraction.

Consistency With Anatomy and Physiology

Waddell's signs are perhaps the best known of numerous indicators of pain behaviors that are more likely to be accounted for by an individual's expectations than by organic pathology.[58,59] One example is that of axial rotation, in which the standing individual's hips are rotated in each direction by the examiner. This essentially affects only the hips and ankles, leaving the pelvis and all above it to move as a unit. Exacerbation of back pain by this maneuver is considered abnormal. It is important, however, when using this method not to rate the individual on only one abnormal test and to place the response in the context of the individual's history and physical examination.

Observer Agreement

Collateral information from relatives and other evaluating professionals is of critical value in determining the consistency of individual behaviors, which helps to confirm that their relationship is to perceived pain and varies little with changes in observers.

Other Inappropriate Illness Behavior

It may be difficult to judge whether or not behavior is compatible with perceived pain. For example, because one cannot know how much leg pain an individual experiences on walking, it is hard to know whether an antalgic gait is exaggerated. Inappropriate illness behavior may be suspected, however, if an individual demonstrates dysfunction in unrelated domains. For example, except in extreme situations, an individual with back pain should not require that the spouse complete the individual's questionnaire—or his or her sentences. Chronic pain rarely precludes making one's own phone calls to the doctor, paying bills, etc. When a person has delegated these functions to others, abnormal illness behavior is likely.

18.4b Incorporating Behavioral Confounders Into Impairment Ratings

Physicians should consider the confounders described in Section 18.4a when they evaluate the pain behaviors of individuals (see Determine if Pain Behaviors Are Present, Section 18.3f) and when they rate the credibility of individuals (see Credibility of the Individual, Section 18.3f).

18.4c Cautions

Although no one would conclude that because an x-ray is of poor quality there is unlikely to be pathology of concern, this non sequitur frequently occurs in cases of aberrant pain behaviors. Such behaviors should properly cause physicians to be uncertain, but not dismissive. Behavior is affected by many factors. The appearance of symptom exaggeration can be created by fear or by having learned that certain actions or positions provoke pain. "Nonphysiologic" signs may occur in dementia. Excessive or exaggerated pain behaviors can be a response to feeling discounted or mistrusted, so that one must emphasize symptoms to persuade physicians of their reality. Anyone might dramatize a problem in an effort to have it taken seriously. Thus, symptom magnification can be an iatrogenic phenomenon that occurs when an individual feels mistrusted or poorly cared for.

18.5 How to Rate Pain-Related Impairment: A Sample Protocol

As the preceding discussion indicates, a physician must rely on a wide range of clinical skills when he or she assesses pain-related impairment. Also, the discussion indicates that several different assessment instruments may be used in the course of the assessments. The plethora of assessment methods available can further complicate the already difficult task facing the examining physician.

The protocol described below selects assessment instruments and procedures that, in the opinion of the authors, permit physicians to reach conclusions about pain-related impairment that are reliable and valid. The specific steps in the protocol are as follows:

1. Determine whether the individual is medically stable.
2. Follow the steps outlined in Figure 18-1.
3. If a formal assessment of pain-related impairment is to be performed:
   a. Have the individual complete the questionnaire shown in Table 18-4.
      (1) This provides information about three domains that are relevant to pain-related impairment: severity of pain, ADL restrictions, and emotional distress.
      (2) Follow the instructions given in Table 18-6 to obtain the person's score for each of these three domains.
   b. Observe the individual's pain behaviors throughout the evaluation. Follow the instructions given in Table 18-5 to obtain the individual's score for the pain behaviors domain.
   c. Make a global assessment of the person's credibility, taking into consideration the factors discussed in the Section 18.4. Assign a score between −10 and +10, where −10 indicates very low credibility and +10 indicates very high credibility. Enter this score in line 5 of Table 18-6. If the credibility score is less than 0, the examiner should consider the possibility of aborting the pain-related impairment assessment on the grounds that the individual does not meet the entry criteria given in Section 18.3b.

d. Follow the instructions given in Table 18-6 to combine scores from each of the above five domains (severity of pain, ADL restrictions, emotional distress, pain behaviors, and credibility) into a total pain-related impairment score. These scores are not impairment ratings but are used only to classify the individual as discussed under c.

e. Follow the instructions given in Table 18-7 to convert this total pain-related impairment score into one of the four categories of impairment described in Table 18-3 (ie, mild, moderate, moderately severe, or severe).

4. Review the material provided in Sections 18.3a and 18.3b to determine whether the pain-related impairment is ratable or unratable.

5. The final impairment rating should include the following:

a. The percentage impairment rating based on the dysfunction in the organ or body part being rated (see step A in Section 18.3d).

b. Additional impairment of up to 3% may be given if an individual has pain-related impairment that increases the burden of illness slightly (see step C in Section 18.3d).

c. If the individual has undergone a formal pain-related assessment:

(1) An indication of the individual's pain-related impairment category (see 3e above).

(2) An indication of whether this impairment is ratable or unratable.

(a) If pain-related impairment is ratable, an indication of whether or not the pain-related impairment is adequately encapsulated by the impairment rating given for organ or body part dysfunction (see Section 18.3a).

Table 18-6 Worksheet for Calculating Total Pain-Related Impairment Score

1. Sum the scores for Section I of Table 18-4, items A-D, and divide by 4; add response to item E. Range is from 0 to 20. _____

2. Total scores for Section II of Table 18-4, items A-P, divide by 16, and multiply by 3. Range is from 0 to 30. _____

3. Sum scores for Section III of Table 18-4, items A-E, and divide by 4. Range is from 0 to 10. _____

4. Global pain behavior rating from Table 18-5 (rating should be −10, 0, or +10). _____

Subtotal steps 1 through 4 (maximum = 70) _____

5. Physician adjustment based on clinical judgment of individual's credibility. Add or subtract 0 to 10. _____

6. Total pain-related impairment score = total of steps 1 through 5 _____

Table 18-7 Determining Impairment Class on the Basis of Total Pain-Related Impairment Score

Total Pain-Related Impairment Score*	Impairment Class
0- 6	No significant impairment
7-24	Mild impairment
25-42	Moderate impairment
43-60	Moderately severe impairment
61-80	Severe impairment

* The impairment rating score is not an impairment rating.

18.6 Psychogenic Pain

Somatoform disorders are a group of conditions characterized by physical symptoms that are not fully explained by a medical condition, the effects of a substance, or another mental disorder.[60] The symptoms are not under voluntary control. *Pain disorder* is diagnosed when pain is a predominant focus of the presentation and causes significant distress or impairment in important areas of functioning. Psychological factors are judged to play a significant role in the onset, severity, exacerbation, or maintenance of the pain. *Pain disorder associated with psychological factors* is diagnosed when psychological factors are judged to have the major role; in this subtype, general medical conditions play little or no role. *Pain disorder associated with both psychological factors and a general medical condition* is indicated when both psychological factors and a general medical condition are judged to have important roles in the onset, severity, exacerbation, or maintenance of the pain. The diagnoses are rather general, and almost any person with persistent pain would meet the inclusion criteria.

These current diagnostic terms appear to refer to conditions previously called *conversion, hysteria,* and **psychogenic pain.** There appears to be no fully satisfactory explanation or conceptualization of these conditions. Since pain is a perceptual *experience,* one could argue that all pain is a psychic phenomenon. Thus, psychogenic pain would be a tautology, much like psychogenic joy. Certainly, those processes in the dorsal horn, spinothalamic tract, and thalamus of an anesthetized person are not considered *pain,* a term reserved for what occurs when these processes access conscious awareness in an aversive fashion.

The concept of psychogenic pain is further complicated by the fact that a variety of conditions formerly considered psychogenic have been found to be neurologically based and that its diagnostic signs have been challenged.[61] Nevertheless, psychogenic pain appears to exist and probably represents several different phenomena. Unlike psychogenic pain, other psychogenic symptoms can be confirmed; for example, conversion blindness preserves the opticokinetic reflex, psychogenic seizures occur during a normal EEG recording, conversion anesthesia does not diminish the sensory evoked potential, and psychogenically paralyzed extremities move during sleep. Such confirmation is unavailable in the case of pain.

Some individuals are seen whose symptoms resemble no organic condition, who have inconsistent and nonphysiologic physical findings, yet who demonstrate great distress with agitation or psychomotor retardation, inability to sleep, and a general misery that is consistent across environments and confirmed by others. Such individuals' suffering is genuine, should not be minimized, and constitutes a risk for suicide. It is most probable that these individuals truly perceive pain, suffer with it, and are impaired.

Chapter 14, which deals with impairment associated with mental disorders, describes a system for assessing impairment among individuals with pain disorders. Examiners will sometimes be uncertain about whether to use the assessment procedures described in this chapter or the ones described in Chapter 14. They should ask the following key question when evaluating an individual whose chronic pain is not fully explained on the basis of organ pathology: Does it appear that psychological factors played a major role in the initiation of the pain syndrome or are playing a major role in its continuation? If the answer to this question is yes, the examiner should use the rating methods described in Chapter 14. If the answer is no, or if the examiner is uncertain, he or she should use the rating methods described in this chapter.

18.7 Malingering

Malingering is conscious deception for the purpose of gain. While most authorities declare that malingering is quite uncommon, there appear to be few data regarding its frequency. Fishbain et al reviewed literature suggesting that malingering is present in 1.25% to 10.4% of individuals with chronic pain; however, they found serious flaws with the methodology and concluded that no conclusions could be drawn from the data.[62]

Other fields provide some limits regarding the prevalence of malingering. In individuals with unexplained intractable diarrhea, 14% had positive stool examinations for laxatives, although all had denied use of laxatives.[63] Among 333 people who claimed compensation for noise-induced hearing loss, the incidence of exaggeration on hearing tests (as determined by cortical evoked response audiometry) was 17.7%.[64] Weintraub cites studies showing that 20% to 46% of people consider purposeful misrepresentation of compensation claims to be acceptable behavior.[65]

These studies suggest that factitious illness and malingering may not be rare, but they do not provide information as to how often these conditions simulate pain. They do suggest that evaluators keep an open mind as to the possibility of these phenomena, which are probably less likely in those seeking treatment than in those seeking compensation.

Confirmation of malingering is extremely difficult and generally depends on intentional or inadvertent surveillance. Anecdotes abound of providers running into wheelchair-bound individuals strolling about a mall or encountering an individual in the parking lot holding a cane in the air and demonstrating a normal gait. By definition, malingering is not a disease but a volitional deception. It thus requires no treatment.

18.8 Conclusion

The assessment of pain-related impairment constitutes a substantial challenge, as it is the most common reason for disability, the most subjective, and perhaps the most multifaceted. Equitable quantification of impairment requires attention to subjective experiences of pain and emotional distress, as well as reports of behavioral impairment, all of which can only be confirmed indirectly. At times, it seems to present the dilemma of being too difficult to perform and too essential to omit.

Despite these obstacles, it appears that each of the components of pain can, in most cases, be assessed with good reliability if a meticulous evaluation is performed that includes observation and collateral information. In this way, the interests of individuals who hope to achieve validation of their symptoms and payers who hope to avoid indiscriminate financial obligations can be fairly addressed.

18.9 Case Examples

Class 1 Mild
Pain severity, based on a combination of intensity and frequency, is mild
Individual's pain is mildly aggravated by performing ADL; is able to perform them with few modifications
Individual demonstrates no or only minimal emotional distress in response to his or her pain
Individual is not receiving treatment for pain on a regular basis
Pain-related limitations during physical examination are mild and appear appropriate; few pain behaviors (overt expressions of pain, distress, and suffering, such as moaning, limping, moving in a guarded fashion, facial grimacing) are observed during examination

Example 18-1

Subject: 28-year-old woman.

History: Individual who is otherwise healthy experiences approximately 20 severe headache events per year.

Current Symptoms: Each headache event begins at night and reaches maximal intensity within 2 to 3 hours. Untreated, average duration is 8 to 12 hours. Headache is associated with severe nausea and vomiting, light-headedness, moderately to severely blurred vision, and diarrhea. Woman is completely asymptomatic between headaches.

Physical Exam: Generally healthy woman. Neurologic examination and past medical history are otherwise normal. Using Table 18-4, the pain intensity score is 6.

Activity Interference (based on protocol described in Table 18-4): Woman is able to perform all ADL, having some difficulties only during the headache episodes. Activity limitations score is 5.

Emotional Distress (based on protocols described in Table 18-4): She reports moderate emotional distress and is concerned about her ability to meet role and responsibilities. The emotional distress score is 4.

Pain Behaviors (based on Table 18-5): No pain behaviors demonstrated; pain behavior score is 0.

Credibility: Credibility score is +5.

Diagnosis: Migraine.

Impairment Rating: Based on the procedures described in Tables 18-4 through 18-7, the individual's total pain-related impairment score is 20. She is therefore classified as having mild pain-related impairment. No ratable impairment based on organ or body part dysfunction.

Comment: During her attacks, this woman is completely impaired by the severity of her pain, its accompaniments, and the treatment that is required to relieve symptoms. Impairment is intermittent, lasting only the duration of the attack and the effects of the medication. She is otherwise unimpaired.

Class 2 Moderate
Pain severity, based on a combination of intensity and frequency, is moderate
Individual has moderate difficulty managing ADL; must make significant modifications in order to perform them (eg, move to a ground floor apartment, buy a car with automatic transmission)
Individual demonstrates mild to moderate affective distress in relation to his or her pain
Individual requires ongoing medical monitoring and is taking medication much of the time
Individual demonstrates significant pain-related limitations on physical examination; relatively few pain behaviors appear during the examination, and they are of indeterminate appropriateness

Example 18-2

Subject: 42-year-old man.

History: Individual developed right carpal tunnel syndrome (CTS) 2.5 years ago while working as a cement mixer. Underwent CTS release 2 months after onset of symptoms. Postoperatively, developed swelling of right hand, along with severe, diffuse pain. Was diagnosed with RSD. Has failed stellate ganglion blocks, numerous medication trials, and a vigorous physical therapy program.

Current Symptoms: Pain in the right hand and forearm, which can extend up to the shoulder. Pain constant at 3-5/10 when inactive. Increased pain and severe swelling of hand with any vigorous right upper extremity (RUE) activity. Based on Table 18-4, pain severity score is 10.

Physical Exam: Dramatic swelling of right hand, along with discoloration and excessive sweating. Range of motion (ROM) of fingers markedly reduced secondary to swelling. Mild hypersensitivity to tactile stimulation of hand. No sensory loss. Demonstrates pain-limited weakness in all muscle groups of distal RUE.

Activity Interference (based on protocol described in Table 18-4): Activity limitation score is 18. Unable to use RUE for any physically demanding activities.

Emotional Distress (based on protocol described in Table 18-4): Severely depressed over ongoing pain and work disability; frequent thoughts of suicide. Emotional distress score is 10.

Pain Behaviors (using the global rating in Table 18-5): A number of pain behaviors that appeared inconsistent with the diagnosis of CTS or RSD were observed, including guarded and protective movements of the lumbar spine and the left upper extremity. These behaviors were judged to be excessive and incongruent with the diagnosed conditions and were rated –7.

Credibility: Moderate; credibility score is +3.

Diagnosis: CTS and RSD.

Impairment Rating: (1) Conventional: 22% whole person impairment due to markedly restricted ROM of all digits of the right hand. (2) Pain related: Using protocol described in Tables 18-4 through 18-7, the individual is assigned a total pain-related impairment score of 28, corresponding to moderate pain-related impairment. The pain-related impairment is felt to be ratable and to be adequately encapsulated within the impairment rating in the conventional impairment rating described above.

Comment: In RSD, impairment is typically secondary to pain and is not easily encompassed by the conventional impairment rating system. This person is unusual in that the swelling and consequent reduced ROM of the fingers was ratable.

Class 3
Moderately Severe
Pain is present most of the time and may reach an intensity of 9-10/10
Individual can perform ADL only with substantial modifications; unable to perform many routine activities (eg, driving a car)
Individual demonstrates moderate to severe affective distress in relation to his or her pain
Individual receives medication to control pain on a maintenance basis
On physical examination, individual demonstrates severe pain-related limitations that may make the examination difficult to perform and results difficult to interpret
A number of pain behaviors are observed during the examination, and they appear to be congruent with organ dysfunction

Example 18-3

Subject: 45-year-old man.

History: History of nine lumbar surgeries over a 15-year period. Started with an L4-5 diskectomy; now is fused from L2 to the sacrum.

Current Symptoms: Low back pain with intermittent radiation into proximal right lower extremity. Also has pain wrapping around his flanks in an L2 distribution and numbness in an S1 pattern in the left lower extremity. Baseline pain is present daily and is described as 4/10 in intensity. About 10 flare-ups per year during which he is confined to bed for several days. On the basis of Table 18-4, pain intensity score is 12.

Physical Exam: Stands leaning forward and to the right; is unable to achieve an erect posture. Palpation reveals significant myofascial pain throughout lumbar and gluteal region. ROM of the lumbar spine is severely restricted in all planes. No sciatic tension signs. Neurologic exam shows signs of a left S1 radiculopathy and diffuse, pain-inhibited weakness in the right lower extremity.

Activity Interference (based on protocol described in Table 18-4): Activity limitation score is 23. Individual is severely limited in sitting, standing, walking, and lifting; he is often unable to travel by car.

Emotional Distress (based on protocol described in Table 18-4): Individual suffers from ongoing depression and experiences acute anxiety during pain flare-ups. Emotional distress score is 6.

Pain Behaviors (based on the rating of global pain behaviors in Table 18-5): Some of the man's pain behaviors seemed ambiguous and somewhat excessive compared to those of others with similar organ dysfuction. The individual was given a global pain behavior rating of −3.

Credibility: Overall credibility is rated as high, based on reports from the individual's treating physician that his activity limitations have been very consistent over a number of years and that he has persevered in work efforts despite his severe lumbar spine condition. He is given a global score of +8 for credibility.

Diagnosis: Lumbar postlaminectomy syndrome.

Impairment Rating: (1) Conventional: 20% whole person impairment based on DRE category IV. (2) Pain related: The total pain-related impairment score is 46, indicating moderately severe pain-related impairment. The impairment is ratable and felt not to be adequately encapsulated in the conventional impairment rating given above.

Comment: The individual has significant impairment by both the conventional and pain-related impairment rating systems. His pain-related impairment, however, is substantially higher than his conventional impairment. He shows a temporal pattern of pain that is typical among people with chronic back pain. He has ongoing pain that is moderately disabling, with frequent superimposed flare-ups that are severely disabling.

Class 4 Severe
Pain is essentially continuous, with intensity reaching 9-10/10 at its worst
Individual must either get help from others for many ADL (eg, preparing food, dressing), modify them drastically (eg, stop bathing), or spend an inordinate amount of time accomplishing them (eg, 2 hours to get out of bed and dressed)
Individual demonstrates severe affective distress in relation to his or her pain and communicates the perception that the pain is completely out of control
Individual is receiving maximal pharmacologic support for his or her pain on an ongoing basis
Physical examination is virtually impossible to perform because individual is intolerant of many examination maneuvers (eg, refuses to ambulate or to allow examiner to palpate symptomatic area); a significant number of pain behaviors are observed during the examination, and they appear to be congruent with organ dysfunction

Example 18-4

Subject: 42-year-old woman.

History: Eight years ago, individual developed bilateral aching forearm pain and numbness of the hands in the context of repetitive wrist/hand motions in her job as an assay technician. Has undergone bilateral carpal tunnel releases, bilateral de Quervain's releases, and bilateral superficial radial neurectomies.

Current Symptoms: Constant burning pain in the dorsal aspect of both forearms and hands, along with aching in the volar aspect of both forearms. This background pain is rated as 6-8/10 in intensity. Even mildly forceful use of either hand (eg, pulling on the doorknob of a heavy door) causes pain to increase to 10/10 and can sometimes provoke flare-ups that last several days. Based on Table 18-4, the pain intensity score is 19.

Physical Exam: Mild swelling of both hands. Multiple scars from the surgeries. No definite temperature or color changes. No abnormal sudomotor activity or trophic changes. ROM of fingers and wrists almost full. Woman recoils with any tactile stimulation of either dorsal forearm or hand. Two-point discrimination is impaired in the distribution of the superficial radial sensory nerve bilaterally. Motor function cannot be tested validly because of severe pain inhibition.

Activity Interference (based on protocol described in Table 18-4): Activities limitation score is 26. Individual is barely able to manage basic ADL, such as dressing herself or maintaining personal hygiene. She cannot type for more than 2 minutes and is unable to drive.

Emotional Distress (based on protocol described in Table 18-4): The individual demonstrates severe anxiety and depression in relation to her pain, despite aggressive antidepressant medication therapy. Emotional distress score is 9.

Pain Behavior (using the global pain behavior score in Table 18-5): The woman appeared quite stoic throughout the evaluation. She demonstrated cutaneous hypersensitivity over the dorsal aspect of both forearms and wrists and significant pain-inhibited weakness of distal upper extremity muscles. However, strength was excellent in proximal muscles. Overall, the pain behaviors observed were judged to be mildly concordant with her medical condition. Pain behavior score is +1.

Credibility: The woman is felt to be sincerely expressing her suffering. Credibility score is +6.

Diagnosis: Bilateral superficial radial neuropathy.

Impairment Rating: (1) Conventional: 5% impairment of the upper extremity due to loss of sensory function in the right superficial radial nerve and 5% impairment of the upper extremity due to loss of sensory function in the left superficial radial nerve. Using the Combined Values Chart (p. 604) yields a total of 10% impairment of the upper extremities, or 6% whole person impairment. (2) Pain related: Using the procedures described in Tables 18-4 through 18-7, the total pain-related impairment score is 69, indicating severe pain-related impairment. It is felt that the impairment is ratable and not adequately encapsulated in the conventional impairment rating provided above.

Comment: The conventional impairment rating is low because the only measurable loss of function the individual has is in sensation of skin innervated by the superficial radial nerve. However, she has neuropathic pain in both upper extremities that causes incapacitating pain. Thus, the pain-related impairment is markedly higher than the conventionally rated impairment.

References

1. Merskey H. Association for the Study of Pain, Subcommittee on Taxonomy. Chronic pain syndromes and definitions of pain terms. *Pain*. 1986(suppl 3):S1.

2. Scarry E. *The Body in Pain*. New York, NY: Oxford University Press; 1985.

3. Covington EC. The biological basis of pain. *Int Rev Psychiatry*. 2000;12:127-146.

4. Deyo RA. The early diagnostic evaluation of patients with low back pain. *J Gen Intern Med*. 1986;1:328.

5. Jensen MC, Brant-Zawadski MN, Obuchowski N, Modic MT, Malkasian Ross JS. Magnetic resonance imaging of the lumbar spine in people without back pain. *N Engl J Med*. 1994;331:69-73.

6. Wiesel SW, Stourmas N, Feffer H. A study of computer assisted tomography: I. The incidence of positive CAT scans in an asymptomatic group of patients. *Spine*. 1984;9:549-551.

7. Woodwell DA. National Ambulatory Medical Care Survey: 1998 Summary. Advance data from Vital and Health Statistics; No. 315. Hyattsville, Md: National Center for Health Statistics; 2000.

8. Guo HR, Tanaka S, Halperin WE, Cameron LL. Back pain prevalence in US industry and estimates of lost workdays. *Am J Public Health*. 1999;89:1029-1035.

9. Guo HR, Tanaka S, Cameron LL, et al. Back pain among workers in the United States: national estimates and workers at high risk. *Am J Ind Med*. 1995;28:591-602.

10. Dionne CE, Koepsell TD, Von Korff M, Deyo RA, Barlow WE, Checkoway H. Predicting long-term functional limitations among back pain patients in primary care settings. *J Clin Epidemiol*. 1997;50:31-43.

11. Rasmussen BK, Jensen R, Olesen J. Impact of headache on sickness absence and utilisation of medical services: a Danish population study. *J Epidemiol Community Health*. 1992;46:443-446.

12. Morris DB. Pain and suffering in history. Symposium at: University of California, Los Angeles; 1999; Los Angeles, Calif.

13. US Commission on the Evaluation of Pain, US Dept of Health and Human Services, Social Security Administration Office of Disability. *Report of the Commission on the Evaluation of Pain*. Washington, DC: US Government Printing Office; 1987. Publication 64-031.

14. Pain and disability: clinical, behavioral, and public policy perspectives. In: Osterwsis M, Kleinman A, Mechanic D, eds. *Institute of Medicine's Committee on Pain and Disability and Chronic Illness Behavior*. Washington, DC: National Academy Press; 1987:28.

15. Rickard K. The occurrence of maladaptive health-related behaviors and teacher-rated conduct problems in children of chronic low back pain patients. *J Behav Med*. 1988;11:107-116.

16. Okifuji A, Turk DC, Kalauokalani D. Clinical outcome and economic evaluation of multidisciplinary pain centers. In: Block A, Kremer E, Fernandez E, eds. *Handbook of Pain Syndromes*. Mahwah, NJ: Lawrence Erlbaum; 1999:77-98.

17. Fordyce WE. *Behavioral Methods for Chronic Pain and Illness*. St Louis, Mo: CV Mosby Co; 1976.

18. Gatchel RJ, Turk DC, eds. *Psychological Approaches to Pain Management*. New York, NY: Guilford Press; 1996.

19. US Commission on the Evaluation of Pain, US Dept of Health and Human Services, Social Security Administration Office of Disability. Appendix C: Summary of the National Study of Chronic Pain Syndrome. In: *Report of the Commission on the Evaluation of Pain*. Washington, DC: US Government Printing Office; 1987.

20. Wilbourn AJ, Porter JM. Thoracic outlet syndromes. *Spine: State of the Art Rev*. 1986;2:597-626.

21. *California Physician's Guide to Medical Practice in the California Workers' Compensation System;* 1994.

22. *Washington Medical Aid Rules and Fee Schedules;* 1999.

23. Jensen MP, Karoly P. Self-report scales and procedures for assessing pain in adults. In: Turk DC, Melzack R, eds. *Handbook of Pain Assessment*. New York, NY: Guilford Press; 1992:152-168.

24. Melzack R, Katz J. Pain measurement in persons in pain. In: Wall PD, Melzack R, eds. *Textbook of Pain*. 3rd ed. New York, NY: Churchill Livingstone; 1994.

25. Tait RC, Chibnall JT, Krause S. The Pain Disability Index: psychometric properties. *Pain*. 1990;40:171-182.

26. Ware JE Jr, Gandek B. Overview of the SF-36 Health Survey and the International Quality of Life Assessment (IQOLA) Project. *J Clin Epidemiol*. 1998;51:903-912.

27. Fairbank JCT, Couper J, Davies JB, O'Brian JP. The Oswestry low back pain disability questionnaire. *Physiotherapy*. 1980;66:271-273.

28. Roland M, Morris R. A study of the natural history of back pain. I. Development of a reliable and sensitive measure of disability in low-back pain. *Spine*. 1983;8:141-144.

29. McDowell I, Newell C. *Measuring Health: A Guide to Rating Scales and Questionnaires*. 2nd ed. New York, NY: Oxford University Press; 1996.

30. Turk DC, Melzack R, eds. *Handbook of Pain Assessment*. New York, NY: Guilford Press; 1992.

31. Turk DC, Malzack R, eds. *Handbook of Pain Assessment*. 2nd ed. New York, NY: Guilford Press; in press.

32. de Bruin AF, de Witte LP, Stevens F, Diederiks JP. Sickness Impact Profile: the state of the art of a generic functional status measure. *Soc Sci Med*. 1992;35:1003-1014.

33. Kerns RD, Turk DC, Rudy TE. The West Haven-Yale Multidimensional Pain Inventory (WHYMPI). *Pain*. 1985;23:345-346.

34. Fernandez E, Turk DC. The scope and significance of anger in the experience of chronic pain. *Pain*. 1995;61:165-175.

35. Turk DC, Okifuji A, Scharff L. Chronic pain and depression: role of perceived impact and perceived control in different age cohorts. *Pain*. 1995;61:93-101.

36. Wesley AL, Gatchel RJ, Garofalo JP, Polatin PB. Toward more accurate use of the Beck Depression Inventory with chronic back pain patients. *Clin J Pain*. 1999;15:117-121.

37. Biggs JT, Wylie LT, Ziegler VE. Validity of the Zung Self-rating Depression Scale. *Br J Psychiatry*. 1978;132:381-385.

38. Knesevich JW, Biggs JT, Clayton PJ, Ziegler VE. Validity of the Hamilton Rating Scale for depression. *Br J Psychiatry*. 1977;131:49-52.

39. Norcross JC, Guadagnoli E, Prochaska JO. Factor structure of the Profile of Mood States (POMS): two partial replications. *J Clin Psychol.* 1984;40:1270-1277.

40. Keefe FJ, Williams DA. Assessment of pain behaviors. In: Turk DC, Melzack R, eds. *Handbook of Pain Assessment.* New York, NY: Guilford Press; 1992:275-283.

41. Turk DC, Kerns RD, Rosenberg R. Effects of marital interaction on chronic pain and disability: examining the downside of social support. *Rehabil Psychol.* 1992;37:357-372.

42. Bigos SJ, Battie MC, Spengler DM, et al. A prospective study of work perceptions and psychosocial factors affecting the report of back injury. *Spine.* 1991;16:1-6.

43. Krause N, Ragland DR, Fisher JM, Syme SL. Psychosocial job factors, physical workload, and incidence of work-related spinal injury: a 5-year prospective study of urban transit operators. *Spine.* 1998;23:2507-2516.

44. Papageorgiou AC, Macfarlane GJ, Thomas E, Croft PR, Jayson MI, Silman AJ. Psychosocial factors in the workplace—do they predict new episodes of low back pain? Evidence from the South Manchester Back Pain Study. *Spine.* 1997;22:1137-1142.

45. van Poppel MNM, Koes BW, Devillé W, Smid T, Bouter LM. Risk factors for back pain incidence in industry: a prospective study. *Pain.* 1998; 77:81-86.

46. Valat JP, Goupille P, Vedere V. Low back pain: risk factors for chronicity. *Rev Rhum Engl Ed.* 1997;64:189-194.

47. Williams RA, Pruitt SD, Doctor JN, et al. The contribution of job satisfaction to the transition from acute to chronic low back pain. *Arch Phys Med Rehabil.* 1998;79:366-374.

48. Gatchel RJ, Polatin PB, Mayer TG. The dominant role of psychosocial risk factors in the development of chronic low back pain disability. *Spine.* 1995;20:2702-2709.

49. Hasenbring M, Marienfeld G, Kuhlendahl D, Soyka D. Risk factors of chronicity in lumbar disc patients. A prospective investigation of biologic, psychologic, and social predictors of therapy outcome. *Spine.* 1994;19:2759-2765.

50. Greenough CG, Taylor LJ, Fraser RD. Anterior lumbar fusion. A comparison of noncompensation patients with compensation patients. *Clin Orthop.* 1994;300:30-37.

51. Penta M, Fraser RD. Anterior lumbar interbody fusion. A minimum 10-year follow-up. *Spine.* 1997;22:2429-2434.

52. Scheman J, Covington EC, Blosser T, Green K. Effects of instructions on physical capacities outcome in a workers' compensation setting. *Pain Med.* 2000;1:in press.

53. Greenough CG, Fraser RD. The effects of compensation on recovery from low-back injury. *Spine.* 1989;14:947-955.

54. Rainville J, Sobel JB, Hartigan C, Wright A. The effect of compensation involvement on the reporting of pain and disability by patients referred for rehabilitation of chronic low back pain. *Spine.* 1997;22:2016-2024.

55. Shechtman O. Using the coefficient of variation to detect sincerity of effort of grip strength: a literature review. *J Hand Ther.* 2000;13:25-32.

56. Lechner DE, Bradbury SF, Bradley LA. Detecting sincerity of effort: a summary of methods and approaches. *Phys Ther.* 1998;78:867-888.

57. Hildreth DH, Breidenbach WC, Lister GD, Hodges AD. Detection of submaximal effort by use of the rapid exchange grip. *J Hand Surg.* 1989;14A:742-745.

58. Waddell G, McCulloch J, Kummel E, Venner RM. Nonorganic physical signs in low-back pain. *Spine.* 1980;5:117-125.

59. Gaines WG Jr, Hegmann KT. Effectiveness of Waddell's nonorganic signs in predicting a delayed return to regular work in patients experiencing acute occupational low back pain. *Spine.* 1999;24:396-400.

60. American Psychiatric Association. *Diagnostic and Statistical Manual of Mental Disorders.* 4th ed. Washington, DC: American Psychiatric Association; 1994.

61. Schweiger A, Parducci A. Nocebo: the psychologic induction of pain. *Pavlovian J Biol Sci.* 1981;16:140-143.

62. Fishbain DA, Cutler R, Rosomoff HL, Rosomoff RS. Chronic pain disability exaggeration/malingering and submaximal effort research. *Clin J Pain.* 1999;15:244-274.

63. Bytzer P, Stokholm M, Andersen I, et al. Prevalence of surreptitious laxative abuse in patients with diarrhea of uncertain origin: a cost benefit analysis of a screening procedure. *Gut.* 1989;30:1379-1384.

64. Rickards FW, De Vidi S. Exaggerated hearing loss in noise induced hearing loss compensation claims in Victoria. *Med J Aust.* 1995;163:360-363.

65. Weintraub MI. Chronic pain in litigation: what is the relationship? *Neurol Clin.* 1995;13: 341-349.

Appendix

Recording Range-of-Motion Measurements

Range-of-motion (ROM) measurements are used in the spine, upper extremities, and lower extremities to identify dysfunction in movement that may result in changes in function in the body part. Physicians have questioned the reproducibility of ROM measurements, as well as their ability to predict aspects of function.[1] Reproducibility may be improved with the use of standardized measurement techniques, proper equipment, trained evaluators, adequate designated warm-up exercises, and uniform recording.[1,2] The purpose of this appendix is to provide further information on factors that can affect reproducibility to lead to greater standardization in technique.

Measurement Devices

The *Guides* refers to the use of goniometers or inclinomers to measure joint motion. Except in the spine, in which the inclinometer is the device of choice, either the inclinometer or the goniometer can be used to reliably measure joint motion, depending on the preference and experience of the examiner. A two-arm goniometer depends on visual assessment of both the stationary and the moving arm. An inclinometer measures gravity and enables the starting position to be consistently recorded with respect to gravity. Some researchers and clinicians believe the inclinometer is easier to use and more accurate, although limited data exist supporting this opinion.[3] Other electronic devices may also yield accurate measurements. Limited data exist concerning how measurements from newer devices compare to the more commonly used goniometers and inclinometers. Before using another measurement device, the evaluator should assess its reproducibility and accuracy compared to established tools and methods.

Measurement Techniques

To increase accuracy, identify anatomic landmarks, properly position and stabilize the body, and use a consistent technique as outlined in the *Guides* to apply the measuring device to the joint. Anatomic landmarks are listed in the *Guides*. It is recommended that the evaluator mark these areas with tape or a marking pencil to ensure the same starting position for repeated measurements. The evaluator should also record the landmarks used in the impairment report; differences in the site of the landmark could result in different findings among examiners.

Prior to obtaining measurements, have the individual perform appropriate warm-up exercises to obtain an accurate assessment of current ability. Include repetitions of extension, flexion, lateral bending, and rotation as listed in the relevant chapters.

Properly position and stabilize the area, taking into account the individual's impairment, level of comfort, and known biomechanical characteristics of the joint.[1] Most optimal positions for measurement are noted in the *Guides*. Obtain proper body alignment and stabilization of the device before recording measurements. Active movements are recommended since they may be more consistent than passive movements, less of a risk to individual injury, and a better approximation of the individual's function.

Figure A-1a Neutral (0°) Starting Positions for ROM Measurements—Frontal Plane

Figure A-1b Neutral (0°) Starting Positions for ROM Measurements——Sagittal Plane

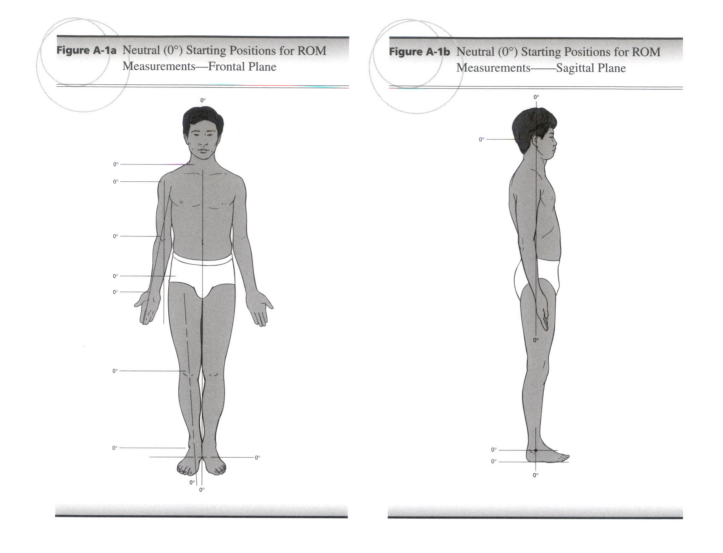

Recording Systems

Differences in recording systems for ROM measurements can contribute to additional errors in interpretation. Ideally, the examiner records the starting point and measurements in reference to the starting point. Subsequent motions are recorded in a reproducible and succinct manner.

ROM measurements can be recorded with text descriptions or with the use of a numeric format. A numeric format has been adopted by some states and a few countries in Europe to facilitate an efficient and uniform way of recording and retrieving data. This numeric format is known as the **SFTR method** of recording joint motion. The SFTR method allows recording of motion with only one letter and a maximum of three numbers. This numeric format is brief and complete, minimizes errors in transcription or understanding, and facilitates communication with the universal language of numbers. The SFTR format also enables easy translation of data from reports to computerized formats and displays.

Several requirements need to be met to use and record measurements according to the SFTR method.

1. All joint measurements are measured from a defined, neutral 0° starting position, as shown in Figure A-1a. This neutral starting position is the generally accepted anatomic position, with the body upright and the upper extremities extended at the side of the body with palms facing anteriorly. If the individual is sitting, supine, or prone, the starting position relates to the upright anatomic position. The starting position for rotation is midway between external and internal rotation or supination and pronation.
2. All joint motion is recorded in three basic planes: sagittal (S), frontal (F), and transverse (T). Rotation (R) crosses multiple planes and receives a separate recording. The planes are depicted in Figure 15-7.
    a. The sagittal (S) plane divides the body into right and left halves. (S) motions include extension and flexion.

b. The frontal (F) plane divides the body into anterior and posterior parts (front and back). (F) motions include abduction, adduction, elevation, depression, radial and ulnar deviation, and lateral bending of the spine to the left and right.

c. The transverse (T) plane divides the body into upper and lower halves. (T) motions include horizontal shoulder extension and flexion, hip horizontal abduction and adduction (hip flexed at 90°), shoulder retraction and protraction, and hallux valgus.

d. Rotation (R) can occur in any of the planes, depending on the limb positions. (R) motions include external and internal rotation, supination and pronation, and spine rotation to the left and right.

3. Record all motions with three numbers in a specific sequence. Record movements to the left or away from the middle of the body first: extension, abduction, external rotation, supination, valgus, eversion, lateral bending, or rotation of the spine to the left. Then record the reference (starting) position, which is normally 0°, in the middle. Record movements toward the middle of the body after the reference 0° (on the right side of 0°): flexion, adduction, internal rotation, pronation, varus, inversion, lateral bending, or rotation of the spine to the right.

4. Record all positions of ankylosis with two numbers, indicating the degree of ankylosis and the reference or starting position of 0°. For example, wrist ankylosis in 20° of extension is recorded as: wrist (S): 20-0 and in 20° of flexion as wrist (S) 0-20.

5. When the neutral 0° position cannot be reached due to limited or restricted motion, the middle number will not be 0 but will be the actual starting position. For example, an elbow flexed at 30° (extension lag of 30°), with further flexion to 90°, is recorded as S: 0-30-90.

Tables A-1, A-2, and A-3 describe a method to record ROM measurements for the upper extremties, lower extremities, and spine, using a standard text description and a numeric recording system, the SFTR method.

Table A-1 Recording ROM Measurements for the Upper Extremities*

Joint	Plane	Normal Active ROM ROM-0-ROM (°)	Clinical Examples	
			Text Description	SFTR Recording (°)
Shoulder	Sagittal	S: Extension -0- flexion (40)-0-(150)	Left extends to 40°, flexes to 150°	Left S: 40-0-150
			Right extends to 30°, flexes to 110°	Right S: 30-0-110
Shoulder	Frontal	Abduction -0- adduction (150)-0-(30)	Left abducts to 100°, adducts to 10°	Left F: 100-0-10
			Right abducts to 150°, adducts to 30°	Right F: 150 -0-30
Shoulder	Rotation	External -0- internal rotation rotation (90)-0-(80)	Left external rotation to 90°, internal rotation to 80°	Left R: 90-0-80
			Right external rotation to 80°, internal rotation to 40°	Right R: 80-0-40
Elbow	Sagittal	Extension -0- flexion (0)-0-(150)	Left extends to 0°, flexes to 150°	Left S: 0-0-150
			Right hyperextends to 0°, flexes to 110°	Right S: 0-0-110
Forearm	Rotation	Supination -0- pronation (80)-0-(80)	Left supinates to 60°, pronates to 80°	Left R: 60-0-80
			Right supinates to 80°, pronates to 80°	Right R: 80-0-80
Wrist	Sagittal	Extension -0- flexion (60)-0-(60)	Ankylosis of left wrist in 20° extension	Left S: 20-0
			Right extends to 20°, flexes to 50°	Right S: 20-0-50
Wrist	Frontal	Radial -0- ulnar deviation deviation (20)-0-(30)	Left radial deviates to 20°, ulnar deviates to 30°	Left F: 20-0-30
			Right radial deviates to 10°, ulnar deviates to 10°	Right F: 10-0-10

* Normal ranges are in parentheses.

Table A-2 Recording ROM Measurements for the Spine*

| Spinal Area | Plane | ROM-0-ROM (°) | Clinical Examples | |
			Text Description	**SFTR Recording (°)**
Cervical	Sagittal	Extension-0-flexion (60)-0-(50)	Extends 30°, flexes 45°	S: 30-0-45
Cervical	Frontal	Left lateral-0-right lateral bend bend (45)-0-(45)	Bends 30° to left, 40° to	F: 30-0-40
Cervical		Left-0-right rotation rotation (80)-0-(80)	Rotates left 40°, right 50°	R: 40-0-50
Thoracic	Sagittal	Extension-0-flexion (0)-0-(45)	Extends 0°, flexes 45°	S: 0-0-45
Thoracic	Frontal	Left lateral-0-right lateral bend bend (45)-0-(45)	Bends left 45°, right 20°	F: 45-0-20
Thoracic		Left-0-right rotation rotation (30)-0-(30)	Rotates left 15°, right 20°	R: 15-0-20
Lumbar	Sagittal	Extension-0-flexion (25)-0-(60)	Extends 25°, flexes 40°	S: 25-0-40
Lumbar	Frontal	Left lateral-0-right lateral bend bend (25)-0-(25)	Ankylosis of the spine in 20° left lateral flexion	F: 20-0
			Ankylosis in 20° right lateral flexion	F: 0-20
			Restricted motion from 20° to 30° of left lateral bending[†]	F: 30-20-0

* Normal ranges are in parentheses.

† A non-0° starting position is noted in the ankylosis table.

Table A-3 Recording ROM Measurements for the Lower Extremities*

Joint	Plane	ROM-0-ROM (°)	Clinical Examples	
			Text Description	SFTR Recording (°)
Hip	Sagittal	Extension-0-flexion (30)-0-(100)	Left extends 30°, flexes 80°	Left S: 30-0-80
			Right extends 10°, flexes 60°	Right S: 10-0-60
Hip	Frontal	Abduction-0-adduction (40)-0-(20)	Left abducts 30°, adducts 10°	Left F: 30-0-10
			Right abducts 20°, adducts 10°	Right F: 20-0-10
Hip	Rotation	External-0-internal rotation rotation (50)-0-(40)	Left external rotation 30°, internal rotation 30°	Left R: 30-0-30
			Right external rotation 20°, internal rotation 15°	Right R: 20-0-15
Knee	Sagittal	Extension-0-flexion (0)-0-(150)	Left extends 0°, flexes 150°	Left S: 0-0-150
			Right hyperextension 10°, flexes 120°	Right S: 0-0-120
Ankle (talocrural)	Sagittal	Extension-0-flexion (20)-0-(40)	Left extends 10°, flexes 10°	Left S: 10-0-10
			Right extends 20°, flexes 40°	Right S: 20-0-40
Ankle (subtalar)	Frontal	Eversion-0-inversion (20)-0-(30)	Left eversion 20°, inversion 30°	Left F: 20-0-30
			Right eversion 10°, inversion 20°	Right F: 10-0-20

* Normal ranges are in parentheses.

References

1. Lea RD, Gerhardt JJ. Current concepts review range of motion measurement. *Bone Joint Surg.* 1995;77:784-798.

2. Mayer T, Kondraske G, Beals S, Gatchel R. Spinal range of motion: accuracy and sources of error with inclinometric measurement. *Spine.* 1997;22:1976-1984.

3. Gerhardt JJ. *Documentation of Joint Motion.* Rev 3rd ed. Portland, Ore: Oregon Medical Association; 1992.

Glossary

Abnormal illness behavior   Behavior that suggests amplification of symptoms for any of a variety of psychological or social reasons or purposes.

Acquired   Developed after birth. Not hereditary or congenital.

Activities of daily living (ADL)   Activities of daily living include those listed in Table 1-2, reproduced below.

Table 1-2 Activities of Daily Living Commonly Measured in Activities of Daily Living (ADL) and Instrumental Activities of Daily Living (IADL) Scales

Activity	Example
Self-care, teeth, personal hygiene	Urinating, defecating, brushing combing hair, bathing, dressing oneself, eating
Communication	Writing, typing, seeing, hearing, speaking
Physical activity	Standing, sitting, reclining, walking, climbing stairs
Sensory function	Hearing, seeing, tactile feeling, tasting, smelling
Nonspecialized hand activities	Grasping, lifting, tactile discrimination
Travel	Riding, driving, flying
Sexual function	Orgasm, ejaculation, lubrication, erection
Sleep	Restful, nocturnal sleep pattern

ADL   See **Activities of daily living (ADL).**

Aggravation   A factor(s) (eg, physical, chemical, biological, or medical condition) that adversely alters the course or progression of the medical impairment. Worsening of a preexisting medical condition or impairment.

Americans with Disabilities Act (ADA)   A civil rights law, signed in 1990, that protects individuals with disabilities against discrimination in such diverse areas as employment, government service entitlement, and access to public accommodations.

Ankylosis   Fixation of a joint in a specific position by disease, injury, or surgery. When surgically created, the aim is to fuse the joint in that position, which is best for improved function.

Apportionment   A distribution or allocation of causation among multiple factors that caused or significantly contributed to the injury or disease and existing impairment.

Assistive devices   Devices that help individuals with a functional loss increase function. Examples include reachers, extended grabbers, hearing aids, and telephone amplifiers.

Blindness   The absence of vision (no light perception, NLP).

Causalgia   See **Complex regional pain syndromes.**

Causation   An identifiable factor (eg, accident or exposure to hazards or disease) that results in a medically identifiable condition.

Chronic pain   Pain that extends beyond the expected period of healing or is related to a progressive disease. It is usually elicited by an injury or disease but may be perpetuated by factors that are both pathogenically and physically remote from the original cause. Because the pain persists, it is likely that environmental and psychological factors interact with the tissue damage, contributing to the persistence of pain and illness behavior.

Combined Values Chart   A method used to combine multiple impairments, derived from the formula A + B(1–A) = *combined* values of A and B, which ensures that the summary value will not exceed 100% of the whole person.

Complex regional pain syndromes (CRPS)
   CRPS I   Reflex sympathetic dystrophy
   CRPS II   Causalgia. Described in Sections 13.8, 16.5e, and 17.2m. Burning pain associated with signs of vasomotor and sudomotor dysfunction and later trophic changes of all tissues from skin to bone. Causalgia follows a lesion of a peripheral nerve, while RSD may follow a sprain, fracture, or nerve or vascular injury.

Congenital condition   Exists at or dates from birth and may be acquired during development in the uterus. A congenital condition is not hereditary.

Contracture   A permanent shortening (as of muscle, tendon, or scar tissue) producing loss of motion, deformity, or distortion.

Contrast sensitivity   The ability to perceive larger objects with low contrast. This ability is important for ADL tasks such as face recognition (see Section 12.4b).

Creatinine clearance   A quantitative measure of the degree of functional impairment of the upper urinary tract.

Cure   Complete recovery from a disease or condition.

Dermatitis   An inflammation of the skin.

Desirable weight   A range of optimal weight given an individual's sex, age, height, and body habitus.

Deterioration or **Decompensation**   An individual's repeated failure to adapt to stressful circumstances.

Diagnostic and Statistical Manual of Mental Disorders, Fourth Edition (DSM-IV)   Published by the American Psychiatric Association, this book lists and describes the criteria necessary to meet a psychiatric diagnosis.

Diffusing capacity   Measurement of gas transfer from the lung tissue into the blood.

Disability   Alteration of an individual's capacity to meet personal, social, or occupational demands or statutory or regulatory requirements because of an impairment. Disability is a relational outcome, contingent on the environmental conditions in which activities are performed.

Disfigurement   An altered or abnormal appearance of color, shape, or structure of the skin or of a body part. Disfigurement may be caused by an injury or illness and may persist after the underlying condition has resolved. Disfigurement may cause social rejection, impairment of self-image, alteration of lifestyle, or other adverse mental and behavioral effects.

Dizziness   A sensation of unsteadiness accompanied by a feeling of movement of the individual.

Dominant extremity   One of a pair of bodily structures that is the more effective or predominant in action.

Dysesthesia   Impairment of sensitivity, especially to touch.

Effects of medication   Medication may impact the individual's signs, symptoms, and ability to function. The physician may choose to increase the impairment estimate by a small percentage (1% to 3%) to account for effects of treatment.

Functional Acuity Score (FAS), Functional Field Score (FFS)   These scores combine the VAS and VFS values from OD, OS, and OU to derive an estimate of the ability to perform generic activities of daily living (see Tables 12-3 and 12-6). Higher values indicate better vision.

Functional limitations   The inability to completely perform a task due to an impairment. In some instances, functional limitations may be overcome through modifications in the individual's personal or environmental accommodations.

Functional Vision Score (FVS)   The *functional vision score* combines the Functional Acuity Score and the Functional Field Score (see Table 12-1*)* with individual adjustments if needed (see Section 12.4b). Higher values indicate better vision.

Handicap   A historical term used to describe disability or a person living with a disability or disabilities. A handicapped individual has been considered to be someone with a physical or mental disability that substantially limits activity, especially in relation to employment or education.

Hernia   A protrusion of an organ or body part through connective tissue or through a wall of the cavity in which it is normally enclosed.

HIV   See **Human immunodeficiency virus (HIV).**

Hormone   A product of living cells that circulates in body fluids and produces a specific effect on the activity of cells remote from its point of origin.

Human immunodeficiency virus (HIV)   Any of a group of retroviruses, and especially HIV-1, that infect and destroy helper T cells of the immune system, causing the marked reduction in their numbers that is one of the diagnostic criteria of AIDS. Also called AIDS virus.

Impairment   A loss, loss of use, or derangement of any body part, organ system, or organ function.

Impairment evaluation   A medical evaluation performed by a physician, using a standard method as outlined in the *Guides,* to determine permanent impairment associated with a medical condition.

Impairment percentages or **ratings**   Consensus-derived estimates that reflect the severity of the impairment and the degree to which the impairment decreases an individual's ability to perform common activities of daily living as listed in Table 1-2.

Independent medical evaluation (IME)   An evaluation performed by an independent medical examiner, who evaluates—but does not provide care for—the individual.

Inherited condition   A condition received from a parent or ancestor by genetic transmission.

Legal blindness   A term used to indicate eligibility for certain benefits. It is a misnomer, since 90% of "legally blind" individuals are not blind. The preferred term, as used in *ICD-9-CM,* is *severe vision loss* (see Section 12.2b.1).

The definition of *legal blindness* varies slightly in different statutes. A common definition is "visual acuity of 20/200 or less." Implementation of this definition depends on the chart used (see Section 12.2b.1). An alternative definition is "visual field loss to a 20° diameter or less." This definition does not address nonconcentric field losses.

Malingering   A conscious and willful feigning or exaggeration of a disease or effect of an injury in order to obtain specific external gain. It is usually motivated by external incentives, such as receiving financial compensation, obtaining drugs, or avoiding work or other responsibilities.

Maximal medical improvement (MMI)   A condition or state that is well stabilized and unlikely to change substantially in the next year, with or without medical treatment. Over time, there may be some change; however, further recovery or deterioration is not anticipated.

Menopause   The period of natural cessation of menstruation, usually occurring between the ages of 45 and 55.

METS   Multiples of resting metabolic energy used for any given activity. Each MET represents 3.5 cc of oxygen consumption per kilogram per minute. One MET equals oxygen uptake at rest. The results of stress testing are expressed in METs.

Motivation   A need or desire that causes a person to act.

Neutral zero measuring method   An approach used by the *Guides* to measure range of motion that defines the neutral or starting position of reference for any joint being measured as the standing anatomic position. The neutral or anatomic position is recorded as the 0° position.

Normal   A range or zone that represents healthy functioning and varies with age, gender, and other factors, such as environmental conditions.

Occupational history   A tool used in a comprehensive clinical assessment to obtain, organize, and assess information about the current and prior workplace environments and exposures and their relationship to illness and injury. An occupational history can provide essential information to improve treatment, prevent further or additional illness or injury, and assist in the determination of whether work directly caused or contributed to the development of the injury or illness.

Pain   An unpleasant sensory and emotional experience associated with actual or potential tissue damage or described in terms of such damage.

Pain behavior   Verbal or nonverbal actions understood by observers to indicate that a person may be experiencing pain, distress, and suffering. These actions may include audible complaints, facial expressions, abnormal postures or gait, use of prosthetic devices, or avoidance of activities.

Paresthesias   A sensation of pricking, tingling, or creeping on the skin, usually associated with injury or irritation of a sensory nerve or nerve root.

Patch test   Patch tests are used to diagnose allergic contact sensitivity. Small patches containing non-irritating concentrations of the allergens to be tested are applied to unbroken skin, usually on the upper back, for 48 hours. A positive test reaction occurs when dermatitis develops at the site of application 48 to 168 hours later.

Permanent impairment   An impairment that has reached maximal medical improvement.

Prosthesis   An artificial device to replace a missing part of the body.

Psychogenic pain   Severe and prolonged pain that is inconsistent with neuroanatomic distribution of pain receptors or without, or grossly in excess of, detectable organic or pathophysiologic mechanisms. As a result, the report of pain is attributed primarily to psychological factors.

Pulmonary function tests   Studies of lung function including such measurements as lung volumes, inspiratory and expiratory flow rates, and efficiency of gas transfer.

Radiculopathy   Any pathological condition of the nerve roots.

Raynaud's phenomenon   A vascular disorder marked by recurrent spasm of the capillaries, especially those of the fingers and toes upon exposure to cold, that is characterized by pallor, cyanosis, and redness in succession and usually accompanied by pain.

Recurrence   A return of the disorder or disease after a remission.

Reflex sympathetic dystrophy   See **Complex regional pain syndromes.**

Reliability   See **Reproducibility.**

Remission   Improvement or a state or period during which the symptoms of a disease are abated.

Replacement medication or **therapy**   Treatment that involves the supply of something (an element, compound, or hormone) lacking or lost to the body's system. Although the person may be fully functional on an everyday basis while taking replacement medication, he or she may be unable to respond properly to stresses such as fever, trauma, or infection. This impaired ability to respond to stress needs careful consideration.

Reproducibility   Synonymous with reliability. Consistency in results when examinations (tests) are repeated.

Sciatica   Pain along the course of a sciatic nerve, especially in the back of the thigh, caused by compression, inflammation, or reflex mechanisms.

Sensitivity   The extent to which individuals with a condition are correctly classified.

SFTR documentation system   A numeric method for recording range-of-motion measurements taken by the neutral zero method.

Social functioning   An individual's ability to interact appropriately and communicate effectively with other individuals.

Somatoform pain disorder   According to *DSM-IV,* this is preoccupation with pain in the absence of physical findings that adequately account for the pain and its intensity, as well as the presence of psychological factors that are judged to have a major role in the onset, severity, exacerbation, and maintenance of pain.

Specificity   The extent to which individuals without a condition are correctly classified.

Spirometry   Measurement by means of a spirometer of the forced vital capacity and its subdivisions, as well as measurement of the speed of airflow achieved in performance of this maneuver.

Stress testing   An electrocardiographic test of heart function before, during, and after a controlled period of increasingly strenuous exercise (as on a treadmill).

Surgically created stoma   An artificial permanent opening, especially in the abdominal wall, created to compensate for anatomic losses and allow either ingress to or egress from the alimentary tract.

Teleroentgenography   A radiographic method used to determine actual limb length.

Tinnitus   A sensation of noise (such as ringing or roaring) in the ear. Tinnitus may be audible or inaudible. Audible tinnitus is usually associated with a muscular tic or vascular bruit. Inaudible tinnitus can be heard only by the person affected and may be associated with an obstruction of the external auditory canal or a disturbance of the auditory nerve and/or the central nervous system.

Treatment   The action or manner of treating an individual, medically or surgically. Medical treatment is the action or manner of treating an individual, medically or surgically by a physician. Treatment may include modalities recommended by a health care provider.

Validity   An accurate measurement apart from random errors. Validity refers to the extent to which a test measures what it is intended to measure.

Vertigo   A sensation of motion (eg, spinning) when there is no motion or an exaggerated sense of motion in response to a given bodily movement.

Vision (low)   A term applied to the large group of individuals who are not blind (hence low *vision*), but who do not have normal vision either (hence *low* vision) (see Section 12.2b.2). In *ICD-9-CM*, low vision is defined as visual acuity loss to less than 20/63 (20/60 if rounded) down to 20/1000 (1/50).

Vision loss (ranges of)   Table 12-2 lists more detailed ranges of visual acuity loss as defined in *ICD-9-CM*.

Range of normal vision	20/25 or better
Mild vision loss (near-normal vision)	Less than 20/25
Moderate vision loss	Less than 20/63 (20/60)
Severe vision loss	Less than 20/160 (20/200 or less)
Profound vision loss	Less than 20/400
Near-blindness	Less than 20/1000
Total blindness	No light perception (NLP)

Table 12-5 defines similar ranges of visual field loss.

Visual acuity   The ability to recognize small objects with high contrast, such as letters on a letter chart (see Section 12.2). This ability is important for ADL tasks such as reading.

Visual Acuity Score (VAS), Visual Field Score (VFS)   Scales used to assign a numeric value to visual acuity and visual field measurements for each eye (see Tables 12-2 and 12-5). They are used for calculation purposes. Higher values indicate better vision.

Visual field   The ability to detect objects in the periphery of the visual environment (see Section 12.3). This ability is important for ADL tasks such as orientation and mobility.

Visual impairment rating   A rating calculated as 100 – FVS. Higher values indicate poorer vision.

VO$_2$ Oxygen consumption or uptake, measured in mL/min.

Whole person impairment   Percentages that estimate the impact of the impairment on the individual's overall ability to perform activities of daily living, excluding work.

Workers' compensation   A compensation program designed to provide medical and economic support to workers who have been injured or become ill from an incident arising out of and in the course of their employment.

Combined Values Chart

The values are derived from the formula A + B(1−A) = combined value of A and B, where A and B are the decimal equivalents of the impairment ratings. In the chart all values are expressed as percents. To combine any two impairment values, locate the larger of the values on the side of the chart and read along that row until you come to the column indicated by the smaller value at the bottom of the chart. At the intersection of the row and the column is the combined value.

For example, to combine 35% and 20%, read down the side of the chart until you come to the larger value, 35%. Then read across the 35% row until you come to the column indicated by 20% at the bottom of the chart. At the intersection of the row and column is the number 48. Therefore, 35% combined with 20% is 48%. Because of the construction of this chart, the larger impairment value must be identified at the side of the chart.

If three or more impairment values are to be combined, select any two and find their combined value as above. Then use that value and the third value to locate the combined value of all. This process can be repeated indefinitely, the final value in each instance being the combination of all the previous values. In each step of this process the larger impairment value must be identified at the side of the chart.

Note: If impairments from two or more organ systems are to be combined to express a whole person impairment, each must first be expressed as a whole person impairment percent.

	1	2	3	4	5	6	7	8	9	10	11	12	13	14	15	16	17	18	19	20	21	22	23	24	25	26	27	28	29	30	31	32	33	34	35	36	37	38	39	40	41	42	43	44	45	46	47	48	49	50
1	2
2	3	4
3	4	5	6
4	5	6	7	8
5	6	7	8	9	10
6	7	8	9	10	11	12
7	8	9	10	11	12	13	14
8	9	10	11	12	13	14	14	15
9	10	11	12	13	14	14	15	16	17
10	11	12	13	14	15	15	16	17	18	19
11	12	13	14	15	15	16	17	18	19	20	21
12	13	14	15	16	16	17	18	19	20	21	22	23
13	14	15	16	16	17	18	19	20	21	22	23	23	24
14	15	16	17	17	18	19	20	21	22	23	23	24	25	26
15	16	17	18	18	19	20	21	22	23	24	24	25	26	27	28
16	17	18	19	19	20	21	22	23	24	24	25	26	27	28	29	29
17	18	19	19	20	21	22	23	24	24	25	26	27	28	29	29	30	31
18	19	20	20	21	22	23	24	25	25	26	27	28	29	29	30	31	32	33
19	20	21	21	22	23	24	25	25	26	27	28	29	30	30	31	32	33	34	34
20	21	22	22	23	24	25	26	26	27	28	29	30	30	31	32	33	34	34	35	36
21	22	23	23	24	25	26	27	27	28	29	30	30	31	32	33	34	34	35	36	37	38
22	23	24	24	25	26	27	27	28	29	30	31	31	32	33	34	34	35	36	37	38	38	39
23	24	25	25	26	27	28	28	29	30	31	31	32	33	34	35	35	36	37	38	38	39	40	41
24	25	26	26	27	28	29	29	30	31	32	32	33	34	35	35	36	37	38	38	39	40	41	41	42
25	26	27	27	28	29	30	30	31	32	33	33	34	35	36	36	37	38	39	39	40	41	42	42	43	44
26	27	27	28	29	30	30	31	32	33	33	34	35	36	36	37	38	39	39	40	41	42	42	43	44	45	45
27	28	28	29	30	31	31	32	33	34	34	35	36	36	37	38	39	39	40	41	42	42	43	44	45	45	46	47
28	29	29	30	31	32	32	33	34	34	35	36	37	37	38	39	40	40	41	42	42	43	44	45	45	46	47	47	48
29	30	30	31	32	33	33	34	35	35	36	37	38	38	39	40	40	41	42	42	43	44	45	45	46	47	47	48	49	50
30	31	31	32	33	34	34	35	36	36	37	38	38	39	40	41	41	42	43	43	44	45	45	46	47	48	48	49	50	50	51
31	32	32	33	34	34	35	36	37	37	38	39	39	40	41	41	42	43	43	44	45	45	46	47	48	48	49	50	50	51	52	52
32	33	33	34	35	35	36	37	37	38	39	39	40	41	42	42	43	44	44	45	46	46	47	48	48	49	50	50	51	52	52	53	54
33	34	34	35	36	36	37	38	38	39	40	40	41	42	42	43	44	44	45	46	46	47	48	48	49	50	50	51	52	52	53	54	54	55
34	35	35	36	37	37	38	39	39	40	41	41	42	43	43	44	45	45	46	47	47	48	49	49	50	51	51	52	52	53	54	54	55	56	56
35	36	36	37	38	38	39	40	40	41	42	42	43	43	44	45	45	46	47	47	48	49	49	50	51	51	52	53	53	54	55	55	56	56	57	58
36	37	37	38	39	39	40	40	41	42	42	43	44	44	45	46	46	47	48	48	49	49	50	51	51	52	53	53	54	55	55	56	56	57	58	58	59
37	38	38	39	40	40	41	41	42	43	43	44	45	45	46	46	47	48	48	49	50	50	51	51	52	53	53	54	55	55	56	57	57	58	58	59	60	60
38	39	39	40	40	41	42	42	43	44	44	45	45	46	47	47	48	49	49	50	50	51	52	52	53	54	54	55	55	56	57	57	58	58	59	60	60	61	62
39	40	40	41	41	42	43	43	44	44	45	46	46	47	48	48	49	49	50	51	51	52	52	53	54	54	55	55	56	57	57	58	59	59	60	60	61	62	62	63
40	41	41	42	42	43	44	44	45	45	46	47	47	48	48	49	50	50	51	51	52	53	53	54	54	55	56	56	57	57	58	59	59	60	60	61	62	62	63	63	64
41	42	42	43	43	44	45	45	46	46	47	47	48	49	49	50	50	51	52	52	53	53	54	55	55	56	56	57	58	58	59	59	60	60	61	62	62	63	63	64	65	65
42	43	43	44	44	45	45	46	47	47	48	48	49	50	50	51	51	52	52	53	54	54	55	55	56	57	57	58	58	59	59	60	61	61	62	62	63	63	64	65	65	66	66
43	44	44	45	45	46	46	47	48	48	49	49	50	50	51	52	52	53	53	54	54	55	56	56	57	57	58	58	59	60	60	61	61	62	62	63	64	64	65	65	66	66	67	68
44	45	45	46	46	47	47	48	48	49	50	50	51	51	52	52	53	54	54	55	55	56	56	57	57	58	59	59	60	60	61	61	62	62	63	64	64	65	65	66	66	67	68	68	69
45	46	46	47	47	48	48	49	49	50	51	51	52	52	53	53	54	54	55	55	56	57	57	58	58	59	59	60	60	61	62	62	63	63	64	64	65	65	66	66	67	68	68	69	69	70
46	47	47	48	48	49	49	50	50	51	51	52	52	53	54	54	55	55	56	56	57	57	58	58	59	60	60	61	61	62	62	63	63	64	64	65	65	66	67	67	68	68	69	69	70	70	71
47	48	48	49	49	50	50	51	51	52	52	53	53	54	54	55	55	56	57	57	58	58	59	59	60	60	61	61	62	62	63	63	64	64	65	66	66	67	67	68	68	69	69	70	70	71	71	72
48	49	49	50	50	51	51	52	52	53	53	54	54	55	55	56	56	57	57	58	58	59	59	60	60	61	62	62	63	63	64	64	65	65	66	66	67	67	68	68	69	69	70	70	71	71	72	72	73
49	50	50	51	51	52	52	53	53	54	54	55	55	56	56	57	57	58	58	59	59	60	60	61	61	62	62	63	63	64	64	65	65	66	66	67	67	68	68	69	69	70	70	71	71	72	72	73	73	74
50	51	51	52	52	53	53	54	54	55	55	56	56	57	57	58	58	59	59	60	60	61	61	62	62	63	63	64	64	65	65	66	66	67	67	68	68	69	69	70	70	71	71	72	72	73	73	74	74	75	75

Combined Values Chart (continued)

	1	2	3	4	5	6	7	8	9	10	11	12	13	14	15	16	17	18	19	20	21	22	23	24	25	26	27	28	29	30	31	32	33	34	35	36	37	38	39	40	41	42	43	44	45	46	47	48	49	50
51	51	52	52	53	53	54	54	55	55	56	56	57	57	58	58	59	59	60	60	61	61	62	62	63	63	64	64	65	65	66	66	67	67	68	68	69	69	70	70	71	71	72	72	73	73	74	74	75	75	76
52	52	53	53	54	54	55	55	56	56	57	57	58	58	59	59	60	60	61	61	62	62	63	63	64	64	64	65	65	66	66	67	67	68	68	69	69	70	70	71	71	72	72	73	73	74	74	75	75	76	76
53	53	54	54	55	55	56	56	57	57	58	58	59	59	60	60	61	61	61	62	62	63	63	64	64	65	65	66	66	67	67	68	68	69	69	69	70	70	71	71	72	72	73	73	74	74	75	75	76	76	77
54	54	55	55	56	56	57	57	58	58	59	59	59	60	60	61	61	62	62	63	63	64	64	65	65	66	66	66	67	67	68	68	69	69	70	70	71	71	71	72	72	73	73	74	74	75	75	76	76	77	77
55	55	56	56	57	57	58	58	59	59	60	60	60	61	61	62	62	63	63	64	64	64	65	65	66	66	67	67	68	68	69	69	69	70	70	71	71	72	72	73	73	73	74	74	75	75	76	76	77	77	78
56	56	57	57	58	58	59	59	60	60	60	61	61	62	62	63	63	63	64	64	65	65	66	66	67	67	67	68	68	69	69	70	70	71	71	71	72	72	73	73	74	74	74	75	75	76	76	77	77	78	78
57	57	58	58	59	59	60	60	60	61	61	62	62	63	63	63	64	64	65	65	66	66	66	67	67	68	68	69	69	69	70	70	71	71	72	72	72	73	73	74	74	75	75	75	76	76	77	77	78	78	79
58	58	59	59	60	60	61	61	61	62	62	63	63	63	64	64	65	65	66	66	66	67	67	68	68	68	69	69	70	70	71	71	71	72	72	73	73	74	74	74	75	75	76	76	76	77	77	78	78	79	79
59	59	60	60	61	61	61	62	62	63	63	64	64	64	65	65	66	66	66	67	67	68	68	68	69	69	70	70	70	71	71	72	72	73	73	73	74	74	75	75	75	76	76	77	77	77	78	78	79	79	80
60	60	61	61	62	62	62	63	63	64	64	64	65	65	66	66	66	67	67	68	68	68	69	69	70	70	70	71	71	72	72	72	73	73	74	74	74	75	75	76	76	76	77	77	78	78	78	79	79	80	80
61	61	62	62	63	63	63	64	64	65	65	65	66	66	66	67	67	68	68	68	69	69	70	70	70	71	71	72	72	72	73	73	73	74	74	75	75	75	76	76	77	77	77	78	78	79	79	79	80	80	81
62	62	63	63	64	64	64	65	65	65	66	66	67	67	67	68	68	68	69	69	70	70	70	71	71	72	72	72	73	73	73	74	74	75	75	75	76	76	76	77	77	78	78	78	79	79	79	80	80	81	81
63	63	64	64	64	65	65	66	66	66	67	67	67	68	68	69	69	69	70	70	70	71	71	72	72	72	73	73	73	74	74	74	75	75	76	76	76	77	77	77	78	78	79	79	79	80	80	80	81	81	82
64	64	65	65	65	66	66	67	67	67	68	68	68	69	69	69	70	70	70	71	71	72	72	72	73	73	73	74	74	74	75	75	76	76	76	77	77	77	78	78	78	79	79	79	80	80	81	81	81	82	82
65	65	66	66	66	67	67	67	68	68	69	69	69	70	70	70	71	71	71	72	72	72	73	73	73	74	74	74	75	75	76	76	76	77	77	77	78	78	78	79	79	79	80	80	80	81	81	81	82	82	83
66	66	67	67	67	68	68	68	69	69	69	70	70	70	71	71	71	72	72	72	73	73	73	74	74	75	75	75	76	76	76	77	77	77	78	78	78	79	79	79	80	80	80	81	81	81	82	82	82	83	83
67	67	68	68	68	69	69	69	70	70	70	71	71	71	72	72	72	73	73	73	74	74	74	75	75	75	76	76	76	77	77	77	78	78	78	79	79	79	80	80	80	81	81	81	82	82	82	83	83	83	84
68	68	69	69	69	70	70	70	71	71	71	72	72	72	72	73	73	73	74	74	74	75	75	75	76	76	76	77	77	77	78	78	78	79	79	79	80	80	80	80	81	81	81	82	82	82	83	83	83	84	84
69	69	70	70	70	71	71	71	71	72	72	72	73	73	73	74	74	74	75	75	75	76	76	76	76	77	77	77	78	78	78	79	79	79	80	80	80	80	81	81	81	82	82	82	83	83	83	84	84	84	85
70	70	71	71	71	72	72	72	72	73	73	73	74	74	74	75	75	75	75	76	76	76	77	77	77	78	78	78	78	79	79	79	80	80	80	81	81	81	81	82	82	82	83	83	83	84	84	84	84	85	85
71	71	72	72	72	72	73	73	73	74	74	74	74	75	75	75	76	76	76	77	77	77	77	78	78	78	79	79	79	79	80	80	80	81	81	81	81	82	82	82	83	83	83	83	84	84	84	85	85	85	86
72	72	73	73	73	73	74	74	74	75	75	75	75	76	76	76	76	77	77	77	78	78	78	78	79	79	79	80	80	80	80	81	81	81	82	82	82	82	83	83	83	83	84	84	84	85	85	85	85	86	86
73	73	74	74	74	74	75	75	75	75	76	76	76	77	77	77	77	78	78	78	78	79	79	79	79	80	80	80	81	81	81	81	82	82	82	82	83	83	83	84	84	84	84	85	85	85	85	86	86	86	87
74	74	75	75	75	75	76	76	76	76	77	77	77	77	78	78	78	78	79	79	79	79	80	80	80	81	81	81	81	82	82	82	82	83	83	83	83	84	84	84	84	85	85	85	85	86	86	86	86	87	87
75	75	76	76	76	76	77	77	77	77	78	78	78	78	79	79	79	79	80	80	80	80	81	81	81	81	82	82	82	82	83	83	83	83	84	84	84	84	85	85	85	85	86	86	86	86	87	87	87	87	88
76	76	76	77	77	77	77	78	78	78	78	79	79	79	79	80	80	80	80	81	81	81	81	82	82	82	82	82	83	83	83	83	84	84	84	84	85	85	85	85	86	86	86	86	87	87	87	87	88	88	88
77	77	77	78	78	78	78	79	79	79	79	80	80	80	80	80	81	81	81	81	82	82	82	82	83	83	83	83	83	84	84	84	84	85	85	85	85	86	86	86	86	86	87	87	87	87	88	88	88	88	89
78	78	78	79	79	79	79	80	80	80	80	80	81	81	81	81	82	82	82	82	82	83	83	83	83	84	84	84	84	84	85	85	85	85	85	86	86	86	86	87	87	87	87	87	88	88	88	88	89	89	89
79	79	79	80	80	80	80	80	81	81	81	81	82	82	82	82	82	83	83	83	83	83	84	84	84	84	84	85	85	85	85	86	86	86	86	86	87	87	87	87	87	88	88	88	88	88	89	89	89	89	90
80	80	80	81	81	81	81	81	82	82	82	82	82	83	83	83	83	83	84	84	84	84	84	85	85	85	85	85	86	86	86	86	86	87	87	87	87	87	88	88	88	88	88	89	89	89	89	89	90	90	90
81	81	81	82	82	82	82	82	83	83	83	83	83	83	84	84	84	84	84	85	85	85	85	85	86	86	86	86	86	87	87	87	87	87	87	88	88	88	88	88	89	89	89	89	89	90	90	90	90	90	91
82	82	82	83	83	83	83	83	83	84	84	84	84	84	85	85	85	85	85	85	86	86	86	86	86	87	87	87	87	87	87	88	88	88	88	88	88	89	89	89	89	89	90	90	90	90	90	90	91	91	91
83	83	83	84	84	84	84	84	84	85	85	85	85	85	85	86	86	86	86	86	86	87	87	87	87	87	87	88	88	88	88	88	88	89	89	89	89	89	89	90	90	90	90	90	90	91	91	91	91	91	92
84	84	84	84	85	85	85	85	85	85	86	86	86	86	86	86	87	87	87	87	87	87	88	88	88	88	88	88	88	89	89	89	89	89	89	90	90	90	90	90	90	91	91	91	91	91	91	92	92	92	92
85	85	85	85	86	86	86	86	86	86	87	87	87	87	87	87	87	88	88	88	88	88	88	88	89	89	89	89	89	89	90	90	90	90	90	90	90	91	91	91	91	91	91	91	92	92	92	92	92	92	93
86	86	86	86	87	87	87	87	87	87	87	88	88	88	88	88	88	88	89	89	89	89	89	89	89	90	90	90	90	90	90	90	90	91	91	91	91	91	91	91	92	92	92	92	92	92	92	93	93	93	93
87	87	87	87	88	88	88	88	88	88	88	88	89	89	89	89	89	89	89	89	90	90	90	90	90	90	90	91	91	91	91	91	91	91	91	92	92	92	92	92	92	92	92	93	93	93	93	93	93	93	94
88	88	88	88	88	89	89	89	89	89	89	89	89	90	90	90	90	90	90	90	90	91	91	91	91	91	91	91	91	91	92	92	92	92	92	92	92	92	93	93	93	93	93	93	93	93	94	94	94	94	94
89	89	89	89	89	90	90	90	90	90	90	90	90	90	91	91	91	91	91	91	91	91	91	92	92	92	92	92	92	92	92	92	93	93	93	93	93	93	93	93	93	94	94	94	94	94	94	94	94	94	95
90	90	90	90	90	91	91	91	91	91	91	91	91	91	91	92	92	92	92	92	92	92	92	92	92	93	93	93	93	93	93	93	93	93	93	94	94	94	94	94	94	94	94	94	94	95	95	95	95	95	95
91	91	91	91	91	91	92	92	92	92	92	92	92	92	92	92	92	93	93	93	93	93	93	93	93	93	93	93	94	94	94	94	94	94	94	94	94	94	94	95	95	95	95	95	95	95	95	95	95	95	96
92	92	92	92	92	92	92	93	93	93	93	93	93	93	93	93	93	93	93	94	94	94	94	94	94	94	94	94	94	94	94	94	95	95	95	95	95	95	95	95	95	95	95	95	96	96	96	96	96	96	96
93	93	93	93	93	93	93	93	94	94	94	94	94	94	94	94	94	94	94	94	94	94	95	95	95	95	95	95	95	95	95	95	95	95	95	95	96	96	96	96	96	96	96	96	96	96	96	96	96	96	97
94	94	94	94	94	94	94	94	94	95	95	95	95	95	95	95	95	95	95	95	95	95	95	95	95	96	96	96	96	96	96	96	96	96	96	96	96	96	96	96	96	96	97	97	97	97	97	97	97	97	97
95	95	95	95	95	95	95	95	95	95	96	96	96	96	96	96	96	96	96	96	96	96	96	96	96	96	96	96	96	96	96	97	97	97	96	97	97	97	97	97	97	97	97	97	97	97	97	97	97	97	98
96	96	96	96	96	96	96	96	96	96	96	96	96	97	97	97	97	97	97	97	97	97	97	97	97	97	97	97	97	97	97	97	97	97	97	97	97	97	98	98	98	98	98	98	98	98	98	98	98	98	98
97	97	97	97	97	97	97	97	97	97	97	97	97	97	97	97	97	98	98	98	98	98	98	98	98	98	98	98	98	98	98	98	98	98	98	98	98	98	98	98	98	98	98	98	98	98	98	98	98	98	99
98	98	98	98	98	98	98	98	98	98	98	98	98	98	98	98	98	98	98	98	98	98	98	98	98	99	99	99	99	99	99	99	99	99	99	99	99	99	99	99	99	99	99	99	99	99	99	99	99	99	99
99	99	99	99	99	99	99	99	99	99	99	99	99	99	99	99	99	99	99	99	99	99	99	99	99	99	99	99	99	99	99	99	99	99	99	99	99	99	99	99	99	99	99	99	99	99	99	99	99	99	100

Combined Values Chart (continued)

	51	52	53	54	55	56	57	58	59	60	61	62	63	64	65	66	67	68	69	70	71	72	73	74	75	76	77	78	79	80	81	82	83	84	85	86	87	88	89	90	91	92	93	94	95	96	97	98	99	100
51	76																																																	
52	76	77																																																
53	77	77	78																																															
54	77	78	78	79																																														
55	78	78	79	79	80																																													
56	78	79	79	80	80	81																																												
57	79	79	80	80	81	81	82																																											
58	79	80	80	81	81	82	82	82																																										
59	80	80	81	81	82	82	82	83	83																																								
60	80	81	81	82	82	82	83	83	84	84																																							
61	81	81	82	82	82	83	83	84	84	84	85																																						
62	81	82	82	83	83	83	84	84	84	85	85	86																																					
63	82	82	83	83	83	84	84	84	85	85	86	86	86																																				
64	82	83	83	83	84	84	85	85	85	86	86	86	87	87																																			
65	83	83	84	84	84	85	85	85	86	86	86	87	87	87	88																																		
66	83	84	84	84	85	85	85	86	86	86	87	87	87	88	88	88																																	
67	84	84	84	85	85	85	86	86	86	87	87	87	88	88	88	89	89																																
68	84	85	85	85	86	86	86	87	87	87	88	88	88	88	89	89	89	90																															
69	85	85	85	86	86	86	87	87	87	88	88	88	89	89	89	89	90	90	90																														
70	85	86	86	86	87	87	87	87	88	88	88	89	89	89	90	90	90	90	91	91																													
71	86	86	86	87	87	87	88	88	88	88	89	89	89	90	90	90	90	91	91	91	92																												
72	86	87	87	87	87	88	88	88	89	89	89	89	90	90	90	90	91	91	91	92	92	92																											
73	87	87	87	88	88	88	88	89	89	89	89	90	90	90	91	91	91	91	92	92	92	92	93																											
74	87	88	88	88	88	89	89	89	89	90	90	90	90	91	91	91	91	92	92	92	92	93	93	93																										
75	88	88	88	89	89	89	89	90	90	90	90	91	91	91	91	92	92	92	92	93	93	93	93	94	94																									
76	88	88	89	89	89	89	90	90	90	90	91	91	91	91	92	92	92	92	93	93	93	93	94	94	94	94																								
77	89	89	89	89	90	90	90	90	91	91	91	91	91	92	92	92	92	93	93	93	93	94	94	94	94	94	95																						
78	89	89	90	90	90	90	91	91	91	91	91	92	92	92	92	93	93	93	93	93	94	94	94	94	95	95	95	95																				
79	90	90	90	90	91	91	91	91	91	92	92	92	92	92	93	93	93	93	93	94	94	94	94	95	95	95	95	95	96																			
80	90	90	91	91	91	91	91	92	92	92	92	92	93	93	93	93	93	94	94	94	94	94	95	95	95	95	95	96	96	96																	
81	91	91	91	91	91	92	92	92	92	92	93	93	93	93	93	94	94	94	94	94	94	95	95	95	95	95	96	96	96	96	96																
82	91	91	92	92	92	92	92	92	93	93	93	93	93	94	94	94	94	94	94	95	95	95	95	95	96	96	96	96	96	96	97	97															
83	92	92	92	92	92	93	93	93	93	93	93	94	94	94	94	94	94	95	95	95	95	95	95	96	96	96	96	96	96	97	97	97	97														
84	92	92	92	93	93	93	93	93	93	94	94	94	94	94	94	95	95	95	95	95	95	96	96	96	96	96	96	96	97	97	97	97	97	97													
85	93	93	93	93	93	93	94	94	94	94	94	94	94	95	95	95	95	95	95	96	96	96	96	96	96	96	97	97	97	97	97	97	97	98	98												
86	93	93	93	94	94	94	94	94	94	94	95	95	95	95	95	95	95	96	96	96	96	96	96	96	97	97	97	97	97	97	97	97	98	98	98	98											
87	94	94	94	94	94	94	94	95	95	95	95	95	95	95	95	96	96	96	96	96	96	96	96	97	97	97	97	97	97	97	98	98	98	98	98	98	98										
88	94	94	94	94	95	95	95	95	95	95	95	95	96	96	96	96	96	96	96	96	97	97	97	97	97	97	97	97	97	98	98	98	98	98	98	98	98	99									
89	95	95	95	95	95	95	95	95	95	96	96	96	96	96	96	96	96	96	97	97	97	97	97	97	97	97	97	98	98	98	98	98	98	98	98	98	99	99	99								
90	95	95	95	95	96	96	96	96	96	96	96	96	96	96	97	97	97	97	97	97	97	97	97	97	98	98	98	98	98	98	98	98	98	98	99	99	99	99	99	99							
91	96	96	96	96	96	96	96	96	96	96	96	97	97	97	97	97	97	97	97	97	97	97	98	98	98	98	98	98	98	98	98	98	98	99	99	99	99	99	99	99	99						
92	96	96	96	96	96	96	97	97	97	97	97	97	97	97	97	97	97	97	98	98	98	98	98	98	98	98	98	98	98	98	98	99	99	99	99	99	99	99	99	99	99	99					
93	97	97	97	97	97	97	97	97	97	97	97	97	97	97	98	98	98	98	98	98	98	98	98	98	98	98	98	98	99	99	99	99	99	99	99	99	99	99	99	99	99	99	100				
94	97	97	97	97	97	97	97	97	98	98	98	98	98	98	98	98	98	98	98	98	98	98	98	98	99	99	99	99	99	99	99	99	99	99	99	99	99	99	99	99	99	100	100	100			
95	98	98	98	98	98	98	98	98	98	98	98	98	98	98	98	98	98	98	98	99	99	99	99	99	99	99	99	99	99	99	99	99	99	99	99	99	99	99	99	100	100	100	100	100	100		
96	98	98	98	98	98	98	98	98	98	98	98	98	99	99	99	99	99	99	99	99	99	99	99	99	99	99	99	99	99	99	99	99	99	99	99	99	99	100	100	100	100	100	100	100	100	100	
97	99	99	99	99	99	99	99	99	99	99	99	99	99	99	99	99	99	99	99	99	99	99	99	99	99	99	99	99	99	99	99	99	99	100	100	100	100	100	100	100	100	100	100	100	100	100	100
98	99	99	99	99	99	99	99	99	99	99	99	99	99	99	99	99	99	99	99	99	99	99	99	99	100	100	100	100	100	100	100	100	100	100	100	100	100	100	100	100	100	100	100	100	100	100	100	100
99	100	100	100	100	100	100	100	100	100	100	100	100	100	100	100	100	100	100	100	100	100	100	100	100	100	100	100	100	100	100	100	100	100	100	100	100	100	100	100	100	100	100	100	100	100	100	100	100	100
	51	52	53	54	55	56	57	58	59	60	61	62	63	64	65	66	67	68	69	70	71	72	73	74	75	76	77	78	79	80	81	82	83	84	85	86	87	88	89	90	91	92	93	94	95	96	97	98	99	100

Index

Index

ISBN 1-57947-085-8

90000>

9 781579 470852